Pediatric Hepatology and Nutrition

Vol-2

Edited by
Suraj Gupte *MD, FIAP*
Professor & Head
Postgraduate Department of Pediatrics
Narayana Medical College/ Narayana General
and Subspeciality Hospitals
Nellore-524002, AP
India
E-mail: surajgupte@rediffmail.com
recentadvances@yahoo.co.uk
Formerly Professor and Head, Department of Pediatrics
MA Medical College, Hisar, Haryana, and Government
Medical College, Jammu, Jammu & Kashmir, India

Hon. Director
Pediatric Education Network

Editor
Recent Advances in Pediatrics (Series), The Short Textbook of Pediatrics, Textbooks of "Pediatric Emergencies", "Neonatal Emergencies", "Pediatric Nutrition". Towards MRCPCH Part II (Theory) Examination Newer Horizons in Tropical Pediatrics (series), Pediatric Yearbook (series), Pediatric Today (Monograph series)
Newer Howons in Tropical Pediatrics

Author
Differential Diagnosis in Pediatrics, Instructive Case Studies in Pediatrics, Pediatric Drug Directory, Infant Feeding, MCQs in Pediatrics, Speaking of Child Care, The Baby Book: Parents Guide from Birth to Infancy

Coeditor
Asian Journal of Maternity and Child Health (Manila, Philippines)

Section Editor/Guest Editor
Pediatrics Today (New Delhi, India)

Editorial Adviser
Asian Journal of Pediatric Practice (New Delhi, India)

Editorial Advisory Board Member/Reviewer
Indian Journal of Pediatrics (New Delhi, India), Indian Pediatrics (New Delhi, India), Journal of Clinical Pediatrics (Patna, India), Indian Journal of Gastroenterology, Hepatology and Nutrition (Jaipur), Synopsis (Detroit) Maternal and Child Nutrition (Preston, UK), Journal of Pediatric Infectious Diseases (Turkey)

Examiner
National Board of Examinations (NBE) for DNB, All India Institute of Medical Sciences (AIIMS), Postgraduate Institute of Medical Education & Research (PGIMER), Sher-i-Kashmir Institute of Medical Sciences (SKIMS), Indira Gandhi Open University (IGNOU), Dr NTR University of Health Sciences (NTRUHS) and several other universities

Pediatric Faculty Selection Expert
All India Institute of Medical Sciences (AIIMS), Union Public Service Commission, Jammu & Kashmir Public Service Commission, Punjab Public Service Commission, Haryana Public Service Commission, etc.

PEEPEE
PUBLISHERS AND DISTRIBUTORS (P) LTD.

Pediatric Gastroenterology, Hepatology and Nutrition

Published by
Pawaninder P. Vij

Peepee Publishers and Distributors (P) Ltd.
Head Office: 160, Shakti Vihar, Pitam Pura, Delhi-110 034 (India)

Correspondence Address: **7/31, First Floor, Ansari Road, Daryaganj**
New Delhi-110 002 (India)

Ph: 41512412, 23246245, 9811156083

e-mail: peepee160@yahoo.co.in

e-mail: peepee160@gmail.com

www.peepeepub.com

First Edition: **2021**

ISBN: 9788184452860 (2 Vols)

to

The fond memory of my parents

and

Everybody contributing to the development of
pediatric gastroenterology, hepatology and nutrition
globally in general and Indian subcontinent in particular

Contributors

Sheffali Abbott
Research Fellow in Pediatric Hepatology
Medical University of Vienna
Vienna, Austria
Ch 70: Clinical Manifestatuions of Liver Disease
Ch 72: Evaluation of Liver Disease
Ch 76: Metabolic Liver Disease: Overview

CE Abraham
Professor
Department of Pediatric Gastroenterology, Hepatology and Nutrition
Institute of Child and Adolescent Health
London, UK
Ch 107: Exclusion Diets

Donald Abraham
Lecturer
Department of Pediatric Surgery
Institute of Child and Adolescent Health
London, UK
Ch 28: Hirschsprung's Disease
Ch 29: Intussusception
Ch 53: Acute Appendicitis
Ch 54: Anorectal Malformations
Ch 56: Hernias

John E Abraham
Lecturer
Department of Pediatric Gastroenterology, Hepatology and Nutrition
Institute of Child and Adolescent Health
London, UK
Ch 26: Remnants of the Omphalomesenteric Duct
Ch 28: Hirschsprung's Disease
Ch 33: Irritable Bowel Syndrome

B Adhisivam
Registrar
Department of Pediatrics
Alo Jahra Hospital
Kuwait
Ch 40: Bloody Diarrhea

Zubair H Aghai
Division of Neonatology
Department of Pediatrics
Cooper University Hospital
Robert Wood Johnson Medical School
Camden, NJ, USA
Ch 47: Necrotizing Enterocolitis

Seema Alam
Reader in Pediatric Gastroenterology
Department of Pediatric Gastroenterology, Hepatology and Nutrition
Institute of Child and Adolescent Health
London, UK
Ch 37: Acute Childhood Diarrhea
Ch 45: Probiotics

RA Anderson
Professor
Department of Pediatric Gastroenterology, Hepatology and Nutrition
Institute of Child and Adolescent Health
London, UK
Ch 42: Persistent Diarrhea
Ch 43: Chronic Diarrhea
Ch 73: Hepatomegaly

George Anthony
Assistant Professor
Department of Pediatric Gastroenterology, Hepatology and Nutrition
Institute of Child and Adolescent Health
London, UK
Ch 25: Intestinal Motility Disorders

Sridhar Arunachalam
Assistant Professor
Department of Pediatrics
Naryana Medical College
Narayana Group of Medical Institutes
Nellore, AP, South India
Ch 48: Recurrent Abdominal Pain

Rosy Aulakh
Senior Resident
Department of Pediatrics/Advanced Pediatric Center
PGIMER, Chandigarh, India
Ch 106: Obesity

Bratati Banerjee
Assistant Professor
Department of Community Medicine
Maulana Azad Medical College
New Delhi, India
Ch 96: Breastfeeding

Akash Bang
Lecturer
Mahatma Gandhi Institute of Medical Sciences
Sewagram, Wardha, India
Ch 113: Nutritional Support in Diarrhea

Sandeep B Bavdekar
Professor
Department of Pediatrics
Seth GS Medical College and KEM Hospital
Mumbai, India
Ch 111: Immunonutrition: A Step Ahead

Lalit Bharadia
Consultant Pediatric Gastroenterologist
Fortis Escorts Hospital,
Jaipur, India
Ch 112: Nutritional Support in Liver Disease

Sunil Bhat
Senior Resident
Department of Pediatrics
University Medical College and
Guru Teg Bahadur Hospital
Delhi, India
Ch 17: Upper Gastrointestinal Bleeding
Ch 50: Lower Gastrointestinal Bleeding
Ch 61: Chronic Pancreatitis

B Vishnu Bhat
Director-Professor
Department of Pediatrics
Jawaharlal Institute of Postgraduate Medical Education and Research (JIPMER), Pondicherry, India
Ch 40: Bloody Diarrhea

MS Bhatia
Professor and Head
Department of Psychiatry
University Medical College
Guru Teg Bahadur Hospital
Delhi, India
Ch 35: Eating Disorders

Shrish Bhatnagar
Consultant Pediatric Gastroenterologist,
Sahara Hospital
Lucknow, India
Ch 37: Acute Childhood Diarrhea

Millie Boetttcher
Division of Pediatric Gastroenterology and Nutrition
Alfred I. duPont Hospital for Children
Wilimington, USA

Charles Brook
Fellow
Department of Pediatric Gastroenterology, Hepatology and Nutrition
Institute of Child and Adolescent Health
London, UK
Ch 65: Peritoneum: Anatomy and Malformations
Ch 66: Peritonitis

Robert S Brown
Assistant Professor
Department of Pediatric Gastroenterology, Hepatology and Nutrition
Institute of Child and Adolescent Health
London, UK
Ch 26: Remnants of the Omphalomesenteric Duct
Ch 33: Irritable Bowel Syndrome

Cynthia Cairo
Lecturer
Department of Pediatric Gastroenterology, Hepatology and Nutrition
Institute of Child and Adolescent Health
London, UK
Ch 30: Foreign Bodies in the Stomach and Intestine
Ch 31: Bezoars in the Stomach and Intestine

Maria Puangco-Curcio
Pediatric Nutritionist
Stony Brook University Hospital
Stony Brook, New York, USA
Ch 118: Nutritional Support in Childhood

Gurmeet K Chaudhry
Assistant Professor
Department of Pediatrics
Christian Medical College and Hospital
Ludhiana, India
Ch 106: Obesity

Anupama Chawla
Director
Division of Pediatric Gastroenterology and Nutrition
Associate Professor of Pediatrics
Stony Brook University Hospital
Stony Brook, New York, USA
Ch 105: Failure to Thrive
Ch 110: Total Parenteral Nutrition (TPN)-Associated Cholestasis
Ch 118: Nutritional Support in Childhood

Stephen Dunn
Professor of Pediatrics Surgery
Chief, General and Transplant Surgery
Division of Transplant Surgery
Alfred I. duPont Hospital for Children
Wilmington, DE, USA
Ch 94: Liver Transplantation

KE Elizabeth
Professor, Consultant Pediatrician and Nutritionist,
Department of Pediatrics
Government Medical College and SAT Hospital
Thiruvananthapuram, India
Ch 115: Nutritional Support in Cystic Fibrosis

Sabeena Farhath
Fellow in Gastroenterology
Division of Pediatric Gastroenterology and Nutrition
Department of Pediatrics
Alfred I. duPont Hospital for Children
Wilmington, DE, USA
Ch 47: Necrotizing Enterocolitis
Ch 117: Nutritional Support in Inflammatory Bowel Disease

Kara Feigenbaum
Clinical Nutritionist
Department of Nutritional Services
Alfred I. duPont Hospital for Children
Wilmington, DE, USA
Ch 116: Nutritional Support in Diabetes Mellitus

Uzma Firdaus
Lecturer Department of Pediatrics
Jawahar Lal Nehru Medical College
Aligarh Muslim University
Aligarh, India
Ch 37: Acute Childhood Diarrhea

Sutapa Ganguly
Professor and Head
In-Charge Liver Clinic
Department of Pediatric Medicine
NES Medical College and Hospital
Kolkata, India
Ch 83: Pyogenic Liver Abscess

Robert Garola
Associate Pathologist
Department of Pathology
Alfred I. duPont Hospital for Children
Wilmington, DE, USA
Ch 121: Pathological Examinations

Ajay Gaur
Associate Professor
Department of Pediatrics
GR Medical College
Gwalior, India
Ch 77: Wilson's Disease

Anil Gautam
Resident
Department of Pediatrics
Dayanand Medical College & Hospital
Ludhiana, India
Ch 109: Parenteral Nutrition in PICU

EE Gomez
Lecturer
Department of Infant and Child Nutrition
Institute of Child and Adolescent Health
London, UK
Ch 99: Protein-Energy Malnutrition

EM Gomez
Associate Clinical Professor
Department of Infant and Child Nutrition
Institute of Child and Adolescent Health
London, United Kingdom
Ch 95: Nutritional Requirements
Ch 99: Protein-Energy Malnutrition
Ch 100: Micronutrients/Minerals and Other Deficiencies

Vani Gopalareddy
Attending Hepatologist
Division of Pediatric Gastroenterology and Nutrition
Department of Pediatrics
Alfred I. duPont Hospital for Children
Wilmington, DE, USA
Ch 86: Autoimmune Hepatitis
Ch 94: Liver Transplantation

Ravi Gupta
Senior Resident
Department of Psychiatry
University College of Medical Sciences
Guru Teg Bhadur Hospital
Delhi, India
Ch 35: Eating Disorders

Ravinder K Gupta
Associate Professor
Department of Pediatrics
Acharya Shri Chandra College of Medical Sciences (ASCOMS)
Sidhra, Jammu, India
Ch 36: Typhoid Fever
Ch 44: Diarrhea-Malnutrition Interaction
Ch 67: Ascites
Ch 87: Drug-Induced Liver Injury

Ritu Gupta
Lecturer
Department of Physiology
Government Medical College
Jammu, India
Ch 36: Typhoid Fever
Ch 44: Diarrhea-Malnutrition Interaction
Ch 67: Ascites
Ch 87: Drug-Induced Liver Injury

Suraj Gupte
Professor and Head
Postgraduate Department of Pediatrics
Narayana Medical College and Hospitals
Nellore, India
Ch 1: Pediatric Digestive System: Clinical Overview
Ch 33: Irritable Bowel Syndrome
Ch 42: Persistent Diarrhea
Ch 43: Chronic Diarrhea
Ch 48: Recurrent Abdominal Pain
Ch 49: Intestinal Parasitic Infestations
Ch 62: Cystic Fibrosis
Ch 66: Peritonitis

Ch 70: Clinical Manifestations of Liver Disease
Ch 72: Evaluation of Liver Disease
Ch 73: Hepatomegaly
Ch 74: Neonatal Cholestasis Syndrome
Ch 76: Metabolic Liver Disease: Overview
Ch 90: Indian Childhood Cirrhosis
Ch 95: Nutritional Requirements
Ch 97: Complementary Feeding
Ch 99: Protein-Energy Malnutrition
Ch 100: Micronutrients/Minerals and Other Deficiencies
Ch 101: Vitamin A Deficiency
Ch 102: Vitamin B-Complex Deficiency States
Ch 103: Scurvy
Ch 104: Nutritional Rickets

Donald Henry
Lecturer
Department of Pediatric Surgery
Institute of Child and Adolescent Health
London, United Kingdom
Ch 68: Congenital Diaphragmatic Hernia

Karoly Horvath
Professor
Division of Pediatric Gastroenterology and Nutrition
Department of Pediatrics
Alfred I. duPont Hospital for Children
Wilmington, DE, USA
Ch 2: Major Manifestions of Gastrointestinal Disease
Ch 3: Clinical Examination of the Gastrointestinal Tract
Ch 13: Gastroesophageal Reflux Disease and Eosinophilic Esophagitis
Ch 34: Food Allergy
Ch 46: Malabsorption Disorders
Ch 51: Gastrointestinal Problems in HIV Infections
Ch 57: Therapeutic Endoscopic Procedures
Ch 59: Pancreas: Anatomy, Physiology and Developmental Anomalies
Ch 60: Acute Pancreatitis
Ch 108: Enteral Nutrition
Ch 114: Nutritional Support in Celiac Disease
Ch 117: Nutritional Support in Inflammatory Bowel Disease
Ch 119: Nutritional Support in HIV/AIDS
Ch 120: Laboratory Tests
Ch 124: Colonoscopy

RS Jaswal
Senior Resident
Department of Pediatrics
Indira Gandhi Medical College
Shimla, India
Ch 39: Oral Rehydration Therapy

RK Kaushal
Professor and Head
Department of Pediatrics
Indira Gandhi Medical College
Shimla, India
Ch 39: Oral Rehydration Therapy

Seema Khan
Associate Professor of Pediatrics
Division of Pediatric Gastroenterology and Nutrition
Department of Pediatrics
Alfred I. duPont Hospital for Children
Wilmington, DE, USA
Ch 27: Constipation
Ch 38: Eosinophilic Gastroenteritis

Rajeev Khanna
Senior Resident
Department of Pediatrics
Aligarh Muslim University
Aligarh, India
Ch 37: Acute Childhood Diarrhea

Jeremy King
Senior Fellow
Division of Pediatric Gastroenterology and Nutrition
Department of Pediatrics
Alfred I. duPont Hospital for Children
Wilmington, DE, USA
Ch 2: Major Manifestations of Gastrointestrinal Disease
Ch 3: Clinical Examination of the Gastrointestinal Tract
Ch 19: Accidental Caustic Ingestions
Ch 57: Therapeutic Endoscopic Procedures
Ch 59: Pancreas: Anatomy, Physiology and Developmental Anomalies
Ch 60: Acute Pancreatitis
Ch 120: Laboratory Tests
Ch 123: Upper Gastrointestinal Endoscopy
Ch 124: Colonoscopy

Girish Kolpuru
Resident,
St Joseph Mercy Oakland
Pontiac, Michigan, USA
Ch 46: Malabsorption Disorders

Swati Kolpuru
Resident
Arizona Children's Gastroenterology,
Banner Desert Children's Hospital,
Mesa, Arizona, USA
Ch 13: Gastroesophageal Reflux Disease and Eosinophilic Esophagitis
Ch 46: Malabsorption Disorders
Ch 51: Gastrointestinal Problems in HIV Infection
Ch 108: Enteral Nutrition
Ch 119: Nutrition Support in HIV/AIDS

Chandra Mohan Kumar
Assistant Professor
Postgraduate Department of Pediatrics
Narayana Medical College and Hospitals
Nellore, South India
Ch 16: Esophageal Perforation
Ch 22: Peptic Ulcer Disease
Ch 69: Liver: Embryology, Anatomy and Physiology
Ch 71: Hepatic Manifestations of Systemic Disease
Ch 85: Reye's Syndrome
Ch 122: Imaging Studies

Renu Kumar
Assistant Professor
Department of Pediatric Surgery
Narayana Medical College and Superspeciality Hospital
Nellore, India
Ch 55: Tumors of the Gut
Ch 63: Pancreatic Pseudocyst
Ch 64: Pancreatic Neoplasms
Ch 91: Diseases Gallbladder
Ch 92: Cystic Diseases of the Liver and Biliary Tract
Ch 93: Liver Tumors

Rameen Lalvani
Senior Resident
LTM Medical College and LTM Hospital
Mumbai, India
Ch 98: Amylase-Rich Foods

E Lee
Consultant
Victoria Hospital
Hong Kong
Ch 14: Non-GERD Esophagitis

Anjali Malkani
Clinical Assistant Professor
Division of Pediatric Gastroenterology and Nutrition
Department of Pediatric
University of Maryland School of Medicine
Baltmone, Maryland, USA
Ch 34: Food Allergy

John Matthai
Pediatric Gastroenterologist-cum-
Professor
Department of Pediatrics
PSG Institute of Medical Sciences and Research
Coimbatore, India
Ch 23: Helicobacter Pylori and Gastrointestinal Disease
Ch 88: Acute Liver Failure

Nitin J Mehta
Chief, Clinical Biochemistry
Sir HN Hospital
Mumbai, India
Ch 98: Amylase-Rich Foods

Meenakshi N Mehta, MD, FIAP
Professor of Pediatrics
Terna Medical College
Navi Mumbai, India
Ch 98: Amylase-Rich Foods

OP Mishra
Professor and Head
Department of Pediatrics
Institute of Medical Sciences
Banaras Hindu University
Varanasi, India
Ch 21: Congenital Anomalies of the Stomach

John Matthai
Pediatric Gastroenterologist-cum-
Professor
Department of Pediatrics
PSG Institute of Medical Sciences and Research
Coimbatore, India
Ch 23: Helicobacter Pylori and Gastrointestinal Disease
Ch 88: Acute Liver Failure

Neelam Mohan
Consultant Pediatric Gastroenterologist and Hepatologist
Center for Child Health
Sir Ganga Ram Hospital
New Delhi, India
Ch 80: Hepatitis B and C

Nalinakshi BM
Resident
Postgraduate Department of Pediatrics
Narayana Medical College and Hospitals
Nellore, India
Ch 4: Dental Issues
Ch 5: Cleft Lip and Cleft Palate
Ch 6: Common Oral Soft Tissues Lesions
Ch 7: Salivary Glands and Jaws
Ch 8: Oral Cavity Problems in Medical Conditions

Sanjay Wazir Pandita
Specialist Registrar
Neonatal Intensive Care Unit
William Harvey Hospital
Ashford, Kent, UK
Ch 74: Neonatal Cholestasis Syndrome (NCS)

Sarah Paul
Professor and Head
Department of Pediatrics
PSG Institute of Medical Sciences and Research
Coimbatore, India
Ch 23: Helicobacter Pylori and Gastrointestinal Disease
Ch 88: Acute Liver Failure

JA Perman
Dean
College of Medicine
University of Kentuchy
Lexington, KY
USA
Ch 13: Gastrointestinal Reflux Vs Eosinohilic Esophagitis

Sumitha Paul
Medical Officer
Department of Pediatric Medicine
NES Medical College and Hospital
Kolkata, India
Ch 83: Pyogenic Liver Abscess

Rajniti Prasad
Senior Lecturer
Department of Pediatrics
Institute of Medical Science
Banaras Hindu University (BHU)
Varanasi, India
Ch 20: Gastrointestinal Tract: Embryology, Anatomy and Physiology
Ch 21: Congenital Anomalies of the Stomach

Ragavan M
Assistant Professor
Department of Pediatric Surgery
Narayana Medical College and Superspeciality Hospital
Nellore, South India
Ch 55: Tumors of the Gut
Ch 63: Pancreatic Pseudocyst
Ch 64: Pancreatic Neoplasms
Ch 91: Diseases of Gallbladder
Ch 92: Cystic Diseases of the Liver and Biliary Tract
Ch 93: Liver Tumors

Sarveshwar Reddy
Assistant Professor
Department of Pediatric Surgery
Narayana Medical College and Superspeciality Hospital
Nellore, India
Ch 52: Acute Abdomen

Rajeev G Redkar
Consultant Paediatric Surgeon
Lilavati, Shushrusha and Wadia Children's Hospital
Mumbai, India
Ch 75: Surgical Jaundice in the Neonates
Ch 89: Portal Hypertension

Priyanka Rohtagi (Rastogi)
Clinical Nutritionist
Monilek Hospital and Research Center
Jaipur, India
Ch 112: Nutritional Support in Liver Disease

Fernando Del Rosario
Assistant Professor
Division of Pediatric Gastroenterology and Nutrition
Department of Pediatrics
Alfred I. duPont Hospital for Children
Wilmington, DE, USA
Ch 19: Accidental Caustic Ingestions
Ch 32: Inflammatory Bowel Disease

Zahira Rushdie
Senior Fellow
Department of Pediatric Gastroenterology, Hepatology and Nutrition
Institute of Child and Adolescent Health
London, UK
Ch 24: Intestinal Obstruction

Verendra Sandur
Assistant Professor of Gastroenterology
Narayana Medical College and Superspeciality Hospital
Nellore, India
Ch 58: Intestinal Transplantation

Anupam Sehgal
Consultant
Sir Gangaram Hospital
New Delhi, India
Ch 80: Hepatitis B and C

Dheeraj Shah
Senior Lecturer
Department of Pediatrics
University Medical College and
Guru Teg Bahadur Hospital
Delhi, India
Ch 17: Upper Gastrointestinal Bleeding
Ch 50: Lower Gastrointestinal Bleeding
Ch 61: Chronic Pancreatitis

Shally Sharma
Senior Fellow in Gastroenterology and Nutrition
Old church Hospital
Essex, UK
Ch 101: Vitamin A Deficiency
Ch 103: Scurvy
Ch 104: Nutritional Riockets

ES Sherlock
Associate Professor
Division of Hepatology
Department of Pediatric Gastroenterology, Hepatology and Nutrition
Institute of Child and Adolescent Health
London, UK
Ch 78: Viral Hepatitis: Overview
Ch 79: Hepatitis A
Ch 81: Hepatitis D
Ch 82: Hepatitis E

Shruti Shrivastava
Resident
Department of Psychiatry
University College of Medical Sciences
Guru Teg Bahadur Hospital
Delhi, India
Ch 35: Eating Disorders

Tejinder Singh
Professor and Head
Department of Pediatrics
Vice-Principal
Director, CMCL-FAIMER Regional Institute
Program Incharge PGDMCH Christian Medical College
Ludhiana, India
Ch 106: Obesity

Utpal Kant Singh
Professor and Head
Department of Pediatrics
Nalanda Medical College
Patna, India
Ch 20: Gastrointestinal Tract: Embryology, Anatomy and Physiology
Ch 21: Congenital Anomalies of the Stomach

SS Slathia
Pediatric Specialist
Directorate of Health
Jammu, India
Ch 84: Amebic: Liver Abscess

Shanthy Sridhar
Medical Director
Neonatal Intensive Care Unit (NICU)
Associate Professor of Pediatrics
Stony Brook University Hospital
Stony Brook, New York, USA
Ch 110: Total Parenteral Nutrition (TPN)-Associated Cholestasis

Praveen C Sobti
Professor and Head of the Unit
Department of Pediatrics
Dayanand Medical College and Hospital
Ludhiana, India
Ch 109: Parenteral Nutrition in PICU

Madhuri Soni
Senior Fellow
Institute of Child and Adolescent Health
London, UK
Ch 11: Esophageal Obstructing Disorders
Ch 12: Esophageal Dysmotility
Ch 15: Hiatal Hernia
Ch 18: Esophageal Foreign Bodies

Raman Sreedharan
Senior Fellow
Department of Pediatric Gastroenterology, Hepatology and Nutrition
Division of Pediatric Gastroenterology and Nutrition
Department of Pediatrics
Alfred I. duPont Hospital for Children
Wilmington, DE, USA
Ch 59: Pancreas: Anatomy, Physiology and Developmental Anomalies
Ch 60: Acute Pancreatitis
Ch 123: Upper Gastrointestinal Endoscopy
Ch 124: Colonoscopy

Jyoti Suvarna
Associate Professor
Department of Pediatrics
Seth GS Medical College and KEM Hospital
Mumbai, India
Ch 41: Antibiotics and Diarrhea
Ch 111: Immunonutrition: A Step Ahead

Satish K Tiwari
Associate Professor
Department of Pediatrics
Medical College
Amravati, India
Ch 113: Nutritional Support in Diarrhea

Anand Venkatarao
Lecturer
Department of Pediatric Gastroenterology, Hepatology and Nutrition
Institute of Child and Adolescent Health
London, UK
Ch 10: Congenital Anomalies of the Esophagus
Ch18: Esophageal Foreign Bodies
Ch 24: Intestinal Obstruction

EA Walker
Lecturer
Department of Pediatric Gastroenterology, Hepatology and Nutrition
Institute of Child and Adolescent Health
London, UK
Ch 9: Esophagus: Embryology, Anatomy and Physiology
Ch 10: Congenital Anomalies of the Esophagus
Ch 11. Esophageal Obstructing Disorders
Ch 12: Esophageal Dysmotility
Ch 15: Hiatal Hernia
Ch 25: Intestinal Motility Disorders

Peter C Wilmot
Senior Fellow
Division of Pediatric Gastroenterology and Nutrition
Department of Pediatrics
Alfred I. duPont Hospital for Children
Wilmington, DE, USA
Ch 27: Constipation

Preface

Time is now ripe to view pediatric gastrointestinal and liver diseases from a perspective with a new depth of insight, particularly the emphasis on nutrition.

Over the past couple of decades, advances in the understanding of gastroenterology, hepatology and nutrition as relevant to infants, children and adolescents have been remarkable, particularly in respect of pathophysiology, genetic basis, and application of basic sciences in the clinical practice, diagnosis and therapy. New information is continuously pouring in, reflecting on the understanding of gastrointestinal and liver diseases.

Concurrently, nutritional support (that is now considered to be the backbone of treatment of gastrointestinal and liver disorders) has also undergone tremendous change in concepts and is beginning to find pride of place in treatment of these disorders. The remarks of the noted author Prof Frederick Suchy that "you can never be a good hepatologist or for that matter gastroenterologist unless you pay enough attention to the nutrition of the patient" describes this concept in the most appropriate terms.

The aim of this book is to provide a framework for a comprehensive and yet-not-exhaustive coverage of various disorders with a special stress on nutritional support in an easy-to-understand way, emphasizing pathophysiology, diagnosis and management. The approach remains by and large applied.

The book is divided into 4 major parts: Part A deals with gastroenterology, Part B with hepatology and Part C with the nutritional support. Finally, Part D dwells on the investigations.

The target readership includes physicians interested in diseases of the digestive tract, pancreas and liver, pediatric residents, pediatricians, and pediatric gastroenterologists, hepatologists and nutritionists.

I express my gratitudes to all the distinguished contributors, drawn from India and abroad, for providing fine material for incorporation in this book and for allowing us to edit it according to the needs of the project and the readers.

Thanks are particularly due to Prof Karoly Horvath, USA, for advising me on editorial matters right from the conception of the project over two years back and also for inspiring his group to contribute a number of excellent chapters to this treatise. Having him as the Guest Editor is a matter of pride.

I acknowledge the contribution of the peer-reviewers for taking pains not only to review the chapters but also putting them in proper perspectives.

Dr Novy Gupte and Manu Gupte deserve my appreciation for their impressive contribution as the Executive Editors of this ambitious project.

Hats of to my wife, Shamma, for her gracious assistance throughout this enterprise in spite of her preoccupation with other academic engagements.

The moral support, motivation and encouragement provided by the Management and Administration of Narayana Medical College and Hospitals, Nellore, India, is gratefully acknowledged. In this behalf, Dr P Narayana, Chairman, Dr CL Venkata Rao, Advisor, Dr S Vijaya Kumar, Coordinator, Dr Ramakrishna, Principal and Dr JN Rao, Medical Superintendent, deserve a special mention.

Hopefully, this textbook shall emerge as a valuable resource for the target audience, especially in India and other Asian countries.

Peepee Publishers and Distributors (P) Ltd and their staff deserve our special gratitude for the excellent get-up and production qualities of the book.

Suraj Gupte, MD, FIAP
Academic Editor

Guest Editor's Introductory Note

Pediatric gastroenterology as a subspecialty started growing over three decades ago in Europe and later in the USA. The establishment of pediatric gastroenterology, hepatology and nutrition societies in individual countries was the next step. This was followed by the introduction of pediatric gastroenterology subspecialty examination. The first examination in the US was held in 1993. This represented the official acceptance of the subspecialty. Now there are pediatric gastroenterology, hepatology and nutrition societies in each continent. The first World Congress in the field was organized in Boston in 2000.

Over this period the clinical practice of gastroenterology has evolved dramatically as the consequence of the significant advances in basic science, drug development and the addition of new diagnostic and therapeutic modalities to our clinical armamentarium.

The last three decades also have provided evidence that spectrum of gastrointestinal diseases is changing. Diseases that were unknown in the third world countries (e.g. celiac disease, cystic fibrosis, inflammatory bowel disease, etc.) now represent new challenges to the practitioners in the developing world. It seems that some of the digestive diseases spread from the western part of the globe to the eastern regions. Around the same time new challenges developed in the western countries, e.g. eosinophilic esophagitis and obesity-related gastrointestinal problems.

Our aim is to present a textbook that focuses on the practical clinical aspects of pediatric gastroenterology, making it useful to the medical students, house officers, residents and all physicians who treat children with gastrointestinal disorders. Primary care providers using this book can access the essential information to diagnose and manage common gastrointestinal and nutritional problems in childhood.

We hope that the clarity and completeness of this textbook will make it a useful practical resource. At the end of each chapter there are "Key Learning Points" for take-home messages and select references ("*Further Readings*") for those who would like to have deeper knowledge of the concerned topic.

Participation in the editing process of this book with Prof Suraj Gupte was indeed a matter of great pleasure. His enthusiasm, expertise and commitment to the pediatric education and improvement of pediatric care in the Indian subcontinent is admirable.

We would like to thank all the contributing authors for their hard work. They were selected because of their expertise in clinical practice and their commitment to excellence in patient care and education that are apparent from their writeups.

Karoly Horvath, MD, PhD
Professor of Pediatrics
Thomas Jefferson University, Philadelphia
Attending Gastroenterologist & Director, Celiac Center
A.1 duPont Hospital for Children
Wilmington DE, USA

Contents

PART A: PEDIATRIC GASTROENTEROLOGY

Section I: Clinical Aspects

Section II: Mouth, Oral Cavity and Salivary Glands

Section III: Esophagus

Section IV: Stomach, Duodenum and Intestine

PART B: PEDIATRIC HEPATOLOGY

PART C: PEDIATRIC NUTRITION

PART D: PEDIATRIC INVESTIGATIONS

Part B

Pediatric Hepatology

Pediatric Hepatology

69 Liver: Embryology, Anatomy and Physiology

Chandra Mohan Kumar

INTRODUCTION

Liver is the largest internal organ of the human body, weighing 1 to 1.5 kg and representing 1.5 to 2.5% of the lean body mass. It has a solid glandular structure. It is located in the right upper quadrant of the abdomen under the right lower ribcage against the diaphragm (right hypochondrium) and epigastrium and projects for a variable extent into the left hypochondrium. It remains anchored in place by ligamentous attachments to the diaphragm, peritoneum, great vessels, and upper gastrointestinal organs.

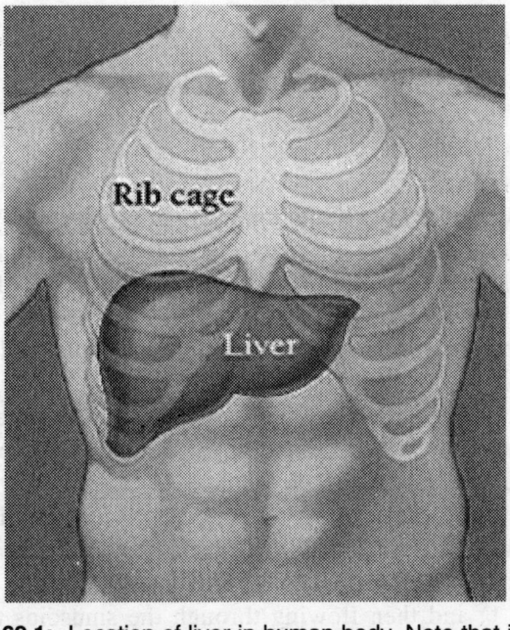

Fig. 69.1: Location of liver in human body. Note that it lies in the right hypochondrium and epigastrium with a projection into the left hypochondrium

EMBRYOLOGY

Liver develops from the hepatic diverticulum, an outgrowth of the ventral wall of the distal foregut (duodenum).

The hepatic diverticulum subsequently divides into a small ventral part, *pars cystica*, the future *gall bladder*, and a larger cranial part, the *pars hepatica,* which differentiates into the parenchyma of the liver and the lining of the biliary ducts. The connection between the hepatic diverticulum and the foregut (duodenum) forms the common bile duct (CBD). The bile duct has a small ventral outgrowth that becomes the *cystic duct* and expands into the gall bladder. The entrance of the bile duct into the small intestine gradually shifts from an initial anterior position to a posterior one and passes behind the duodenum.

The hepatocytes arrange into a series of branching and anastomosing plates in the mesenchyme of the transverse septum. These plates subsequently intermingle with vitelline and umbilical veins to form *hepatic sinusoids*. Besides contributing to the sinusoids, the splanchnic mesenchyme in the transverse septum also forms the *stroma*, the fibrous and serous coverings; the hepatic capsule, the *falciform ligament*, and the hematopoietic tissue (*Kupffer cells*) of the liver. The *connective tissue* and *smooth muscle* of the biliary tract also develops from this mesenchyme.

By the sixth week, the liver performs hematopoiesis (the formation of blood cells).

Gross Anatomy

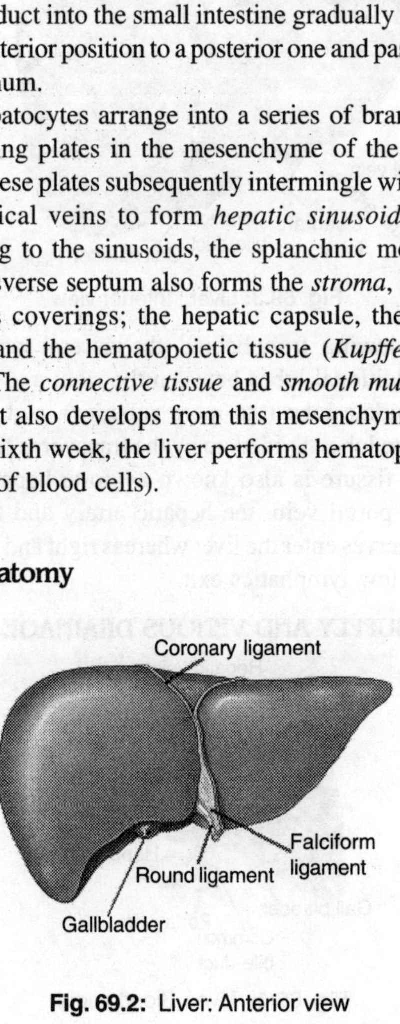

Fig. 69.2: Liver: Anterior view

Liver appears reddish-brown in color and resembles a four-sided pyramid laid on one side in shape.

It has five surfaces and one border. The surfaces are:

1. Anterior
2. Posterior
3. Superior
4. Inferior
5. Right.

The border is inferior border; a sharp border separating anterior surface from inferior surface.

It comprises four anatomical lobes:

- Left lobe
- Right lobe
- Caudate lobe, and
- Quadrate lobe

On viewing from the front, the dominant right and left lobes can be seen. These are separated by the falciform ligament. The right lobe is much larger than the left lobe and accounts for the 5/6th of the liver in volume.

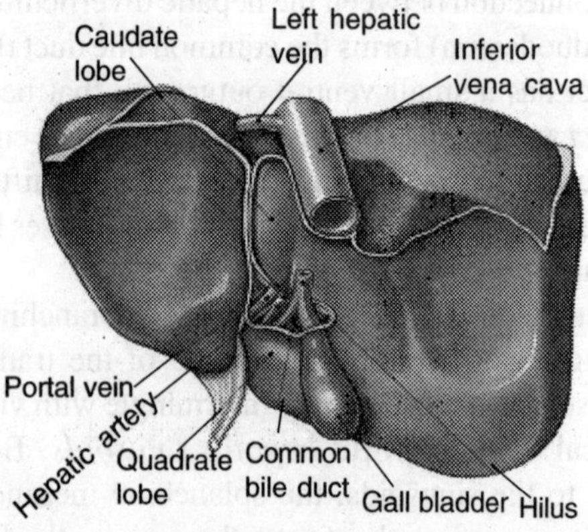

Fig. 69.3: Liver: Inferior view

While viewing from behind (the visceral surface), there are two additional lobes between the right and left. These are the caudate lobe (the more superior), and below this the quadrate lobe, divided up by the transverse fissure. This transverse fissure is also known as porta hepatis through which the portal vein, the hepatic artery and the hepatic plexus of nerves enter the liver whereas right and left hepatic ducts and few lymphatics exit.

BLOOD SUPPLY AND VENOUS DRAINAGE

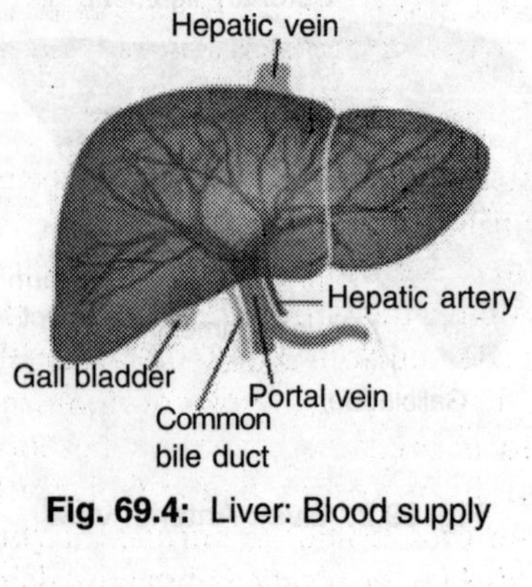

Fig. 69.4: Liver: Blood supply

It receives a dual blood supply from portal as well as systemic circulation. Approximately 20% of the blood flow is oxygen-rich blood from the hepatic artery, and 80% is nutrient-rich blood from the portal vein arising from the stomach, intestines, pancreas and spleen. Before entering the liver both the hepatic artery and portal vein divide into right and left branches and within the liver the subdivided into segmental to interlobular vessels running in the portal canals and then finally to hepatic sinusoids where the bloods of both the systems mix.

Hepatic sinusoids drain into interlobular veins which join to form sublobular veins. These in turn unite and form the hepatic veins draining directly into inferior vena cava.

LOBULAR ARCHITECTURE

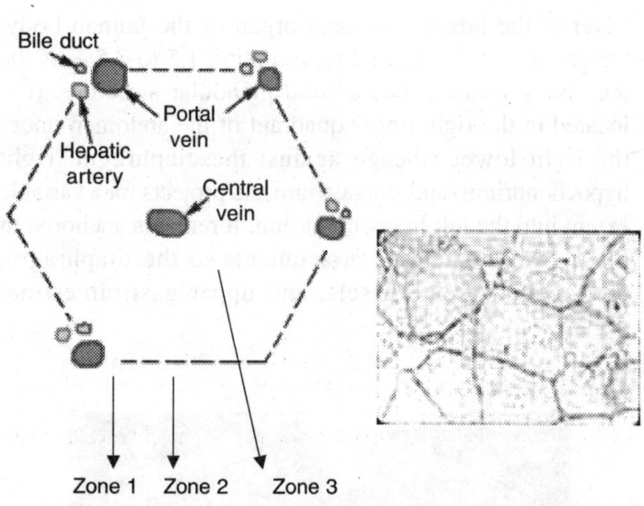

Fig. 69.5: Normal hepatic architecture

The majority of cells in the liver are hepatocytes, which constitute 2/3rds of the mass of the liver. The remaining cell types are Kupffer cells (members of the reticuloendothelial system), stellate (fat-storing) cells, endothelial cells and blood vessels, bile ductular cells, and supporting structures.

On light microscopy, the liver appears to be organized in lobules, with portal areas at the periphery and central veins in the center of each lobule.

However, from a functional point of view, the liver is organized into acini, with both hepatic arterial and portal venous blood entering the acinus from the portal areas (zone 1) and then flowing through the sinusoids to the terminal hepatic veins (zone 3), the intervening hepatocytes constituting zone 2. The advantage of regarding the acinus as the physiologic unit of the liver is that it helps to explain the morphologic patterns and zonality of many vascular and biliary diseases not explained by the lobular arrangement. Portal areas of the liver consist of small veins, arteries, bile ducts, and lymphatics organized in a loose stroma of supporting matrix and small amounts of collagen. Blood flowing into the portal areas is distributed through the sinusoids, passing from zone 1 to zone 3 of the acinus and draining into the terminal hepatic veins ("central veins"). Secreted bile flows in the opposite direction, in a counter-current pattern from zone 2 to zone 1. The sinusoids are lined by unique endothelial cells that have prominent fenestrae of variable size, allowing the free flow of plasma but not cellular elements. The plasma is thus in direct contact with hepatocytes in the subendothelial space of Disse.

Hepatocytes have distinct polarity. The basolateral side of the hepatocyte lines the space of Disse and is richly lined with microvilli. It demonstrates endocytotic and pinocytotic activity, with passive and active uptake of nutrients, proteins, and other molecules. The apical pole of the hepatocyte forms the cannicular membranes through which bile components are secreted. The canniculi of hepatocytes form a fine network, which fuses into the bile ductular elements near the portal areas.

Kupffer cells occupy sinusoidal vascular space and represent the largest group of fixed macrophages in the body.

Red blood cells stay in the sinusoidal space as blood flows through the lobules, but white blood cells can migrate through or around endothelial cells into the space of Disse and from there to portal areas, where they can return to the circulation through lymphatics.

PHYSIOLOGY

Liver performs numerous and vital roles in maintaining homeostasis.

The functions of liver are summarized in Table 69.1.

Table 69.1: Functions of the liver

Homeostasis	Glucose Proteins Fat and cholesterol Hormones Vitamins, in particular fat-soluble ones (A, D, E, K)
Synthesis	Proteins including the clotting factors (~50g/day) Bile acids (important in fat digestion) Heparin (anti-coagulant) Somatomedins (hormones that promote growth in bone, soft tissues) Estrogen Angiotensinogen Cholesterol Acute phase proteins
Storage	Vitamins Glycogen Cholesterol Iron, copper Fats
Excretion	Cholesterol, bile acids, phospholipids Bilirubin Drugs Poisons including heavy metals Hormones
Filtering	Poisons Nutrients including amino acids, sugars, and fats Bilirubin, bile acids IgA Drugs Dead or damaged cells in circulatory system
Immune	Excretes IgA into digestive tract Kupffer cells (macrophages) filter out antigens

The functions include the synthesis of most essential serum proteins (albumin, carrier proteins, coagulation factors, many hormonal and growth factors), the production of bile and its carriers (bile acids, cholesterol, lecithin, phospholipids), the regulation of nutrients (glucose, glycogen, lipids, cholesterol, amino acids), and metabolism and conjugation of lipophilic compounds (bilirubin, anions, cations, drugs) for excretion in the bile or urine. Measurement of these activities to assess liver function is complicated by the multiplicity and variability of these functions.

The most commonly used liver "function" tests are measurements of serum bilirubin, albumin, and prothrombin time. The serum bilirubin level is a measure of hepatic conjugation and excretion, and the serum albumin level and prothrombin time are measures of protein synthesis. Abnormalities of bilirubin, albumin, and prothrombin time are typical of hepatic dysfunction.

Frank liver failure is incompatible with life, and the functions of the liver are too complex and diverse to be subserved by a mechanical pump, dialysis membrane, or concoction of infused hormones, proteins, and growth factors. One of the liver's most remarkable abilities is self-repair and the regeneration of damaged tissues.

KEY LEARNING POINTS

- Largest organ, developing from the hepatic diverticulum of the distal foregut.
- Dual blood supply from portal and systemic circulation.
- Two-third mass constituted by hepatocytes, remaining cells being Kupffer cells (members of the RES).
- Microscopically, organized in lobules with portal veins at the periphery and central veins in the center of each lobule.
- Functionally, organized into acini that should be regarded as its physiologic unit.
- Among its many vital functions, ranging from homeostasis through storage to immune, rank the synthesis of serum proteins.
- Self repair and regeneration of damaged tissue a remarkable ability.
- Frank failure incompatible with life.

FURTHER READINGS

1. Bates MD, Balistreri WF. The gastrointestinal tract: Development of the human digestive system. In: Fanaroff AA, Martin RJ (eds): *Neonatal-Perinatal Medicine: Diseases of the Fetus and Infant*, 7th edn. St. Louis: Mosby 2002:1255-1263.
2. Chaurasia BD. The liver in: *Human Anatomy*, 4th edn. New Delhi: CBS 2004: 288-293.
3. Karpen SJ, Suchy FJ. Structural and functional development of the liver. In Suchy FJ, *et al.* (editors): Liver Disease in Children, 2nd edn. Philadelphia: Lippincott; Williams and Wilkins: 2001;3-21.
4. Zakim D, Boyer TD. *Hepatology: A Textbook of Liver Disease*, 4th edn. Philadelphia: Saunders 2003.
5. Zaret KS: Hepatocyte differentiation from the endoderm and beyond. *Curr Opin Genet Dev* 2001;11:568-574.

70 Clinical Manifestations of Liver Disease

Suraj Gupte • Sheffali Abbott

INTRODUCTION

Manifestations of liver disease, a life-threatening state, may be clinical and pathologic. A good knowledge of these manifestations adds up to our high index of suspicion which is essential for identifying it.

JAUNDICE

Also termed *icterus*, it denotes yellow discoloration of sclera, skin and mucous membranes as a result of hyperbilirubinemia. Clinically obvious jaundice beyond neonatal period points to serum bilirubin >2 to 3 mg/dL (34-51 mcmol/L). The corresponding bilirubin in neonates is >5 mg/dL (85 mcmol/L).

Jaundice may well be the first and the solitary pointer to liver dysfunction.

In an infant, jaundice with clay or light-colored (acholic) stools and dark urine is a sign of cholestasis (conjugated hyperbilirubinemia) warranting evaluation without delay. Usually, it indicates decreased excretion of bile by dysfunctional hepatic parenchymal cells or obstruction of the biliary tract. Additional causes of cholestasis in relation to biliary tract include sepsis, inflammation, toxins and metabolic or genetic diseases.

Unconjugated hyperbilirubinemia points to increased production, hemolysis, reduced hepatic removal or altered metabolism of bilirubin.

HEPATOMEGALY

Enlarged liver may well be an important sign of liver disease, especially when accompanied by jaundice. It is, therefore important to know how to determine whether the size is beyond the acceptable limit.

Liver is normally palpable upto 2 cm below the right costal margin in the right midclavicular line. In a neonate, palpability beyond 3.5 cm should be considered abnormal.

Just dependence on palpability of liver can, at times is, be misleading. As for example, downward displacement of liver by the diaphragm (visceroptosis in rickets, hyperinflation of lungs) or thoracic organs may give the erroneous impression of hepatomegaly. Furthermore, in some normal subjects, the lower edge of the right lobe may extend downward, giving the false impression of enlargement of the liver.

Measurement of *liver span* is, therefore, more relevant and reliable than its palpability below the costal margin. It is measured by first percussing the upper border of dullness and then palpating the lower border in the right midclavicular line. The span measures 4.5 to 5.0 cm at 1 week of age, 7 to 8 cm in boys and 6.0 to 6.5 cm in girls by 12 years of age.

Over and above the size of the liver, examination should note its consistency (whether firm, soft), feel of the border (whether leafy, sharp or rounded), presence of tenderness, and surface (smooth, nodular). Also important is to detect a bruit.

The size of spleen and presence of ascites and other stigmata of liver disease should also be ascertained.

In addition to the physical examination, now it is considered important to have a more objective assessment of the liver and gall bladder size and consistency by ultrasonography. In fatty liver secondary to malnutrition, obesity, hyperalimentation and chronic steroid therapy as well as in metabolic liver disease (glycogen storage disease), hyperchogenic liver parenchyma is seen on ultrasonography.

PRURITUS

Intense pruritus, at times accompanied by skin excoriation is a sign of cholestasis. Though it is believed to be the result of deposition of bile salts in the skin, it appears that its etiology is multifactorial. Its intensity is in no way related to magnitude of hyperbilirubinemia. It responds to treatment with:

- Antihistamines (lordatidine).
- Bile-acid binding agents (cholestyramine).
- Choleretic agents (ursodeoxycholic acid).
- Opiate antagonists.
- Antibiotics.

PORTAL HYPERTENSION

The child with cirrhosis is said to have developed the complication of portal hypertension when the portal pressure difference between the portal vein and the systemic veins (inferior vena cava or hepatic veins) exceeds a threshold of 10 mmHg (normal 3-6 mmHg).

Further complications of portal hypertension include ascites and variceal hemorrhage, which should be considered potentially lethal.

Ascites

Presence of ascites in a known case of chronic liver disease (usually cirrhosis) signals development of portal hypertension and liver insufficiency.

Variceal Hemorrhage

In portal hypertension, there is a tendency for development of significant portosystemic collaterals, the so-called *gastroesophageal varices.* These varices may rupture because of increased pressure within the varix with resultant changes in the diameter of the varix and increased wall tension exceeding the strength of the wall, causing life-threatening bleeding. Such a bleeding can be enormous on account of two factors, namely:

- Massive blood flow and pressure in the portosystemic collateral system.
- Absence of a natural mechanism to temponade variceal hemorrhage.

SPIDER ANGIOMAS (TELANGIECTASIAS)

Predominantly over the face and chest of children with chronic liver disease may be seen vascular spiders. These are the central pulsating arterioles from which small, wiry venules radiate. The altered estrogen metabolism appears to be the cause.

PALMAR ERYTHEMA

As a consequence of enhanced blood flow and vasodilation, children suffering from chronic liver disease may show blotchy erythema predominantly over the thenar and hypothenar eminences.

XANTHOMAS

Chronic cholestasis couple with hypercholesterolemias may cause deposition of lipid in the dermis and subcutaneous tissue in the form of brown nodules over the extensor surfaces of the limbs followed by the eyelids.

ENCEPHALOPATHY

Depending on the presence of portosystemic shunting, alteration in the blood-brain barrier and the interaction of toxic metabolites with CNS, encephalopathy may develop in a child with progressive liver disease.

Encephalopathy may be present in a sheer subtle form rather than an acute outstanding manifestation. The manifestations of subtle encephalopathy include:

- Deterioration of school performance.
- Depression.
- Emotional outbursts.

Its precipitation may follow:

- Intercurrent illness.
- Drugs.
- Bleeding.
- Dehydration, dyselectrolytemia and acid-base disturbance.

The exact modus operandi of hepatic encephalopathy remains speculative. The hypotheses are:

- Altered ammonia metabolism.
- Synergestic neurotoxins.
- False neurotransmitters with plasma amino acid imbalance.

ENDOCRINAL ABNORMALITIES

Occurrence of endocrinal abnormalities is less common in children than in adults with liver disease.

RENAL DYSFUNCTION

Hepatorenal syndrome (HRS) is defined as functional renal failure in patients with end-stage liver disease. Intense renal vasoconstriction is the hallmark of the syndrome.

HEPATOPULMONARY SYNDROME

Liver disease may be accompanied by hypoxemia and intrapulmonary vascular dilation. This triad is termed *hepatopulmonary syndrome.* Manifestations include shortness of breath or exercise intolerance, cyanosis, digital clubbing and oxygen saturation < 96%.

Following timely liver transplantation, the pulmonary signs and symptoms subside.

RECURRENT CHOLANGITIS

Chronic cholestatic liver disease is prone to ascending infection of the biliary system from time to time. The causative pathogens are gram-negative enteric organisms (*E. coli, Klebsiella, Pseudomonas, Enterococcus*). When medical therapy fails, liver transplantation is the only remedy.

MISCELLANEOUS

- Anorexia (anicteric hepatitis, cirrhosis associated with chronic cholestasis).
- Abdominal distention/pain due to ascites, spontaneous peritonitis, visceromegaly, etc. (Table 70.1).
- Malnutrition/vitamin deficiencies.
- Growth failure.
- Bleeding (biliary obstruction with vitamin K deficiency, excessive liver damage).
- Portal hypertension with hypersplenism, causing decreased synthesis of clotting factors, production of qualitatively abnormal proteins or alterations in platelet number and function.
- Altered drug metabolism, prolonging the biologic half-life of commonly used drugs.

Table 70.1: Causes of abdominal discomfort/pain in liver disease

- Stretch of liver capsule from its distention
- Viral hepatitis
- Congestive hepatomegaly
- Liver abscess
- Perihepatitis
- Cholangitis
- Ascites
- Peritonitis

KEY LEARNING POINTS

- Clinical jaundice denotes a serum bilirubin > 5 mg/dL in neonates and > 2-3 mg/dL in subsequent age groups.
- Hepatomegaly, especially in association with jaundice, is an important sign of liver disease.
- Intense pruritus points to cholestasis.
- Ascites and variceal bleeding are signs of Ch portal hypertension (> 10 mmHg against the normal of 3-6 mmHg).
- Hepatic encephalopathy may be present is a subtle form rather than an acute remarkable manifestation.
- Renal dysfunction (hepatorenal syndrome) and pulmonay dysfunction (hepatopulmonary syndrome) are serious manifestations.
- Remaining manifestations include recurrent anorexia, bleeding, growth retardation and nutritional deficiencies, cholangitis, spider angiomas, palmar erytema, xanthomas, etc.

FURTHER READINGS

1. Balistereri WF. Pediatric hepatomegaly: A half-century of progress. *Clin Liver Dis* 2000;4:191-210.
2. Boamah L, Balistreri WF. Manifestations of liver disease. In: Kligman RM, Behrman RE, Jenson HB, Stanton BF (eds): *Nelson Textbook of Pediatrics*, 18th edn. Philadelphia: Saunders 2008: 1661-1665.

71 Hepatic Manifestations of Systemic Diseases

Chandra Mohan Kumar

INTRODUCTION

Liver is a major site of metabolic activities in human body. It is one of the most important organs taking part in various synthetic, regulatory, storage, detoxification and excretory activities. It is more vulnerable to systemic disorders since:

1. It is a part of digestive system, hepatobiliary system and reticuloendothelial system. The systemic disorders having effects on any of these systems are likely to ultimately affect hepatic functions.
2. It is a highly vascular structure having dual blood supply in the form of systemic and portal circulation.

Hence, a large number of diseases like PEM, anemias, cardiac failure, infectious diseases, rheumatic diseases, pulmonary disorders and infiltrative storage diseases, which primarily affect systems other than liver, have noteworthy hepatic manifestations.

FATTY LIVER IN PROTEIN-ENERGY MALNUTRITION

Protein-energy malnutrition is still a very common and serious problem in developing world. Mild to moderate enlargement of liver due to diffuse accumulation of neutral fat is a common manifestation of kwashiorkor. The pathogenesis of fatty liver in PEM has been a controversial issue. It is believed to be due to decreased production of apolipoprotein B-100 (apoB-100); which is responsible for carrying fat in plasma out of the liver in combination with VLDL. Also, there is increased flux of free fatty acids from adipose depots to liver. On biochemical examination aminotransferases like ALT and AST remain elevated whereas alkaline phosphatase (ALP) levels are found to be lower than normal controls.

HEPATIC INVOLVEMENTS IN ANEMIAS

Many types of hemolytic anemias including homozygous sickle cell anemia, compound heterozygosity for sickle cell anemia and β-thalassemia, glucose-6-phosphate dehydrogenase (G6PD) deficiency, hereditary spherocytosis, hemolysis, elevated liver enzymes, and low platelets (HELLP) syndrome, congenital erythropoietic porphyria in infancy and late-onset erythropoietic porphyria, and pseudohemolytic uremic syndrome may manifest with liver dysfunction.

The most important among them is sickle cell anemia. In sickle cell anemia when a large number of erythrocytes becomes sickled within the hepatic circulation, blood flow through the liver may become impaired. A large volume of blood may become pooled in the liver, causing acute hepatic enlargement and pain and decreased hematocrit. This situation is known as *veno-occlusive hepatic sequestration crisis*. It has been reported that intrahepatic sickling crisis can cause acute hepatic failure in upto 10% of patients with hepatic sequestration crises. Such crises may even prove fatal in children younger than 10 years. Conjugated hyperbilirubinemia is the only biochemical marker in individuals with hepatic sickling crisis. It may be confirmed by liver biopsy.

Jaundice and hyperbilirubinemia may be caused by hemolysis plus transfusion-related viral hepatitis. In one study among the cases of SCD, 50% had hepatomegaly, and 11% had hepatitis. The edge of an enlarged liver in patients with sickle cell anemia usually is smooth and tender to palpation. In a study of 100 patients with sickle cell disease in USA, about one third had liver dysfunction. In another series cirrhosis has been observed in upto 16% to 29% of patients with sickle cell disease. Patients with HELPP syndromes have elevated liver enzymes as a part of the disease spectrum.

LIVER IN CONGESTIVE CARDIAC FAILURE

Liver, very frequently, bears the brunt of CCF as it lies close to the right atrium as well as it gets ¼th of the cardiac output. So it may have various types of presentations described as *ischaemic hepatitis* and *congestive hepatopathy* or *cardiac cirrhosis*. Various studies have documented hepatic involvements in congestive cardiac failure. In a large series of 175 patients with both acute and chronic congestive heart failure, hepatomegaly was present in 90% to 95% and ascites in 17% to 25%. Although overt jaundice is uncommon in congestive heart failure (seen only in 5% in patients with acute congestive heart failure) mild elevation of the serum bilirubin level occurs in up to 70% of patients. The total serum bilirubin levels are usually less than 3 mg/dL, with a predominantly unconjugated fraction. However, in patients with chronic, severe heart failure, jaundice may be so deep as to suggest biliary obstruction. But, fortunately, in these cases, even in the presence of deep jaundice, the level of serum alkaline phosphatase is usually normal or minimally elevated, a finding that helps to distinguish cardiac jaundice from obstructive jaundice.

Serum aminotransferase levels are elevated mildly, usually two to three times the normal value, in upto 1/3rd of patients with chronic heart failure. In patients with severe acute heart failure complicated by hypotension, however, the serum aminotransferase levels may be greatly elevated, simulating acute viral hepatitis.

The congestive cardiac failure affects the liver by three pathogenic mechanisms: Decreased hepatic blood flow, increased hepatic venous pressure, and decreased arterial oxygen saturation. The most important structural changes occur due to the effect of passive congestion on the liver. Electron microscopic studies of congested livers have documented that this increased pressure can cause the atrophy of hepatocytes in zone 3 (areas around central vein). Increased hepatic venous pressure also results in sinusoidal congestion and enlargement of the sinusoidal fenestrae leading to exudation of protein-rich fluid into the space of Disse. The resulting perisinusoidal edema may impair diffusion of oxygen and nutrients to hepatocytes. Continued ischemic insults or chronic passive congestion can result in liver fibrosis in the zone 3 and in the space of Disse, leading to further impairment of the blood-to-hepatocyte diffusion of oxygen and nutrients. A significant degree of necrosis in zone 3 (that is caused by acute left-sided heart failure) has been documented even in the absence of right-sided heart failure, suggesting that reduced cardiac output may be the predominant determinant of hepatic ischemia and fibrosis in some patients. Thus, all these factors contribute to development of perivenular necrosis and fibrosis, called *cardiac cirrhosis.*

Cardiac cirrhosis classically is seen in patients with constrictive pericarditis or prolonged mitral valve disease and secondary tricuspid regurgitation.

HEPATIC INVOLVEMENT IN TROPICAL INFECTIOUS DISEASES

Enteric Fever

Enteric fever, is a common infectious disease caused by *Salmonella typhi* and *Salmonella paratyphi,* is encountered in children in tropical countries including India. It is not an uncommon finding to have a soft hepatomegaly in the physical examination of the child. Incidence of hepatomegaly is believed to be 2-3 times more common in typhoid fever than paratyphoid fever and has been reported between 23-90% in children with typhoid fever. A higher incidence of hepatomegaly has been reported in children suffering from multidrug resistant (MDR) typhoid fever.

Hepatic manifestations of typhoid fever are known for more than a century now, first reported by William Osler in 1899. Since then a lot of work has been done in this regard and now we have quite a reasonable information and evidence regarding various hepatic manifestations of enteric fever. They include mild elevation of aminotransferases and alkaline phosphatases seen quite frequently during the second and third weeks of their illness to a picture indistinguishable from acute viral hepatitis. In various studies the incidences of deranged hepatic enzyme levels have been estimated to be in the range of 23% in first week which increases to more than 50 percent of cases in the second and third weeks. However, 4-5 percent of children may present with elevated serum bilirubin levels, 10 fold increases in aminotransferases and abnormally prolonged PT, making it difficult to distinguish from acute viral hepatitis. Jaundice associated with typhoid fever tends to occur at the peak of fever which differentiates it from viral hepatitis in which case fever usually comes down after the appearance of jaundice.

Liver biopsies demonstrate focal Kupffer cell hyperplasia and mononuclear cell infiltration of the portal space. The Kuppffer cells tend to aggregate and the aggregations have been called "typhoid nodules". Focal necrosis of liver cells is common.

Malaria

Hepatomegaly is a common feature of malaria. The liver is enlarged early, usually after the first paroxysms and is usually firm and may be tender. On gross appearance it is edematous, colored brown, gray or even black as a result of deposition of malaria pigment. Biopsy shows dilated hepatic sinusoids containing hypertrophied Kupffer cells and parasitized red cells. Small areas of centrilobular necrosis may be seen in severe cases due to shock or disseminated intravascular coagulation. Prolonged infection may be associated with stromal induration and diffuse proliferation of fibrous connective tissue. However, changes of cirrhosis are not seen.

In falciparum malaria, in addition to the involvement of the mesenchyma, the hepatocytes may also be involved, causing functional changes as well (malarial hepatitis). Malarial hepatitis is characterized by hyperbilirubinemia, increased levels of transaminases and alkaline phosphatase. Liver involvement in severe falciparum malaria is due to impairment of local microcirculation associated with hepatocellular damage.

In patients with repeated attacks of malaria, liver also enlarges significantly along with a large and hard spleen. However, there is no functional abnormality of the liver in these patients.

HEPATIC DYSFUNCTIONS IN RHEUMATOLOGIC DISEASES

Systemic Lupus Erythematosus

SLE is an important autoimmune rheumatic disorder manifested by rash, photosensitivity, arthritis, renal, hematological and neuropsychiatric manifestations. Liver involvement in SLE is not an uncommon finding. Various studies have documented that the incidence of jaundice is 3-10%. Hepatomegaly has been seen in as high as 20-40% of the patients with SLE. On examination, the liver may be found to be slightly enlarged and tender on palpation. Frequently, routine biochemical evaluations show a slightly raised enzymes (AST, ALT, alkaline phosphatase and GGT) although patients may remain asymptomatic. Lupus involvement of the liver is usually mild and does not progress to severe hepatitis or cirrhosis. An important entity to distinguish from lupus hepatitis is lupoid hepatitis, now better known as *autoimmune hepatitis*. An important but rare manifestation of lupus in liver is hepatic vasculitis, which responds to corticosteroids therapy. In neonates, maternal lupus manifests as transient elevation of hepatic enzymes.

Rheumatoid Arthritis

Rheumatoid arthritis is a chronic polyarthritis, associated with many extraarticular features. Elevated levels of serum aminotransferases have been reported in patients with RA who do not have an alternate diagnosis that explains the increased levels of liver enzymes.

Kendall and colleagues in 1970 observed that 26% of patients with RA had elevated levels of alkaline phosphatase that were confirmed to be of hepatic origin by correlation with serum 5-nucleotidase concentrations. This observation prompted them to coin a new term "*rheumatoid liver*" but additional markers of liver function, including levels of serum bilirubin, aspartate aminotransferase (AST), and alanine aminotransferase (ALT), were all within normal limits. Similarly liver biopsy findings in patients with RA does not suggest a consistent structural abnormality. Most biopsy reports suggest only minor nonspecific changes. Thus, it can be concluded that with existing evidence, except for mild elevation in levels of serum aminotransferases, liver abnormalities are not common in RA.

Systemic Sclerosis

Systemic sclerosis (SSc) is a rare autoimmune inflammatory abnormality characterized by excessive deposition of collagen in several organs and in the blood vessels. The hepatic manifestation in cases of SSc is primary biliary cirrhosis (PBC), which is an autoimmune disorder characterized by chronic cholestatic liver disease, progressive inflammatory destruction of the interlobular and septal bile ducts with development of periportal inflammation, fibrosis and cirrhosis.

Ankylosing Spondylitis

Liver enzyme abnormalities are observed in 26% of patients, correlating directly with ESR elevations. Elevations in levels of serum alkaline phosphatase and gamma-glutamyl transpeptidase (GGT) are also detected suggesting a hepato biliary origin. Management with NSAIDs improve LFT abnormalities, thus documenting these liver enzymes abnormalities as direct evidence of AS.

These rheumatic diseases may have hepatic dysfunctions in another way also. The treatment of these disorders has a significant toll on the hepatic functions. NSAIDs may have direct hepatotoxicity or idiosyncratic hepatotoxicities. They cause an increase in liver enzymes. Sulfasalazine, a commonly used drug for ulcerative colitis and rheumatoid arthritis is also a known hepatotoxic drug.

Methotrexate, another second line drug for RA causes hepatic fibrosis and cirrhosis.

Hence, elevation in liver enzymes is not an uncommon finding in rheumatic diseases which may be a primary non-articular manifestation or a complication of treatment of these diseases.

HEPATIC MANIFESTATIONS OF PULMONARY DISEASES

Cystic Fibrosis

Cystic fibrosis is an autosomal recessive disease primarily of the lungs, exocrine pancreas, liver and intestines. Its incidence is estimated to be 1 of 2000 live births among Caucasians. It is not frequent in India and other Asian countries. It is due to a defect in expression of CFTR protein. Although the CFTR protein is not located on hepatocytes, its absence have an impact on the function as well as architecture of the liver. One role of the CFTR protein, which is located on the apical surfaces of the intrahepatic and extrahepatic bile ducts, is to regulate chloride secretion into bile. Dysfunction or absence of this protein results in a decrease in the water and sodium content of bile, leading to an increase in bile viscosity. This subsequently decreases the bile flow with resultant obstruction of intrahepatic bile ducts. The most frequent hepatic complication is focal biliary-type cirrhosis (FBC). In most of the cases with cystic fibrosis, clinical evidence of liver disease may not be obvious. Factors that have been identified as risk factors for liver disease in CF include pancreatic insufficiency, HLA haplotype B7-DR 15-DQ6, male sex, and presence of meconium ileus. About 2% of neonates with cystic fibrosis present with neonatal jaundice. In half of these patients, jaundice is accompanied by meconium ileus. The clinical and biochemical presentation can be confused with biliary atresia. The cholestasis resolves with time, but residual fibrosis may remain. Elevated levels of AST or ALT also may be the initial clue to liver involvement. An elevated bilirubin level is a late finding and suggests significant liver disease.

The incidence of FBC increases with the age of the child. Studies that involved autopsies of patients with cystic fibrosis have reported evidence of FBC in 10% of infants less than 3 months, in 27% of children older than 1 year, and in 72% of adults. The incidence of cirrhosis with evidence of portal hypertension was reported to be 0.1% in CF patients 2 to 5 years old.

Alpha-1- Antitrypsin Deficiency

Alpha-1-antitrypsin deficiency is an autosomal recessive metabolic disorder that can affect the lungs, liver, kidneys, and pancreas. It affects 1 in 1600 to 1800 live births. Alpha-1-antitrypsin is a glycoprotein that is produced in the liver and is encoded by a single gene, Pi, which is located on chromosome 14. The normal variant is PiMM, and the most common abnormal alleles, PiZZ, PiSS and PiNull, produce 15%, 60%, and 0% of the normal levels of a1 AT, respectively.

The PiZZ phenotype accounts for over 95% of a1 AT deficiency-induced pulmonary and liver diseases. Neonatal jaundice, elevated liver enzymes, bile duct reduplication and severe fibrosis and cirrhosis are the hepatic manifestations in cases of alpha-1- antitrypsin deficiency. Prolonged neonatal jaundice is observed in 86% of PiZZ phenotype.

LIVER IN STORAGE/INFILTRATIVE DISEASES

Lipid storage diseases such as Gaucher's disease and Niemann-Pick disease, other storage diseases like abetalipoproteinemia and Fabry's disease present with hepatomegaly due to abnormal deposition of fats or glycogen. Similarly in Hurler's syndrome, an uncommon genetic condition, liver enlarges due to deposition of mucopolysaccharides, *chondroitin sulphate B* and *heparan sulphate*. A relatively common genetically inherited disorder is hemochromatosis (HHC) in which there is deposition of excessive iron in hepatocytes. Iron deposition in macrophages of RE system is also seen in secondary hemosiderosis.

KEY LEARNING POINTS

- Being the major site of metabolic activities in human body, liver is an innocent sufferer in various diseases of different organs and organ systems.
- Disordered liver function does not necessarily mean primary hepatic pathology.
- Noteworthy systemic diseases involving liver include anemias, CCF tropical infections (enteric fever, malaria), rheumatologic disorders (SLE, RA, ankylosing spondylitis), pulmonary disease (CF, A-1-antitrypsin deficiency) and storage disorders (Gaucher's, Niemann-Pick, Hurler's).
- In PEM, hepatomegaly resulting from fatty change, causes only subtle liver dysfunction.

FURTHER READINGS

1. Truswell AS. Malnutrition and carbohydrate and lipid metabolism. In: Suskind RM, Lewinter Suskind L (eds): *The Malnourished Child.* New York: Raven Press 1990:95-118.
2. Johnson CS, Omata M, Tong MJ, *et al.* Liver involvement in sickle cell disease. *Medicine (Baltimore)* 1985;64:349-356.
3. Corwin Q. Edwards, Anemia and the liver hepatobiliary manifestations of anemia *Clin Liver Dis* 2002;6: 891-907.
4. Rasoolinejad M, Esmailpoor Bazaz N and Mogbel Alhosein B. Salmonella ahepatitis (analysis of hepatic involvement in 107 patients with typhoid fever) *Acta Medica Iranica* 2003;4: 161-163.
5. Srivastava A, Khanduri A, Lakhtakia S. Falciparum malaria with acute liver failure *Trop Gastroenterol* 1996; 17:172-174.
6. Jagadish K, Patwari AK, Sarin SK, Prakash C, Srivastava DK, Anand VK. Hepatic manifestations in typhoid fever. *Indian Pediatr* 1994;31:807-811.
7. Seeto RK, Fenn B, Rockey DC. Ischemic hepatitis: Clinical presentation and pathogenesis. *Am J Med* 2000;109:109-113.
8. Walker Nancy J. Zurier Robert B. Liver abnormalities in rheumatic diseases *Clin Liver Dis* 2002;66:933-946.
9. Thomas J. Layden, Laura Kulik, Hepatic manifestations of pulmonary diseases *Clin Liver Dis* 2002;6:969-979.

72 Evaluation of the Liver Disease

Suraj Gupte • Sheffali Abbott

INTRODUCTION

Over and above a carefully recorded history and physical examination, evaluation of suspected liver disease involves a judicious selection out of a battery of screening and diagnostic tests, including liver biopsy and imaging studies.

AIMS AND OBJECTIVES OF EVALUATION PROCESS

1. Is liver dysfunction present?

If yes

2. Its nature?
3. Its magnitude?
4. Is it treatable?
5. Monitoring of response to treatment?
6. Prognosis?

COMPONENTS OF THE EVALUATION OF LIVER FUNCTION STRATEGY

- Good, focused history and physical examination.
- Careful interpretation of information (symptoms and signs) obtained therefrom.
- Biochemical liver function tests.
- Imaging studies.
- Liver biopsy.

Biochemical Tests

The typical liver profile tests includes serum bilirubin (total and fractionated), transaminases (ALT, AST), alkaline phosphatase, GGTP, prothrombin time, LDL, protein (total, albumin and globulin).

Serum Bilirubin

This is the main bile pigment in humans which, when elevated, causes jaundice. Bilirubin is formed primarily from the breakdown of "heme". It is taken up from blood processed through the liver, and then secreted into the bile by the liver. Normal individuals have only a small amount of bilirubin circulating in blood (<1.2 mg/dL). Conditions, which cause increased formation of bilirubin, such as destruction of red blood cells, or decrease its removal from the blood stream, such as liver disease may result in an increase in the level of serum bilirubin. Levels greater than 3 mg/dL are usually noticeable as jaundice. The bilirubin may be elevated in many forms of liver or biliary tract disease, and thus it is also relatively nonspecific. However, serum bilirubin is generally considered a true test of liver function (LFT), since it reflects the liver's ability to take up, process, and secrete bilirubin into the bile.

Determination of serum bilirubin in conjugated and unconjugated forms assists in differentiating hyperbilirubinemia of hepatic origin from that of hemolytic origin. A predominant conjugated hyperbilirubinemia points to hepatocellular dysfunction and hepatic excretory dysfunction.

Serum Transferases/Transaminases

Alanine amino transferase (ALT). Previously popular as serum glutamate pyruvate transaminase (**SGPT**), it is supposed to be a liver-specific enzyme. Its normal range is 5-40 IU/L. A level above 50 IU/L points to liver dysfunction, more specifically hepatocellular dysfunction.

Aspartate aminotransaminase (AST). Previously popular as serum glutamic-oxaloacetic transaminase (**SGOT**), it is supposed to be abnormal not only in liver disease but also in involvement of heart and other organs. The normal range is 5-40 IU/L. A level > 50 IU/L is considered abnormal.

In acute hepatocellular failure, both ALT and AST show remarkable rise. The rise in their level is less marked in chronic liver disease.

Serum Alkaline Phosphatase (AP)

The serum level of enzyme, *alkaline phosphatase (AP),* is elevated in a large number of disorders that affect the drainage of bile, such as a gallstone or tumor blocking the common bile duct, or drug-induced hepatitis, blocking the flow of bile in smaller bile channels within the liver. Serum AP is also found in other organs, such as bone, placenta, and intestine. Hence, GGT (*vide infra*) is utilized as a supplementary test to be sure that the elevation of alkaline phosphatase is indeed related to the liver or the biliary tract.

Gamma Glutamyl Transpeptidase (GGT or GGTP)

The GGT enzyme level is specifically elevated in case of liver disorders only in contrast to the alkaline phosphatase that tends to be elevated in diseases of bone, placenta and intestine as well.

Different cells have different enzymes inside them, depending on the function of the cell. Liver cells happen to have lots of AST, ALT and GGTP inside them. When cells die or are damaged, the enzymes leak out causing the blood level of these enzymes to rise. That is why the levels of these enzymes in the blood are considered good indicators of liver cell damage. ALT is more specific for liver disease than AST because AST is found in more types of cell (e.g. heart, intestine, muscle). AST, for instance, will rise after a heart attack or bruised kidney. GGTP and AP are said to be more specific for evaluating biliary disease since they are made in bile duct cells. In liver disease caused by excess alcohol ingestion, the AST tends to exceed the ALT, while the reverse is true for viral hepatitis. However, this particular generalization is often wrong. There are several things to remember:

- These tests have a meaning, but they generally cannot be interpreted without clinical information. They are probably most useful to track, or follow a particular problem, but even then they often "bounce around" greatly.
- These numbers are not linear. An AST that is 300 is not twice as bad as 150 (normal is less than 40), and an AST of 94 and 80 are essentially the same to a liver specialist.
- These numbers do not always detect all liver disease. Some patients with severe advanced liver disease will have normal or nearly normal enzyme levels.

Though serum transaminases and alkaline phosphates are often called "liver function tests" ("LFTs"), these tests do not, in fact, measure the liver function *per se*. In order to assess the liver function, they must be corroborated with other tests, including albumin, bilirubin, and prothrombin time. Clinical factors should be considered as well.

Albumin

It is a major protein produced by the liver. The chronic liver disease causes a decrease in the amount of albumin thus produced. For this reason, in liver disease, and particularly in more advanced liver disease, the level of the serum albumin is reduced (less than 3.5 mg/dL).

Prothrombin Time

The prothrombin time is a useful test. There is a good correlation between abnormalities in coagulation measured by the prothrombin time and the degree of liver dysfunction. It is usually expressed in seconds and compared to a normal control patient's blood.

Other Blood Tests

- Over and above these tests, specific and specialized tests may be used to make a precise diagnosis of the cause of liver disease.
- Elevations in serum iron, the percent of iron saturated in blood, or the storage protein ferritin may indicate the presence of hemochromatosis, a liver disease associated with excess iron storage.
- In abnormal metabolism of metals, Wilson's disease, there is an accumulation of copper in the liver, a deficiency of serum ceruloplasmin and excessive excretion of copper into the urine.
- Low levels of serum alpha-1-antitrypsin may indicate the presence of lung and/or liver disease in children or adults with alpha-1-antitrypsin deficiency.
- A positive antemitochondrial antibody indicates the underlying condition of primary biliary cirrhosis.
- Striking elevations of serum globulin, another protein in blood.
- The presence of antinuclear antibodies or antismooth muscle antibodies are clues to the diagnosis of autoimmune chronic hepatitis.
- There are specific blood tests that allow the precise diagnosis of hepatitis A, hepatitis B, hepatitis C, and hepatitis D.

In summary, blood tests are used to diagnose or monitor liver disease. They may be simply markers of disease (e.g., ALT, AST, alkaline phosphatase and GGT), more true indicators of overall liver function (serum bilirubin, serum albumin, and prothrombin time) or specific tests that allow the diagnosis of an underlying cause of liver disease. Interpretation of these liver tests is a sophisticated process that the physician should utilize in the context of medical history, physical examination, and other tests such as X-rays or other imaging studies of the liver.

LIVER IMAGING MODALITIES

These include:

- Plain X-ray.
- Ultrasonography.
- CT scanning.
- Radionuclide scanning.
- Cholangiography.

- Endoscopic retrograde cholangiopancreatography (ERCP); and
- Selective angiography of celiac, hepatic artery or superior mesenteric for visualizing the hepatic or portal circulation.

Table 72.1 gives characteristics of different imaging procedures in relation to evaluation of liver dysfunction.

Table 72.1: Liver imaging modalities and their important features

Plain X-ray
- Enlargement which may not otherwise be apparent on clinical examination
- Hepatic or biliary tract mass may displace an air-filled loop of bowel
- Calcification in liver in case of parasitic or neoplastic disease
- Calcification in vasculature in case of portal vein thrombosis
- Calcification in gall bladder or biliary tree in case of gall stones
- Collection of gas within liver in case of liver abscess
- Collection of gas within biliary tract, or portal circulation in case of necrotizing enterocolitis.

Ultrasonography (US)
- Information about size, composition and blood flow of liver
- Increased echogenicity in fatty infiltration
- Small mass lesions (1-2 cm)
- Stones in gall bladder or biliary tract (US is better than cholangiography)
- Choledochal cyst
- Biliary atresia
- US assisted liver biopsy, aspiration or cholangiography
- Doppler US evaluates patency of portal vein, demonstrate collateral circulation, assess size of spleen and even small amount of ascitic fluid, vascular patency after liver transplantation.

CT Scan
- Useful for children >2 years only
- Gives similar information as by US though it is more useful in detecting focal lesions e.g. tumors, cysts or abscesses
- Enhance by contrast medium, it may reveal a neoplastic mass density slightly different from that seen in normal liver
- Best modality in hepatic tumor for defining its anatomic extent, solid or cystic nature and vascularity
- Differentiation of obstructive from nonobstructive cholestasis.

MRI
- MR cholangiography useful in differentiating biliary tract lesions
- More accurate than US in detecting focal lesions e.g. tumors, cysts, abscesses.

Radionuclide Scanning

The technique employs selective uptake of radio-pharmaceutical agent such as:

Contd.

Contd.

- Technetium 99m-labelled sulfur colloid, which can detect focal lesions like tumors, cysts and abscesses > 22-3 cm in diameter
- 99m Tc–iminodiacetic acid agents which can differentiate intrahepatic cholestasis from extrahepatic obstruction in neonates
- Gallium 67 which can detect inflammatory and neoplastic conditions.

Cholangiography
- Percutaneopus transhepatic cholangiography with a fine needle is the choice.

ERCP
- Endoscopic retrograde cholangiopancreatography (ERCP) is an endoscopic method of reexamining the bile ducts in older children.

Selective Angiography
- SA of the celiac, superior mesenteric or hepatic artery may be employed to visualize the hepatic or portal circulation (both arterial and venous) in evaluation of portal hypertension, before shunting procedure and define blood supply of tumors before surgery.

LIVER BIOPSY

It may be employed for:

- **Diagnosis**
  - Neonatal cholestasis (histologic diagnosis).
  - Enzyme analysis in inborn errors of metabolism.
  - Analysis of stored material e.g. iron, copper, specific metabolites.
- **Follow-up**
  - Response to therapy.
  - Detection of complications of therapy.

Table 72.2 lists selected indications of liver biopsy.

Table 72.2: Important indications of liver biopsy

- Neonatal cholestasis
- Chronic active hepatitis
- Reye syndrome
- Metabolic liver disease
- Intrahepatic cholestasis
- Congenital hepatic fibrosis
- Unidentified portal hypertension
- Enzyme analysis in inborn errors of metabolism
- Analysis of stored material e.g. iron, copper, some metabolites

KEY LEARNING POINTS

- Components of evaluation include clinical workup and careful interpretation, biochemical tests, imaging studies and liver biopsy.
- Typical biochemical tests include serum ALT, AST, AP, GGPT, PT, LDL and proteins; these tests are

employed to diagnose and also monitor the progress/recovery of the disease process.
- Imaging studies include plain X-ray, US, CT scan, MRI radionuclide screening, cholangigraphy, ERCP, selective angiography.
- Liver biopsy may be employed both for diagnosis and follow-up.

FURTHER READINGS

1. Balistreri W F. Pediatric hepatology. A half century of progress. *Clin Liver Dis* 2004;4:191-210.
2. Balistreri W, Ng VL. Evaluation of patients with possible liver dysfunction. In: Kliegman RM, Behrman RE, Jenson HB, Stanton BF (eds): *Nelson Textbook of Pediatrics*, 18th edn. Philadelphia: Saunders 2008:1665-1668.
3. Batres LA, Maller ES. Laboratory assessment of liver function and injury in children. In: Suchy PS, Sokel RJ, Balistreri WF (eds); *Liver Disease in Cholestasis,* 2nd edn. Philadelphia: Lippincott, Williams and Wilkins 2001:155-170.
4. Moyer V, Freese Dk, Whitington PF, *et al.* Guidelines for the evaluation of cholestatic jaundice in infants. Recommendations of the North American Society for Pediatric Gastroenterology, Hepatology and Nutrition. *J Pediatr Gastroenterol Nutr* 2004;39:115-128.

73 Hepatomegaly

Suraj Gupte • RA Anderson

INTRODUCTION

Hepatomegaly, usually accompanied by splenomegaly, in infancy and childhood is a frequent clinical finding. Not always it is a manifestation of the liver disease. In fact, in a large proportion, the etiology may be elsewhere.

Various mechanisms involved in its development are:

1. Inflammation/infection: Viral hepatitis.
2. Storage: Inborn errors of metabolism.
3. Infiltrations: Tumors.
4. Vascular congestion.
5. Increased size of biliary space: Extrahepatic obstruction, fibrosis.

ETIOLOGY

Table 73.1 lists causes of hepatomegaly in different pediatric age groups.

Table 73.1: Differential diagnosis of pediatric hepatomegaly

Newborn

Infections: Intrauterine STORCH group of infections, neonatal hepatitis, septicemia/sepsis, malaria

Metabolic/Storage: Galactosemia, fructosemia, glycogenosis IV, alpha-1-antitrypsin deficiency, cystic fibrosis, hypothyroidism, hypopituitarism, Gaucher disease, Niemann-Pick disease, Wolman disease, tyrosinemia

Zellweger (cerebrohepatorenal) syndrome, bile acid metabolic defects, neonatal iron storage disease, copper overload (ICC), arginase deficiency, mitochondrial DNA depletion

Genetic/Chromosomal: Down syndrome, Trisomy E, leprechaunism

Intrahepatic: Idiopathic neonatal hepatitis, intrahepatic cholestasis, intrahepatic biliary hypoplasia

Extrahepatic: Extrahepatic biliary atresia, choledochal cyst, inspissated bile syndrome (bile/mucus plug, bile duct stenosis

Miscellaneous: CCF, drugs, TPN, histiocytosis, shock, enteritis, intestinal obstruction, neonatal lupus erythematosus

Infants

All of above plus viral hepatitis A, B and C and ICC

Contd.

Childhood and Adolescence

Infections: Hepatitis A, B, C, D and E, chronic hepatitis, liver abscess (both amebic and pyogenic), typhoid fever, malaria, hydatid cyst, infectious mononucleosis

Metabolic/Storage: ICC Mucopolysaccharidosis, glycogen storage disease, lipidosis, alpha-1-antitrypsin deficiency, Wilson's disease

Fatty Change/infiltration: Kwashiorkor, Reye syndrome, tuberculosis, cystic fibrosis, tetracycline toxicity

Malignancy: Lymphomas, hepatoblastoma, histiocytosis, metastases

Congestive: CCF, constrictive pericarditis, Budd Chiari syndrome, VOD of liver

Miscellaneous: Congenital cyst, drugs

In the following situations hepatomegaly is associated with massive splenomegaly:

- Infections: Chronic malaria/tropical splenomegal, kala-azar.
- Chronic myeloid leukemia.
- Myelofibrosis.
- Thalassemia.
- Hypersplenism.
- Portal hypertension (extrahepatic).
- Gaucher's disease.

In the following situations, massive hepatomegaly is associated with splenomegaly:

- Cysts: Hydatid disease.
- Infection: Abscess (pyogenic or amebic).
- Tumors: Hepatoblastoma, secondary metastasis.
- Chronic cholestasis (extrahepatic).
- Congenital hepatic fibrosis.
- Glycogen-storage disease.

EVALUATION

Clinical

It should include a good history and clinical examination. Box 73.1 gives helpful clues in the evaluation of pediatric hepatomegaly. More important than sheer palpability of the liver is the measurement of liver span. Additional information needed is the shape, consistency, surface characters, border, tenderness, murmurs, bruit and accompanying splenomegaly.

Box 73. 1 gives the clues that are helpful in the evaluation and differential diagnosis of hepatomegaly.

Box 73. 1: Helpful clues in evaluation of pediatric hepatomegaly

H/o sibling/familial involvement	ICC, Wilson's disease, thalassemia
H/o transfusions/ needle pricks	HBV, HCV
Fever	Enteric fever, malaria, viral hepatitis, leptospirosis (in acute cases) tuberculosis, kala-azar, chronic active hepatitis (in chronic cases)
Jaundice	Viral hepatitis, cirrhosis, enteric fever
Edematous PEM	Kwashiorkor
Anemia	Thalassemia, leukemia, portal hypertension
Lymphadenopathy	Hematogenous tuberculosis, malignancy
Engorged neck veins/ raised JVP	Constrictive pericarditis, congestive cardiac failure (CCF)
Rash	Histiocytosis
Cataracts with mental retardation and splenomegaly	Galactosemia
Hazy or cloudy cornea	Mucopolysaccharidosis type 1
Kayser-Fleischer ring	Wilson's disease
Microcephaly/ hydrocephalus	TORCH/ STORCH group of intrauterine infections
Neurologic manifestations	Wilson's disease
Refractory rickets	Cystinosis, tyrosinosis, Wilson's disease
Cystic kidneys	Congenital hepatic fibrosis
Mental retardation	Galactosemia, lipid storage disease
Movement disorder	Wilson's disease

Investigative

Over and above the tests routinely carried out for evaluation of liver status, the following further investigations may well be in order depending on the individual merits of the case:

- TORCH/STORCH titers in case of intrauterine infections.
- Viral markers in case of viral hepatitis (A, B, C, D, E).
- Autoimmune markers in case of chronic hepatitis.
- Alpha-fetoprotein in case of hepatoblastoma.
- Sweat chloride in case of cystic fibrosis.
- Metabolic studies:
  - Copper studies in case of Wilson's disease, Indian childhood cirrhosis (ICC).
  - Enzyme studies in case of galactosemia, Gaucher's disease, Niemann-Pick disease.
  - Urine succinyl-acetone in case of tyrosinemia.

INTERPRETATION

Hepatomegaly accompanying infections or inflammations, including viral hepatitis, is a transient phenomenon that resolves within a few weeks.

Persistent hepatomegaly, especially when accompanied by evidence of progressive liver dysfunction, is usually indicative of a chronic liver disease that may end up as cirrhosis. Aggressive investigative evaluation is mandatory in such cases.

KEY LEARNING POINTS

- May be a manifestation of either liver disease or a disease process elsewhere in the body.
- Frequently accompanied by splenomegaly, the predominance of the size of liver or spleen assisting in reaching the diagnosis.
- Evaluation should include clinical workup, measurement of the liver span being more important than its sheer palpability.
- Clues that assist in the etiologic diagnosis must be borne in mind.
- In addition to the routine tests, certain special investigations may be warranted depending on the merit of each case e.g. TORCH/STORCH titers in case of intrauterine infections, sweat chloride in case of CF, metabolic studies, say Cu in case of Wilson's disease.

FURTHER READINGS

1. Balistereri WF. Pediatric hepatomegaly: A half century of progress. *Clin Liver Dis 2000;*4:191-210.
2. Gupte S, Anderson RA. Pediatric hepatology. In: Gupte S (ed): *The Short Textbook of Pediatrics,* 11th edn. New Delhi: Jaypee 2008 (in press).
3. Gupte S. Mass in abdomen. In: Gupte S (ed): *Differential Diagnosis in Pediatrics* 5th edn. New Delhi: Jaypree 2008.

74 Neonatal Cholestasis Syndrome (NCS)

Suraj Gupte • Sanjay Wazir Pandita

INTRODUCTION

By definition, it is a prolonged and pathologic elevation of serum levels of conjugated bilirubin beyond first 14 days of life. In India, it is estimated to constitute 30% of the hepatobiliary disorders. Since cholestasis often extends beyond neonatal period, the term *cholestasis of infancy* may well be more appropriate.

CLASSIFICATIONS

NCS may be classified as per Table 74.1.

Table 74.1: Classifications of neonatal cholestasis

Classification I

I. Intrahepaatic (Hepatocellular)
- Neonatal hepatitis (NH)
- Paucity of intrahepatic bile ducts (PIBD)

II. Extrahepatic

Classification II

I. Neonatal hepatitis

II. Obstructive cholestasis (cholangiopathy)
- Extrahepatic
- Intrahepatic

ETIOPATHOGENESIS

Predisposing factors for neonatal cholestasis include:
- Immaturity of excretory function.
- Insufficient intrahepatic circulation.
- Inborn errors of metabolism.

Etiologic conditions are listed in Table 74.2. Experience in India and other countries of S-E Asia indicates that around 67% cases are equally distributed between extrahepatic and intrahepatic etiology. The left over 33% cases are of idiopathic neonatal hepatitis. Two most likely mechanisms are virus-induced hepatic insult and metabolic liver disease. Irrespective of the cause, clinical manifestations of all forms of cholestasis are by and large similar.

Table 74.2: Etiology-cum-differential diagnosis of neonatal cholestasis syndrome

Infections: Hepatitis A, B and C, TORCH /STORCH group of infections, septicemia/sepsis

Metabolic: Galactosemia, fructosemia, glycogenosis IV, alpha-antitrypsin deficiency, cystic fibrosis, hypothyroidism, hypopituitarism, Gaucher disease, Niemann-Pick disease, Wolman disease, tyrosinemia, Zellweger (cerebrohepatorenal) syndrome, bile acid metabolic defects, neonatal iron storage disease, copper overload (ICC), arginase deficiency, mitochondrial DNA depletion

Genetic/Chromosomal: Down's syndrome, Trisomy E, leprechaunism

Intrahepatic: Idiopathic neonatal hepatitis, intrahepatic cholestasis, intrahepatic biliary hypoplasia

Extrahepatic: Extrahepatic biliary atresia, choledochal cyst, inspissated bile syndrome (bile/mucus plug, bile duct stenosis, mass (neoplasia, stone)

Miscellaneous: Drugs, total parenteral nutrition (TPN), histiocytosis, shock, enteritis, intestinal obstruction, neonatal lupus erythematosus, myeloproliferative disease

Prolonged cholestasis leads to serious consequences in the form of biliary cirrhosis with portal hypertension. Over and above this, the infant develops hepatotoxicity and pruritus from regurgitation of the retained bile and wide spectrum of malnutrition and growth retardation.

CLINICAL FEATURES

Manifestations of neonatal cholestasis include persistent icterus with high-colored urine and clay-colored or light (alcholic) stools and hepatomegaly (Fig. 19.8) as a result of poor bile flow because of liver cell injury or bile duct obstruction, and bleeding diathesis as a result of vitamin K insufficiency and hypoprothrombinemia because of hepatic synthetic dysfunction.

DIAGNOSIS

Since clinical features hardly provide any concrete clues regarding the underlying cause of cholestasis, a recourse to investigations becomes mandatory (Table 74.3). Nevertheless, the following important points in history and clinical workup must be borne in mind:

- Presence of cataract and cherry-red spots point to galactosemia and lipid storage disease, respectively.
- Detection of chorioretinitis means an intrauterine infection like toxoplasmosis, rubella, cytomegalovirus (CMV).
- Higher birth weight, earlier onset of icterus with clay-colored stools, coexistence of congenital malformations and absence of familial occurrence are points in favor of EHBA rather than neonatal hepatitis.

Table 74.3: Investigative workup for suspected neonatal cholestasis syndrome (NCS)

Blood: Total and fractional bilirubin, transaminases, alkaline phosphatase, prothrombin time
Serology: Evidence of infections (HBsAg, specific viral serology, VDRL)
Blood, urine, spinal fluid cultures: For bacteria, herpes simplex, CMV, enteroviruses
Abdominal ultrasonography is particularly of value in identifying such surgically correctable conditions as choledochal cysts
Radionuclide hepatobiliary scintography is of great value in excluding EHBA. During this procedure, 24-hour duodenal intubation may be done to determine the radioactivity in stomach and duodenal fluid
Liver biopsy is vital in differentiating between surgical and nonsurgical cases of cholestasis.

Contd.

Contd.

Magnetic resonance cholangiopancreatography (MRCP)
Endoscopic retrograde cholangiopancreatography (ERCP)
Intraoperative/Perioperative cholangiography (IOC/POC) is the most confirmatory tool for the diagnosis of EHBA.

MANAGEMENT

Nutritional support is central to any treatment offered to infants with cholestasis. It is advisable to provide medium-chain triglycerides (coconut oil) for enhancing fat and energy assimilation and fat soluble vitamins to makeup for their poor absorption. Anorexic infants should receive nasogastric feeding.

Replacement therapy may be warranted in the form of fat-soluble vitamins (A, E, D, K), water-soluble vitamins and micronutrients (calcium, phosphate, zinc).

Treatment of pruritus is in the form of phenobarbital, choleretics (ursodeoxycholic acid), or bile acid binders (cholestyramine), rifampicin, naloxene, terfemadine, or 3-4 minute/day phototherapy with ultraviolet or infrared rays.

Chemotherapy for sepsis, especially in the presence of ascites and end-stage liver disease.

Appropriate treatment of associated complications such as variceal bleed (endoscopic sclerotherapy, ascites, hepatic encephalopathy, renal failure.

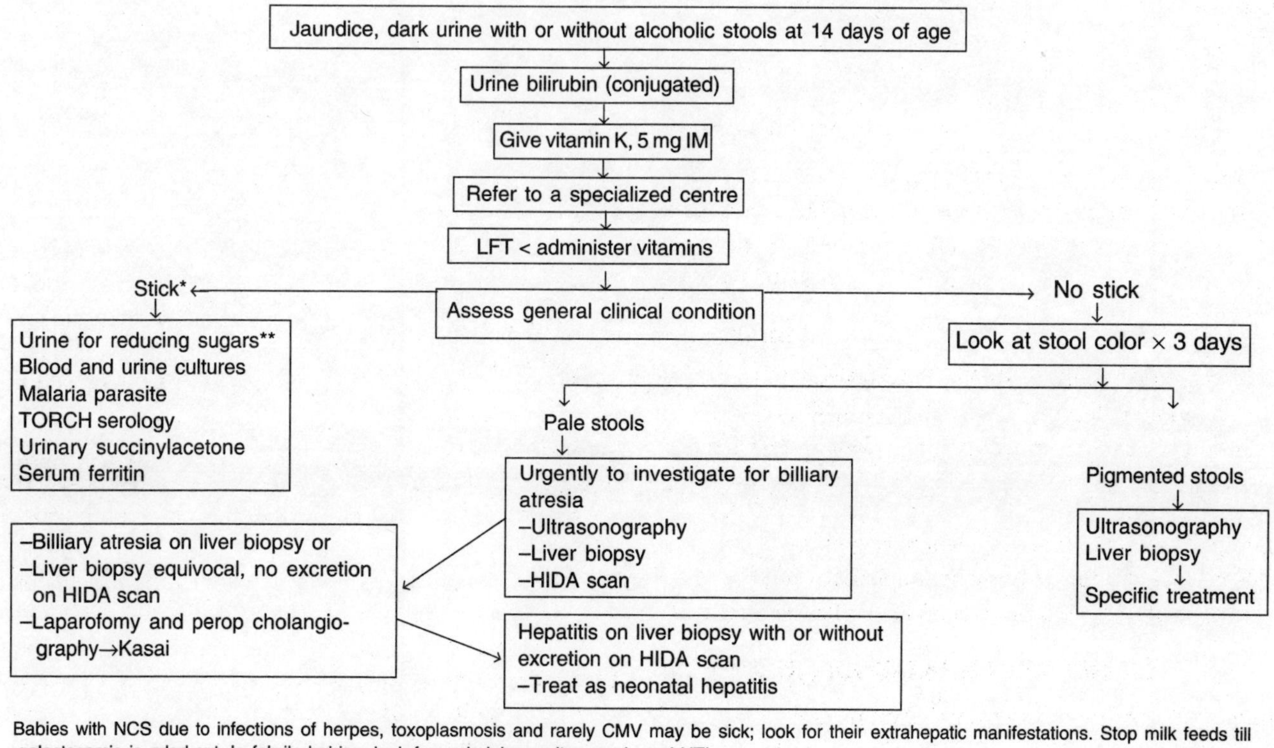

* Babies with NCS due to infections of herpes, toxoplasmosis and rarely CMV may be sick; look for their extrahepatic manifestations. Stop milk feeds till galactosemia is ruled out. In febrile babies, look for malarial parasite, sepsis and UTI.

** This is to look for galactose in urine while on milk feeds. If reducing substances are positive, check urine samples with glucose stick. If negative, most likely reducing substances in urine are due to galactose. Treat as galactosemia.

Fig. 74.1: Algorithmic approach to neonatal cholestasis syndrome (NCS)

Surgical treatment is indicated in EHBA and choledochal cyst, provided that liver damage has not advanced to the stage of cirrhosis.

Liver transplantation may be done in end-stage liver disease (liver failure) in case the family can afford it.

A practical algorithm is given in Fig. 74.1.

PROGNOSIS

On account of delayed diagnosis and referral in a vast majority of infants with NCS, prognosis is unfavorable. In idiopathic neonatal hepatitis of sporadic variety, around 60-70% cases recover whereas in the familial variety recovery occurs in only 20-30% cases, the remaining cases ending up as chronic liver disease with cirrhosis.

KEY LEARNING POINTS

- Defined as conjugated serum bilirubinemia > first 14 days of life, as a result of neonatal hepatitis or cholangiopathy secondary to either extrahepatic or intrahepatic obstructive cholestasis.
- Left unattended, leads to serious consequences in the form of biliay cirrhosis with portal hypertension.
- An algorithmic approach for investigative workup and early management is important for good results.
- Supportive therapy, including nutritional correction, is important in all cases.
- Surgical treatment is indicated in EHBA and choledochal cysts, provided that liver damage is not to the xtent of cirrhotic changes.
- Liver transplantation is the only treatment in end-stage liver disease.

FURTHER READINGS

1. Balistereri WF, Bove KE, Ryckman FC. Biliary atresia and other disorders of the extrahepatic bile ducts. In: Suchy FJ, Sokol RJ, Balistereri WF (eds): *Liver Disease in Children*, 2nd edn. Philadelphia: Lippincott Williams and Wilkins 2001: 253-274.
2. Gupte S, Anderson RA. Hepatology. In: Gupte S (ed): *The Short Textbook of Pediatrics*, 11th edn. New Delhi 2008: 423-449.
3. Pediatric Gastroenterology Subchapter of the Indian Academy of Pediatrics. Consensus Reoport on Neonatal Cholestasis Syndrome (NCS). *Indian J Pediatr Gastroenterol, Hepatol Nutr* 2000;1:20-23.
4. Shah HA, Spivak W. Neonatal cholestasis: New approaches to diagnostic evaluation and therapy. *Pediatr Clin North Am* 1994;41:943-966.
5. Tomar BS. Infantile cholestasis. In: Gupte S (ed): *Recent Advances in Pediatrics (Special Vol 6: Gastroenterology, Hepatology and Nutrition).* New Delhi: Jaypee 200: 246-255.

75 Surgical Jaundice in the Neonates

Rajeev G Redkar

INTRODUCTION

Neonatal cholestasis is defined as a pathological state of the liver whereby there is reduction in the excretion of bile from the biliary tree into the intestines. Neonatal cholestasis syndrome (NCS) is diagnosed when newborn babies have jaundice beyond 14 days of age accompanied by dark urine and, at times, pale or chalky white stools. The conjugated bilirubin in such patients is more than 1.5 mg % or 20% of the total serum bilirubin.

A neonate could develop cholestasis in response to a wide variety of insults, hepatic or systemic. Mainly, the disorders, which affect the extrahepatic biliary tree are essentially amenable to surgical treatment. These may present in a manner which may be indistinguishable clinically from the other varieties of infective, metabolic or endocrine causes of neonatal jaundice.

Amongst the surgical causes of jaundice in neonates, a condition that has a probability of occurrence of nearly 3 out of 4 cases is "biliary atresia". This condition is discussed in greater details in this chapter. Besides this, there are other rare causes like choledochal cysts, inspissated bile plug syndrome and spontaneous perforation of bile ducts, which also contribute to the list of conditions causing surgical jaundice in neonates. A significant proportion of these, if untreated, may evolve into chronic liver disease and ultimately may require liver transplantation.

BILIARY ATRESIA

Biliary atresia implies absence of extra and intrahepatic bile ducts in a neonate (Fig. 75.1). This is the result of a progressive, destructive, sclerosing inflammatory process affecting the biliary tree. The children affected are either jaundiced since birth or they become so within the first week or two of life. However, they are otherwise healthy and well-nourished. Uncorrected cases suffer a progressive obliteration of the bile ducts and biliary cirrhosis rapidly develops. Surgical correction has to be done prior to 10 weeks of age for better results. A delay in surgical treatment causes a poorer outcome. Hence, it is imperative that one does not waste valuable time in repeating investigations for neonatal jaundice but refer to appropriate centers for early diagnosis and management.

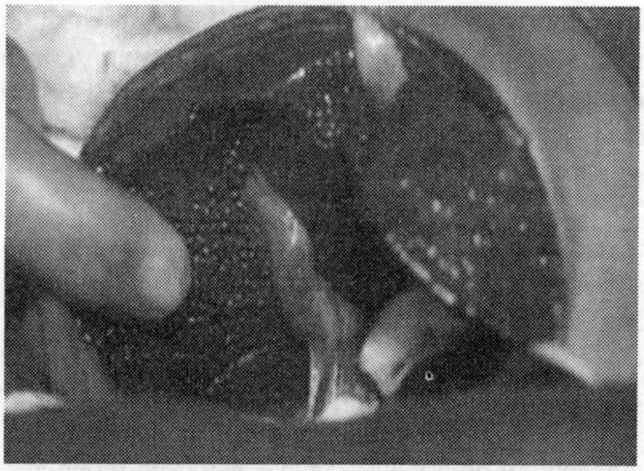

Fig. 75.1: Biliary atresia (See for colour figure Plate 8)

Historical Aspects

Single case reports of infants with biliary atresia were documented in the 19th century. Most of these reports were collected together by Thomson in 1892. The major advance in treatment came with the work of Dr. Morio Kasai (Fig. 75.2) in Sendai, Japan, who observed that dissection of the porta hepatis in a female infant with biliary atresia produced a flow of bile. He anastomosed an intestinal conduit to the raw area in the porta hepatis (area on the under surface of the liver between the left and the right portal vein). Details of his operation were published in 1959. Improvements in the technical aspects of the operation followed rapidly. Anastomosing a Roux-en-Y loop of jejunum to the porta hepatis is now known as "Kasai's porto-enterostomy".

Etiology

The incidence of this pathology is similar throughout the world ranging from 0.8 to 1.0 per 10,000 live births. The true etiology of biliary atresia is unknown although a large number of factors have been implicated.

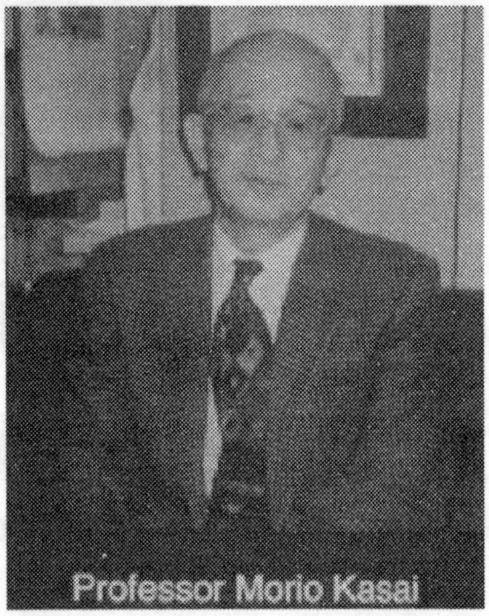

Fig. 75.2: The propounder of the Kasai's operation

1. *Congenital factors:* About 10% of cases of biliary atresia have other extrahepatic anomalies (polysplenia, asplenia, malrotation of intestines, situs inversus, absent inferior vena cava) which has been termed as biliary atresia splenic malformation (BASM) syndrome. The critical period of early development for all the affected components of this syndrome (bile ducts, IVC, portal vein, spleen) is from 25-40 days of gestation. Hence, an "embryopathic insult" at this early stage of development helps to explain this. A small number of biliary atresia cases have been detected antenatally on maternal ultrasound scans.
2. *Genetic factors:* There are isolated cases of biliary atresia associated with Trisomy 18 and other chromosomal anomalies. Affected individuals with a definite familial tendency to biliary atresia have also been reported.
3. *Viral studies:* Some clinical studies have suggested that there is a high incidence of positive serology against *Reovirus type III* in infants with biliary atresia.
4. *Anatomical factors:* Although common pancreato-biliary channel is demonstrated in 5% of the normal population, it has been demonstrated in 60% in the cases of biliary atresia. Experimental studies have also shown that prenatal direct ligation of the common bile duct can reproduce some features of biliary atresia.
5. *Metabolic factors:* A number of metabolic abnormalities like changes in monohydroxy bile acids and in the amino acid L-proline have been recognized in the bile of infants with satisfactory biliary drainage after operation.

Clinical Features and Investigations

Infants with biliary atresia present with conjugated hyperbilirubinaemia, dark urine and pale, acholic stools. Birth weight and gestation are usually normal and initially the infants feed and thrive appropriately. The liver is enlarged and in older infants there is commonly ascites and splenomegaly.

A diagnosis of biliary atresia is made preoperatively by excluding medical causes of conjugated hyperbilirubinaemia and observing the characteristic histological appearance of a percutaneous liver biopsy.

Liver biochemistry is nonspecific but shows raised total and direct serum bilirubin, elevated alkaline phosphatase and gamma glutamyl transpeptidase levels.

Hepatobiliary ultrasound scan excludes other surgical cause of jaundice such as choledochal cysts and obstructed extrahepatic ducts due to inspissated bile.

Radionucleide hepatobiliary imaging (HIDA scan) fails to show bile excretion in cases of biliary atresia and can discriminate between this condition and neonatal hepatitis.

Endoscopic retrograde cholangio-pancreatography (ERCP) and magnetic resonance cholangio-pancreatography (MRCP) have recently been tried when the diagnosis remains unclear even after liver biopsy. However, there are not only technically difficult to perform but also difficult to interpret in this age group. A simpler alternative is provided by a formal laparotomy and an intraoperative cholangiography.

Surgery (Fig. 75.3)

The biliary tree is approached *via* a right-sided transverse incision extended usually across the midline. If the diagnosis has not been established preoperatively, an operative cholangiogram is obtained *via* a catheter in the gall bladder. Only complete visualization of the whole biliary tree excludes biliary atresia at this stage. The obliterated biliary tract is divided distally and elevated to help separate it from the underlying portal vein and the adjacent hepatic artery. It is then dissected free and transected high at the level of the porta hepatis. Biliary continuity is restored using a loop of jejunum, which is anastomosed to the transected porta hepatis as a portoenterostomy (Fig. 75.4).

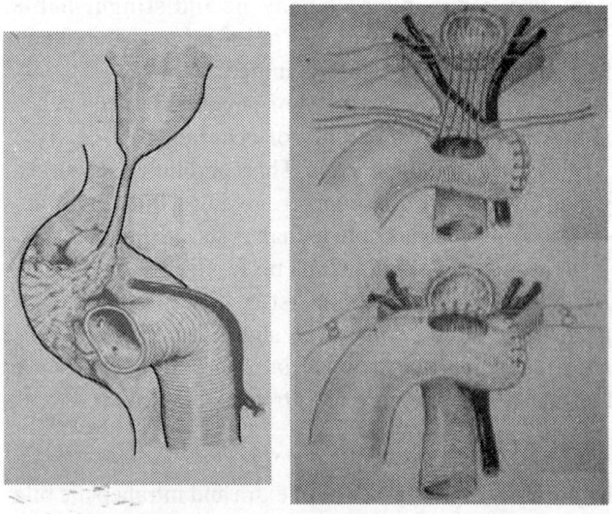

Fig. 75.3: Steps in Kasai's operation

Infants tolerate this operation very well. Early complications are unusual but may include bleeding from the portal dissection or a persistent ascitic fluid leak from the abdominal drain.

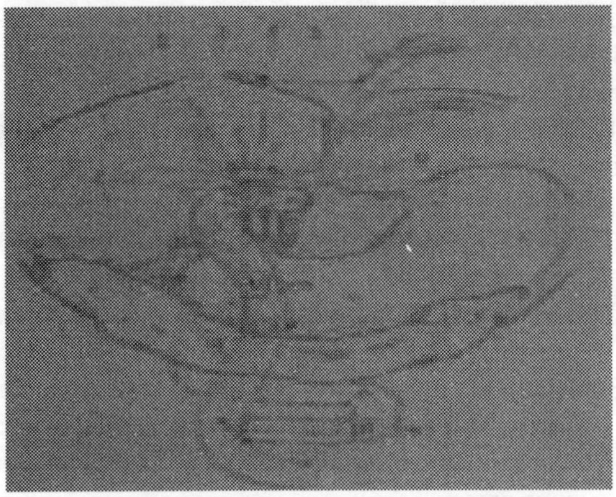

Fig. 75.4: Kasai's protoenterostomy

Results of Kasai's Portoenterostomy Operation

A number of variables have been shown to be useful in predicting the effectiveness of portoenterostomy. Age at surgery has been the most widely quoted prognostic criteria and it is stated that infants operated within 10 weeks of age have a reasonably better chance of successful operation. Uncorrected biliary obstruction causes progressive intrahepatic disease and the longer this is allowed to persist the more irreversible is the outcome. Macroscopic appearances of the bile ducts at operation and microscopic analysis of the resected biliary tree specimen are also thought to help prognosticate the outcome of the operation.

Almost 50% of infants have bile flow following surgery. However, about 30 to 40% of the children may survive to reach 10 years of age with their native liver intact. Biliary atresia is the most common indication for liver transplantation during childhood. Initially transplantation was used for survivors of the Kasai operation with life-threatening complications e.g. variceal bleeding and chronic liver failure. However, with the increasing experience of transplantation in the western world, early liver replacement has been undertaken in infants who have had no response to portoenterostomy.

Specific Complications Following Portoenterostomy

All survivors after portoenterostomy for biliary atresia develop some degree of chronic liver disease. Commonly, this is manifested by hepatomegaly and marginal elevation of liver enzymes. Some may have signs of more overt liver damage such as ascites, intermittent jaundice, failure to thrive and portal hypertension. Complications in these children include:

1. *Ascending bacterial cholangitis:* This is recorded in 40 to 50% of cases and almost always occurs in children with some degree of bile flow. It is characterized by worsening jaundice, fever and acoholic stools. The diagnosis may be confirmed by blood cultures but it is important to treat suspected cases early with broad-spectrum antibiotics.
2. *Portal hypertension:* About 60% of children who survive to age of 2 years have endoscopic evidence of esophageal varices, although only approximately half of those will ever bleed. The average age of first bleed is about three years and is manifested by sudden hematemesis and melena. After initial supportive therapy, endoscopic sclerotherapy is the mainstay of treatment using sclerosants.
3. *Metabolic and nutritional consequences of cholestasis:* All infants treated for biliary atresia have a degree of liver impairment and diminished liver reserve. Persistent cholestasis and diminished bile flow may cause fat and fat-soluble vitamin malabsorption. Vitamin K-dependent coagulopathy and rickets may occur.
4. *Miscellaneous:* Intrapulmonary shunting and hypoxia may develop in anicteric children following Kasai operation. The mechanism for this is unknown. This complication is resistant to conventional treatment and liver transplantation appears to be the only specific treatment. Large intrahepatic cysts may occur occasionally in long-term survivors after portoenterostomy. These may be associated with attacks of cholangitis.

CHOLEDOCHAL CYSTS

This implies a fusiform or cystic dilatation of the extrahepatic bile ducts (Fig. 75.5). The incidence has been estimated as 1 in 150,000 live births. A local abnormality of the wall of the bile duct or a long common pancreatobiliary channel is thought to be the cause of this anomaly. There are various types of choledochal cysts like cystic, fusiform, diverticular and entire dilatation of the extra and intrahepatic biliary tree.

Clinical presentation may involve a classic triad of symptoms of jaundice, pain and a mass in the right hypochondrium, which is noted in about 30% of the cases. A complication of the choledochal cysts such as a perforation or portal hypertension may be the presenting feature.

Ultrasonography is the diagnostic modality for identifying the problem. A CT scan of abdomen may be useful in very large lesions. An ERCP or MRCP may help in structural identification of a common pancreatobiliary channel.

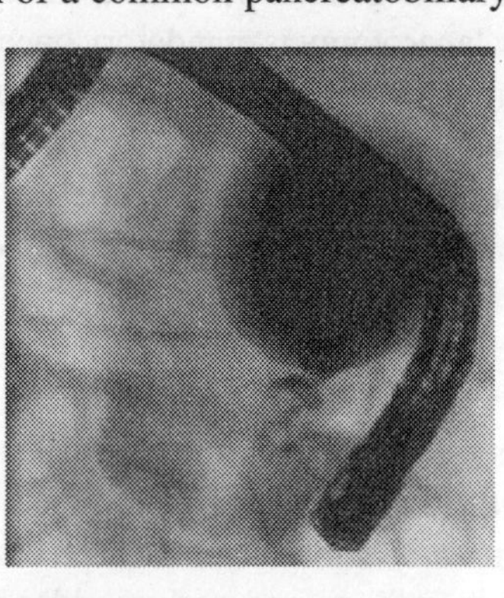

Fig. 75.5: Choledochal cyst (See for colour figure Plate 8)

It is now clear from long-term studies that the treatment of choice is radical excision of the cyst and anastomosing a loop of intestine at the residual normal bile duct. This has the advantages of removing the fibrous duct walls and reducing the chances of malignancy of the bile ducts in later life.

This implies precipitation of bile crystals or sludge in the lumen of the bile ducts. The pigment that forms the debris with the ducts is mainly calcium bilirubinate. This disorder in the past has been associated with hemolysis secondary to blood group incompatibility. Recent reports suggest a relationship between parenteral nutrition, prematurity, bowel dysfunction and dehydration and the occurrence of inspissated bile.

Inspissated bile syndrome may be difficult to differentiate clinically from the biliary atresia. Jaundice and acholic stools are usual and liver function tests show an obstructive picture with an elevation of conjugated bilirubin, alkaline phosphatase and gamma glutamyl transferase. Ultrasonography may reveal a dilated proximal biliary tree and bile sludge or stones and radionucleide scans show an absence of hepatic excretion in the intestines.

Inspissated bile may disappear spontaneously in the neonatal period. Severe bile duct obstruction must be treated surgically with either saline irrigation of the common bile duct or occasionally with duodenotomy, ampullary sphincterotomy and removal of any impacted mass of bile pigment.

SPONTANEOUS PERFORATION OF THE BILE DUCT

This is a rare condition where the bile duct perforates and the bile leaks in the peritoneal cavity. If undiagnosed, this may have a fatal outcome. These infants present with jaundice and abdominal distention. The biliary ascitis may cause inguinal herniae or hydroceles, which may show bile staining. This may also be accompanied by vomiting due to duodenal compression. The jaundice is of the conjugated type with pale stools and dark urine.

USG may identify a complex echogenic mass around the common bile duct representing a localized collection of bile. HIDA nuclear scan may show a leakage of bile from the bile duct into the general peritoneal cavity.

Exploratory laparotomy is mandatory once the diagnosis is made. At surgery, it is usually identified that the bile duct is perforated at the junction of the cystic duct with the common hepatic duct. Suturing of the perforation with decompression of the biliary tree usually resolves the problem in most of the cases.

CHOLELITHIASIS

Cholelithiasis in children appears to have a bimodal distribution with a small peak in infancy and a steadily rising incidence from early adolescence. There could be a male predominance in infancy and early childhood but a clear female predisposition emerges during adolescence. In children all types of stones are noted but black pigment stones are more common.

The etiologic factors for the stone formation in the gall bladder include:

1. Hemolytic disorders like sickle cell anemia, hereditary spherocytosis, thalassemia, G-6-PD deficiency, ABO incompatability.
2. Gall bladder hypomotility due to total parenteral nutrition or lack of enteral feeding.
3. Structural problems with the extrahepatic biliary system like choledochal cyst or biliary strictures.
4. Ileal resection or necrotising enterocolitis or short gut syndrome.
5. Medications like ceftriaxone, somatostatin, cyclosporine.

The presentation of cholelithiasis in infants is very variable. Gallstones are frequently asymptomatic, but they may cause nonspecific symptoms such as poor feeding, vomiting and irritability, or give rise to acute cholecystitis, choledocholithiasis with obstructive jaundice and/or cholangitis, or rarely bile duct perforation. The diagnostic modality of preference is an ultrasound scan of abdomen while a CT scan is useful in choledocholithiasis. A functional study with radioactive isotope (HIDA or DISIDA) is a sensitive investigation in acute cholecystitis.

Many authors have reported spontaneous resolution of gallstones. Resolution presumably occurs as a result of dissolution or flushing of the debris through the biliary tree. Both increased bile flow and changes in its composition are likely to be the curative factors.

Surgical management is necessary for symptomatic or complicated gallstone disease. Cholecystectomy is the standard treatment for gallstones but rarely cholecystostomy may be appropriate in severely ill patients. In hereditary spherocytosis, cholecystectomy is indicated for patients with asymptomatic calculi who are undergoing splenectomy for hematological reasons. Cholecystectomy can be done by laparoscopic technique or by a small subcostal incision.

KEY LEARNING POINTS

Extrahepatic Biliary Atresia (EBA)

- Kasai's portoenterostomy is the surgery of choice though it is known to predispose to such complications as ascending cholangitis, portal hypertension, intrapulmonary shunting and hypoxia, and nutritional deficiencies.
- Poor response to portoenterostomy is an indication for liver transplantation.

Choledochal Cysts

- A fusiform or cystic dilatation of the extrahepatic bile duct, presenting with a triad of symptoms of

jaundice, pain and a mass in the right hypochondrium.
- US is the diagnostic modality of choice.

Cholelithiasis

- Predisposing factors include chronic hemolytic disease, TPN, NEC and choledochal cyst.
- US is the diagnostic modality of preference.
- Though spontaneous resolution may occur, surgical management is necessary for symptomatic or complicated cases.

FURTHER READINGS

1. Davenport M, Savage M, Mowat AP, Howard ER. The biliary atresia and splenic malformation syndrome. *Surgery* 1993;113: 662-668.
2. Howard ER. Biliary atresia: Etiology, Management and complications. In: Howard ER (ed): *Surgery for Liver Diseases in Children*. Oxford: Butterworth-Heinemann 1991:39-59.
3. Karrer FM, Price MR, Bensard DD *et al*. Long-term results with the Kasai operation. *Arch Surg* 1996;131:493-496.
4. Mieli-Vergani G, Howard ER, Portmann B, Mowat AP Later referral for biliary atresia: Missed opportunities for effective surgery. *Lancet* 1989;i :421-423.
5. Parashar K, Taplow MJ, McCrae MA. Experimental Reovirus type III induced murine biliary tract disease. *J Pediatr Surg* 1992;27:843-847.
6. Redkar RG, Davenport M, Howard ER Antenatal diagnosis of biliary tract abnormalities. *J Pediatr Surg* 1998; 33: 700-704.
7. Spitz L. Ligation of the common bile duct in foetal lamb. An experimental model for the study of biliary atresia. *Pediatr Res* 1980;14:740-748.

76 Metabolic Liver Diseases: Overview

Suraj Gupte • Sheffali Abbott

INTRODUCTION

In view of the indispensable role of liver in metabolism, metabolic diseases of liver may follow:

- When absence of enzymes produces a block in a metabolic pathway.
- When unmetabolized substrate accumulates proximal to a block.
- When deficiency of an essential substance produced distal to an aberrant chemical reaction develops.
- When synthesis of an abnormal metabolite occurs.

Clinical manifestations that point to possible existence of a metabolic liver disease include:

- Recurrent vomiting, failure to thrive, short stature, dysmorphic features, edema/anasarca.
- Jaundice, hepatomegaly, splenomegaly, fulminant hepatic failure.
- Hypoglycemia, organic academia, lactic academia, hyperammonemia, bleeding, coagulopathy.
- Developmental delay, psychomotor retardation, hypotonia, progressive neuromuscular deterioration, seizures.
- Cardiac dysfunction/failure, unusual odors, rickets, cataracts.

Though a large number of metabolic liver disorders are known (some being in the process of identification), the broad categories are:

A. Inherited unconjugated hyperbilirubinemia.
B. Inherited conjugated hyperbilirubinemia.
C. Hepatolenticular degeneration (Wilson's disease).
D. Indian childhood cirrhosis.
E. Neonatal iron storage disease.
F. Miscellaneous: Alpha-1-antitrypsin deficiency.

INHERITED UNCONJUGATED HYPERBILIRUBINEMIA

Failure of conjugation (glucuronidation) of serum bilirubin before excretion into bile by the enzyme, bilirubin-uridinediphosphoglucuranate glucuronosyltransferase (UDPGT) causes three disorders:

1. *Crigler-Najjar syndrome type I:* Due to complete absence of enzyme activity.
2. *Crigler-Najjar syndrome type II:* Due to poor enzyme activity.
3. *Gilbert syndrome:* Relatively more common but benign; due to polymorphism in promoter region of UGTIAI that also decreases normal gene activity to 30%.

Crigler-Najjar Syndrome Type I

Also called *glucuronyl transferase deficiency,* it is inherited as an autosomal recessive trait.

Clinical Manifestations

It is characterized by persistence of unconjugated hyperbilirubinemia (> 20 mg/dL) beyond first week of life with risk of kernicterus.

Diagnosis

In any neonate with very high unconjugated hyperbilirubinemia without hemolysis, Crigler-Najjar type I should be seriously considered.

Bilirubin level in bile is <10 mg / (normal 50-100 mg/dL. Phenobarbital (5 mg/kg/24 hours (O) response test may be employed to differentiate type I and II. In type II there is remarkable fall in serum bilirubin level following therapy with phenobarbital secondary to an inducible phenobarbital response element on the UGTIOAI promotor.

Confirmation of diagnosis is by measurement of hepatic glucuronyl transferase activity in liver biopsy sample.

DNA diagnosis is now available.

Identification of heterozygous state in parents strongly suggests this diagnosis.

Treatment

- Repeated phototherapy/exchange transfusion(s) to keep unconjugated serum bilirubin < 20 mg/dl.

- Phenobarbital therapy is recommended to find response plus to differentiate type I from II is the mainstay of treatment.
- As the subject grows, response to phototherapy gradually reduces. Therefore, alternative measures like agar, cholestyramine or calcium phosphate need to be considered to interfere with enterohepatic recirculation of bilirubin.
- Prompt treatment of superadded infections, febrile episodes and other illnesses to prevent kernicterus. Remember, dangerous levels for development of kernicterus are 75 mg/dL beyond neonatal period and 45-55 mg/dL in adolescents.
- Plasmopheresis and limitation of bilirubin production by inhibition of heme oxygenase using metalloporphyrin therapy.
- Curative treatment is in the form of orthotopic liver transplantation.
- Genetically engineered enzymatic replacement therapy and liver-directed gene therapy are yet in experimental stage though their role as potential therapeutic options for future appears to be promising.

Prognosis

Despite, all available preventive measures, the subject sooner or later develops kernicterus.

Crigler-Najjar Syndrome Type II

As is the case with CN type I, CN type II is an autosomal recessive disease caused by homozygous missense mutations in UGTIAI leading to somewhat decreased enzymatic activity.

Clinical Manifestations

During neonatal period, it causes unconjugated hyperbilirubinemia in first 3 days of life, serum bilirubin ranging between 1.5-22 mg/dL after third week of life. There is no hemolysis and kernicterus is unusual.

Diagnosis

Bilirubin level in bile is almost normal.

Main problem is of differentiating from type I by employing phenobarbital therapeutic test (vide infra).

Treatment

Continued phenobarbital therapy is central to long-term reduction in serum bilirubin levels.

Prognosis

Risk of kernicterus, though very small, remains.

INHERITED CONJUGATED HYPERBILIRUBINEMIA

A small number of rare autosomal recessive disorders (Dubin-Johnson syndrome, Rotor syndrome) may cause mild conjugated hyperbilirubinemia, resulting in slight jaundice, usually manifesting in adolescence or later. Liver function remains normal. Jaundice may be exacerbated by:

- Infection
- Drugs
- Alcohol
- Contraceptives
- Pregnancy.

Dubin-Johnson syndrome has a defect in hepatocyte secretion of bilirubin glucuronide. Liver cells characteristically are laden with black pigment resembling melanin.

Rotor syndrome has an additional deficiency in organic anion uptake. An important difference from DJS lies in elevated urinary coproporphyrin excretion with relative elevation of coproporphyrin 1 isomer. No black is not seen here.

HEPATOLENTICULAR DEGENERATION

Also termed Wilson's disease, this is an autosomal recessive disorder characterized by degenerative changes in brain, liver disease and Kayser-Fleischer rings in the cornea. Abnormal gene is localized in the long arm of chromocome 13 (13q14.3). The detailed description follows in a separate chapter (Ch. 77).

INDIAN CHILDHOOD CIRRHOSIS

Now widely believed to be secondary to high copper content, probably secondary to its excess dietary ingestion, this disease is characterized by jaundice, hepatosplenomegaly, ascites and malnutrition predominantly in infants from rural India (though similar cases are seen in Middle East, West Africa, North and Central America). The disease is only infrequently encountered now. It is discussed in details in Chapter 36.

NEONATAL IRON STORAGE DISEASE

Also termed neonatal hemochromatosis, this rapidly progressive and fatal disease, affecting neonates in first few days of life, is characterized by hepatomegaly, hypoglycemia, hypoprothrombinemia, hypoalbumuinemia, hyperferritenemia, hyperbilirubinemia, and coagulopathy refractory to vitamin K.

Etiology appears to be a gestational insult that also causes prematurity and/or IUGR. Associated renal agenesis may be present.

Diagnosis is established by documentation of extrahepatic siderosis (iron inclusion) in biopsy material from buccal mucosal glands. MRI shows iron-laden pancreas and other organs.

Treatment may be in the form of:

- Intravenous immunoglobulins (IVI) administered to the mother once a week from 18th week of gestation until therapy.
- Iron chelating agents (desferioxamine) along with aggressive antioxidant therapy.
- Liver transplantation.

ALPHA-1-ANTITRYPSIN DEFICIENCY

Alpha-1-antitrypsin-deficient neonates present with jaundice, acholic stools and hepatomegaly in first week of life. Jaundice usually disappears in 2nd-4th month.

When complete resolution fails, persistent liver disease or cirrhosis may follow.

When presentation first occurs in older children, manifestations are asymptomatic hepatomegaly, chronic liver disease or cirrhosis.

Liver transplantation proves curative.

KEY LEARNING POINTS

- Follows, among other defects, absence of an enzyme, producing a block in the metabolic pathway.
- Well-known examples include inherited hyperbilirubinemia (unconjugated or conjugated), Wilson's disease, ICC, neonatal iron storage disease and alpha-1-antitrypsin deficiency.
- The most important conditions causing unconjugated hyperbilirubinemia, Crigler-Najjar type I and II are differentiated by phenobarbital response test.
- Conditions causing inherited conjugated hyperbilirubinmia (Dubin-Jonson syndrome, Rotor syndrome) cause mild conjugated hyperbilirubinemia, usually manifesting in adolescence or later.
- Wilson's disease is characterized by degenerative changes in brain, liver disease and Kayse-Fleischer rings in the cornea.
- Neonatal iron storage disease, characterized by siderosis (iron inclusion), is a rapidly progressive and fatal disease.
- Alpha-1-antitrypsin deficiency has a tendency to cause persistent liver disease or cirrhosis.

FURTHER READINGS

1. Bosma PJ. Inherited disorders of bilirubin metabolism. *J Hepatol* 2003;38:107-117.
2. Grabhorn E, Richter A, Burdelski M, *et al.* Neonatal hemochromatosis: Long-term experience with favorable outcome. *Pediatrics* 2006;118:2060-2065.
3. Perlmutter DH. Alpha-1-antitrypsin deficiency: Diagnosis and treatment. *Clin Liver Dis* 2004;8:839-859.
4. Tao TY, Gitlin JD. Hepatic copper metabolism: Insights from genetic disease. *Hepatology* 2003;37:1241-1247.

77 Wilson's Disease

Ajay Gaur

INTRODUCTION

Wilson's disease is an autosomal recessive disorder of copper metabolism leading to excessive accumulation of copper in the liver, brain, kidneys and many other organs in the body. It is characterized by degenerative changes in the brain, liver disease, and Kayser-Fleischer rings in the cornea. Kinnear Wilson, a neurologist, who described it in 1912, considered it a primary degenerative disorder of the brain, while Hall in 1921 associated it with liver disease and introduced the term "hepatolenticular degeneration".

The basic defect appears to reside in impaired intracellular transport of copper into a hepatocytes pool essential for biliary excretion of copper and for incorporation of copper into ceruloplasmin. It is estimated that the worldwide prevalence of the disorder is 1 in 30,000, while the carrier frequency is 1 in 180. The gene recently has been identified to be a copper-binding membrane spanning protein with P-type ATPase motifs that characterize metal transport proteins.

PATHOPHYSIOLOGY

Copper is an essential trace element. Its dietary sources include liver, shellfish, chocolate, peas and unprocessed wheat. Normally, 50 percent of the ingested copper is unabsorbed, 30 percent is lost through the skin and the remaining 20 percent is retained by the body for maintaining homeostasis.

The highest concentrations are in the liver, brain, heart and kidneys, 50% of total body copper is in the large mass of muscle and bone. In humans, 20-30% of ingested copper is absorbed by an energy-requiring mechanism in the stomach and upper small intestine. Copper is transported from the intestine bound to albumin at a specific binding site on the protein. In the liver, the copper undergoes reaction crucial to total body metal homeostasis. Copper is incorporated into an oxidase, ceruloplasmin, synthesized in the liver; 90 to 95% of total plasma copper is bound to ceruloplasmin. In addition, there is a high capacity excretory pathway in hepatocytes by which copper is excreted into the bile as amino acid and bile acid complexes. This last sequence is the major excretory pathway for copper, and the metal so processed is not available for resorption. The copper transported as ceruloplasmin is not readily dissociated and is probably exchanged in extrahepatic tissues following a ceruloplasmin-receptor interaction at cell surfaces.

In addition to cuproenzymes, another copper binding protein has been described in liver, intestine, and other tissues, i.e. low-molecular-weight metalloproteins (8000-10000 d) of high sulfhydryl content, capable of binding other metals (zinc, cadmium, mercury and silver) as well as copper. This family of proteins, termed metallothioneins, is ubiquitous in distribution among tissues and species and its members have been identified as the major intracellular metal-binding proteins in a variety of tissues. Metallothioneins are coded on autosomes, metallothioneins likely function in a storage-detoxification capacity. Although a role in intracellular transport has been postulated.

In Wilson's disease, there is no increase in copper absorption from the gut. The basic defect seems to be the inability of the liver to incorporate copper into apoceruloplasmin, as well as secrete copper into the bile. It has been shown that in patients with Wilson's disease, copper concentrations are very high in the lysosomes of the hepatocytes and very low in the bile. ATP 7B protein deficiency impairs biliary copper excretion, resulting in positive copper balance; copper accumulated in the hepatocytes induces cell damage through reactive oxygen radicals. Excess hepatic copper is initially bound to metallothionein, but as this storage capacity is exceeded, liver damage begins as early as 3 years of age. Defective copper incorporation into apoceuloplasmin leads to excess catabolism and low blood levels of ceruloplasmin. Serum copper levels are usually lower than normal because of low blood ceruloplasmin, which normally binds > 90% of serum copper. As the disease progresses, non ceruloplasmin serum copper (free copper) levels increase, resulting in copper buildup in other parts of the body, such as brain, leading to neurologic and psychiatric disease. At the same time relentless accumulation of copper in the liver reaches the point at which the retention capacity exceeded. Copper than escapes the liver to damage other organs, particularly the brain and kidneys, and accumulates in the cornea, visible as Kayser-Fleischer rings. Release of copper from necrotic hepatocytes leads to damage of other tissues all over the body including the brain, kidneys and red blood cells. The underlying mechanism of liver damage in Wilson's disease is presumably oxidant injury to the hepatocytes mitochondria, which is the target organelle in copper, induces toxicity. Lipid peroxidation of the mitochondria resulting from copper overload leads to functional alterations. Ionic copper inhibits pyruvate oxidase in brain and ATPase in membrane, leading to decreased ATP phosphocreatine and potassium content of tissue. The glycolytic pathway and microsomal membrane ATPase are inhibited.

The role of ceruloplasmin, an alpha 2 globulin produced exclusively by the liver, in the pathogenesis of Wilson's disease is unclear. In most patients with Wilson's disease, ceruloplasmin levels are low in the serum. In addition, lower than normal levels are found in heterozygotes with no manifestation of the disease.

GENETICS

Wilson's disease is inherited as an autosomal recessive trait. The disease has been reported in diverse population groups, with estimates of incidence varying from 1/35,000 to 1/100,000. The gene locus for Wilson's disease is on the long arm of chromosome 13 at 14q 21, with tight linkage to the esterase D gene and to a number of flanking restriction-fragments-length polymorphisms (RFLPs). The disease-associated gene (ATP 7B) encodes a copper-transporting P type ATPase, the WND protein, structurally similar to the Menkes disease protein. Mutation analysis indicates that Wilson's disease is caused by a large number of different mutations, and that many of these will be rare. Such heterogeneity will make molecular diagnostic screening by direct mutation detection problematic. It is likely that there are numerous mutations of the gene, and most patients have 2 different mutations, having acquired one from each parent. The two most frequently observed mutations are a point mutation resulting in C to A transversion or a frame-shift.

Studies using the recently-cloned ceruloplasmin gene indicates that the underlying abnormality is a defect in both translation and transcription of the ceruloplasmin mRNA. However, a genetic defect in the processing of ceruloplasmin does not completely explain the pathogenesis of Wilson's disease. In addition, the gene for ceruloplasmin is on chromosome 3 while the Wilson's disease gene has been linked to chromosome 13. RFLP analysis has been applied in the identification of heterozygotes, the presymptomatic diagnosis of homozygotes for the Wilson's disease gene, and the prenatal diagnosis of Wilson's disease in families at risk.

CLINICAL MANIFESTATIONS

Clinical manifestations are related to the deposition of copper in various organs; and rarely presents before 5 years of age. Most patients present with either liver or CNS involvement, even though other organs can also be affected. (Table 77.1). About 25 percent of patients have multiple organs involved at presentation. In children, hepatic manifestations usually precede neurologic manifestations by many years.

Table 77.1: Clinical manifestations of Wilson's disease

Hepatic
Acute self-limited hepatitis
Chronic active hepatitis
Fulminant hepatic failure
Cirrhosis
Neurologic
Psychiatrics
Ophthalmologic
Renal
Miscellaneous
Coomb's negative hemolytic anemia
Skeletal: Bone demineralization
Cholelithiasis

Hepatic Manifestations

An episode of hepatitis may occur, with elevated blood transaminase enzymes, with or without jaundice and then spontaneously regress, Hepatitis often reoccurs, and most of these patients eventually develop cirrhosis. Hepatic decompensation is associated with elevated serum bilirubin, reduced serum albumin and coagulation factors, ascites, peripheral edema, and hepatic encephalopathy. In severe hepatic failure, hemolytic anemia may occur because large amounts of copper are released into the blood stream. The association of hemolysis and liver disease makes Wilson's disease a likely diagnosis.

Patient with Wilson's disease may also present as fulminant hepatic failure with rapid progression and death. Without a positive family history, diagnosis is difficult in these patients, even with investigations. Rarely, cirrhosis with portal hypertension may be a presenting feature. Any patient between the ages of 5 and 20 years of age presenting with liver disease of unknown etiology should be evaluated for Wilson's disease, especially if evidence of Coombs negative hemolytic anemia is present.

CNS Manifestations

The age range for neurologic presentation is from 6 years

onwards. It occurs predominantly in young adults. However, as many as 50% of teenagers may have some evidence of neurologic involvement. CNS involvement in Wilson's disease is extensive and not limited to the basal ganglia as was earlier thought. SPECT studies have shown that in addition to striatal injury, there is also significant damage to the substantia nigra. However, the damage is limited exclusively to the motor system, with the sensory system being totally spared. Symptoms are gradual in onset and progression is slow. Characteristic findings include resting and intention tremors, a flapping tremor of the hands and shoulder brought out by abducting the arms and holding the forearms horizontal in front of the body (the so-called wing-beating tremor), irregular oscillations of the eyeballs, infrequent blinking, difficulty with fine motor functions, and an ataxic unsteady gait are common initial presentations. These patients may not be able to dress, drink out of a cup. Dysarthria, dystonia, gait disturbances and mask-like frozen facies with an almost pathognomonic retracted upper lip, drolling, athetoid or choreic movements, with asymmetric posture of the limbs with the wrist in flexion and hand fisted, and rather frequent myoclonus become apparent much later (signs of progressive basal ganglia destruction). Seizures, including focal seizures, have been reported. In some patients, the signs may be as asymmetric as to present as a dystonic hemiparesis. Intellect is normal. Neurologic disease is almost always associated with the presence of Kayser-Fleischer rings (KF rings). Kayser-Fleischer rings may be absent in young patients with liver disease but are always present in patients with neurologic symptoms.

Psychiatric Manifestations

Psychiatric signs may range from inattentiveness, poor school performance, depression, aggressive outbursts, neurosis and even psychosis to behavior disorders. Severe personality changes have been reported in Wilson's disease. These signs are believed to be caused by storage of copper in the cortex as well as in the basal ganglia.

Ophthalmologic Manifestations

Kayser-Fleischer (KF) rings have long been considered the hallmark of Wilson's disease. It is important to remember that they may not be seen in children with only hepatic manifestations of Wilson's disease. In addition, KF rings may also be seen in other conditions, most notably chronic active hepatitis, primary biliary cirrhosis, long standing intrahepatic cholestatic syndromes, multiple myeloma, and intraocular foreign bodies containing copper alloys. KF rings appear as golden brown or bronze or greenish yellow discoloration (depending on the color of the iris) in the limbic region of the cornea (Fig. 77.1). A slit lamp biomicroscopy examination is necessary for detection, even though it can occasionally be visible to the naked eye. The rings are first noted in the upper part at 11 to 1 O' clock, then in the lower part and finally extend laterally to complete the ring. This ring of copper granules deposited in the Descemet's membrane is only a small fraction of the total corneal copper. Most of the copper is deposited in the stromal layers, which does not cause any color change and hence is not visible even under slit-lamp. Copper diffuses into the cornea from the aqueous humor; and this movement is inversely related to the evaporation of tears from the surface of the cornea. Since evaporation is less at the superior poles of the cornea, a KF ring is first visible at the upper part of the limbus.

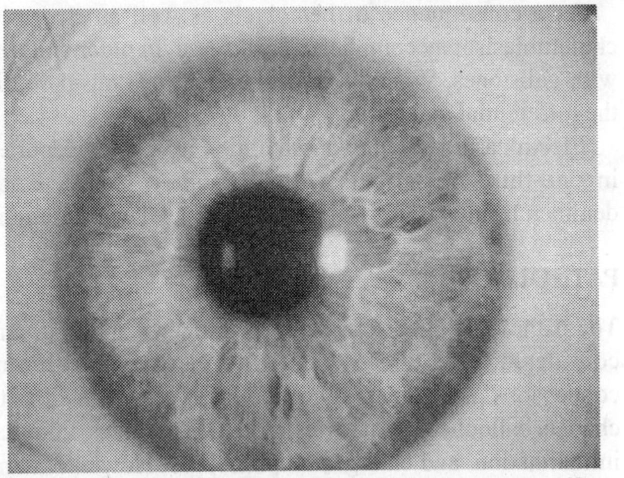

Fig. 77.1: Kayser-Fleischer rings in Wilson's disease (See for colour figure Plate 8)

Sunflower cataracts are occasionally seen in association with KF rings. They appear as a golden disc with radiating spokes, in the anterior capsule of the lens. They resolve with therapy.

Renal Manifestations

Renal involvement is common and is characterized by proximal tubular dysfunction and a decrease in glomerular filtration rate. Sign of renal involvement include hematuria and evidence of Fanconi syndrome, generalized amino-aciduria, and reduced specific gravity. A urinary acidification defect due to distal tubular dysfunction can also occur. Glycosuria, uricosuria, hypercalciuria, hyperphosphaturia, and renal tubular acidosis. The renal tubular dysfunction may be related to a direct toxic effect of copper granules deposited within the tubular epithelium. Renal function must be delineated in every patient prior to the institution of therapy because the therapeutic agent generally used can be nephrotoxic.

Other Manifestations

Acute hemolytic anemia with jaundice can occur prior to hepatitis and neurologic symptoms. The hemolysis occurs due to oxidative injury to the red blood cell membranes from excess serum copper.

As a consequence of hemolysis as well as cirrhosis, cholelithiasis may complicate the disease. In older children with gallstones, Wilson's disease should be considered in the differential diagnosis.

Electrocardiographic abnormalities have been reported in one-third of patients with Wilson's disease. Bone demineralization is the most common skeletal manifestation.

PATHOLOGY

The pathologic effects on the liver, kidneys, and brain are considered to be directly related to the accumulation of copper ions. All grades of hepatic injury occur, with fatty change, ballooned hepatocytes, glycogen granules, minimal inflammation, and enlarged Kupffer cells. However, none can be considered pathognomonic. Although the lesions are not specific, they are strongly supportive of the diagnosis of Wilson's disease, in combination with the clinical and laboratory findings. Fat deposition is the earliest change seen. Fine lipid droplets of triglycerides are dispersed throughout the cytoplasm. This progress gradually to hepatic steatosis. In the precirrhotic stage of Wilson's disease, the changes resemble a chronic, active hepatitis with focal necrosis, scattered acidophilic bodies, and moderate to severe steatosis. Glycogenated nuclei in periportal hepatocytes are a typical finding in Wilson's disease (Fig. 77. 2). Kupffer's cells are hypertrophied and may contain hemosiderin. Electron microscopy shows mitochondrial changes. As the hepatic lesion progresses collagen deposition occurs, leading on to cirrhosis. In later stages, periportal fibrosis, portal inflammation, along with fibrous bands and finally cirrhosis occur. The cirrhosis is often macronodular but may be of mixed type, with periportal fibrosis, cholangiolar proliferation and lymphocytic infiltration. Cholangiolar proliferation and lymphocytic infiltration is also seen. The presence of copper may not be cytochemically demonstrable in the precirrhotic stage. In young, asymptomatic patients, the copper is diffusely present in the cytoplasm but later accumulates in lysosomes. Rhodamine and rubeanic acid stains specifically detect the presence of copper. Copper associated protein can be stained with orcein or aldehyde fuchsin.

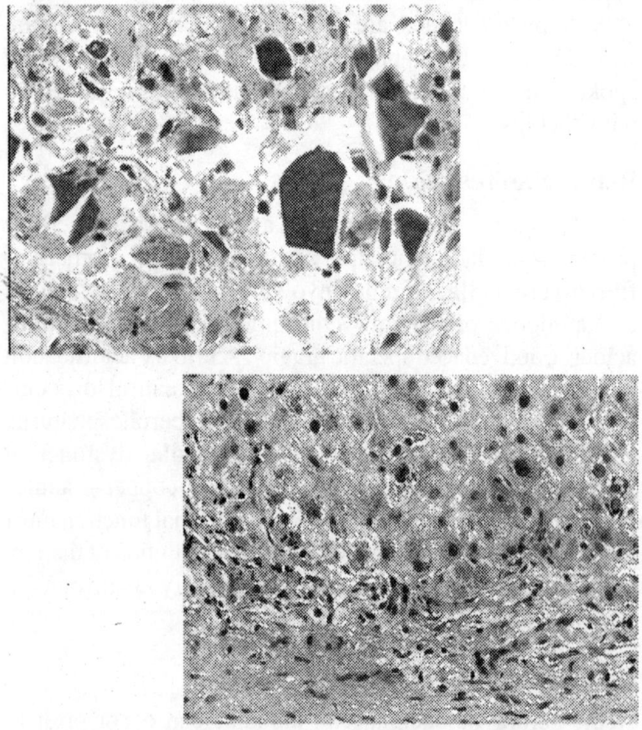

Fig. 77.2: Hepatolenticular degeneration-glycogenated nuclei in periportal hepatocytes, fatty changes and piecemeal necrosis (See for colour figure Plate 9)

ULTRASONOGRAPHIC CHANGES

The ultrastructural changes in Wilson's disease are pathognomonic. The large, dense mitochondria with altered smooth endoplasmic reticulum shows pronounced pleomorphism, intracristal spaces widen, and microcysts from at the tips of the cristae. Copper deposits are extremely electron dense.

PATHOPHYSIOLOGIC STAGING

A staging system that explains the progression of the disease has been devised by Desis *et al.*

Stage I: Progressive accumulation of copper in the cytosol of hepatocytes (usually asymptomatic).

Stage II: Redistribution of copper from the cytosol to the lysosomes of the hepatocytes and simultaneously copper is released from the liver (Patient develops features of liver disease).

Stage III: Lysosomal copper storage progress leading to stimulation of fibro genesis and gradual progression to cirrhosis (Progression to clinical disease).

Stage IV: The onset of hepatic or neurologic manifestation occurs.

Stage V: Irreversible liver or brain damage signifies.

DIAGNOSIS

A high index of suspicion is the key to early diagnosis. Wilson's disease should be considered in children and teenagers with unexplained acute or chronic liver disease, neurologic symptoms of unknown cause, acute hemolysis, psychiatric illnesses, behavioral changes, Fanconi syndrome, or unexplained bone disease.

Diagnosis is based on clinical and family history with a few key investigations. The classical triad of hepatic disease, neurologic involvement and KF rings represents a late stage in the disease process.

The best screening test is to measure the serum ceruloplasmin level. Seventy-five percent of children presenting with hepatic manifestations of Wilson's disease have decreased ceruloplasmin levels. The normal ceruloplasmin concentration in children aged 2-10 years is 22-54 mg/dL with some variation among laboratories. Adult concentrations (19-66 mg/dL) are reached by about 12 years. However, a number of other conditions can also be associated with low serum ceruloplasmin levels (Table 77.2). Moreover, heterozygote with no manifestation of Wilson's disease may also have low levels. Ceruloplasmin should, therefore, not be the sole criterion for the diagnosis of Wilson's disease.

Table 77.2: Conditions associated with low serum ceruloplasmin

- Malnutrition
- Protein losing enteropathy
- Chronic active hepatitis with or without hepatic failure
- Nephrotic syndrome
- Hereditary hypoceruloplasminemia

Twenty-four hours urinary copper excretion (usually <40μg/day) is increased to greater than 100 μg/day and often upto 1,000 μg or more per day in patients who present with fulminant hepatitis. A 24-hour urine collection should be obtained, and care taken to avoid contaminating the specimen with copper. However, elevated urinary copper concentration can also occur in other disease as well (Table 77.3). In equivocal cases, the response of urinary copper output to chelation may be of diagnostic help; after challenge with penicillamine in doses of 750 mg/square metre body surface area per day in two divided doses is considered by many as diagnostic of Wilson's disease.

Table 77.3: Conditions associated with increased urinary copper levels

- Fulminant hepatic failure
- Chronic active hepatitis
- Primary biliary cirrhosis
- Cholestatic syndrome of infancy

Total serum copper levels are unreliable in diagnosis. The crucial measurement of free toxic copper (copper not bound to ceruloplasmin) is technically difficult. The total serum copper concentrations are low in most patients. Rarely, a patient may have serum copper concentrations in the normal range, or even above normal, reflecting a normal ceruloplasmin concentration. The normal serum copper ranges from 72 to 186 mg/dL. The copper content of liver, brain, kidneys and cornea is increased. The hepatic content can be severe as a discriminant in diagnosis. Hepatic copper concentration in symptomatic and presymptomatic patients with the disease ranges from 94 to 1825 μg/g dry weight as compared with the normal 20-45 μg/g. It has been suggested that concentrations greater than 400 μg/g, in the absence of prolonged cholestasis, are strongly indicative of Wilson's disease, whereas concentrations below 94 μg/g dry weights exclude it. (For comparison, hepatic copper content in chronic active hepatitis is generally less than 300 μg/g dry weights) while increased levels may be seen in other conditions like Indian childhood cirrhosis, primary biliary cirrhosis and cholestatic syndromes of infancy.

Liver biopsy is of value for examination of the histology and for measurement of the hepatic copper content (normally <10 μg/g dry weight). In Wilson's disease, hepatic copper content exceeds 250 μg/g dry weights. In healthy heterozygotes, levels may be intermediate. Percutaneous liver biopsy should always be performed if there are no contraindications. There are no pathognomonic features on routine histopathology. Rubeanic acid staining demonstrates copper granules in the hepatocytes. Quantitative assay of the hepatic copper concentration should be done whenever possible.

When liver biopsy is contraindicated, radioactive copper studies are useful. Incorporation of radio copper into ceruloplasmin is defective in Wilson's disease. This can be performed by the kinetic analysis of plasma and ceruloplasmin radioactive copper concentrations after an intravenous dose of ^{64}Cu. Patients with Wilson's disease do not have a normal secondary rise in plasma radioactivity or incorporation of ^{64}Cu into ceruloplasmin is decreased compared with normal, but is still measurable. Unfortunately, only a few centers in the world perform this test. All asymptomatic relatives especially siblings should be screened, using slit-lamp examination, and measurement of serum ceruloplasmin level and 24-hour urine copper, if any one of the test is abnormal, a liver biopsy should be performed. The "gold standard" for diagnosis remains liver biopsy with quantitative copper assays.

Imaging studies of the brain may be helpful in diagnosis. CT abnormalities include ventricular dilatation, cortical atrophy, basal ganglia hypodensity and posterior fossa atrophy (Fig. 77.3).

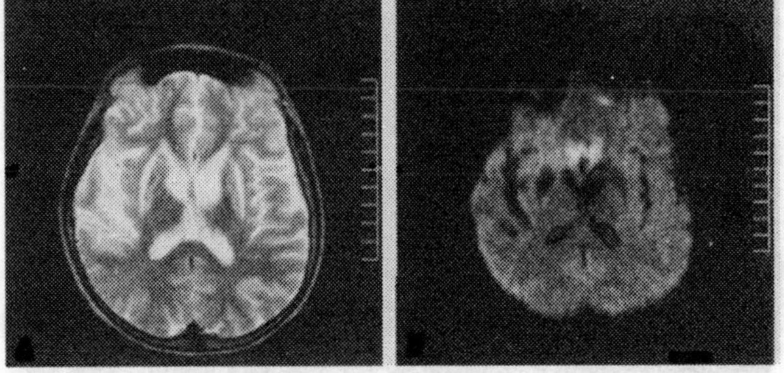

Fig. 77.3: Imaging abnormalities: Ventricular dilatation cortical and basal ganglia hypodensity

Even though CT findings are more likely in older patients with neurological involvement, it may be abnormal in children who are asymptomatic or have only hepatic involvement. The severity of CT findings does not correlate with clinical symptoms and is of little prognostic value. MRI may be more useful than CT in assessing the extent of involvement. The diagnosis by genetic studies and mutation screening are not practical as large number of inactivating mutations have been reported in the ATP 7B gene, but DNA haplotype analysis can be used to genotype siblings of an affected patients. All diagnostic tests for Wilson's disease are listed and compared in Table 77. 4.

TREATMENT

Wilson's disease is fatal if untreated, but successful outcome can be achieved with early effective therapy (Table 77. 5).

The objectives of the treatment are preventing intake of copper-containing foods (Table 77. 6), prevent copper from accumulating in tissues, chelating excess tissues copper for urinary excretion, preventing copper absorption, and rendering tissue copper nontoxic.

The mainstay of medical therapy is the use of copper binding agent D-penicillamine. It is a derivative of penicillin, which chelates copper and enhances urinary excretion. It is administered orally in 4 divided doses about 30 to 45 minutes before food. The daily dose is 20 mg per kg body weight in young children and 0.5-0.75 g/day for patients younger than 10 years. Therapy should be initiated with small doses, and then gradually increased. The usual maintenance dose is 1 g/d in divided doses for children overage 10 years. If treatment is begun in a presymptomatic patient, the development of symptoms is prevented. If treatment is begun early in the course of the disease, neurologic and hepatic function can be normalized. Side effect of D-penicillamine include early and late reactions in 25% of patients, there is a mild hypersensitivity reaction with morbilliform or urticarial rash, lymphadenopathy, fever, leucopenia, and thrombocytopenia. The reaction occurs within 10 days of the onset of treatment and clears with cessation of therapy. If it is necessary to begin treatment again, the dose should be increased gradually from 10 to 50 mg/d until the therapeutic range is again achieved. Concurrent treatment with corticosteroids and antihistamines may be necessary during this period. More severe later reactions include immune complex nephritis (nephritic syndrome). Drug-induced lupus erythematosus, Goodpasture syndrome, oral ulcerations, and agranulocytosis. If the drug must be withdrawn in the face of severe complications, it can often be reinstituted slowly and carefully, with or without corticosteroids. As D-penicillamine is a pyridoxine antagonist, Pyridoxine supplementation (25 mg thrice weekly) is recommended to offset the antipyridoxine effect of penicillamine. There is a dramatic increase in urinary copper excretion, about 48 hours after therapy is begun and values upto 100 times normal may be obtained. Urinary copper levels may be used as a good indicator of response to therapy in Wilson's disease.

Table 77.5: Treatment options in Wilson's disease

Dietary	Restriction of copper containing foods
Drugs :	Penicillamine
	Trientene
	Zinc
Orthotopic liver transplantation	

Table 77.4: Useful diagnosis tests for Wilson's disease

Test	*Usefulness*	*Normal value*	*Heterozygous*	*Wilson's disease*
Serum Ceruloplasmin	+	180-350 mg/L (18-35 mg/dl)	Absent	Low in 85%, present in 99% + if neurologic or psychiatric symptoms present.
		Low in 20%		
KF rings	+ +	Absent		Present in 30-50% in hepatic presentation and presymptomatic state
24-h urine Cu	+ + +	0.3-0.8µmol (20 -50 µg)	Normal to 1.3 µmol (80 µg)	>1.6 µmol (>100 µ in symptomatic patients 0.9 to > 1.6 µmol (60 to >100 µg) in presymptomatic patients
Liver Cu	+ + + +	0.3-0.8 µmol/g (20-50 µg) tissue	Normal to 2.0 µ (125 µg)	> 3.1 µmol (200 µg) (obstructive liver disease can cause false-positive results)
Haplotype Analysis	+ + + + (Siblings only)	0 Matches	1 Match	2 Matches

Usefulness: + somewhat useful, to + + + +, very useful

Abbreviations: KF, Kayser Fleischer; Cu, Copper.

Ceruloplasmin serum copper ("free" copper) levels increase, resulting in copper buildup in other parts of the body, such as the brain, leading to neurologic and psychiatric disease.

Table 77.6: Copper content of various foods

Food	*Copper Concentration (μg/g wet)*	*Size of Typical Serving (g)*	*Copper/Serving (mg)*
Meats			
Fish	0.61	120	0.07
Chicken	0.34	120	0.04
Dairy			
Egg	0.8	40	0.03
Single Sliced Cheese	0.43	120	0.05
Bread			
Whole Wheat	1.07	30	0.03
Chocolate			
Candy Bar	1.18	15	0.02
Milk	0.33	120	0.04
Vegetables			
Peas	2.38	120	0.29
Soya Beans	109	120	0.13
Fruits			
Applesauce (can)	0.20	120	0.02
Applesauce (bottle)	0.30	120	0.04
Nuts			
Walnuts	6.51	30	0.20
Soups			
Onion	1.49	15	0.02
Mushrooms			
Dry	2.12	50	0.11
Beverages			
Tea	0.025	120	0.03
Cola (bottle)	0.001	356	0.00

Biochemical improvement is slow and may take many months. Improvement in clinical symptoms may, however, be seen within a few weeks of therapy. Occasionally, the neurological symptoms initially worsen with treatment, but subsequently steady improvement occurs. Kayser-Fleisher rings may disappear completely or atleast partially fade with treatment. The dose of penicillamine may be increased further if symptomatic improvement is not obtained after a few weeks. Liver biopsy findings show gradual improvement, with decrease in portal fibrosis and inflammation; but normalization is rare.

Adequacy of therapy may be assessed by serial determination of 24-hour urinary copper excretion. Calculated free serum copper has also been recommended. [Serum Copper- (S Ceruloplasmin x 3)]. Values less than 20 indicates adequate therapy.

Trientine (triethylene tetramine dihydrochloride) is the alternative chelating agent in patients who do not tolerate penicillamine. Cupriuresis is lesser than with penicillamine but is therapeutically adequate. It is given 1 hour before food and the dose is 20 mg per kg per day in children below 10 years of age. Older children and adults require 1.0 to 1.5 g daily in divided doses. Drugs toxicity includes bone marrow suppression, nephrotoxicity, skin and mucosal lesions and iron deficiency anemia.

Elemental zinc (zinc acetate 50 mg thrice daily), an antagonist of copper absorption is another alternative. Zinc has also been used as adjuvant therapy or as maintenance therapy owing to its unique ability to impair the gastrointestinal absorption of copper. It is most effective when taken on an empty stomach. Zinc acetate is given in adults at a dose of 25 to 50 mg three times a day. Pediatrics dosing guidelines have not been established. Its efficacy is based on induction of both gut and liver metallothionein.

Copper is absorbed in the proximal small intestine, and once it crosses the intestinal brush border, it binds to and saturates the metallothionein inside the enterocytes. Zinc induces metallothionein synthesis in the enterocytes. Metallothinoein bound copper cannot move out of the cells to reach the blood stream. The intestinal cells therefore become loaded with this complexed copper and are then eliminated by desquamation into the intestinal lumen. Zinc must not be given with penicillamine or trientene, since it chelates with these drugs and forms complexes that are therapeutically inactive. However zinc act very slowly and may take months for therapeutic benefit. It is currently recommended that zinc may be tried in patients with Wilson's disease in whom both penicillamine and trientine are contraindicated or ineffective. Disadvantages include its potential delayed benefit to neurologic disease.

High copper containing food should be avoided, but a low copper diet is not a substitute for chelation therapy. A major attempt should be made to restrict copper intake to less than 1 mg/day. The drinking water should be tested because patients with Wilson's disease can tolerate only 0.02 ppm, if the copper content of the water exceeds 0.1 mg/L, it may be necessary to demineralize the water. Treatment must be continual and life long. No long-term adverse effects have been noted after continuous chelation therapy for over 30 years.

Improvements in the morbidity and mortality of orthotopic liver transplantation have made hepatic transplantation a therapy of significant choice in Wilson's disease. Orthotopic liver transplantation (OLT) is indicated only in the following situations:

- Fulminant hepatic failure.
- Severe hepatic decompensation and cirrhosis, with no improvement after 2-3 months of chelation therapy.
- Severe progressive hepatic insufficiency in a patient who discontinued treatment.

OLT has also been performed for neurological manifestations of Wilson's disease, which was unresponsive to chelation therapy. Post-transplant patients do not require D-penicillamine, and no recurrence of Wilson's disease in a transplanted liver has been reported.

PROGNOSIS

Wilson's disease is progressive and fatal if untreated. Death follows the hepatic, neurologic, renal, or hematological complications. Among children who present as chronic active hepatitis, almost 50 percent respond to treatment. Fulminant hepatitis is frequently fatal despite chelation therapy. Patients who present as an acute hepatitis or are asymptomatic do very well with treatment. Prognosis is poor in the acute neurological form of Wilson's disease. Among patients with gradual neurological involvement, 75 percent respond to treatment. In asymptomatic siblings of affected patients, early institution of chelation therapy can prevent expression of the disease.

KEY LEARNING POINTS

- An autosomal recessive disorder of copper metabolism, causing degenerative changes in brain, liver disease and Kayser-Fleischer rings in the cornea.
- Clinical manifestations are secondary to deposition of copper in various organs.
- Diagnosis is based on clinical presentation with family history and few investigations, the best screening test being serum ceruloplasmin level.
- Mainstay of treatment is the copper-binding agent, D-penicillamine, trientine and zinc being the alternatives for subjects with poor tolerance to it.
- OLT is recommended in subjects with neurologic diseases not responding to chelation therapy.
- Left untreated, it is uniformly progressive and fatal.

FURTHER READINGS

1. Schwarxenberg SJ, Sharp HL. Update on metabolic liver diseases. *Pediatr Clin North Am* 1996;43:27-56.
2. Rudolph JA, Balistreri WF. Metabolic disease of the liver. In: Behrman RE, Kliegman RM, Jenso HB (eds): *Nelson Textbook of Pediatric 17th edn.* Philadelphia: Saunders 2004;1321-1324.
3. Yamaguchi Y, Heinz ME, Gitlin JD: Isolation and characterization of a human liver cDNA as a candidate gene for Wilson's disease. *Biochem Biophys Res Com* 1993; 197: 271.
4. Chelly J, Monaco HP: Cloning the Wilson's diseases gene. *Nat Genet* 1993;5: 317.
5. Sokol RJ. Wilson's disease an Indian childhood cirrhosis. In: Suchy FJ: *Liver disease in children.* St. Louis: Mosby 1994: 747-757.
6. Jeon B, Kim JM, Jeon. Dopamine transporter imaging with C 1231 D-beta–CIT Demonstrates presynaptic nigrostriatal dopaminergic damage in Wilson's diseases. *J Neurol Neurosurg Psych* 1998;65:60-64.
7. Ghosh JB, Chakrabarty S, Singh AK, Gupta D. Wilson disease—Unusual features. *Indian J Pediatr* 2004; 71:937-938.
8. Jain S, Scheuer PJ, Archer BB. Histological demonstration of copper and copper-associated protein in chronic liver diseases. *J Clin Pathol* 1998;31:784.
9. Dacosta CM, Baldwin D, Portman B. Value of urinary copper excretion after penicillamine challenge, in the diagnosis of Wilson's disease. *Hepatology* 1992;15:609.
10. DaCosta CM, Baldwin D, Portmann B. Value of urinary copper excretion after penicillamine challenge in the diagnosis of Wilson's disease. *Hepatology* 1992;15:609.
11. Merli M, Patriaca M, Loudianos G. Use of the stable isotope 65 cu test for the screening of Wilson's disease in a family with two affected members. *Ital J Gastro Hepat* 1998; 30:270-275.
12. Cutbert JA: Wilson's disease. Update of a systemic disorder with protean manifestations. *Gastroenterol Clin North Am* 1998; 27:655-681.
13. Pleskow RG, Grand RJ: Wilson's disease. In Walker AW, Durie PR, Hamilton JR (eds): *Pediatric Gastrointestinal Disease.* Philadelphia: BC Dekker Inc 1991;1014-1025.
14. Siafakas CG, Jonas GM, Alexander S. Early onset of nephrotic syndrome after treatment with D-Penicillamine in a patient with Wilson's disease. *Am J Gastroenterol* 1998; 93:2344-2346.
15. Scheinberg IH, Sternlieb I. *Wilson's Disease.* Philadelphia: Saunders 1984.
16. Dubois RS, Roderson DO, Hambridge KM. Treatment to Wilson's disease with triethylene tetramine hydrochloride (Trientene). *J Pediatr Gastroenterol Nutr* 1990;10:77-80.
17. Hill GM, Brewer GJ, Prasad AS. Treatment of Wilson's disease with zinc. I, Oral zinc therapy regimens. *Hepatology* 1987; 7:522-528.
18. Berwer GJ, Dick RD, Johnson VD, *et al.* Treatment of Wilson's disease with zinc: Long-term follow-up studies. *J Lab Clin Med* 1998: 132264-132278.
19. Schilsky ML, Scheinberg IH, Sternlieb I: Liver transplantation for Wilson's disease: Indications and outcome. *Hepatology* 1994; 19:583-588.
20. Kalra V, Khurana D, Mittal R. Wilson's disease—Early onset and lessons from a pediatrics cohort in India. *Indian Pediatr* 2000;37:595-601.
21. Pandit A, Bavdekar A, Bhave S. Wilson's disease. *Indian J Pediatr* 2002;69:785-791.

78 Viral Hepatitis: Overview

ES Sherlock

INTRODUCTION

Generally speaking, the term, *hepatitis*, denotes a constellation of symptoms and signs resulting from hepatic inflammation and hepatic cell necrosis. Though viruses are the most important causative agents, toxins and alcohol may also cause acute hepatitis in which insult is acute and occurs in a previously asymptomatic subject. Such diseases as Wilson's disease, leukemias and lymphomas may lead to a clinical picture mimicking acute hepatitis.

Viral hepatitis is defined as an infection by hepatropic viruses (at least 5 are well recognized now, namely hepatitis A (HAV), hepatiis B (HBV), hepatitis C(HCV), hepatitis D (HDV) (previously non A, non B) and hepatitis E (HEV)) characterized by diffuse liver cell necrosis and inflammation leading to a characteristic constellation of clinical, biochemical and pathologic alterations.

In some subjects, Epstein-Barr Virus (EBV) or cytomegalovirus (CMV) may also cause acute hepatitis (Table 78.1).

Today, viral hepatitis is the most common cause of liver disease globally. In India and many other countries it is a public health problem.

HEPATOTROPIC VIRUSES

A large number of hepatotropic viruses are responsible for causing hepatitis in children, in many instances the infection remaining asymptomatic or causing only mild and transient manifestations.

Table 78.1: Viruses causing hepatitis

Most recognized hepatotropic viruses: Hepatitis A, B, C, D and E viruses

Hepatotropic viruses causing coinfection: Hepatitis G viruses

Non-hepatotropic viruses causing hepatitis as a part of multisystem involvement: Hepatitis simplex virus (HSV), cytomegalovirus (CMV), Epstein-Barr virus (EBV), Varicella-Zoster virus (VZV), HIV, rubella, adenoviruses, enteroviruses, parvovirus B_{19}, and arboviruses.

Table 78.2 summarizes the salient features of the five hepatotropic viruses.

Table 78.2: Salient features of 5 hepatotropic viruses

- *Hepatitis A virus* (HAV) is an RNA virus, which is very much identical to enteroviruses. It measures 27 nm and produces raised titer of anti-HAV IgM antibody in the serum, which is important for its serologic diagnosis as also anti-HAV IgG antibody which persists virtually for ever, thereby preventing reinfection. Chronic infection seldom occurs.
- *Hepatitis B virus* (HBV, Dane particle) is a DNA virus, measuring 42 nm with complex structure consisting of surface antigen (HBsAg), a central or core antigen (HBcAg), and DNA polymerase. Another antigen, HBHAg, appears to be a part of HBcAg. Its presence in serum points to highly contagious stage; beyond 3 months in children and 6 months in adults to a chronic infection.
- *Hepatitis C virus* (HCV) is an RNA virus, measuring 60 to 70 nm. It was formerly designated post-transfusion non-A, non-B hepatitis virus. Its serum marker is anti-HCV (IgG, IgM).
- *Delta virus* (HDV) is an RNA virus, measuring 36 nm, which is associated with a nucleoprotein (delta antigen) and covered with HBsAg. It needs the HBsAg for its replication and expression. The HDV presence and spread is, therefore, closely linked with HBsAg.
- *Hepatitis E virus* (HEV) is an RNA virus, measuring 32 to 34 nm. It was formerly designated as eternal non-A, non-B hepatitis virus. Its serum marker is anti-HEV.

PATHOGENESIS

Following invasion by a hepatotropic virus, liver suffers by two mechanisms:

1. Direct cytopathic insult.
2. Immune-mediated insult.

The involvement of the liver is total though lobular architecture remains intact. The prominent pathologic changes are:

- Necrosis most marked in centrilobular areas.
- Acute mixed inflammatory infiltrate in portal areas (maximal) and lobules.
- Balloon degeneration and necrosis of single or group of parenchymal cells frequent.

- Fatty change rare, except in HCV infection.
- Diffuse Kupffer cell hyperplasia in sinusoids.
- Giant cells in neonates.

CLINICAL PROFILE

All forms of acute viral hepatitis present clinically in more or less three stages.

The ***prodromal stage*** (lasting 2-7 days) is characterized by nausea, vomiting, high-colored urine, pyrexia and right hypochondral pain/tenderness. As the icteric stage approaches, these symptoms tend to decline and even disappear.

The ***icteric stage*** (lasting 7-14 days) is characterized by clinically manifest icterus, light pale stools and tender hepatomegaly. It may persist in grown-up children for several weeks.

The ***convalescent stage*** is characterized by subsiding icterus. In due course, the child reverts to normal health.

DIFFERENTIAL DIAGNOSIS

Differential diagnosis is from other causes of acute onset jaundice. These causes vary in neonatal period and rest of childhood (Table 78.3).

Table 78.3: Differential diagnosis of viral hepatitis

Neonates	
Bacterial (E.coli, Listeria)	
Nonhepatotropic viruses (HSV, enteroviruses, CMV)	
Metabolic:	Tyrosinemia
Anatomic:	Biliary atresia, choledochal cyst
Later Childhood	
Anatomic:	Extrahepatic obstruction (gallstone, primary sclerosing cholangitis, pancreatic pathology)
Inflammatory:	Autoimmune hepatitis, juvenile rheumatoid arthritis, Kawasaki disease, immune dysregulation)
Infiltrative:	Malignancies
Toxins:	
Metabolic:	Wilson's disease, cystic fibrosis
Infection:	EBV, varicella, malaria, leptospirosis, syphilis

BIOCHEMICAL PROFILE

Three categries of profiles are described:

Profile 1: Raised serum alanine aminotransferase (ALT) and aspartate transferase (AST).

Profile 2: Cholestasis demonstrated by high conjugated bilirubin levels, serum alkaline phosphatase (ALP), 5-nucleotidase, gamma-glutamyl transpeptidase (GGT) and urobilinogen.

Profile 3: Altered synthetic function as reflected by prolonged prothrombin time, high INR, low serum albumin, hypoglycemia, lactic acidosis, hyperammonemia or clinical signs like poor clearance of medications (dependent on liver function), altered sensorium with exaggerated deep tendon reflexes.

ADVANCES HAVING INFLUENCE ON THERAPY OF VIRAL HEPATITIS

- Definition of molecular structure of classic viral hepatitis viruses.
- Elucidation of genetic structure/cloning of new forms of viral hepatitis.
- Epidemiologic studies providing incidence of various forms.
- Epidemiologic studies identifying high-risk situations for each etiologic virus.
- Institution of anti-HCV screening to cut down incidence of post-transfusion hepatitis.
- Immunoprophylaxis aimed at interruption of spread of hepatotropic viruses, particularly in preventing maternal-to-infant passage of hepatitis B virus.
- Development of hepatitis B and A vaccines.
- Employment of interferon in chronic hepatitis B and C and development of alternative forms of therapy.

KEY LEARNING POINTS

- A constellation of symptoms and signs resulting from hepatic inflammation and hepatic cell necrosis, secondary to insult usually by the hepatotropic viruses (A, B, C, D, E and G).
- Liver suffers via two mechanisms, namely direct cytopathic and immune-mediated insults.
- Clinical profile comprises prodromal, icteric and convalescent stages.
- Biochemical profile too comprises three categories.

FURTHER READINGS

1. Avunduk C. Viral hepatitis. In: *Manual of Gastroenterology*, 3rd edn. London: Lippincott Williams and Wilkins 2001:351-375.
2. Yazigi N, Balistreri WF. Viral hepatitis. In: Kliegman RM, Behrman RE, Jenson HB, Stanton BF (eds): *Nelson Textbook of Pediatrics*, 18th edn. Philadelphia: Saunders 2008: 1680-1690.
3. Sherlock S, Dooley J. Viral hepatitis: General features, hepatitis A, hepatitis E and other viruses. In: *Diseases of Liver and Biliary Tract*, 11th edn. London: Blackwell 2002:267-284.
4. Yazigi NA, Balistreri WF. Acute and chronic viral hepatitis. In: Suchy FJ, Sokol RJ, Balistreri WF (eds): *Liver Disease in Children*, 2nd edn. London: Lippincott Williams and Wilkins 2001:365-428.

79 Hepatitis A

ES Sherlock

INTRODUCTION

Globally, Hepatitis A is the most common viral hepatitis with highest incidence in the developing world where it may well account for 75% cases of viral hepatitis (Fig. 79.1). On an average, 33% of HAV infection is seen in children. It is believed that the actual figures may well be yet higher since many children, especially, aged 3 to 5 years, with this infection have minimal manifestations and are missed. Earlier it was held that a large proportion of Indian children develop natural immunity by age 10 years. Observations made recently have contradicted this impression.

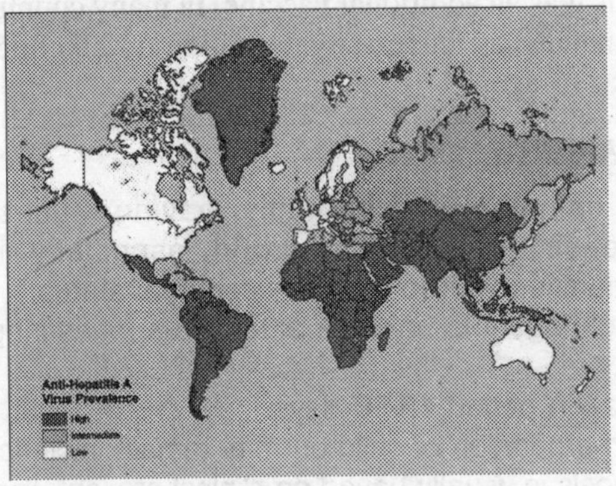

Fig. 79.1: Geographical prevalence of HAV

ETIOPATHOGENESIS

HAV is an RNA enterovirus, a member of the picornaviridea family measuring 27 nm by immune electron microscopy (Fig. 79.2) and infecting only the humans and the other primates. It belongs to hepatovirus group of picornovirus. It is relatively resistant to disinfection.

Major modus operandi of hepatic insult is through host immune response.

The growth of the etiologic agent, hepatitis A virus in tissue culture and subsequent development of highly sensitive immunoassay for detecting antibody against this virus (anti-HAV) has led to a better understanding of HAV infection.

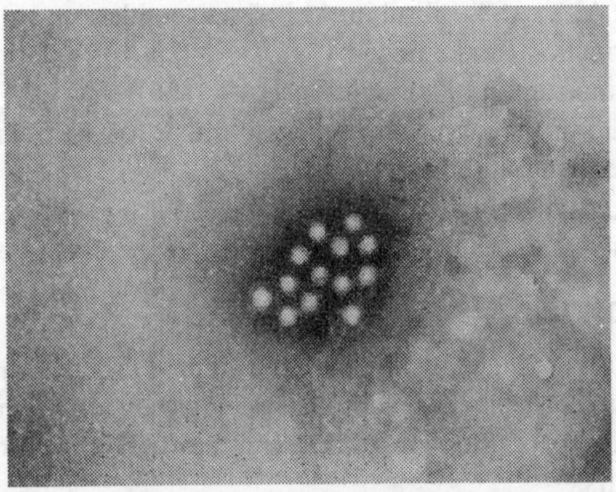

Fig. 79.2: Microscopic picture of HAV

EPIDEMIOLOGY

Hepatitis A has the highest prevalence in communities with low socioeconomic status on account of substandard hygiene and/or sanitary practices. A very contagious state, hepatitis A infection usually occurs through orofecal route. Overcrowding, poor sanitation, poor water and food hygiene, poor personal hygiene, improper sanitation, etc play significant role in its spread.

Outstanding risk factors include:

- Close contact with hepatitis a patient, including sexual contact.
- Travel to endemic areas.
- Intravenous drug abuse (during incubation period).
- Day-care centers.

CLINICAL MANIFESTATIONS

Incubation period is 15 to 50 days. Following a short prodrome, the child develops an acute febrile illness with sudden anorexia, nausea, vomiting, malaise (manifestations mimicking acute gastroenteritis or gastritis) and, in a proportion of children (usually older ones), jaundice. Generally, speaking the illness lasts 7-14 days.

Extrahepatic manifestations include regional lymphadenopathy, splenomegaly, hypoplasia/aplasia of marrow, GIT ulceration, arthritis, nephritis, vasculitis, acute pancreatitis, myocarditis, thrombocytopenia and cryoglobinemia.

Hepatitis A is usually self-limited, the severity being age dependent. It may well be inapparent in infants and preschool children (anicteric).

Fulminant hepatic failure (FHF) secondary to HAV infection is rare. When it occurs, there usually is an underlying chronic hepatitis. Incidence of FFH is more in developing countries.

DIAGNOSIS

Though the diagnosis is usually clinical with support from raised ALT, AST, bilirubin, ALP, 5-nucleotidase and GGT, confirmation can be done by:

- Demonstrating antibodies to HAV (anti-HAV IgM) by radioimmunoassay. It remains positive for 4-6 months after acute infection.
- Identifying viral particles in stools.

For research purpose, a viral PCR may be employed.

PROGNOSIS

Hepatitis A is usually an acute, self-limited illness, usually resolving both biochemically and histologically in due course without any progression to AFH, chronic carriage or chronic hepatitis.

Yet, in a small proportion of cases, a biphasic, relapsing or protracted course may be encountered. These are the subjects in whom anti-HAV IgM may persist over 12 to 14 months – of course at a low titer.

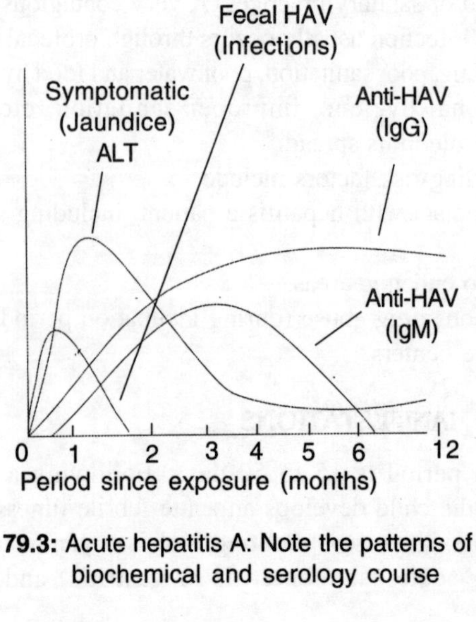

Fig. 79.3: Acute hepatitis A: Note the patterns of clinical, biochemical and serology course

COMPLICATIONS

1. Acute liver failure (ALF) especially when there is coinfection with HBV or HEV.
2. Cholestatic syndrome.

TREATMENT

It is by and large supportive, comprising:

- Maintenance of nutrition (particularly fat-soluble vitamins) and hydration (at times IV fluids).
- Antipruritic agents in case of disturbing itching.
- Monitoring for acute liver failure, and preparedness for its management.

PREVENTION

Conservative/General Measures

- Improvement in water and food hygiene.
- Handwashing after handling the patient.
- Restraining school attendance by the child for 1 week after onset of jaundice.

Immunoglobulins

Immune globulin administration to exposed individuals for, at least temporary protection, may be considered.

Vaccination

Hepatitis A vaccine is recommended after 1 year of age in two doses given IM at 6 months interval. The dose is 720 IU until 19 years of age and 1440 IU after that age.

At present, the Indian Academy of Pediatrics (IAP) recommends it as an additional vaccine. In many countries, it is recommended as universal vaccination for all children above 1 year of age.

KEY LEARNING POINTS

- Most common viral hepatitis, having highest incidence in developing world, especially in communities with low socio-economic status.
- Etiologic agent is an RNA enterovirus measuring 7 nm.
- Incubation period 15-50 days.
- A high proportion of children may remain inicteric.
- Diagnosis is usually based on clinical presentation plus LFT.
- Usually a self-limited disease, warranting only supportive treatment.
- Hepatitis A vaccine, after first year of life, provides a dependable prophylaxis.

FURTHER READINGS

1. Centers for Disease Control and Prevention (CDC). Multistate outbreak of hepatitis A among young adult concert attendees – United States, 2003 *Morb Mort Wkly Rep* 2003;52:844-845.
2. Temte JL. Should all children be immunized against hepatitis A ? *Br Med J* 2006;332:715-718.
3. Wheeler C, Vogt TM, Armstrong GL. An outbreak of hepatitis A-associated with green onions. *N Engl J Med* 2005;353: 890-897.

80 Hepatitis B and C

Neelam Mohan • Anupam Sehgal

HEPATITIS B

Five percent of the earth's population have hepatitis B, making it one of the most common infective diseases in the world today. There are estimated 400 million causes of hepatitis B virus (HBV) worldwide 80% of whom reside in Asia and western pacific. Effective vaccines have been available for more than 20 years now, but perinatal exposure continues in high prevalence areas.

Clinical Outcome of HBV Infection

Patients in whom hepatitis B surface antigen (HbsAg) persists in serum for more than 6 months are referred to as "chronic HBsAg carriers". In common usage, the term "carrier" is often employed to refer to persistently infected individuals with normal serum aminotransferase levels (sometimes also referred to as healthy HBV carriers). The term "healthy carrier" seems to be a poor one in that these patients may have evidence for hepatic inflammation on biopsy, particularly when serologic markers of viral replication are evident. Because of potentially confusing nomenclature, it has been proposed that the carrier state be categorized as inactive or active, with the former referring to patients who have evidence for HBV replication by PCR-based assay only and normal or only mildly abnormal serum aminotransferase levels. Long-term follow-up of inactive carriers suggests that the majority of patients do not have progressive liver disease and do not develop complications. However, there are major exceptions to this rule. Some of these patients have periodic reactivations of their liver disease in association with an increase in viremia and immunologic responses. Some patients with the inactive carrier state may develop hepatocellular carcinoma. Active carriers, in contrast, have evidence for HBV replication by standard hybridization assays, abnormal serum aminotransferase levels, and evidence for chronic hepatitis, with or without concomitant cirrhosis.

The age at which the individual becomes infected with HBV correlate with clinical outcome and the possible route of exposure. Liver injury and extrahepatic disorders are caused by cell-mediated and humoral patterns of response of HBV infection. The severity of the liver injury reflects the activity of the immune response: the strongest response causes the greatest hepatocellular injury and higher likelihood of viral clearance. Thus, HBV infection in adults with intact immune systems is likely to cause clinically apparent acute hepatitis B, with only 1 percent to 5 percent of cases becoming chronically infected. By contrast, as much as 95 percent of infected neonates become chronic HBV carriers and generally develop subclinical infection because of their immature immune systems. Spontaneous survival in acute liver failure resulting from hepatitis B is between 20 and 30 percent. Liver transplantation has resulted in 50 percent to 60 percent survival rate, and recurrent disease in the allograft is infrequent in this situation. Anti-viral therapy has little rationale for fulminant hepatitis B because most of the immunologically mediated liver damage and elimination of HBV has already occurred by the time of presentation. Patients in whom the diagnosis of acute fulminant hepatitis B is suspected are often HBe-Ag-negative and may be HBs-Ag-negative when first seen. Thus, the accurate diagnosis of fulminant liver failure resulting from hepatitis B may require testing with immunoglobulin (Ig) M antibody to HBc antigen (HBcAg).

Between one third and one quarter of people chronically infected with HBV are expected to develop progressive liver disease (including cirrhosis and primary liver cancer). An estimated 15 percent to 25 percent of all age groups with chronic HBV infection die prematurely from these conditions.

Patients who lack evidence for HBeAg and have normal serum aminotransferase levels rarely transmit the infection to others and usually do not have progressive liver disease even after prolonged follow-up.

Several large cohort studies have demonstrated that the presence of active viral replication and long-standing necro-inflammatory liver disease, resulting from HBV infection, strongly influence the rate of progression to cirrhosis. Cirrhosis is associated with decreased survival and higher frequency of complications, including hepatocellular carcinoma.

Serologic Markers of HBV infection

HBsAg is the serologic hallmark of HBV infection. HBsAg appears in serum 2 to 10 weeks after exposure to the virus and before the onset of symptoms or the elevation of serum aminotransferase levels. In patients who subsequently recover, HBsAg usually becomes undetectable after 4-6 months. Persistence of HBsAg for more than 6 months implies progression to chronic HBV infection.

The disappearance of HBsAg is followed by the appearance of anti-HBs. In most patients, anti-HBs persist for life, conferring long-term immunity. In some patients anti-HBs may not become detectable, but these patients do not appear to be susceptible to recurrent infection. **Anti-HBs** may not be detectable during a window period of several weeks to months after the disappearance of HBsAg. During this period, diagnosis of HBV infection is made by detection of IgM antibodies against HBcAg. Anti-HBc is detectable in acute and chronic HBV infection. During acute infection anti-HBc is predominantly of the IgM class. **IgG anti HBc** persists in those who recover from acute hepatitis B.

Isolated presence of anti-HBc in the absence of HBs Ag and anti-HBs may occur in the following four settings:

a. During the window period of acute hepatitis B when it is predominantly of the IgM class.
b. Many years after recovery from acute hepatitis B when anti-HBs has fallen to undetectable levels.
c. False positive serologic test and after.
d. Many years of chronic infection when the HBs Ag titer has decreased below the level of detection.

HbeAg is a soluble viral protein that is found in serum early during acute infection. HbeAg positive 3 or more months after the onset of illness indicates a high likelihood of transition to chronic infection. HbeAg is an indication of viral replication and infectivity. In general seroconversion

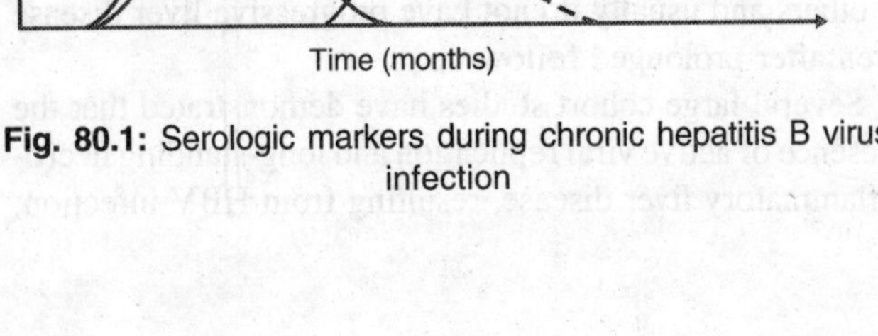

Fig. 80.1: Serologic markers during chronic hepatitis B virus infection

from HbeAg to anti-Hbe is associated with disappearance of HBV DNA in serum and remission of liver disease. Some patients however, continue to have active liver disease and detectable HBV DNA in serum resulting from either low levels of wild-type virus or the presence of precore mutation that impairs e antigen secretion.

HBV DNA Tests

HBV DNA can be measured in serum using **qualitative or quantitative assays.** PCR assay are more popular than non-PCR based assay. Quantitation of serum HBV DNA is useful in several situations such as candidacy for antiviral treatment, response to antiviral treatment, determining etiology of biochemical flares, detection of phenotypic and genotypic resistance to lamivudine and other nucleosides etc.

Qualitative HBV DNA testing is useful in cryptic HBV infection (i.e. HBs Ag negative patients) and determining the infectivity of anti-HBc positive donor and in patients with fulminant hepatitis B who frequently have cleared HBsAg by the time they obtain medical attention.

HBV Genotypes

HBV has 8 genotypes. Each genotype has its distinct geographical and ethnic distribution. Genotypes A and D occur frequently in Africa, Europe and India. Genotypes B and C are prevalent in Asia.

Several studies have shown that compared with genotype C, genotype B is associated with spontaneous HBeAg seroconversion at a younger age less active liver disease slower progression to cirrhosis and less frequent development of HCC. A study from India indicated that genotype D is more often associated with HBeAg negative chronic hepatitis B and more severe disease and may predict the occurrence of HCC in your patients.

The diagnosis of acute hepatitis B is based on the detection of HBsAg and IgM anti-HBc. During the initial phase of infection, the markers of HBV replication (HBeAg and HBV DNA) are present. Recovery is accompanied by the disappearance of HBV DNA, seroconversion from HBeAg to anti-HBe, and subsequently seroconversion from HBsAg to anti-HBs. Rarely, patients may have entered the window period at the time of presentation; IgM anti-HBc is the sole marker of acute HBV infection in these cases. This situation is more common in patients with fulminant hepatitis B, in whom virus clearance tends to be relatively rapid.

Past HBV infection is diagnosed by the detection of anti-HBs and IgG anti-HBc. Immunity to HBV infection after vaccination is indicated by the presence of anti-HBs only.

The diagnosis of chronic HBV infection is based on the detection of HbsAg. Additional tests for HBV replication (HBeAg and serum HBV DNA) should be performed to

Table 80.1: Diagnosis of hepatitis B virus infection

	HBsAg	*HBeAg*	*IgM anti-HBc*	*IgG anti-HBc*	*Anti-HBs*	*Anti-HBe*	*HBV DNA*	*Interpretation*
Acute HCV infection	+	+	+		-		+	Early phase
	-	-	+		-	+	+/-	Window phase
	-	-	-	+	+	+	-	Recovery phase
Chronic HBV infection	+	+	-	+	-	-	+	Replicative phase (HBeAg positive chronic hepatitis)
	+	-	-	+	-	+	-	Low/non-replicative phase
	+	-	-	+	-	+	+	Precore mutant variants (HBeAg negative chronic hepatitis)
	+	+/-	+/-	+	-	+/-	+/-	Exacerbations of chronic hepatitis

HBV DNA detected by unamplified assay.
HbsAg, hepatitis B surface antigen; HbeAg, hepatitis B e antigen; HBc, hepatitis B core; IgM immunoglobulin.

determine if the patient should be considered for antiviral therapy. PCR assays are more sensitive. However, the pathogenic significance of minute amounts of HBV DNA that can be detected only by PCR but not by hybridization or signal amplification assays is uncertain. HBeAg-negative patients who have normal ALT levels do not have to be evaluated further, but those with elevated ALT levels should be tested for serum HBV DNA to determine if the liver disease is related to persistent HBV (wild type or variant) replication. Additional tests for hepatitis C and hepatitis D should be performed to rule out super infection with other hepatitis virus(es).

Management

The main aim of the treatment of chronic hepatitis B is to suppress HBV replication before irreversible liver damage occurs. Currently, IFN-α and lamivudine are the only approved treatments. Many new antiviral and immunomodulatory therapies are being evaluated. Some of these have shown promise and may play a key role in the treatment of chronic HBV infection.

Treatment of Chronic Hepatitis B

- Interferon α.
- Antiviral agents:
  - Lamivudine.
  - Adefovir.
  - Emtricitabine.
  - Entecavir.
  - Clevudine.
  - β-L-Thymidine (L-dT).
- Immunomodulatory therapy:
  - Interleukin 12.
  - Thymosin.
- HBV-specific:
  - DNA vaccination.
- Combination treatment:
  - Interferon + Lamivudine.
  - Lamivudine + adenofovir dipivoxil.

Aims of Treatment

The initial goals are to suppress HBV replication and induce a remission of liver disease. The ultimate goals are to eliminate HBV, prevent progression to cirrhosis and HCC, and improve survival. Response is usually defined as sustained clearance of HBeAg with or without detectable anti-HBe, failure to detect HBV DNA in serum (with unamplified assays), and regression of liver disease (normalization of ALT levels and decrease in necrotic inflammation on liver biopsy). At a recent National Institute of Health workshop on the management of hepatitis B, it was proposed that the definitions and criteria of the response to antiviral therapy of chronic hepatitis B be standardized. The proposal categorized responses as biochemical (BR), virologic (VR), or histologic (HR), and as on-therapy or sustained off-therapy.

Table 80.2: Definition of response to antiviral therapy of chronic hepatitis B

Category of response	
Biochemical (BR)	Decrease in serum level to within the normal range.
Virological (VR)	Decrease in serum HBV DNA to undetectable levels in unamplified assays (< 10 ^{5} copies/Ml) and loss of HbeAg in patients who were initially HbeAg-positive.
Histologic (HR)	Decrease in histology activity index by at least 2 points in comparison with value on pretreatment liver biopsy.
Complete (CR)	Fulfillment of criteria of biochemical and virological response and loss of HbsAg.
Time of assessment	
End-of-treatment	At the end of a defined course of treatment.
Sustained response (SR-6)	Six months after discontinuation of therapy.
Sustained response (SR-12)	Twelve months after discontinuation of therapy.

HBV-Hepatitis B virus; HbeAg-Hepatitis B e antigen; HbsAg-Hepatitis Bs antigen.

ANTIVIRAL THERAPY

Interferon

At present the standard therapy of chronic HBV infection among children is interferon-alpha (IFN). As per the consensus advice of 1999, the indications for treatment of children with IFN are HBsAg positivity, HbeAg positivity more than 6 months, active viral replication (HBV DNA positivity) and elevated serum alanine aminotransferase (ALT) more than twice the normal value in children older than two years. These criteria, however, excluded a majority of Asian children with normal serum ALT levels, who have perinatally acquired disease.

Side Effects of interferon include:

- Flu-like illness.
- Fatigue.
- Anorexia, nausea.
- Emotional lability, anxiety, irritability, depression.
- Bone marrow suppression: Neutropenia, thrombocytopenia.
- Sleep disturbance.
- Unmasking or exacerbation of autoimmune disorders, thyroid dysfunction.

It is contraindicated in case of decompensated liver disease, cytopenia, autoimmune disease and severe renal or cardiac disease. Results of IFN in trails vary from 20%-60% success. It is found to be higher in European children as compared to Asian population, probably because of perinatal transmission and young age at infection acquisition in the latter. Israeli experience in children with chronic hepatitis B is 31.5% response rate. They concluded that IFN treatment is to be given only for children with HBV and significantly elevated liver enzymes.

Interferon is available as 3 MU and 5 MU and is given as a subcutaneous injection, is available as single injection or multidose injection as in pen-interferon. Bortolotti *et al.* have examined the long-term effects of IFN treatment in children with HBV and have seen HBeAg clearance rates of 60% versus 65% in the control group and HBsAg loss in 25% of the cases after a 5-year follow-up.

PEG Interferon

Shortcomings of interferon treatment are its fast absorption, large volume of distribution, short serum half life (2-5 hours), rapid renal clearance, limited efficacy, acute and chronic side effects. To achieve optimum results, constant viral suppression is needed. Polyethylene glycol or PEG is an inert, non-toxic and water-soluble polymer which when linked to interferon results in increase in its *in vivo* biological activity. PEG-Interferon is interferon linked to polyethylene glycol moiety, which is given as weekly injections and provides constant viral suppression during that time (Fig. 80.2).

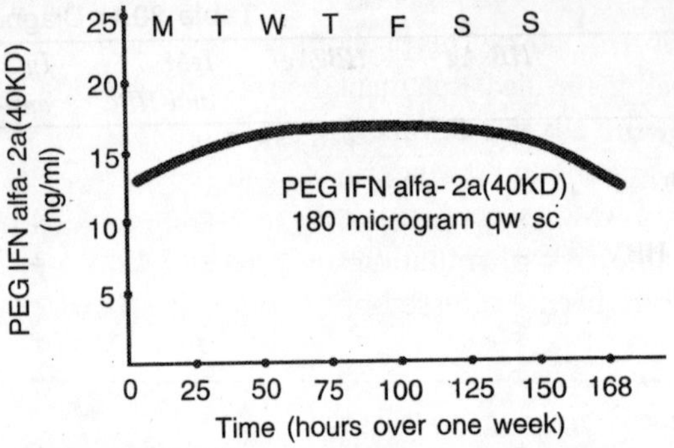

Fig. 80.2: Outcome of PEG interferon treatment in hepatitis B

Characteristics of PEG interferon are rapid and sustained absorption, increased half life, improved antiviral activity, reduced frequency of dosing, reduce clearance, less side effects and improved patient compliance. Studies of PEG interferon in chronic hepatitis B infection in adults have shown definite advantages over interferon therapy (SVR ~ 30-40%), though results are not as good as compared to chronic hepatitis C infection. However studies with PEG interferon are children are still undergoing and therefore data from children is not available.

Lamivudine

Lamivudine (LAM) is a nucleoside analogue that prevents HBV DNA synthesis by competitively inhibiting the viral reverse transcriptase and DNA-polymerase stages of virus replication and by termination of proviral DNA chain extension. Clinical trials have been performed among children with a recommended dose of 3 mg/kg with a maximum dose of 100 mg, which have shown a satisfactory tolerability profile. Kocak *et al.* has shown HBV DNA clearance of 64.8% but HbeAg clearance of 7.4% with less than 6% seroconversion of anti-HbeAg, when used in children with low viral replication (low HBV DNA levels). Patients with severe histologic activity and high baseline ALT seem to show better results in terms of seroconversion after treatment with lamivudine. However, in majority of the cases there is reappearance of HBV DNA replication on stopping lamivudine. Another major concern with the use of lamivudine is development of resistance to LAM treatment with the emergence of mutant HBV species. Certain HBV species show mutations in the tyrosine-methionine-aspartate-aspartate (YMDD) locus of the HBV-RNA-dependent DNA polymerase and therefore develop resistance to therapy with LAM after 6-9 months. Studies suggest that the incidence of YMDD mutations increases with the duration of treatment, from 22% after 24 weeks to 38-40% and 67% after 2 and 4 years respectively. The initial positive response to LAM treatment may then be followed by virological rebound and exacerbation of hepatitis and seroconversion to low-level viral conversion (Fig. 80.3).

There is no consensus on how to manage patients who develop a mutation. This phenomenon poses a great difficulty in deciding the ideal treatment time and in balancing positive response to adverse effects. This uncertainty of treatment is of paramount importance in pediatrics, as children may require LAM therapy for an indefinite length of time with an inevitable risk of mutation and relapse. Concerns have, therefore, been expressed about the use of LAM outside research trials and LAM has not been licensed for use in hepatitis B in children universally. Experience in adults has shown that adefovir may be effective in patients who develop lamivudine resistant mutant.

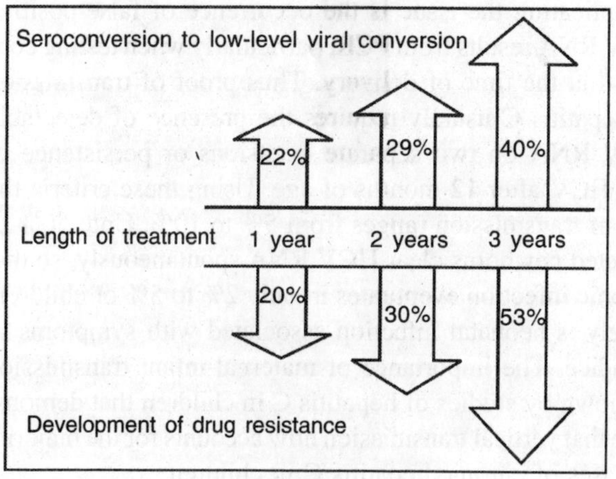

Fig. 80.3: Outcome of prolonged treatment with lamivudine in hepatitis-B

Adefovir Dipivoxil

Adefovir Dipivoxil is a synthetic acyclic adenine nucleotide analogue. It is a potent inhibitor of HBV reverse transcriptase of the wild-type HBV, famciclovir-resistant and lamivudine-resistant mutants.

Two large international multicentric double-blinded, placebo-controlled studies in adults have shown that 10 mg oral. Adefovir dipivoxil daily given for 40 weeks is effective in terms of histologic improvement, HBV DNA suppression, ALT normalization and HBsAg loss (1.6-2% vs. 0%) in both HBeAg positive and HBeAg negative CHB. In HBeAg positive patients, HBeAg loss and HBeAg seroconversion also increased as compared with controls (12% vs. 6%). The development of resistance was 2% after 2 years of therapy. There is a lot of interest generated presently with the use of the drug in chronic hepatitis and trials are underway in children.

Famciclovir

Famciclovir is known to induce seroconversion, but seems to show weaker suppression than LAM and therefore might be useful only in combination with LAM or other antiviral agents.

Entecavir

Entecavir is a guanosine nucleoside analogue and has been tested in clinical trials among adults. With a safety profile similar to LAM, it has shown to be more effective in viral suppression compared to LAM, in wild type and in LAM resistant infections with HBV. Both entecavir and adefovir may play an important role in the further development of antiviral treatment of HBV.

Other antiviral therapy agents include thymosin, clevudine, etc.

Combination Therapy

There has been interest in using a combination of IFN or PEG-IFN with LAM hoping that the combination might have additional antiviral effects. What remains to be identified is the most appropriate regimen, i.e. whether LAM is to be used before or along with IFN or after initial dose IFN etc. Studies are still undergoing in pediatrics on PEG interferon in children and on newer antiviral agents. The only pediatric studies on combination therapy have used IFN and LAM. While Selimoglu *et al.* compared a combination treatment to IFN monotherapy, Dikici *et al.* compared different regimens of IFN and LAM combination.

Hepatitis B Vaccination

The use of hepatitis B vaccination and need for universal hepatitis B vaccine cannot be overemphasized.

HEPATITIS C

Hepatitis C is the result of infection with hepatitis C virus (HCV). Though common cause of both acute and chronic liver disease in adults, it is an uncommon infection in children. It is estimated to affect 170 million people worldwide and approximately 1% of the population based on studies carried out in blood donors. The incidence is probably lower in children although there is no sufficient data on HCV in children.

Hepatitis C virus is a double RNA shelled virus, approximately 50 to 50 nm. The virus genome has structural and non-structural protein genes. A distinctive feature of HCV is its sequence diversity or heterogeneity. This variability is called species diversity. HCV can be classified into genotypes, subtypes and isolates based on sequence diversity of the genome.

Genomic Organization and Viral Proteins

HCV consists of a 9.6-kb, positive (sense), single-strand RNA genome that comprises a highly conserved 341-base 5' noncoding region, a single long open reading frame (ORF) of 9,033 to 9,099 bases, and a 3' noncoding region. The ORF encodes a polyprotein precursor of approximately

3,000 amino acids. This polyprotein is cleaved cotranslationally and posttranslationally by both cellular and viral proteases to produce at least 10 polypeptides with various functions in replication and virus assembly (Fig. 80.4).

Table 80.3: Heterogeneity of HCV

Classification	*Average degree of diversity**
Quasispecies	<1%-5%
Isolate	2% -15%
Subtype a, b, c	10%-30%
Genotype 1,2,3,4,5,6	>30%

* *Variability in nucleotide sequence in representative regions of the viral ribonucleic acid.*

Genotypes 1 and 2 are found worldwide; genotype 3 is common in the Indian subcontinent and Southeast Asia. The clinical importance of genotypes is related to the response to antiviral therapy. Patient with genotypes 1 and 4 are more likely to be resistant to interferon-based therapy than are patients with genotypes 2 or 3.

Table 80.4: The modes of transmission of hepatitis C

- Blood transfusion
- Administration of blood products (anti-hemophilic factor, factor IX, intravenous immunoglobulin)
- Injection drug use
- Cocaine snorting
- Accidental occupational exposure (i.e. needlestick)
- Exposure to contaminated medical equipment (reusable syringes, inadequately sterilized medical instruments, contamination of intravenous fluids or injectable medications)
- Tattooing or body piercing
- Sexual spread
- Maternal-infant spread.

Hepatitis C can be spread from HCV-positive mother to newborn, but such spread is uncommon. In large prospective studies, 5% to 10% of infants born to anti-HCV-positive mothers acquire hepatitis C during the first 1 to 2 years of life. The transmission appears to occur in the postnatal period, although instances of HCV infection detected at the time of birth have been reported. All infants born to anti-HCV-positive mother have anti-HCV in serum as a result of passive transfer of immunoglobulin in utero. The passively transferred anti-HCV can persist for 12 months and possibly longer, which makes anti-HCV testing unreliable for documenting transmission. Most studies have relied upon HCV RNA testing to detect transmission, but HCV RNA intermittent positivity may be transient. Also complicating the issue is the occurrence of false-positive HCV RNA results from PCR, particularly when testing cord blood at the time of delivery. Thus proof of transmission of hepatitis C usually requires the presence of detectable HCV RNA on two separate occasions or persistence of anti-HCV after 12 months of age. Using these criteria the rate of transmission ranges from 5% to 10%. Upto 50% of infected newborns clear HCV RNA spontaneously, so that chronic infection eventuates in only 2% to 5% of children. Rarely is neonatal infection associated with symptoms or jaundice. The importance of maternal-infant transmission is shown by studies of hepatitis C in children that demonstrate that vertical transmission now accounts for the majority of cases of chronic hepatitis C in children.

Maternal-infant transmission of hepatitis C occurs only if the mother has HCV RNA in addition to anti-HCV in serum. Other factors that are reported to correlate with a higher likelihood of transmission of hepatitis C are high maternal titers of HCV RNA, co-infection with HIV, a prolonged or difficult delivery, and the use of internal fetal monitoring during delivery.

Transmission of HCV has not been associated with breastfeeding. If breastfeeding is elected, careful breast hygiene and avoidance of feeding if there are cracks in the nipples are appropriate.

Clinical Course of Hepatitis C

The clinical, biochemical, and serologic course of a "typical"

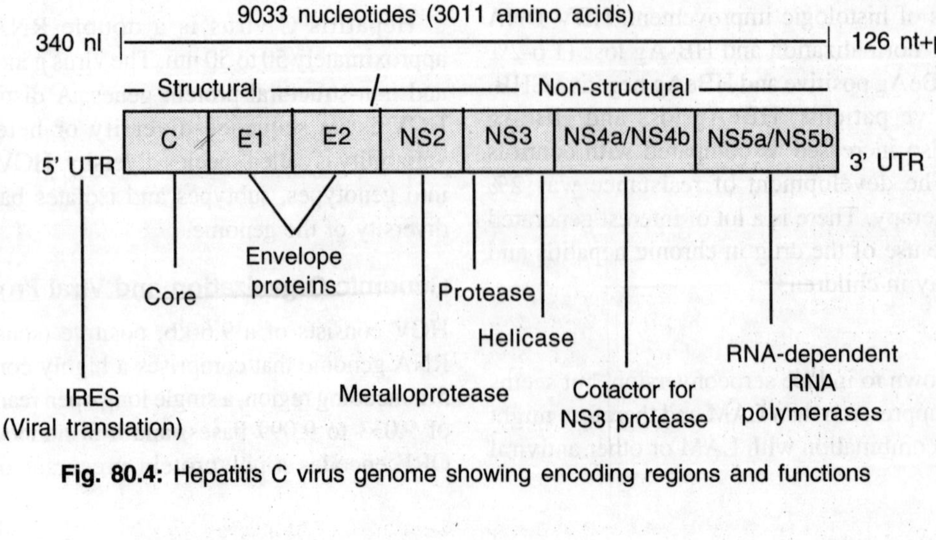

Fig. 80.4: Hepatitis C virus genome showing encoding regions and functions

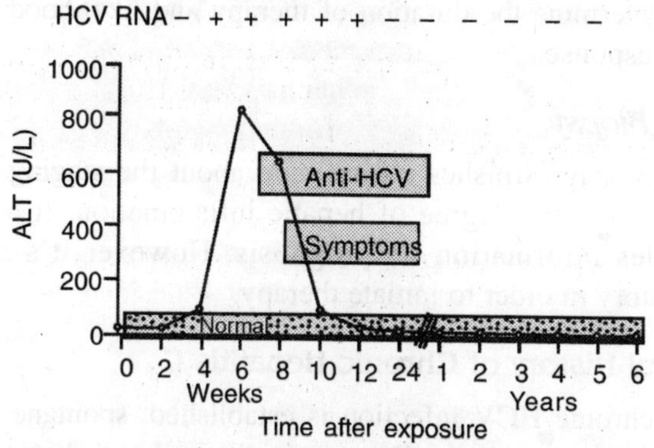

Fig. 80.5: Typical course of acute hepatitis C. HCV RNA is detectable by polymerase chain reaction within 2 weeks of exposure. ALT levels rise thereafter, and symptoms appear 6-8 weeks after viremia. Anti-HCV generally arises late, after onset of ALT elevations and symptoms. In self-limited disease HCV RNA is cleared and ALT returns to normal levels with resolution of the clinical disease. HCV, hepatitis C virus; RNA, ribonucleic acid; ALT, serum alanine aminotransferase

case of acute hepatitis C is shown in Figure 1.5. The incubation period of acute hepatitis C lasts for 15 to 75 days, averaging 50 days. During this period and within a week or two of exposure, HCV RNA becomes detectable in serum and levels of virus gradually rise.

Diagnosis of Acute Hepatitis C

The diagnosis of acute hepatitis C is suggested by the presence of clinical or biochemical evidence of acute hepatitis accompanied by anti-HCV or HCV RNA in serum.

The presence of anti-HCV or HCV RNA in a patient with biochemical evidence of acute hepatitis is suggestive but not completely diagnostic of acute hepatitis C. Neither anti-HCV nor HCV RNA testing can reliably distinguish between acute and chronic hepatitis C with a superimposed form of acute liver injury or acute exacerbation.

A more common issue in managing patients with acute hepatitis is the need to rule out hepatitis C as a cause of acute liver injury in a patient who lacks other serologic markers for hepatitis A (IgM anti-HAV) and B (hepatitis B surface antigen [HbsAg] and IgM anti-HBc). In this situation testing for HCV RNA during the acute illness or testing for anti-HCV both during the acute illness and during convalescence effectively rules out acute hepatitis C.

Clinical Course of Chronic Hepatitis C

The course of a patient developing chronic hepatitis C is shown in Figure 80.6.

Diagnosis of Chronic Hepatitis C

The diagnosis of chronic hepatitis C is generally made on the basis of persistence of ALT elevation or HCV RNA in serum for 6 months or longer.

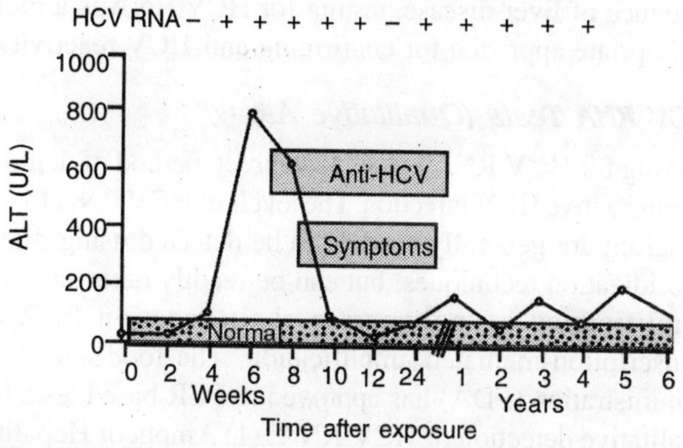

Fig. 80.6: Typical course of chronic hepatitis C HCV RNA is detectably by polymerase chain reaction within 2 weeks of exposure. ALT levels rise thereafter and symptoms appear 6 to 8 weeks after viremia. Anti-HCV generally arises late, after onset of ALT elevations and symptoms. With development of chronic disease, serum ALT and HCV RNA levels fluctuate, being intermittently normal or undetectable. Chronic infection is shown by persistence of HCV RNA positivity with or without ALT elevations. HCV, hepatitis C virus; RNA, ribonucleic acid; ALT, serum alanine aminotransferase

Table 80.5: Hepatitis C virus peptides in immunodiagnostic assays

	EIA-1	*EIA-2*	*EIA-3*	*RIBA-1*	*RIBA-2*	*RIBA-3*
5-1-1(NS4)	-	-	-	+	+	-
C 100-3(NS3-4)	+	-	-	+	+	+
C33c (NS 3)	-	-	-	-	+	+
C200 (fusion C100/C 3)	-	+	+	-	-	-
C22-3 (core)	-	+	+	-	+	+
NS5	-	-	+	-	-	+

EIA- Enzyme immunoassay; RIBA- recombinant immunoblot assay.

Table 80.6: Sensitivity and predictive value of enzyme immunoassay (EIA) for HCV infections
Positive predictive value (%)

Assay	*Sensitivity(%)*	*Time for positivity after infection (wks)*
EIA–1	70 - 80	16
EIA–2	92- 95	10
EIA–3	97	7-8

Serologic and Virologic Markers of Hepatitis C

Anti-HVC Assays

The most widely used tests for anti-HCV are EIAs (Elisa immune assays). Several third generation EIAs are commercially available and approved for use in screening blood. Current assays have a high degree of sensitivity and specificity.

Immunoblot Assays

Immunoblot assays for anti-HCV are available for confirmation of EIA test results. In patients with biochemical evidence of liver disease, testing for HCV RNA is a more appropriate approach for confirming anti-HCV reactivity.

HCV RNA Tests (Qualitative Assay)

Testing for HCV RNA is the most direct method of demonstrating active HCV infection. The levels of HCV RNA found in serum are generally too low to be detected using direct hybridization techniques, but can be readily detected after amplification by polymerase chain reaction PCR or transcription-mediated amplification. The food and drug administration (FDA) has approved to PCR based tests for qualitative detection of HCV-RNA; (1) Amplicor Hepatitis C Virus Test, version 2.0, and (2) Cobas Amplicor Hepatitis C Virus Test, version 2.0 (Roche Molecular Systems, Branchburg, NJ), which have limits of detection of approximately 50 IU/mL. A third approved test is the VERSANT® HCV RNA Qualitative Assay.

HCV RNA Levels (Quantitative Assays)

Testing for the level of HCV RNA can be helpful in assessing the likelihood of a response before or during therapy. Two major commercial assays are widely available, one being based upon competitive qualitative PCR (qPCR) and one using signal amplification of branched DNA (bDNA). The level of HCV RNA in blood helps in predicting the likelihood of response to treatment, and the change in the level of HCV RNA during treatment can be used to monitor response.

HCV Genotyping

There are 6 major HCV genotypes although genotype does not predict the outcome of infection, it does predict the likelihood of treatment response, and in many cases, determines during the treatment. Genotyping can be done by sequence analysis of various regions of the virus, by restriction fragment length polymorphism analysis, by probe-specific hybridization, or by line probe assay (LiPA). These tests are expensive. Common Genotypes in Indian patients are Genotype 2 and 3.

AASLD recommendations for testing with HCV RNA assays are:

1. Patients suspected of having chronic HCV infection should be tested for HCV antibodies.
2. HCV RNA testing should be performed in:
   a. Patients with a positive anti-HCV Test.
   b. Patients for whom antiviral treatment is being considered, using a quantitative assay.
   c. Patients with unexplained liver disease whose anti-HCV test is negative and who are immune-compromised or suspected of having acute HCV infection.
3. HCV genotype should be determined in all HCV-infected persons prior to treatment in order to determine the duration of therapy and likelihood of response.

Liver Biopsy

Liver biopsy furnishes information about the staging of fibrosis and the degree of hepatic inflammation. It also provides information on prognosis. However it's not mandatory in order to initiate therapy.

Natural History of Chronic Hepatitis C

After chronic HCV infection is established, spontaneous resolution is uncommon. Disease activity in chronic hepatitis C may improve or worsen spontaneously, but loss of viremia is rare.

The relatively benign natural history of chronic hepatitis C in young individuals are supportive of studies of children infected with hepatitis C as a result of maternal-infant exposure or blood transfusion. In a large study from Germany 10 to 20 years follow-up was available on a cohort of children who underwent open-heart surgery in the 1980s. It usually progresses to cirrhosis after 15-20 years. The progression is more severe or rapid in the presence of excess iron in liver or associated HIV. Unlike hepatitis B infection hepatocellular carcinoma does not develop in the absence of cirrhosis, with chronic hepatitis C infection.

Treatment Objectives and Outcomes

The goal of treatment is to prevent complications of HCV infection; this is principally achieved by eradication of infection. Infection is considered eradicated when there is sustained virologic response (SVR), defined as the absence of HCV RNA in serum by a sensitive test at the end of treatment and 6 months later. Persons in whom HCV RNA levels remain stable on treatment are considered non-responders, while those whose HCV RNA levels decline (e.g. by >2 logs), but never become undetectable, are referred to as partial responders.

Therapy of Children

There have been substantial improvements in the success of HCV treatment, and there are currently several treatments approved by the FDA. In randomized clinical trials in adults, the highest overall SVR rates have been achieved with the combination of weekly subcutaneous injections of long-acting peg interferon alfa and oral ribavirin, which represents the current standard of care. The response is better for non-genotype 1 (65-70% as compared to< 40%). Response to therapy is measured by estimating the number of patients who are HCV RNA negative by PCR 6 months after stopping therapy. Present recommendation is to use the combination therapy for a period of 1 year in genotype 1 as compared to 6 months in other genotypes.

Interferon and ribavarin are approved by FDA for use in treatment of hepatitis C in children. The drug has been used in the dose of 3MU/M^2 three times a week for 6-12 months, along with a dose of 15 mg/kg bid of ribavarin. Interferon is contraindicated in children less than 2 years of age due to its negative effect on growth and possible role in the development of spastic diplegia. Preliminary uncontrolled studies suggest that children have a better rate of response to interferon therapy than adults and that they tend to have fewer side effects. A meta-analysis of 10 studies of IFN use in children has shown a response rate as high as 70% in non-type 1 and 27% in type 1 patients. One of largest group of children in India with HCV are those who have been multi-transfused. These children often have high ferritin levels and excess iron load results not only in more liver damage but also poorer response to therapy. Also, the most common adverse effect of ribavarin is anemia and this translates to increased blood transfusion requirement. Our study of interferon therapy for treatment of chronic hepatitis C in thalassemia children in India (n=11) has shown that the response to interferon is good. Chronic hepatitis C rarely resolves spontaneously: and children with this disease are likely to have the infection for life. For these reasons, early treatment may be appropriate and is often requested. Recently FDA has also approved PEG interferon therapy for use in chronic hepatitis C infection in children.

Children who should be treated include:

1. Acute HCV infection that has not resolved (HCV viremia present) after 12 weeks.
2. Progressive HCV infection with or without elevated transaminases and biopsy showing necro-inflammatory changes.

Liver Transplantation

Liver transplantation has been performed in children with end-stage HCV disease. Like in adults, the reinfection of the graft with HCV is almost universal.

Hepatitis C Vaccine

There has been some progress made in developing a vaccine against hepatitis C, which is still in experimental stages.

The rapid advances in knowledge of HCV and availability of new tools to evaluate virus replication and inhibition promise to provide new, more effective, and better tolerated approaches to the treatment and prevention of this important liver disease.

KEY LEARNING POINTS

Hepatitis B

- One of the most common infective diseases worldwide.
- HBsAg is its serologic hallmark; anti-HBs usually persists for life, conferring long-term immunity; HBc.
- Treatment of chronic hepatitis B is aimed at suppression of HBV replication before irreversible liver damage occurs, currently IFN-alpha and lamivudine being the only approved drugs.
- Universal hepatitis B vaccination is the key to prevention.

Hepatitis C

- An uncommon infection in children.
- Etiologic agent, hepatitis C virus, is a double RNA shelled virus, around 50-? nm in size, known for its species diversity.
- Diagnosis is suggested by presence of clinical or biochemical evidence of acute hepatitis accompanied by anti-HCV RNA.
- Diagnosis of chronic hepatitis C is generally made on the basis of persistence of ALT elevation or HCV RNA in serum for 6 months or longer.
- Currently, therapeutic treatment is by a combination of long-acting interferon alpha and ribaviron.
- Liver transplantation is indicated in subjects with end-stage HCV disease.
- Hepatitis C vaccine remains in experimental stage.

FURTHER READINGS

1. Alexopoulos CG, Vaslamatizis M, Hatzidimitriou G: Prevalence of hepatitis B virus marker positivity and evolution of hepatitis B virus profile, during chemotherapy, in patients with solid tumors. *Br J Cancer* 1999: 81:69.
2. Bortolotti F, Jara P *et al.* Long term effect of alpha interferon in children with chronic hepatitis B, *Gut* 2000;46:715-718.
3. Bortolotti F, Lorio R, Resti M, *et al.*: An epidemiological survey of hepatitis C virus infection in Italian children in the decade 1990-1999. *J Pediatr Gastroenterol Nutr* 2001; 32:562.
4. Ceci O, Margiotta M, marello F, *et al.*: Vertical transmission of hepatitis C virus in a chohort of 2,447 HIV-seronegative pregnant women: A 24-month prospective study. *J Pediatr Gastroenterol Nutr* 2001; 33:570.
5. Choo QL, Richman KH, Han JH, *et al.* Genetic organization and diversity of the hepatitis C virus. *Proc Natl Acad Sci USA* 1991;88:2451-2455.
6. Chu CJ, Hussain M, Lok A S. Hepatitis B virus genotype B is associated with earlier HBEAg seroconversion compared with hepatitis B virus genotype C. *Gastroenterology* 2002; 122: 1756-1762.
7. Chu CJ, Keeffe EB, Han SH, Perrillo R P, Min A D, Soldevila - Pico C, Carey W, Brown R S Jr, Luketic V A, Terrault N, Lok A S. Hepatitis B virus genotypes in United States: Results of a nationwide study. *Gastroenterology* 2003; 125:444-451.
8. Conte D, Fraquelli M, Prati D, *et al.*: Prevalence and clinical course of chronic hepatitis C virus (HCV) infection and rate of HCV vertical transmission in a cohort of 15,250 pregnant women. *Hepatology* 2000; 31:751.
9. Dikici B, Bosnak M, Bosnak V, Dagli A, Davutoglu M, Yagci RV, Haspolat K. Comparison of treatments of chronic hepatitis B in children with lamivudine and alpha-interferon combination and alpha-interferon alone. *Pediatr Int* 2002; 44(5): 517-521.
10. Fried MW, Shiffman M, Reddy RK, *et al.*: Pegylated (40kDa) itnterferon alfa -2a (PegasysTM) in combination with ribavirin:

efficacy and safety results from a phase III, randomized, actively-controlled, multicenter study. *Gastroenterology* 2001; 120:289A.
11. Hadziyannis SJ, Sette H, Morgan TR, Balan V, Diago M, Marcellin P, Ramadori G, *et al.* Peginterferon alfa-2a (40 kilo daltons) and ribavirin combination therapy in chronic hepatitis C; randomized study of the effect of treatment duration and ribavirin dose. *Ann intern Med* 2004; 140;346-355.
12. Hadziyannis SJ, Tassopoulos NC, heathote EJ *et al.* For the adevofir Dipivoxil 438 study group *et al.* Adefovir dipivoxil for the treatment of Hepatitis B e antigen–negative chronic hepatitis B. *N Engl J Med.* 800-07:348;2003.
13. Hadziyannis, S *et al.* Entecavir in patients with chronic hepatitis B failing lamivudine. AASLD. *Hepatology* 2001; 34:340A.
14. Hepatitis C Virus infection. *N Engl J Med* 2001; 345:41-52.
15. Jacobson KR, Murray K, Zellos A, Schwarz KB: An analysis of published trials of interferon monotherapy in children with chronic hepatitis C. *J. Pediatr Gastroenterol Nutr* 2002;34: 52-58.
16. Jara P, Bortolotti F. Interferon-alpha treatment of chronic hepatitis B in childhood: A consensus advice based on experience in Europoean Children. *J Pediatr Gastroenterol Nutr* 1999; 920:163-170.
17. Jonas MM, Kelly DA, Mizerski J, Badia IB, Areias JA, Schwarz KB, Little NR, Greensmith MJ, Gardner SD, Bell MS, Sokal EM; International pediatric lamivudine investigator Group. Clinical trail of lamivudine in children with chronic hepatitis B. *N Engl J Med* 2002; 346 (22):1706-1713.
18. KAO J H. Hepatitis B viral genotypes: Clinical relevance and molecular characterstics. *J Gastroenterol Hepatol* 2002;17: 643-650.
19. Kao JH, Chen PJ, Lai MY, Chen DS. Hepatitis B genotypes correlate with clinical outcomes in patients with chronic hepatitis B. *Gastroenterology* 2000;118:549-554.
20. Keam SJ, Scott LJ. Lamivudine: In children and adolescents with chronic hepatitis B virus infection. *Pediatr Drugs 2002*; 4 (10): 687-94; discussion 695-696.
21. Kocak N, Ozen H, Saltuk IN, Gurakan F, Yuce A. Lamivudine for Children With Chronic Hepatitis B. *Am J Gastroenterol* 2000; 95:2989-2990.
22. Lai CL *et al.* Entecavir vs lamivudine in chronic hepatitis B. *J.Hepatol* 2001; 34(Suppl):24.
23. Lai CL, Yuen MF, Hui CK, Garrido-Lestache S, Cheng CT, Lai YP. Comparison of the efficacy of lamivudine and famciclovir in Asian patients with chronic hepatitis B: Results of 24 weeks of therapy. *J Med Virol* 2002; 67(3): 334-38.
24. Leung N. Clinical experience with Lamivudine. *Semin Liver Dis* 2002; 22 Suppl 1:15-22.
25. Liang TJ, Rehermann B, Seeff LB, Hoofnagle JH: Pathogenesis, Natural History, treatment, and prevention of hepatitis C. *Ann intern med* 2000; 132:296-305.
26. Liaw YF. Management of YMDD mutations during lamivudine therapy in patients with chronic hepatitis B. *J Gastroenterol Hepatol* 2002; 17 Suppl 3:S333-S337.
27. Lok AS, Heathcote EJ, Hoofnagle JH. Management of hepatitis B 2000—Summary of a workshop. *Gastroenterology* 2001; 20:828-1853.
28. Manns MP. McHutchison JG, Gordon SC, Rustgi Vk, Shiffman M, Reindollar R, Goodma ZD, *et al.* Peginterferon Alfa-2b plus ribavirin compared with interferon alfa 2b plus ribavirin for initial treatment of chronic hepatitis C: A randomized trial. *Lancet* 2991;358;958-965.
29. Marcellin P, Chang TT, Lim SG, *et al.* For the adevofir Dipivoxil 437 study croup. *et al.* Adefovir dipivoxil for the treatment of Hepatitis B e antigen-positive chronic hepatitis B. *N Engl J Med* 2003;348:808-816.
30. Mohan N.; Prevalence of hepatitis C infection and response of treatment to interferon alpha in beta thalassemia patients: 2004; 39: 100-105.
31. NI YH, Chang MH, Wang KJ, Hsu HY, Chen HL, Kao j H, Chen D S. Clinical relevance of hepatitis B virus genotype in children with chronic infection and hepatocellular carcinoma. *Gastroenterology* 2004;127:1733-1738.
32. Orito E, Mizokami M, Sakugawa H, Michitaka K, Ishikawa K, Ichida T, *et al.* A case-control study for clinical and molecular biological differences between hepatitis B viruses of genotypes-B and C. Hapna HBV Genotype Research Group. *Hepatology* 2001;133:218-223.
33. Selimoglu MA, Aydogdu S, Unal F, Zeytinoglu A, Yuce G, Yagci RV. Alpha interferon and lamivudine combination therapy for chronic hepatitis B in children. *Pediatr Int* 2002; 44: 404-08.
34. Shapira R, Daudi N, Klein A, Shouval D, Mor E, Tur-Kaspa R, Dinari G, Ben-Ari Z. Seroconversion after the addition of famciclovir therapy in a child with hepatitis B virus infection after liver transplantation who developed lamivudine resistance. *Transplantation* 2002; 73: 820-822.
35. Simmonds P. Viral heterogeneity of the hepatitis C virus. *J hepatol* 1999;31 (suppl 1):54-60.
36. Sumi H, Yokosuka O, Seki N, Arai M, Imazeki F, Kurihara T, Kanda T, Fukai K, Kato M, Saisho H. Influence of hepatitis B virus genotypes on the progression of chronic type B liver disease. *Hepatology* 2003;37:19-26.
37. Thakur V, Guptan RC, Kazim SN, Malhotra V, Sarin SK. Profile, spectrum and singificance of HBV genotypes in chronic liver disease pateints in Indian subcontinent. *J Gastroenterol Hepatol* 2002; 15 (Suppl.):E34-40.
38. Vogt M, Lang T, Frosner G, *et al.*: Prevalence and clinical outcome of hepatitis C infection in children who underwent cardiac surgery before the implementation of blood-donor screening. *N Engl J Med* 1999; 341: 866.
39. Yokosuka O, Kojima H, Imazeki F, *et al.*: Spontaneous negativation of serum hepatitis C virus RNA is a rare event in type C chronic liver diseases: Analysis of HCVRNA in 320 patients who were followed for more than 3 years. *J Hepatology* 1999; 31:394.
40. Zucker SD. All kidding aside with the use of lamivudine in children with chronic hepatitis B. *Gastroenterology* 2002; 123:1741-1743; discussion 1743.

81 Hepatitis D

ES Sherlock

INTRODUCTION

Delta hepatitis, caused by the delta agent (an incomplete virus that employs the synthetic apparatus of hepatitis B virus for its own replication), is known for an epidemiology that correlates well with that of chronic hepatitis B.

ETIOPATHOGENESIS

The causative agent, HDV, is capable of producing infection only in the presence of HBV infection. In other words, it cannot produce infection without HBV as a helper virus. Hence, it is considered a "defective" virus. It is 36 nm in diameter and unable to produce its own coat protein. Whereas its outer coat is composed of excess HbsAg from HBV, the inner core is a single-stranded circular RNA. It is here that HDV antigen is expressed.

Pathologic hepatic damage is directly secondary to cytopathic injury and more severe compared to HBV. In fact, in all very severe cases of HBV, coinfection with HHDV must be considered.

EPIDEMIOLOGY

HDV can cause infection in two ways:

- First, simultaneously with HBV infection, the so-called "coinfection".
- Secondly, subsequent to the HBV infection that is already present, the so-called "superinfection".

In areas of high prevalence i.e. developing countries, transmission usually is either intrafamilial or through intimate contact.

In areas of low prevalence, i.e. prosperous Europe and USA, it is uncommon in children.

CLINICAL MANIFESTATIONS

Though the incubation period for HDV coinfection remains same as that of HBV, it is 2 to 8 weeks in case of its superinfection.

Clinical presentation, though more severe, is on the same pattern as in a in case of other hepatropic viruses. However, there is only a low risk of developing chronic hepatitis.

In coinfection, acute hepatitis is common and much more severe than HBV alone.

In superinfection, though acute hepatitis is rare, risk of developing both acute liver failure and chronic hepatitis is significant.

COMPLICATIONS

- ALF.
- Chronic hepatitis in case of coinfection.

DIAGNOSIS

Since HDV has not yet been isolated and no circulating antigen is so far identified, the diagnosis is by:

- Detecting IgM antibody to HDV 2-4 weeks after coinfection and 10 weeks after superinfection.
- PSR assays for viral RNA.

MANAGEMENT

Since no HDV-targeted therapy is yet available, treatment is by and large supportive. In addition, attempts are made to treat the HBV infection which is an essential prerequisite for HBV infection.

PREVENTION

There being no vaccine available for HD, HB vaccine and HBIG are given for the indications in HB.

KEY LEARNING POINTS

- A defective virus, able to cause infection only in the presence of hepatitis B.
- Infection is more severe than hepatitis B as such.
- Infection may be "coinfection" or "superinfection".
- Diagnosis is by IgM antibody to HDV.
- Treatment is by and large supportive.
- In the absence of any vaccine, prevention is by HB vaccine and HBIG.

FURTHER READINGS

1. Chang MH, Hadzie D, Rouassant AH, *et al.* Acute and chronic hepatitis. Working Group Report of the Second World Congress of Pediatric Gastroenterology, Hepatology and Nutrition. *J Pediatr Gastroenterol Nutr* 2004;39:5584-5588.
2. Kelly D, Skidmore S. Hepatitis C-Z: Recent advances. *Arch Dis Child* 2002;86:339-343.

82 Hepatitis E

ES Sherlock

INTRODUCTION

Hepatitis E, notorious for high mortality in pregnant women, is now being implicated for major epidemics of viral hepatitis in the Indian subcontinent and some other S-E Asian countries.

ETIOPATHOGENESIS

The causative agent is a cytopathic virus, causing pathologic changes that mimic those of other hepatitis viruses, both hepatotropic and nonhepatotropic.

The viral particles are 27 to 34 nm in diameter, are non-enveloped and contain a single-strand of positive-sense RNA that is approximately 7300 bases in length. The virus particle was first visualized in 1983[2] but was only molecularly cloned in 1990.

It was previously classified family Caliciviridae. However, its genome more closely resembles the rubella virus. It is now classified as the only member of the genus Herpevirus. Notably, this genus has not yet been assigned to a family.

EPIDEMIOLOGY

Hepatitis E is prevalent in most developing countries. In fact, it is common in any country with a hot climate. It is widespread in Southeast Asia, northern and central Africa, Middle-East and Central America.

It is spread mainly through fecal contamination of water supplies or food (fecal-oral transmission). Person-to-person transmission is uncommon.

Outbreaks of epidemic HE most commonly occur after heavy rainfalls and monsoons because of the disruption of water supplies.

CLINICAL MANIFESTATIONS

Incubation period is 15 to 60 days (mean 40 days).

HEV manifestations are the protype of HAV with the following differences:

1. Its attack rates are highest in adolescents and adults regardless if it is an epidemic form or sporadic form.
2. It is usually subclinical or anicteric but is capable of causing more severe illness.
3. Mortality rate due to fulminant hepatitis, usually in adolescents and young adults (especially pregnant women), is quite high (upto 20% compared to <1% in HAV).
4. It does not cause chronic liver disease.
5. Histologic picture is characterized by ballooning degeneration, cholestasis and pseudoglandular change.
6. Intrauterine infection may occur.

Complications occur only in pregnant women.

DIAGNOSIS

Hepatitis E should be suspected in outbreaks of waterborne hepatitis occurring in developing countries, especially if the disease is more severe in pregnant women, or if hepatitis A has been excluded. Epidemiologic evidence can help in establishing a diagnosis.

Laboratory tests for establishing the diagnosis include:

- *Blood tests* which detect elevated antibody levels of specific antibodies to HE in the body or by reverse transcriptase polymerase chain reaction (RT-PCR). Serum anti-HEV demonstration by enzyme immunoassay is the most frequently employed test. Recently, its value in endemic areas has been questioned. After one week of onset of illness, IgM antibody to viral antigen becomes positive.
- *PCR* for demonstration of viral RNA in stools and serum.

Since cases of HE are not clinically distinguishable from other types of acute viral hepatitis, confirmation of diagnosis needes these tests . Unfortunately, these tests are not widely available.

MANAGEMENT

HE is a self-limiting disease. Since no specific treatment is presently available, supportive care is important.

PREVENTION

Based on the existing knowledge, the best management of HAV lies in its prevention through:

- Improved sanitation.
- Provision of potable drinking water; and
- Proper sewage disposal.

HE vaccine, based on recombinant viral proteins, has been developed. The vaccine appears to be highly effective and safe. Nevertheless, further studies are needed to assess the long-term protection and the cost-effectiveness of hepatitis E vaccine.

Immunoglobulin (pooled from sufferers from HEV) may be somewhat effective.

Surveillance and Control

Surveillance and control procedures should include:

- Provision of safe drinking water and proper disposal of sanitary waste.
- Monitoring disease incidence.
- Determination of source of infection and mode of transmission by epidemiologic investigation.
- Detection of outbreaks.
- Spread containment.

KEY LEARNING POINTS

- A self-limiting disease caused by a cytopathic virus, the pathologic changes mimicing hepatitis viruses, both hepatotropic and nonhepatotropic.
- Manifestations are prototype of hepatitis A.
- Diagnosis in suspected cases is by blood tests that detect elevated antibody titer of specific antibodies: HE, RT-PCR, serum anti-HEV, or PCR.
- Prevention is through improved sanitation, proper sewage disposal and availability of potable drinking water.
- HE vaccine, though developed, needs further evaluation.

FURTHER READINGS

1. Emerson SU, Purcell RH. Hepatitis E virus. *Rev Med Virol* 2003;13:145-54.
2. Emerson SU, Purcell RH. Running like water: The omnipresence of hepatitis E. *N Engl J Med* 2004;351:2367-2368.
3. Amon JJ, Drobeniuc J, Bower WA, Magana JC, Escobedo MA, Williams IT, *et al.* Locally acquired hepatitis E virus infection, El Paso, Texas. *J Med Virol* 2006;78:741-746.

83 Pyogenic Liver Abscess

Sutapa Ganguly • Sumitha Paul

INTRODUCTION

Pyogenic liver abscess is a rare and life-threatening disease in children. It is often associated with immunocompromised conditions.

The development of new radiologic techniques, the improvement in microbiologic identification, advancement of drainage techniques and launching of higher generation of antibiotics have decreased mortality rates to 5-30%. Yet, the prevalence has remained relatively unchanged. Left untreated, the infection remains uniformly fatal.

PATHOPHYSIOLOGY

The liver receives blood from both systemic and portal circulation. Consequently, there is increased exposure to bacteria and increased chance of infection. However, the Kupffer cells lining the sinusoids clear the bacteria so efficiently that infection rarely occurs. Liver may become infected by different routes.

Biliary tract disease remains the most common source of pyogenic liver abscess (PLA) and accounts for 60% cases. There are obstructions of bile flow resulting in stagnation and bacterial proliferation. Through pressurization, portal tributaries and lymphatics are infected with subsequent pylephlebities and abscess formation.

Stricture, malignancies and congenital stenosis are inciting factors. Abscesses are generally multiple.

Infection of abdominal organs may result in septic embolization of the portal vein, resulting in pylephlebitis. Septic emboli are ultimately trapped in the liver resulting in abscess formation. Appendicitis was a very common source of infection in the preantibiotic era through the incidence is declining presently. Microabscesses in liver coalesce to from a single abscess.

Microabscess formation may complicate bacteremia secondary to endocarditis, pyelenephritis and pyoderma. Cases are reported in the immunocompromised children e.g. with leukemia, granulomatous disease or on immunosuppressive therapy.

This accounts for 15% of cases of liver abscesses.

Penetrating hepatic trauma can inoculate organisms directly into the liver resulting in PLA. Non-penetrating trauma can cause localized tissue necrosis and create an environment favoring bacterial growth with resulting PLA.

PLA has rarely been reported as a secondary infection in amebic abscess, hydatid cyst cavity or hepatic tumors.

The predeliction of infection of right hepatic lobe to left hepatic lobe is 2:1. Bilateral involvement occurs in 5% cases. The prediction for right lobe can be attributed to its blood supply from both the superior mesenteric and portal veins, whereas left lobe receives inferior mesenteric and splenic drainage.

It also contains denser network of biliary canaliculi and overall accounts for more hepatic mass. Studies have suggested that a more streaming effect in the portal circulation is causative.

ETIOLOGY

Microabscesses are most commonly secondary to bacteremia or candidermia. *Staphylococcus aureus, Escherechia coli, Salmonella* and anaerobic organisms are common offenders.

There are increasing number of reports of anerobic involvement, probably due to increased and improving awareness and improving culturing techniques. The most frequent anerobes are *Bacterioides species, Fuso-bacterium, microaerophilic* and *anerobic streptococci*. A colonic source is the initial focus of infection.

Staphylococcus aureus abscesses usually result from hemotogenous spread of organisms involved with distant infections such as endocarditis. *S milleri is neither anerobic* nor micro aerophilic. It has been associated with both monomicrobial and polymicrobial abscesses in patients with Crohn's disease, as well as other patients with PLA.

Fungal abscesses primarily are due to *candida albicans* and occur in individuals with prolonged exposure to antimicrobials, hematologic malignancies and in children with congenital or acquired immunodeficiency. There are published reports on abscesses caused by *Actinomyces species*, *Yersinia enterocolitica*, *Salmonella typhi* and *Brucella melitensis*.

CLINICAL FEATURES

Fever with chills, pain and tenderness in the right hypochondrium, anorexia, malaise and weight loss are the common mode of presentation. Child may present with hacking cough or hiccup due to diaphragmatic irritation. Pain may be referred to the right shoulder. Individuals with solitary abscess may have indolent presentation and those with microabscesses an acute mode of presentation.

On examination, there is a tender hepatomegaly with or without palpable cystic mass. Tenderness in the epigastrium is suggestive of left lobe involvement. Decreased breath sounds in the right lung base with shifting of mediastinum to the same side signify collapse involving the lower lobe of right lung.

A pleural or hepatic friction rub can be associated with diaphragmatic irritation or inflammation of the liver capsule. Jaundice may be an accompaniment in 25% cases and is usually associated with bile duct inflammation.

LABORATORY INVESTIGATIONS

- *Routine blood test* may reveal anemia of chronic disease, neutrophilic leukocytisis and raised ESR.
- *Blood culture* is positive in approximately 50% of cases.
- *Culture of abscess* fluid helps in giving microbiologic diagnosis.
- *Liver function tests:* Jaundice is uncommon; serum aminotransferases may be slightly elevated. Hypoalbuminemia and elevation of alkaline phosphatase are most common abnormalities.
- *Imaging techniques:* Chest X-ray may show elevation of the right dome of diaphragm and fluoroscopic screening will reveal decreased mobility. Right pleural reaction is found in 50% cases Bisilar atelectasis may also be found.
- *Ultrasound evaluation* reveals hypoechoic masses with irregularly-shaped borders. It allows close evaluation of the biliary tree and simultaneous aspiration. The major benefit of this technique is portable machines, which can be transported to bedside of acutely ill patients. But the technique is very much operator-dependent.
- *CT scan* (sensitively is 95-100%): On CT evaluation the abscesses are revealed as hypodense areas surrounded by a capsule and a contract enhancement. Gases can be seen in as many as 20% lesions. Abscesses less than 1 cm in diameter can be detected by scan. This technique is useful to defect underlying pathology.

PROCEDURES

Percutaneous needle aspiration of the cavity material under USG or CT scan guidance. This can be performed during initial diagnostic procedure.

Percutaneous catheter drainage was introduced into the seventh decade. Overal success rate is equal to or more than surgical drainage. The advantage are reduced cost and recovery time. Catheter is flushed daily unless the output is less than 10 cc/day or cavity collapse is documented. Even multiple abscesses have been drained successfully by this method.

Contraindications include coagulopathy, difficult access path to the cavity and sometimes abscesses with viscous pus.

MEDICAL MANAGEMENT

Antibiotic therapy as the sole treatment modality is indicated only when the child is too ill to undergo any invasive procedure or in those with multiple abscesses not amenable to either drainage technique. In these instances, child may require many months of antibiotic therapy with serial imaging and close monitoring of associated conditions.

Treatment of choice is percutaneous aspirations or catheter drainage with antibiotic therapy.

Until cultures are available, the choice of antimicrobial agents should be directed towards the most commonly involved pathogens. Regimens using betalactam/betalactamase inhibitor combinations, carbapenems, or second-generation cephalosporins with anaerobic coverage are the preferred mode of treatment to cover entero-pathogens and anaerobics. Metronidazole or clindamycin needs to be added when *Bacterioides fragilis* is the offender. If fungal pathogens are a possibly, empirical antifungal therapy should be considered. Initial therapy for fungal abscesses should be amphotericin B. Fluconazole, though not considered to be the first line of antifungal therapy, may be used when amphotericin B fails.

Ultimately, culture sensitivity report will guide the therapy. Short courses (on an average 2 weeks) of therapy after percutaneous drainage have been successful in a small series of patients but there are reports of recurrences in other. Currently 4 to 6 weeks of therapy has been recommended for adequately drained solitary lesions. Multiple abscesses may require upto 12 weeks of therapy.

Surgical Management

Current indications for surgical management of PLA include signs of peritonitis; failure of drainage procedure or the abscesses with viscid pus. Surgery can be performed by two approaches:

- A transperitonial approach allows drainage of abscess and abdominal exploration. It sometimes helps in the location of an etiologic source.
- For high posterior bisans, a posterior transpleural approach can be utilized. Although this allows easier access to the

abscess, the identification of multiple lesions or a concurrent intra-abdominal pathology is lost. Postoperative complications are higher.

COMPLICATIONS

An untreated hepatic abscess is uniformly fatal due to complications that include rupture into pleural and peritoneal spaces and retroperitoneal extension, sepsis and endopathalmitis when an abscess is associated with *Klebsiella pneumoniae* bacteremia.

KEY LEARNING POINTS

- Usually accompanies immunocompromised states.
- Most frequently secondary to bacteremia, S. aureus, E. coli, Salmonella and anaerobic organisms being the common offenders.
- Common mode of presentation is chills, pain and tenderness in the right hypochondrium, anorexia, malaise and weight loss.
- Ultrasound and CT scan are the most important investigations.
- Treatment of choice is percutaneous or catheter drainage with broad-spectrum antibiotics that includes anaerobic coverage.
- Indications for surgery include peritonitis, failure of drainage procedure or the abscess with viscid pus.
- Untreated cases end up fatally.

FURTHER READINGS

1. Arslan N, Unal N, Uzuner N, *et al.* Pyogenic liver abscesses in a child spreading to pulmonary and subcutaneous tissues. Case report. *Turkish J Pediatr* 2004;46:279-282.
2. Low T, Wang CC, Hsu ML, *et al.* Pyogenic liver abscesses caused by *Pseudomonas aeruginosa* in a previously healthy child: Report of one case. *Acta Paediatr Taiwanica* 2000; 41: 98-100.
3. Kumar A, Srinivasan S, Sharma AK. Pyogenic liver abscess in children: South Indian experiences. *J Pediatr Surg* 1998;33: 147-421.
4. Agarwal S, Mathur NB, Gang A. Portal vein thrombosis complicating on neonatal hepatic abscess. *Indian Pediatr* 2003;40:997-1001.
5. Taguchi T, Ikeda K, Yakabe S, *et al.* Percutaueous drainage of post-traumatic hepatic abscess in children under ultrasound imaging. *Pediatr Radiol* 1998;18 :85-87.
6. Pizybyszewska D, Kolcun-Penkowska T. Post traumatic hepatic abscess in 5 years old girl. *Wiadomosci Lekarskie* 1992; 45: 916-919.
7. Chou FF, Sheen-Chen SM, Lee TY. Single and multiple pyogenic liver abscesses: Clinical course, etiology and results of treatment *World J Surg* 1997;21: 384-388.
8. Chu KM, Fan ST, Hai EC Pyogenic liver abscess. An audit of experience over past decade. *Arch Surg* 1996;131: 148-152.
9. Kar P, Kapoor S, Jain A Pyogenic liver abscess: Etiology, clinical manifestation and management. *Trop Gastroenterol* 1998;19: 136-140.
10. Seeto RK, Rockey DC. Pyogenic liver abscess. Changes in etiology, management and outcome. *Medicine* 1996; 75 : 100-103.
11. Corredoria J, Casariego E, Moreno C, Prospective study of *Streptococcus milleri* hepatic abscesses. *Eur J Clin Microbio Infect Dis* 1998;17; 556-560.
12. Sani PN, Hoosen AA, Piloy DE. Hepatic abscess caused by *Salmosulla typlis*. A case report and review of literature. *Dig Dis Sci* 1994;39: 1694-1696.
13. Strungs I, Farrell DJ, Mater LD: Multiple hepatic abscesses due to Yersinia enterocolitica. *Pathology* 1995; 27: 374-377.
14. Sugano S, Matuda T, Suzuki T. Hepatic actinomycosis: Case report and review of the literature. *Japan J Gastroenterol* 1997; 32: 672- 676.

84 Amebic Liver Abscess

SS Slathia

INTRODUCTION

The liver acts as an initial filter of absorbed contents of intestine and is, thus, at risk to contamination with microbial agents of all varieties. Other than hepatotropic viruses, the liver can be affected by:

a. Spread of bacterial/parasitic infection from outside liver
b. Primary infection by spirochetes, protozoa, tubercular or fungal infections
c. Systemic effects of bacterial or granulomatous infection.

Liver abscess, generally regarded a rare condition in the Western world, is not an uncommon problem in children residing in tropical countries. Bacterial and parasitic invasion of liver are the two common etiological factors. Clinical features are variable depending upon the cause, size of abscess, general health, the features of associated disease and complications.

Among investigations, role of ultrasound in diagnosing liver abscess and role of IHA in diagnosing cause of liver abscess are very important.

Treatment of patient is either medical or surgical, depending upon the size, location, toxicity and response to antimicrobials. Surgical procedure depends upon surgeon's previous experience and facilities available. The best mode of management is yet not clear.

The various types of abscesses encountered in children are:

a. Amebic liver abscess (ALA).
b. Pyogenic liver abscess (PLA).
c. Fungal liver abscess.
d. Tubercular liver abscess.

AMEBIASIS AND AMEBIC LIVER ABSCESS (ALA)

Amebic infection is common throughout the world; about 10% of the world's population is infected with *E.histolytica.* Amebiasis may also cause systemic manifestations. In a majority of cases infection is asymptomatic. It is prevalent more so in regions with poor standards of personal and food hygiene and inadequate sanitation. Young, immunocompromised and malnourished children and those on steroids are at a higher risk of severe E. histolytica infection. *E. histolytica* is estimated by the World Health Organization to be second only to malaria as a protozoal cause of death.

Liver abscess is the most frequent complication of amebiasis. There are two species of Entameba that commonly infect humans. *E.dispar* causes only asymptomatic infection while *E.histolytica* is pathogenic species and may produce symptomatic disease in 10% of infected persons. Infection with *E.dispar* is 10 times more common than *E. histolytica.*

Among all cases of amebiasis, the incidence of ALA has been reported to vary between 3-9%.

ALA has highest rate of incidence in developing countries including India and Pakistan. About 80% of abscesses are solitary, more than 83% are located in right lobe and about 17% are in left lobe. The pleuropulmonary complications of ALA are reported in 20% of cases. Rupture into peritoneal cavity or into an intra-abdominal viscus occurs in 6-9% of patients.

Majority of ALA occurs between the ages 21 and 50. Below 20 years of age, the incidence is less than 7% and above the age of 50, it is less than 21%. It must, therefore, be noted that no age is exempt and cases have been encountered in infants. The highest incidence is between the ages of 1-3 years. This is perhaps because at this age children tend to swallow things indiscriminately. It may occur even in early infancy.

Male predominance as in adults, has not been observed in children. Table 84.1 presents clinical syndromes associated with E. histolytica infection.

Table 84.1: Clinical syndromes associated with E. histolytica lesions

Intestinal amebiasis
Asymptomatic cyst passers
Acute amebic colitis
- Mucosal disease

Contd.

Contd.

- Transmural disease
- Ulcerative postdysenteric colitis

Appendicitis
Ameba
Amebic stricture

Extraintestinal amebiasis

Amebic liver abscess (ALA)
Perforation and peritonitis
Pleuropulmonary amebiasis
Amebic pericarditis
Cutaneous amebiasis.

PATHOGENESIS

Amebiasis is the third leading cause of death from parasitic disease worldwide. The causative protozoan parasite, *Entamoeba histolytica,* is a potent pathogen. Secreting proteinases that dissolve host tissues, killing host cells on contact, and engulfing red blood cells, *E. histolytica* trophozoites invade the intestinal mucosa, causing amebic colitis. In some cases amebae breach the mucosal barrier and travel through the portal circulation to the liver, where they cause abscesses consisting of a few *E. histolytica* trophozoites surrounding dead and dying hepatocyte and liquefied cellular debris. Amebic liver abscesses grow inexorably and, at one time, were almost always fatal, but now even large abscesses can be cured by antibiotic.

DIAGNOSIS

Amebic liver abscess is more common than pyogenic abscess. Diagnosis is through clinical findings, serology and hepatic imaging.

Since diagnosis of a liver abscess in children is often difficult, awareness of the condition, especially in endemic areas, may aid in early detection. It presents as an acute process in a majority of the cases or as a chronic indolent disease.

The complaints are often nonspecific, thus delaying the diagnosis. The most common symptoms are fever, abdominal discomfort or pain (more in the right upper quadrant of the abdomen). Epigastric pain is commonly seen in left lobe abscesses. At times, pain is referred to the right shoulder or right lower quadrant of the abdomen. Cough with or without expectoration and pleuritic chest pain is also seen in ALA. Jaundice is seen in about 10% of amebic abscesses and usually is mild, but it can be severe with large abscesses. The child is very irritable and may present with vomiting. A preceding history of dysentery may be elicited in these children.

On examination, a slight fullness in the right hypochondrium may be detected.The right lobe of the liver is involved more often than the left.

Elevated right dome of diaphragm is a common X-ray finding. Color of pus, anchovy sauce-like, is seen only infrequently. This may be because of superadded infection with pyogenic organisms.

The most difficult differential diagnosis is pyogenic liver abscess Chapter 83.

Investigations

Amebic liver abscess in children may be diagnosed by the presence of leukocytosis, moderate anemia high ESR and raised liver enzymes, particularly alkaline phosphatase.

Trophozoites in stool are seen in <50% of ALA patients. Microscopic examination of a fresh specimen of stools is necessary for the diagnosis of intestinal infection with *E. histolytica.* Light microscopy cannot distinguish between *E.histolytica* and *E.dispar* unless ingested erythrocytes are seen within trophozoites, a finding pathognomic for *E.histolytica*. Microscopy is now an obsolete technique (unable to distinguish the more frequent nonpathogenic *E. dispar* from *E. histolytica*) in advanced countries. In addition, microscopy misses up to two-thirds of the infections detcted by antigens tests or PCR. Presence of *E. histolytica* in stools only supports the diagnosis.

Serum antibodies to amebae develop only during *E. histolytica* infection and not during *E. dispar* infection.

Positive amebic serology like ELISA, indirect hemagglutination, counter current immunoelectrophoresis and latex fixation are helpful.

PCR and detection of antigen by monoclonal antibodies are newer techniques. Indirect hemagglutination is highly sensitive. If it is negative, ALA can be safely ruled out. However, 10% patients with acute ALA may have negative serology. Antibodies to *E. histolytica* become positive after one week of onset of symptoms and may remain positive upto 6 months. Recently, it has been reported that serological test based on recombinant *E. histolytica* antigens may help in differentiating active infection from past exposure to parasite.

In most cases, US, CT, MRI or isotope scans can localize and delineate the size of abscess. Aspiration of typical pus from the liver, its examination and amebic serology are often required to diagnose amebic etiology.

MANAGEMENT

Majority of the cases are treated conservatively. However some advocate needle aspiration along with antiamebic drugs in management of ALA.

Drugs

Nitroimidazoles, chloroquin and dehydroemetine are effective drugs.

Metronidazole, a tissue amebicidal is given in a dose of 30-50 mg/kg/in three divided doses (maximum 500-750 mg/dose) per day orally for 10 days. Other two nitroimidazoles, tinidazole and ornidazole, are also effective.

Dehydremetine1-2 mg/kg SC or IM (never IV) per day for ten days is preferred to emetine as it may be more effective and safer even when administered in high doses. Tachycardia, T wave depression, arrhythmias, or proteinuria while giving drug warrants stoppage of drug.

Chloroquine may be useful but it is toxic to children if given in large doses.

Iodoquinol 30-40 mg/kg/24 hours orally divided in 3 doses for 20 days is drug of choice for asymptomatic cyst carriers.

Paromomycin and diloxanide are also used.

COMPLICATIONS AND UNUSUAL PRESENTATIONS

ALA usually occurs in right lobe of liver and is solitary (30-70%). Unusual presentations include multiple abscesses, left lobe abscesses, abscesses presenting as compressive lesion, and abscesses rupturing into viscera. Pus can rupture into pleuro-pulmonary area, subphrenic space, peritoneal cavity, and pericardial space. The last is usually due to left ALA and may result in pericardial temponade. Other less common complications are rupture or compression or thrombosis of hepatic veins or inferior vena cava, ALA may coxist with hepatitis A and hepatitis E infection, or HbsAg carriers.

VARIANTS

Multiple Abscesses

Fifteen percent of the patients may have multiple abscesses, presenting with fever, toxemia, deep jaundice and encephalopathy. Toxemia suggests added bacterial infection. These may present with symptoms indistinguishable from hepatic encephalopathy due to acute hepatocellular failure.

Left Lobe Abscess

Thirty-five percent of patients present with a left lobe abscess. Half of these have associated lesions in right lobe while remaining have solitary left lobe abscess. These patients have longer duration of symptoms (3-4 weeks). Fever is less commonly observed as compared to right lobe. It presents as a large epigastric mass and may be confused with pseudocyst of pancreas. Comlications like peritonitis and toxemia are more common

Compression Lesions

A posteriorly located ALA in the right lobe may present as inferior vena cava obstruction or hepatic outflow obstruction. In fact ALA has been reported as cause of Budd Chiary syndrome in few patients from Indian subcontinent.

Extension of the Abscess

It may extend to pleural cavity, with empyema thoracis, peritoneal cavity presenting as peritonitis and shock in about 7% of cases. Rupture into biliary tree and colon has also been reported. A subhepatic collection may also occur.

KEY LEARNING POINTS

- Most frequent complication of amebiasis.
- Diagnosis is though clinical suspicion, serology, radiology and hepatic drainage, the most difficult differential diagnosis being pyognic live abscess.
- Unusual presentations include multiple abscesses, left lobe abscess, compression lesions and extension of the abscess to pleural or peritoneal cavity and rupture into the biliary tree and colon.
- Majority of cases respond to conservative antiamebic therapy (nitroimidazole, chloroquine, dehydroemetine); only some cases need needle aspiration.

FURTHER READINGS

1. Ahsan T, Jehangir MU, Mahmood T, *et al*. Amebic vs pyogenic liver abscess. *J Pak Med Assoc* 2002;52:497-501.
2. Balistreri WF. Liver abscess. In: Kliegman RM, Behrman Re, Jenson HB, Staton BF (eds): *Nelson Textbook of Pediatrics*, 18th edn. Philadelphia: Saunders 2008:1690-1692.
3. Stanley SI, Jackson TF, Foster L, Singh S. Longitudinal study of the antibody response to recombinant *Entameba histolytica* antigen in patients with amebic liver abscess. *Am J Trop Med Hyg* 1998;58:414-416.
4. William Ap. Amebiasis. In: Rudolph CD, Rudolp AM (eds): *Rudolph's Pediatrics*. New York: McGraw-Hill 2003:1122-1124.

85 Reye's Syndrome

Chandra Mohan Kumar

INTRODUCTION

Reye's syndrome (RS), now a rare clinical condition affecting children following a viral illness like influenza or chickenpox, has been a dreaded disease in 7th through 9th decade of last century. It is an acute encephalopathy with fulminant hepatic failure. Although it bears the name of R KD Reye who first described it as a distinct clinical entity in Australia in 1963, descriptions of similar clinical entities were made elsewhere earlier than that. A notable among them was "Jamshedpur fever'' reported from India by Dr. Najib Khan in1956.

Over last few decades, there has been a significant fall in the incidence of this potentially fatal disease. Although etiology of RS is not known, the condition typically appeared after an episode of viral illness, most commonly upper respiratory tract infection (URTI), gastroenteritis, influenza or chickenpox. It commonly followed the use of asprin as an antipyretic during the illness. Now use of aspirin has reduced drastically in pediatric practice; Reye's syndrome too has become a rare entity.

Nevertheless, recognition and prevention remains a very important aspect to safeguard against its resurgence. The fact that manifestations of Reye's syndrome are in no way unique to it and given that no test is specific for Reye syndrome, the diagnosis is to be made by exclusion. A high index of suspicion is critical for its recognition. It should be considered in any child with vomiting and altered sensorium.

DIAGNOSTIC CRITERIA

Diagnostic criteria from the Centers for Disease Control and Prevention (CDC) are as follows:

- Acute noninflammatory encephalopathy with an altered level of consciousness.
- Hepatic dysfunction with a liver biopsy showing fatty metamorphosis or a more than 3-fold increase in alanine aminotransferase (ALT), aspartate aminotransferase (AST), and/or ammonia levels.
- No other explanation for cerebral edema or hepatic abnormality.
- CSF with 8 or fewer WBCs per cubic millimeter (8 X 10^9/L or fewer).
- Brain biopsy with cerebral edema without inflammation.

Some inborn errors of metabolism such as fatty-acid oxidation defects, amino and organic acidopathies, urea-cycle defects, and disorders of carbohydrate metabolism are also known to present similar clinical features hence need to be excluded before reaching to a diagnosis of Reye's syndrome.

Early recognition and treatment are essential to prevent death and to optimize the likelihood of recovery without neurologic impairment.

PATHOPHYSIOLOGY

The pathogenesis is not clear, but it appears to involve mitochondrial dysfunction that inhibits oxidative phosphorylation and fatty-acid beta-oxidation in a virus-infected, sensitized host. The host has usually been exposed to mitochondrial toxins, like salicylates in most of the cases. The other hypothesis suggests that salicylates stimulate the expression of inducible nitric oxide synthase (iNOS) because of findings of iNOS stimulation in African children with fatal malaria. Malaria causes symptoms similar to those of Reye syndrome and is often treated with aspirin.

Histologic changes include cytoplasmic fatty vacuolization in hepatocytes, astrocyte edema and loss of neurons in the brain, and edema and fatty degeneration of the proximal lobules in the kidneys. All cells have pleomorphic, swollen mitochondria that are in reduced number, along with glycogen depletion and minimal tissue inflammation. Hepatic mitochondrial dysfunction results in hyperammonemia, which is thought to induce astrocyte edema, resulting in cerebral edema and increased intracranial pressure (ICP).

CLINICAL PRESENTATIONS

Age

The peak ages are 5-14 years, with a median of 6 years and

a mean of 7 years. Reye syndrome rarely occurs in newborns or in children older than 18 years.

Sex

Seen equally in both sexes.

History

Almost all the affected children have history of at least 1 viral illness in the 3 weeks preceding the onset of Reye syndrome. The other important aspects in history are:

1. Illnesses include viral URTI or influenza, varicella, gastroenteritis and other illness with exanthem.
2. Salicylates were detectable in the blood of a vast majority of patients.
3. Influenza B (most common), influenza A, and varicella-zoster virus are most often involved.
4. Parainfluenza, adenovirus, coxsackieviruses A and B, echovirus, Epstein-Barr virus, rubella virus, measles virus, cytomegalovirus, herpes simplex virus, parainfluenza viruses, and poliomyelitis viruses are less commonly involved than the pathogens listed above.
5. Reye syndrome can occur after vaccination with live viral vaccines.
6. Abrupt onset of pernicious vomiting occurs 12 hours to 3 weeks after viral illness; the mean is 3 days.
7. Neurologic symptoms usually occur 24-48 hours after onset of vomiting. Lethargy is usually the first neurologic manifestation.
8. Diarrhea and hyperventilation may be the first signs in children younger than 2 years.
9. Irritability, restlessness, delirium, seizures, and coma occur.
10. Obtain an appropriate history in any child who presents with symptoms similar to those of Reye syndrome to determine whether an IEM should be considered.

Signs and Symptoms

- Signs and symptoms of Reye syndrome include protracted vomiting, with or without clinically significant dehydration, encephalopathy in afebrile patients with minimal or absent jaundice and hepatomegaly.
- For children younger than age 2, the first signs of Reye's syndrome may be diarrhea and rapid breathing. For older children and teenagers, early signs of Reye's syndrome may include:
  - Persistent or continuous vomiting.
  - Unusual sleepiness or lethargy.

As the condition progresses, signs and symptoms may become more serious:

- Irritable, aggressive or irrational behavior.
- Confusion.
- Weakness or paralysis in the arms and legs.
- Seizures.
- Loss of consciousness.

The clinical stages of RS are as follows:

a. Stage 0–Alert, abnormal history and laboratory findings conversant with Reye syndrome, no clinical manifestations.
b. Stage 1–Vomiting, sleepiness and lethargy.
c. Stage 2–Restlessness, irritability, combativeness, disorientation, delirium, tachycardia, hyperventilation, dilated pupils with sluggish response, hyperreflexia, positive Babinski sign, and appropriate response to noxious stimuli.
d. Stage 3–Obtunded, comatose, decorticate rigidity, and inappropriate response to noxious stimuli.
e. Stage 4–Deep coma, decerebrate rigidity, fixed and dilated pupils, loss of oculovestibular reflexes, and dysconjugate gaze with caloric stimulation.
f. Stage 5–Seizures, flaccid paralysis, absent deep tendon reflexes (DTRs), no pupillary response, and respiratory arrest.
g. Stage 6–Patients who cannot be classified because they have been treated with curare or other medication that alters level of consciousness.

DIFFERENTIAL DIAGNOSIS

Following conditions may resemble RS, hence needs to be excluded before a diagnosis of Reye's syndrome is made:

- Encephalitis.
- Meningitis.
- Hepatitis with hepatic encephalopathy.
- Subdural and epidural hematoma.
- Poisonings and toxins like Aflatoxin, Organophosphorus, Amatoxin and Carbamates.
- Inborn errors of metabolism of fatty-acid oxidation, amino and organic acidurias, urea-cycle defects, and disorders of carbohydrate metabolism.

LABORATORY STUDIES

- Liver function tests (LFT) – Elevated ammonia levels is the most important laboratory finding of RS. Ammonia levels are elevated as much as 1.5 times normal (upto 1200 mcg/dL) 24-48 hours after the onset of mental status changes. Ammonia levels may return to the reference range in stages 4 and 5. Levels of transaminases, ALT and AST increase to 3 times normal but may return to the reference ranges by stages 4 or 5.
- Bilirubin levels are > 2 mg/dL (usually < 3 mg/dL) in 10-15% of patients. Usually serum bilirubin remains in anicteric range. If direct bilirubin is more than 15% of total or the total is >3 mg/dL, RS is unlikely.
- The prothrombin time (PT) and activated partial thromboplastin time (aPTT) are prolonged >1.5-fold in majority of the cases.
- Assay of coagulation factors ii, vii, ix, x and fibrinogen to assess the synthetic function of liver.

- Hypoglycemia is a common finding in children with RS.
- Lipase and amylase levels are elevated.
- Serum bicarbonate levels are decreased secondary to vomiting.
- BUN and creatinine levels are elevated.
- Lactic dehydrogenase (LDH) levels may be high or low.
- Metabolic acidosis is present.
- Urine specific gravity is increased; 80% of patients have ketonuria.
- CSF examination should be done to rule out other causes likely to present with similar clinical picture. The CSF opening pressure remains high suggesting raised ICP.
- An extensive metabolic workup to exclude IEM must be performed and should include evaluation for defects of fatty-acid oxidation, amino and organic acidurias, urea-cycle defects, and disorders of carbohydrate metabolism.
- Liver biopsy after correction of coagulation profile can help in diagnosis of toxic liver disease as well as IEMs.

Imaging Studies

CT or MRI imaging of brain reveals cerebral edema but may remain normal in RS. However these studies are indicated to rule out other conditions likely to present with behavior changes and decreased level of conciousness like RS.

EEG

An electroencephalogram (EEG) may reveal slow-wave activity in the early stages and flattened waves in advanced stages.

MANAGEMENT

Successful management of Reye's syndrome needs a coordinated team work of pediatrician, neurologist, neurosurgeon and gastroenterologist.

Resuscitation and maintenance of airway, breathing and circulation and correction of hypoglycemia, hyperammonemia , electrolyte imbalance and prevention and/or control of cerebral edema are of prime importance in management of a case of RS.

Supportive care is based on the stage.

Care by stage is as follows:

Stages 0-1

Patient is kept in quiet environment.

Frequent monitoring of vital signs and laboratory values. Correction of fluid and electrolyte abnormalities, acidemia and hypoglycemia. If the patient is initially hypoglycemic, dextrose 25% is administered as an intravenous (IV) bolus at a dose of 1-2 mL/kg. If the initial pH is less than 7.2, bicarbonatis given upto 1 mEq/kg/h.

Maintenance of fluids, electrolytes, serum pH, albumin, serum osmolality, urine output, and glucose values is important. Overhydration may precipitate cerebral edema. Use colloids (e.g., albumin) as necessary to maintain intravascular volume. Dehydration may compromise cardiovascular volume and reduce cerebral perfusion.

Stage 2

Continuous cardiorespiratory monitoring, placement of arterial lines and urine catheters to monitor urine output, and ECG and/or EEG are standard care.

Prevent increased ICP. Elevate the head of the bed and avoid overhydration and use of hypo-osmotic fluids.

Correction of hyperammonemia. Sodium phenylacetate/sodium benzoate (Ammonul), a medication that treats hyperammonemia is the treatment of acute hyperammonemia and associated encephalopathy in patients with deficiencies in enzymes of the urea cycle may be used for this purpose.

Diuretics to control fluid overload and insulin to maintain euglycemia should be employed. In addition, administer ondansetron 0.15 mg/kg during the first 15 minutes of the initial dose. If the ammonia level is more than 500 mcg/dL or if the patient's condition fails to respond to the initial dose of sodium phenylacetate/sodium benzoate, preferably hemodialysis should be performed.

Stages 3-5

Continuous monitoring of ICP, central venous pressure, arterial pressure, and/or end-tidal carbon dioxide. Manage the airway with rapid-sequence intubation and ventilation as appropriate for raised ICP.

Treat increased ICP by following standard guidelines.

Treat seizures with phenytoin 10-20 mg/kg IV as a loading dose followed by 5 mg/kg/d IV divided every 6 hours or fosphenytoin dosed as 10-20 mg/kg phenytoin equivalents (PEs).

Correct coagulopathy (PT >16 seconds), particularly if an intracranial bolt and/or liver biopsy is required. In rare cases, an exchange transfusion is required.

COMPLICATIONS

Though RS is itself a very complex illness it may be further complicated by

- Brain herniation, status epilepticus, syndrome of inappropriate secretion of antidiuretic hormone (SIADH), and diabetes insipidus.
- Acute respiratory failure, aspiration pneumonia.
- Cardiovascular collapse.
- GI bleeding, pancreatitis.
- Acute renal failure.
- Sepsis.

PROGNOSIS

1. Mortality rate has decreased in recent years from 50%

to less than 20% with more effective and vigorous case management.

2. Markers of poor prognosis are:
   a. Patients younger than 5 years.
   b. Serum ammonia levels >300 mcg/dL are associated with poor prognosis.
   c. Rapid progression from stage 1 to stage 3 or presentation with stage 4 or 5 is associated with a poor prognosis. The death rate based on stage at time of admission is 18% for stage 0 and 90% for stage 5.
   d. The prognosis is worse with liver and muscle involvement (i.e., AST/ALT >1, LDH isoenzymes 1-5, elevated creatine kinase–MM [CK-MM] and creatine kinase–MB [CK-MB]) than with either involvement alone.
   e. Hypoproteinemia unresponsive to fresh frozen plasma (FFP) and vitamin K indicates a poor prognosis.
3. Survivors have an increased risk of long-term neurologic sequelae, particularly if ammonia levels are >300 mcg/dL, if they have stage 2-5 disease, and/or if they are younger than 2 years.
   a. The ammonia level is the best predictor.

KEY LEARNING POINTS

- Now a rare illness, Reye's syndrome is characterized by acute encephalopathy together with fulminant hepatic failure following a viral illness, especially chickenpox, triggered by the use of aspirin. Clinical icterus is conspicuous by its absence.
- Clinically, it has been categorized into six stages.
- Differential diagnosis is from encephalitis, meningitis, hepatitis with encephalopathy, subdural and epidural hematoma, etc.
- High ammonia level is the most important laboratory finding.
- Success treatment, needing a coordinated team work involving pediatrician, neurologist, neurosurgeon and gastroenterologist, varies with the clinical stage.
- The prognosis is worsened with superimposed complications, including ARF, sepsis, acute respiratory failure, aspiration pneumonia, GI bleeding, pancreatitis and CNS problems.
- Survivors have an increased risk of long-term neurologic sequelae.

FURTHER READINGS

1. Belay ED, Bresee JS, Holman RC, *et al.:* Reye's syndrome in the United States from 1981 through 1997. *N Engl J Med* 1999;340: 1377-1382.
2. Casteels-Van Daele M, Van Geet C, Wouters C, Eggermont E: Reye syndrome revisited: A descriptive term covering a *group of heterogeneous disorders. Eur J Pediatr* 2000;159: 641-648.
3. Chang PF, Huang SF, Hwu WL, *et al.:* Metabolic disorders mimicking Reye's syndrome. *J Formos Med Assoc* 2000;99: 295-299.
4. Clark I, Whitten R, Molyneux M, Taylor T: Salicylates, nitric oxide, malaria, and Reye's syndrome. *Lancet* 2001; 357(9256): 625-627.
5. Cohen J, Powderly WG. *Infectious Diseases*, 2nd edn. New York: Elsevier 2004:310-311.
6. Goetz, CG. *Textbook of Clinical Neurology*. 2nd edn. St. Louis: Saunders 2003: 656-657.
7. Gupte S. Reye's syndrome (Annotation). *Indian J Pediatr* 1975;42:176-178.
8. Hall SM, Lynn R, Johnson GM, Belay ED, Schonberger LB, Monto, AS. Reye's syndrome. *NEJM* 1999; 341: 845-847.
9. Lovejoy FH Jr, Smith AL, Bresnan MJ, *et al.:* Clinical staging in Reye syndrome. *Am J Dis Child* 1974;128: 36-41.
10. Monto AS. The Disappearance of Reye's syndrome — A public health triumph. *NEJM* 1999;340: 1423-1424.
11. Noble J. *Textbook of Primary Care Medicine*. 3rd edn. St. Louis: Mosby 2001:46-47.

86 Autoimmune Hepatitis

Vani Gopalareddy

DEFINITION

Autoimmune liver disease comprises a group of disorders of the liver with demonstrable circulating antibodies. The antibodies vary, and define the type of autoimmune liver disease. The chronic inflammatory reaction can target the liver parenchyma autoimmune hepatitis (AIH) or the biliary tree (sclerosing cholangitis) or both (overlap syndrome). Upto 20% of patients do not have any detectable antibodies (antibody-negative AIH).

Autoimmune hepatitis is an unresolving inflammation of the liver of unknown cause. It is characterized by the presence of hepatitis (piecemeal necrosis or interface hepatitis) that is periportal or more widespread on histologic examination, hypergammaglobulinemia, autoantibodies in serum and complete response to immunosuppressive therapy.

TYPES OF AIH

- **Type 1:** Synonyms: Autoimmune chronic active hepatitis, lupoid hepatitis, plasma cell hepatitis, chronic active hepatitis.
- **Type 2.**
- **Type 3:** Anti-SLA (soluble liver antigen).
- **Drug-induced.**
- **Overlap syndromes** (Variant forms).
- **AIH with APECED** syndrome (Autoimmune polyendocrinopathy, candidiasis, ectodermal dystrophy).
- **Giant cell hepatitis** with autoimmune hemolytic anemia.

ETIOPATHOGENESIS

AIH develops because of loss of self-tolerance by the host immune system. Cytotoxic lymphocytes are then directed against normal liver cells. Following activation of inflammatory response, the resulting cytokine production leads to continued macrophage activation, enhanced HLA expression and B-cell autoantibody production leading to continued hepatocellular injury.

Genetic predisposition is suggested by the increased frequency of HLA haplotypes HLA B8/DR3/DR4 and coexistence of other autoimmune disorders.

Proposed triggers for initiation of inflammatory response include drug and viral agents. The common drugs implicated to trigger AIH are methyldopa, isoniazid, minocycline, sulphasalazine, dihydralazine, nitrofurantoin, pemoline and infliximab. Drug-induced liver disease with autoantibodies is not truly autoimmune hepatitis since the syndrome is caused by a specific agent whose removal terminates the disease.

Viruses such as measles, Epstein-Barr, cytomegalovirus, human herpes virus 6, hepatitis A, B and C are known to trigger AIH. Similarly, vaccination, especially with multiple antigenic preparations, can overcome self-tolerance and produce a self-perpetuating illness.

CLINICAL MANIFESTATIONS AND PRESENTATION (TABLE 86.1)

Autoimmune hepatitis affects all age groups and ethnic groups. Disease expression and behavior in turn may vary greatly according to the geographical region and ethnicity of the susceptible population. 30-40% of newly diagnosed AIH cases occur in patients younger than 20 years of age. Although the peak incidence in pediatrics is in pubertal girls, it has been diagnosed in infants as young as 6 months. Concurrent immune diseases are found in 30-40% of patients with autoimmune hepatitis. There is often a family history of autoimmune disease (first degree relative in 40% cases). Inflammatory bowel disease, diabetes and thyroiditis are the most frequently noted conditions. Celiac disease is noted in about 6% of patients. Other associated conditions described include hemolytic anemia, glomerulonephritis, Sjögren's syndrome, idiopathic thrombocytopenia. AIH may also occur with autoimmune polyglandular syndrome type 1 (APECED), which is characterized by hypothyroidism, Addison's disease, ectodermal dystrophy and chronic mucocutaneous candidiasis.

The presentation of AIH may be quite variable with following predominant types:

- Acute presentation resembling viral hepatitis with

Table 86.1: Clinical and immunologic features of AIH

Clinical Features	*Type 1*	*Type 2*	*Type 3*
Diagnostic antibodies	*Anti-SMA, ANA	*Anti-LKM1	*Anti-SLA
Age	Bimodal (10-20 y and 40-70y)	Pediatric (2--14 y); rare in adults	Adults (30-50 y)
Women (%)	78	89	90
Concurrent immune disease (%)	41	34	58
Gamma globulin elevation	+++	+	++
Low immunoglobulin A (IgA)	No	Occasional	No
HLA association	B8,DR3, DR4	B14,DR3, C4AQO	Uncertain
Steroid response	+++	++	+++
Progression to cirrhosis (%)	45	82	75

*ASMA: anti-smooth muscle antibody; ANA: antinuclear antibody; anti-LKM: anti-liver-kidney microsomal antibody; anti-SLA: anti-soluble liver antigen.

anorexia, malaise abdominal discomfort and jaundice in about 50% of cases.

- Fulminant hepatic failure in about 11% cases, more so with type 2.
- Insidious onset with nonspecific symptoms, intermittent jaundice for many years prior to presentation.
- Complications of cirrhosis and portal hypertension.
- Incidental finding of elevated transaminases.

Variant Forms of Autoimmune Hepatitis (Table 86.2, Fig. 86.1)

Patients with variant forms of autoimmune hepatitis have autoimmune features but do not satisfy the criteria for a definite or probable diagnosis of autoimmune hepatitis. In addition, they cannot be placed in another diagnostic category. Such patients have features associated with both autoimmune hepatitis and another type of chronic liver disease (overlap syndromes) or have findings that are incompatible with the diagnosis of autoimmune hepatitis

Table 86.2: Variant forms of autoimmune hepatitis

Syndrome	*Distinguishing features*
Overlap syndromes	
Autoimmune hepatitis and primary biliary cirrhosis	Mitochondrial antibodies Histologic cholangitis Hepatic copper deposition Cholestatic laboratory changes Responsiveness to corticosteroid therapy
Autoimmune hepatitis and primary sclerosing cholangitis	Chronic ulcerative colitis Histologic cholangitis Cholestatic laboratory changes No responsiveness to corticosteroid therapy Abnormal cholangiogram
Autoimmune hepatitis and chronic viral infection: Autoimmune predominant	Titer of ASMA or ANA > 1: 320 Titer of ASMA and ANA > 1: 40 Piecemeal necrosis (interface hepatitis), lobular hepatitis and portal plasma cell infiltrates
Autoimmune heapatitis and chronic viral infection: Viral predominant	Titer of ASMA or ANA <1:320 Antibodies to LKM 1 and HCV viremia Portal lymphoid aggregates, steatosis or bile duct injury
Outlier syndromes	
Autoimmune cholangitis	Absence of mitochondrial antibodies ANA and SMA common Histologic feature of bile duct injury Concurrent cholestatic laboratory changes Antibodies to carbonic anhydrase Normal cholangiogram
Cryptogenic chronic hepatitis	Absence of ASMA, ANA, LKM or microsomal antibody at presentation Histologic findings identical to those of autoimmune hepatitis HLA-B8,HLA-DR3 or HLA-B8-DR3 common Possible antibodies to SLA or liver pancreas Possible late appearance of conventional antibodies Responsiveness to corticosteroid therapy.

*ASMA: Anti-smooth muscle antibody; ANA: Antinuclear antibody; Anti-LKM: Anti-liver-kidney microsomal; Anti-SLA: Anti-soluble liver antigen.

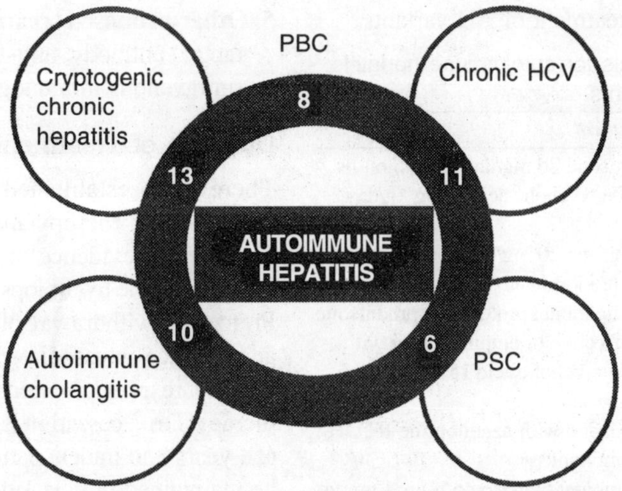

Fig. 86.1: Variant forms of autoimmune hepatitis. The numbers represent percentages (%)

according to the criteria codified by the international panels (outlier syndromes).

Differential Diagnosis

- Chronic hepatitis B.
- Chronic hepatitis C.
- Chronic drug induced hepatitis.
- Primary sclerosing cholangitis.
- Alpha-1–antitrypsin deficiency.
- Wilson's disease.
- AIDS-related cholangiopathy.
- Graft-versus-host disease.
- Nonalcoholic steatohepatohepatitis.
- Alcoholic steatohepatitis.

DIAGNOSIS/ INVESTIGATIONS

Autoimmune hepatitis has been recognized since the 1950s, but its diagnostic criteria have only recently been proposed. No particular sign, symptom or liver test abnormality is specific for diagnosis of AIH. The suspicion of autoimmune hepatitis depends largely on the detection of autoantibodies. International Autoimmune Hepatitis Group has promulgated criteria for definite and probable diagnosis for AIH and also a scoring system has also been proposed.

Factors Used in the Scoring System of AIH

- Gender (female predominance).
- Alkaline phosphatase: Alanine aminotransferase < 3:1.
- Autoantibodies present.
- Viral markers absent.
- Other etiologies excluded.
- Minimal alcohol consumption (<25g/day in women and < 30g/day in men).
- Other autoimmune diseases in patient or close relative.

The definitive diagnosis of autoimmune hepatitis requires the presence of compatible laboratory and histologic findings, the absence of viral markers, denial of excessive alcohol consumption, lack of exposure to blood products and hepatotoxic medications, and the presence of hypergammaglobulinemia (globulin level >1.5 times the upper limit of normal). Antinuclear antibodies (ANA), smooth-muscle antibodies (ASMA), or antibodies to liver/kidney microsome (anti-LKM) are required for the diagnosis and must be present in titers of at least 1:80 in adults and 1:20 in children.

Lobular hepatitis is part of the histologic spectrum of autoimmune hepatitis if it is present in conjunction with periportal hepatitis but biliary lesions, copper deposits, granulomas and other changes suggestive of another cause of lobular hepatitis preclude the diagnosis of autoimmune hepatitis.

MANAGEMENT

Treatment of AIH relies on immunosuppressive therapy. It is typically responsive to therapy and should be commenced even in those with fulminant presentation or cirrhosis. Response to therapy is defined as marked improvement in either or both clinical symptoms along with laboratory features (transaminases, immunoglobulin levels) within 1 month of starting treatment and continued response and/or histological improvement wherein liver biopsy within 1 year of starting treatment showing only minimal activity.

In general prednisone is utilized initially at a dose of 1-2 mg/kg/day and tapered gradually over 2-3 months to a daily low dose (5-10 mg) regimen. Azathioprine (AZA) in the dose of 2 mg/kg/day or 6-mercaptopurine (6-MP) in the dose of 1-1.5 mg/kg/day is introduced either at the beginning of treatment or as steroids are tapered within the first 2 months. Addition of AZA may allow steroids to be reduced or even withdrawn completely. The goal of therapy is to have minimal or no elevation of transaminases on the lowest possible doses of medication.

Table 86.3 gives emperic treatment of AH variants.

Table 86.3: Empiric treatments for autoimmune hepatitis variants

Variants	*Treatment*
Autoimmune hepatitis and primary biliary cirrhosis	Prednisone 20 mg/day for 6 months Ursodeoxycholic acid 15mg/kg/day
Autoimmune hepatitis and primary sclerosing cholangitis	Prednisone 20 mg/day for 6 months if AIH predominant Investigational protocols if prednisone is ineffective or empirical trial with ursodeoxycholic acid 15 mg/kg/day
Autoimmune hepatitis and chronic viral hepatitis	Prednisone with azathioprine if AIH predominant Recombinant interferon if viral-predominant
Autoimmune cholangitis	Prednisone 20 mg/day for 6 months Ursodeoxycholic acid 15 mg/kg/day for 6 months
Cryptogenic chronic hepatitis	Prednisone with azathioprine until remission, treatment failure, drug toxicity or response

First-line Medications

1. **Prednisone**:
   Dosage: 1-2 mg/kg/day (initially) in 1-2 divided doses (maximum 60 mg/day).
   Adverse effects: Acne, hirsutism, hypertension, hyperglycemia, cataract, osteoporosis, obesity, cushingoid features.
2. **Azathioprine** (AZA) or 6-Mercaptopurine (6-MP).
   Dosage: AZA at 2-3 mg/kg/day, 6-MP at 1-1.5 mg/kg/day.
   Adverse effects: Cholestatic hepatotoxicity, bone marrow suppression, idiosyncratic pancreatitis, teratogenicity.

Second-line Medications

Shown to be effective in those who fail to respond to azathioprine/low dose prednisone.

1. Cyclosporine
   Dosage: 3-5 mg/kg/day in 3 divided doses.
   Adverse effects: Nephrotoxicity, gingival hyperplasia, hirsutism, hyperlipidemia.
2. Tacrolimus
   Dosage: 0.1mg/kg/day in 2 divided doses.
   Adverse effects: Nephrotoxicity, tremor, seizures, hyperglycemia, cardiomyopathy.
3. **Mycophenolate mofetil (MMF):** Promising drug.
   Dosage: 600 mg/square meter body surface area in 2 divided doses.
   Adverse effects: Gastrointestinal disturbance, bone marrow toxicity.
4. **Other medications:** Sirolimus, Budesonide, ursodiol.
5. **Other proposed treatments:** Anti-TNF (tumor necrosis factor) antibody, anti-IL2 (interleukin2) antibody, IVIG (intravenous immunoglobulin) among others.

Duration of Treatment

There is no established optimal duration of treatment. Cessation of therapy may be considered if there is no biochemical evidence of liver dysfunction for at least 1-2 years and if the liver biopsy shows no inflammatory activity. Premature withdrawal of treatment or withdrawal during adolescence is associated with relapse and most relapses usually respond to reinstitution of immunosuppressive therapy. Drug cessation is effective in only 20% of pediatric (18 years and under) patients. Remission is more likely to be maintained in type 1 than in type 2 AIH.

PROGNOSIS/OUTCOME

Without treatment, nearly 50-90% of patients with severe AIH die within 5-10 years. On the contrary, the odds for transplant-free survival are greater than 80% for treated patients. Failure of serum aminotransferase abnormalities to improve by at least 50% within 6 months of conventional treatment is highly predictive of the need for liver transplantation or an alternative management strategy. Similarly, sustained normalization of the serum alanine aminotransferase level prevents progression of the disease and decompensation of cirrhosis.

Despite an initial good response to immunosuppression, gradual histological progression may continue over years towards end-stage liver disease warranting a liver transplant for survival. Failure of medical treatment is more likely when cirrhosis is present at diagnosis, long standing disease prior to starting treatment and in early onset AIH. Recurrence after transplantation despite immunosuppression occurs in about 50% of children, compared to 17% of adults.

AIH may lead to consideration for liver transplantation Table 86.3.

Table 86.3: Indications for liver transplantation

- Fulminant hepatic failure.
- Intolerable side-effects.
- Complications of cirrhosis.
- Failure of medical therapy.
- Hepatic decompensation occurring while on treatment.

UNRESOLVED ISSUES IN AIH

- Need for endoscopic retrograde cholangiopancreatography (ERCP) at initial diagnosis.
- Best treatment of overlap syndromes.
- Role of follow-up liver biopsies.
- Duration of therapy.
- Long-term prognosis.

KEY LEARNING POINTS

- Autoimmune hepatitis (AIH) is a severe progressive liver disease that often leads to cirrhosis and significant morbidity.
- The presentation of AIH may be quite variable and can present at any age and rarely in infants as well.
- The diagnosis of AIH depends largely on the detection of autoantibodies. The antibodies vary, and define the type of autoimmune liver disease.
- Concurrent immune diseases are found in 30-40% of patients with autoimmune hepatitis.
- Excellent response to immunosuppressive therapy.

FURTHER READINGS

1. Choudhuri G, Somani SK, Baba CS, Alexander G. Autoimmune hepatitis in India: Profile of an uncommon disease. *BMC Gastroenterol* 2005; 5:27-34.
2. Czaja AJ. Current concepts in autoimmune hepatitis. Important review of the diagnostic criteria, pathogenic mechanisms, and treatment strategies of autoimmune hepatitis. *Ann Hepatol* 2005; 4:6-24.
3. Czaja AJ, Bianchi FB, Carpenter HA, *et al.* Treatment challenges and investigational opportunities in autoimmune hepatitis. *Hepatology* 2005; 41:207-215.
4. Czaja AJ, Carpenter HA. Empiric therapy of autoimmune hepatitis with mycophenolate mofetil: Comparison with conventional treatment for refractory disease. *J Clin Gastroenterol* 2005; 39:819-825.
5. Czaja AJ. Autoantibodies in autoimmune liver disease. *Adv Clin Chem* 2005; 40:127-164.
6. Floreani A, Rizzotto ER, Ferrara F, *et al.* Clinical course and outcome of autoimmune hepatitis/primary sclerosing cholangitis overlap syndrome. *Am J Gastroenterol* 2005; 100:1516-1522.
7. Santos RG, Alissa F, Reyes J, *et al.* Fulminant hepatic failure: Wilson's disease or autoimmune hepatitis? Implications for transplantation. *Pediatr Transpl* 2005; 9:112-116.

87 Drug-Induced Liver Injury

Ravinder K Gupta • Ritu Gupta

INTRODUCTION

Liver is particularly concerned with drug metabolism, especially of drugs given orally. The drugs must be lipid soluble to have passed the membrane of the intestinal cell. These must then be presented to the liver and converted to water-soluble (more polar) compounds for excretion via the urine or bile.

Liver is the main site of drug metabolism and is particularly susceptible to structural and functional injury after ingestion, parenteral administration, or inhalation of chemical agents, drugs, plant derivative (home remedies), or environmental toxins. The possibility of drug use or toxin exposure at home in the parental workplace should be explored for every child with liver dysfunction.

The clinical spectrum of illness may vary from asymptomatic biochemical abnormalities of liver function to fulminant failure.

DRUGS AND LIVER DISEASE

Drugs can cause toxic effects, mimicking almost every naturally occurring liver disease in man (Table 87.1). About 2% of all cases of jaundice in hospitalized patients are drug induced. About one-quarter of cases of fulminant hepatic failure in the USA are thought to be medicament-related. In any patient with liver disease it is essential to know all drugs that have been taken over the last 3 months. The physician may have to be a detective to identify them all.

Early suspicion of a drug-related hepatic reaction, and, if possible, accurate diagnosis, are essential. Severity is greatly increased if the drug is continued after symptoms develop or after serum transaminases rise. This provides grounds for negligence claims.

The response of the liver to drugs depends on interplay between absorption, environmental factors and genetics.

An individual drug may cause more than one type of reaction. There may be an overlap between hepatic, cholestatic and hypersensitivity reactions. Halothane, for instance, can cause zone 3 necrosis and also an acute hepatitis-like picture. The promazines overlap between the hepatic and cholestatic types. Methyl dopa can cause acute or chronic hepatitis, cirrhosis, hepatic granulomas or cholestasis.

Drugs are an important cause of liver injury. More than 900 drugs, toxins, and herbs have been known to cause liver injury, and drugs account for 20-40% of all instances of fulminant hepatic failure approximately 75% of the idiosyncratic drug reactions result in liver transplantation or death. Drug induced hepatic injury is the most common reason cited for withdrawal of an approved drug. Pediatricians must be vigilant in identifying drug-related liver injury because early detection can decrease the severity of hepatotoxicity if the drug is discontinued. The manifestations of drug-induced hepatotoxicity are variable, ranging from asymptomatic elevation of liver enzymes to fulminant hepatic failure. Knowledge of the commonly implicated agents and a high index of suspicion are essential in diagnosis.

MORTALITY/MORBIDITY

In the United States, approximately 2000 cases of acute liver failure occur annually and drugs account for over 50% of them (39% are due to acetaminophen, 13% are idiosyncratic reactions due to other medications). Drugs account for 2-5% of cases of patients hospitalized with jaundice and approximately 10% of all cases of acute hepatitis.

PHARMACOKINETICS

The hepatic clearance of drugs given by mouth depends on the efficiency of the drug metabolizing enzymes, the intrinsic clearance, the liver blood flow and the extent of plasma protein binding. Drugs vary in their pharmacological effects according to the relative importance of these different pharmacokinetic factors.

Drugs which are avidly taken up by the liver (high intrinsic clearance) are said to have a high first-pass metabolism. The rate-limiting factor in their hepatic uptake

Table 87.1: Classification of hepatic drug reaction

Type	*Features*	*Examples*
Zone 3 necrosis	Dose dependent, Organ failure	Carbon tetrachloride Paracetamol Halothane
Mitochondrial cytopathies	Affects children Reye's-like syndrome Cirrhosis	Valproate
Steato-hepatitis	Long half-life Cirrhosis	Perhexilline Amiodarone
Acute hepatitis	Bridging necrosis Short term, acute Long term, chronic Active – hepatitis	Methyl dopa Isoniazid Halothane Ketoconazole
General hypersensitivity	Often with granulomas	Sulphonamides Quindine Allopurinol
Fibrosis	Portal hypertension Cirrhosis	Methotrexate Vinyl chloride Vitamin A
Cholestasis Canalicular	Dose dependent, reversible Reversible 'obstructive'	Sex hormones Chlorpromazine
Hepatocanalicular	Jaundice	Erythromycin Nitrofurantion Azathioprine Benoxprofen
Ductular Vascular	Age related Renal failure	
Veno-occlusive disease	Dose dependent	Irradiation Cytotoxics
Sinusoidal dilatation and Peliosis		Azathioprine Sex hormones
Hepatic vein obstruction	Thrombotic effect	Sex hormones
Portal vein obstruction Biliary	Thrombotic effect	Sex hormones
Sclerosing cholangitis	Cholestasis	Hepatic arterial FUDR
Gall bladder sludge Neoplastic	Biliary colic	Ceftriaxone
Focal nodular hyperplasia	Benign. Presents space-occupying lesion	Sex hormones
Adenoma	May rupture Usually regress	Sex hormones
Hepato-cellular carcinoma	Very rare Relatively benign	Danazol Sex and anabolic Hormones

is liver blood flow and indeed their clearance can be used to measure liver blood flow. Indocyanine green is one such drug. These drugs are usually highly lipid soluble. If liver blood flow falls, for instance due to cirrhosis or heat failure, the systemic effect of the high first-pass rate drug will be enhanced. Administration of drugs such as propranolol or cimetidine which lower hepatic blood flow will have a similar effect.

Because of its high first-pass uptake, a drug such as glyceryl trinitrate has to be given sublingually to avoid entry into the portal vein. Similarly, lignocaine has to be given intravenously.

Drugs with a low intrinsic clearance, such as theophylline, depend on enzyme function. Changes in hepatic blood flow have little effect. Plasma protein binding limits the presentation of the drug to hepatic enzymes. This will be affected by changes in the synthesis and degradation of plasma proteins.

METABOLISM OF DRUGS

The liver metabolizes virtually every drug or toxin introduced in the body. Most drugs are lipophilic soluble), enabling easy absorption across cell membranes. In the body, they are rendered hydrophilic (water soluble) by biochemical processes in the hepatocytes to enable inactivation and easy excretion. Metabolism of drugs occurs in 2 phases. In the phase 1 reaction, the drug is made polar by oxidation and hydroxylation. All drugs may not undergo this step, and some may directly undergo the phase 2.

The cytochrome P-450 enzymes catalyze phase 1 reactions. Most of these intermediate reactions are transient and highly reactive. These reactions may result in the formation of metabolites that are more toxic than the parent substrate and may result in liver injury. As an example, the metabolite of acetaminophen is N-acetyl-p-benzoquinone-imine (NAPQI) and is produced with ingestion of high doses of acetaminophen. NAPQI is responsible for the liver injury in such cases of toxicity. Cytochrome P-450 enzymes are hemoproteins located in the smooth endoplasmic reticulum of the liver. At least 50 enzymes have been identified, and based on structure; they are categorized into 10 groups; with groups 1, 2 and 3 b most important in drug metabolism. Each P-450 enzyme can metabolize many drugs. Drugs have the same P-450 specificity for biotransformation may competitively inhibit each other, resulting into interactions. Several drugs can induce and inhibit the P-450 enzyme.

Phase 2 reactions may occur within or outside the liver. They involve conjugation with a moiety (acetate, amino acid, sulfate, glutathione, glucuronic acid) that further increases solubility. Subsequently excrete the smaller molecules.

Drugs that induce and inhibit the P-450 enzymes are as follows:

- **Inducers**
  Phenobarbital, phenytoin, carbamazepine, primidone, ethanol, glucocorticoids, rifampin, griseofulvin, quinine, omeprazole - induced P-450.
- **Inhibitors**
  Amiodarone, cimetidine, erythromycin, grape fruit,

isoniazid, ketoconazole, metronidazole, sulfonamides, quinidine, omeprazole - inhibits P-450.

Hepatic Drug Metabolism

The main drug-metabolizing system resides in the microsomal fraction of the liver cell (smooth endoplasmic reticulum). The enzymes concerned are mixed function mono-oxygenases, cytochrome c-reductase and cytochrome P-450. Reduced NADPH in the cytosol is a co-factor. The drug is rendered more polar by hydroxylation or oxidation. Alternative phase I drug metabolizing reactions include the conversion of alcohol to acetaldehyde by alcohol dehydrogenases found mainly in the cytosolic fraction.

Enzyme inducers include barbiturates, alcohol, anesthetics, hypoglycemic and anticonvulsant agents, griseofulvin, rifampicin, glutethimide, phenylbutazone and meprobamate. Enlargement of the liver following the introduction of drug therapy can be related to enzyme induction.

This biotransformation involves conjugation of the drug or drug metabolite with a small endogenous molecule. The enzymes concerned are usually not confined to the liver, but are present there in high concentration.

Active transport: This system is located at the biliary pole of the hepatocyte. The mechanism is energy dependent and can be saturated.

Biliary and urinary excretion: Factors determining whether the metabolized drug will be excreted ultimately in bile or urine are multiple and many are unclear. Highly polar substances are excreted unaltered in the bile and also those which become more polar after conjugation. Those with a molecular weight exceeding 200 tend to be excreted in the bile. As the molecular weight falls, the urinary route becomes more important.

The P-450 System

Drug metabolism and the production of toxic metabolites are performed by the P-450 system of hemoproteins situated in the endoplasmic reticulum of the hepatocyte. At least 50 P-450s have been identified and there are undoubtedly more. Each P-450 protein is encoded by a unique gene. The human P-450s concerned with drug metabolism are members of the three families, P-450-I, P-450-II, and P-450-II. Each P-450 has a unique substrate binding site, capable of binding some, but not all, drugs. Each P-450 can metabolize many drugs. Genetic differences in the catalytic activity of the P-450s may determine idiosyncratic, untoward reactions to drugs. This is exemplified by the poor metabolism and debrisoquine (an anti-arrhythmic drug) due to abnormal expression of P-450-II-D6. This enzyme system also metabolizes most β-blockers and neuroleptics. Poor metabolism of debrisoquine can be identified by PCR amplification of parts of the mutant genes for cytochrome P-450-II-D6. This raises the possibility that in the future patients who will react abnormally to a drug can be identified.

P-450-II-E1 is involved in the production of electrophilic metabolites of acetaminophen.

P-450-III-A is concerned with the metabolism of cyclosporine and other drugs, especially erythromycin, steroids and ketoconazole. P-450-II-C polymorphism affects the metabolism of mephenytoin, diazepam and many other drugs.

Enzyme Induction and Drug Interactions

Enzyme induction, by increasing the P-450 enzymes leads to enhanced production of toxic metabolites. Expression of P-450s and induction by phenobarbitone are maintained in transplanted hepatocytes without reference to acinar position or zonal sinusoidal microenvironment.

Two active drugs competing for an enzyme binding site may lead to the drug with the lower affinity being metabolized more slowly and thus having a more prolonged action.

Table 87.2: Characteristics of some human liver P-450s

P-450	Drug substrates	Probable inducers
I-A1	Carcinogens	Omeprazole
I-A2	Caffeine Theophylline	Cigarette smoke Acetaminophen
II-C*	Mephenytoin Tienylic acid Diazepam Tolbutamide Phenylbutazone	None identified
II-D*	Debrisoquine Most beta-blockers Many neuroleptics Encainide Codeine	None identified
II-E1	Acetaminophen Ethanol	Ethanol Isoniazid
III*	Cyclosporin A Erythromycin Ketoconazole Nifedipine Estrogens Midazolam/triazolam Lidocaine	Anti-seizure medications Rifampicin Glucocorticoids

** Multiple subfamily members exist which may have differing catalytic properties and regulation.*

Ethanol induces P-450-II-E1 and so enhances the toxicity of acetaminophen similarly, patients treated with isoniazid which also induces P-450-II-E1 have increased acetaminophen toxicity.

P-450-III-A which metabolizes cyclosporine is induced by rifampicin and steroids. This explains the reduced blood cyclosporine levels when these drugs are given. Cyclosporin, F506, erythromycin and ketoconazole compete for binding and metabolism by P-450-III-A and cyclosporine levels rise after they are given.

Omeprazole induces P-450-I-A. This is important in the biotransformation of procarcinogens, carcinogens and many drugs. An increased tendency to malignancy after omeprazole is possible.

In the future, it should be possible to determine P-450 profiles and detect those likely to develop an adverse drug reaction. Selective inhibitors or inducers may be used to alter the P-450.

Risk Factors for Drug-Induced Liver Injury

- *Race:* Some drugs appear to have different toxicities based on race. For example, blacks Hispanics may be more susceptible to isoniazid (INH) toxicity. The rate of metabolism is control of P-450 enzymes and can vary from individual to individual.
- *Age:* Apart from accidental exposure, hepatic drug reactions are rare in children. Elderly are at increased risk of hepatic injury because of decreased clearance, drug-to-drug inter; reduced hepatic blood flow, variation in drug binding, and lower hepatic volume. In addition diet, infections, and multiple hospitalizations are important reasons for drug-induced hepatotoxicity.
- *Sex:* Although the reasons are unknown, hepatic drug reactions are more common in females.
- *Alcohol ingestion:* Alcoholic persons are susceptible to drug toxicity because alcohol induced injury and cirrhotic changes that alter drug metabolism. Alcohol causes depletion of glutathione (hepatoprotective) stores that make the person more susceptible to toxicity by drugs.
- *Liver disease:* In general, patients with chronic liver disease are not uniformly at increased risk to hepatic injury. Although the total cytochrome P-450 is reduced, some may be affected more others. The modification of doses in persons with liver disease should be based on the knowledge of the specific enzyme involved in the metabolism. Patients with HIV infection who are co-infected with hepatitis B or C virus are at increased risk for hepatotoxic effects when treated with antiretroviral therapy. Similarly, patients with cirrhosis are at increased risk of decompensation to toxic drugs.
- *Genetic factors:* A unique gene encodes each P-450 protein. Genetic differences in the P-450. Enzymes can result in abnormal reactions to drugs, including idiosyncratic reactions. Debrisoquine is an antiarrhythmic drug that undergoes poor metabolism because of abnormal expression of P-450-II-D6. This can be identified by polymerase chain reaction amplification mutant genes. This has led to the possibility of future detection of persons who can have abnormal reactions to a drug.
- *Other co-morbidities:* Persons with AIDS, persons who are malnourished, and persons who are fasting may be susceptible to drug reactions because of low glutathione stores.
- *Drug formulation:* Long-acting drugs may cause more injury than shorter-acting drugs.
- Host factors that may enhance susceptibility to drugs, possibly inducing liver disease:
  - Female - Halothane, Nitrofurantion, sulindac
  - Male - Amoxicillin-clavulanic acid (Augmentin)
  - Old age - Acetaminophen, halothane, INH, amoxicillin-clavulanic acid
  - Young age Salicylates, valproic acid
  - Fasting or malnutrition - Acetaminophen
  - Large body mass index/obesity - Halothane
  - Diabetes mellitus - Methotrexate, niacin
  - Renal failure - Tetracycline, allopurinol
  - AIDS-Dapsone, trimethoprim-sulfamethoxazole
  - Hepatitis C - Ibuprofen, ritonavir, flutamide
  - Preexisting liver disease - Niacin, tetracycline, methotrexate.

PATHOPHYSIOLOGY AND MECHANISMS OF DRUG-INDUCED LIVER INJURY

- *Pathophysiologic mechanisms:* The pathophysiologic mechanisms of hepatotoxicity are explored and include both hepatocellular and extracellular mechanisms. The following are the list of mechanisms that have been described.
- *Disruption of the hepatocytes:* Covalent binding of the drug to intracellular proteins cause a decrease in ATP levels, leading to actin disruption. Due to disassembly of actin the surface of the hepatocytes causes blebs and rupture of the membrane.
- *Disruption of the transport proteins:* Drugs that affect transport proteins at the canalicular membrane can interrupt bile flow. Loss of villous processes and interruption of transmembrane pumps such as multidrug resistance-associated protein 3 prevent the excretion of bile causing cholestasis.
- *Cytolytic T-cell activation:* Covalent binding of a drug to the P-450 enzyme acts as an immunogen, activating T cells and cytokines and stimulating a multifaceted immunological response.
- *Apoptosis of hepatocytes:* Activation of the apoptotic pathways by the tumor necrosis factor-alpha receptor of fats may trigger the cascade of intercellular cascades, which results in programmed cell death.
- *Mitochondrial disruption:* Certain drugs inhibit mitochondrial function by a dual effect both beta-oxidation energy production by inhibiting the synthesis of nicotinamide and dinucleotide and flavin adenine dinucleotide, resulting in decreased ATP production.
- *Bile duct injury:* Toxic metabolites excreted in bile may cause injury to the bile duct epithelium.

- **Drug toxicity mechanisms:** The classic division of drug reactions is into at least 2 major groups (1) drugs that directly affect the liver and (2) drugs that mediate an immune response.
  - *Intrinsic or predictable drug reactions:* Drugs that fall into this category cause reproduction injuries in animals, and the injury is dose related. The injury can be due to the drug or to a metabolite. Acetaminophen is a classic example of a known intrinsic or predicted hepatotoxin at supertherapeutic doses. Another classic example is carbon tetrachloride.
  - *Idiosyncratic drug reactions:* Idiosyncratic drug reactions can be classified as hypersensitivity or immunoallergic and those that are metabolic idiosyncratic.
    i. *Hypersensitivity:* Phenytoin is a classical example, if not common, cause of hypersensitivity reactions. The response is characterized by fever, rash, and eosinophilia and immune-related response with a typical short latency period of 1-4 weeks.
    ii. *Metabolic-idiosyncratic:* This type of reaction occurs through an indirect method of the offending drug. Unlike intrinsic hepatotoxins, the response rate is varied and can occur within a week or up to one year later. It occurs in a minority of patients taking the drug, and no clinical manifestations of hypersensitivity are noted.

Immunological Hepatotoxicity

The metabolite may act as a hapten with cell protein so inducing immunological liver injury. The P-450s can be involved. Several P-450 isoenzymes are present and inducible on the membranes of hepatocytes and immunization against them might lead to immunological destruction of the liver cell.

Patients with halothane hepatitis have serum antibodies that recognize halothane-altered liver microsomal proteins.

An idiosyncratic reaction to the diuretic, tienilic acid is associated with auto antibodies that react with both liver and kidney microsomes (anti-LKM-II). The antigen recognized is within the P-450-II-C family which is also involved in the metabolism of tienilic acid.

Mitochondrial Cytopathies

Some drugs seem to have a predominant effect on mitochondrial function causing inhibition of respiratory chain enzymes. Clinically they are marked by vomiting and apathy. Lactic acidosis, hypoglycemia and metabolic acidosis are seen. Mitochondrial β-oxidation of fatty acids is associated with micro vesicular fatty liver. Electron microscopy shows mitochondrial damage. The diseases are multi-system.

Steato-Hepatitis

The reaction termed non-alcoholic steato- hepatitis (NASH) histologically resembles acute alcoholic hepatitis with sometimes, in addition, electron microscopical evidence of lysosomal phospholipidosis. Mallory's hyaline is found in zone 3 in distinction to true alcoholic hepatitis.

Fibrosis

Fibrosis forms part of most drug reactions, but in some it may be the predominant feature. The fibrous tissue is deposited in the Disse space, where it obstructs sinusoidal blood flow, causing non-cirrhotic portal hypertension and hepato-cellular dysfunction. The lesion is related to toxic drug metabolites and is usually in zone 3, an exception being methotrexate where the damage is in zone 1.

Vascular

Sinusoidal dilatation

Focal dilatation of zone 1 sinusoids may complicate contraceptive or anabolic steroid therapy. This can cause hepatomegaly and abdominal pain with rises in serum enzymes. Hepatic arteriography shows stretched, attenuated branches of the hepatic artery with a patchy parenchymal pattern where areas of contrast alternate with areas not well filled. The condition regresses on stopping the hormone.

A similar change may complicate azathioprine given after renal transplantation and this may be followed 1-3 years later by fibrosis and cirrhosis.

Peliosis hepatitis

The large blood-filled cavities may or may not be lined with sinusoidal cells. They are distributed randomly, the diameter varying from 1 mm to several cm. Electron microscopy shows passage of red blood cells through the endothelial barrier and perisinusoidal fibrosis may develop. These alterations might constitute the primary event.

Veno-occlusive disease (VOD)

Small, zone 3 hepatic veins are particularly sensitive to toxic damage, reacting by sub endothelial edema and subsequent collagenization. The disease was originally described from Jamaica due to toxic injury to the minute hepatic veins by pytrolizidine alkaloids taken as senesced in medicinal bush teas. It has since been described from India, Israel, Egypt and even Arizona. It has been related to contamination of wheat.

The disease is marked by an acute stage with painful hepatomegaly, ascites and inconspicuous jaundice. The patient may recover, die or pass into a sub-acute stage of hepatomegaly and recurrent ascites. The chronic type resembles any other cirrhosis. Diagnosis is made by liver biopsy.

Azathioprine induces endothelialitis. Its long-term use in kidney and liver transplant recipients is associated with sinusoidal dilatation, peliosis, VOD and nodular regenerative hyperplasia. *Cytotoxic therapy* especially with cyclophosphamide BNCU, azathioprine, busulphan, VP-16 and total body irradiation exceeding 12 Gy are associated with VOD. VOD follows high-dose cytoreductive therapy in bone marrow recipients. There is widespread damage to zone 3 structures including hepatocytes, sinusoids and particularly small hepatic venules. It is marked by jaundice, painful hepatomegaly and weight gain (ascites). In 25% of patients it is severe with death occurring within 100 days.

Hepatic irradiation: The liver has a low tolerance to radiotherapy. Radiation hepatitis increases when doses reach or exceed 35 Gy to the whole organ delivered as 10 Gy a week. VOD appears 1-3 months after completion of therapy. It may be transient or death may ensue from liver failure. Histologically, zone 3 hemorrhage is seen with hepatic venules showing fibrosis and obliteration.

Hepatic vein occlusion (Budd-Chiari syndrome) has been reported following oral contraceptive, and after azathioprine in a renal transplant patient.

Acute Hepatitis

Only a very small proportion of patients taking the drug will have the reaction. There is usually no method of predicting who would be susceptible. The reaction is unrelated to dose but is more common after multiple exposures. The onset is delayed about 1 week after exposure.

The pre-icteric period of gastrointestinal symptoms resembles acute hepatitis and is followed by jaundice associated with pale stools and dark urine and an enlarged tender liver. Biochemical tests indicate hepatocellular damage. Serum γ-globulins are increased.

In those who recover, maximum serum bilirubin levels are reached after 2-3 weeks. The more seriously affected show a shrinking liver and die of hepatic failure. The mortality is high for those that are clinically recognized, higher than for sporadic virus hepatitis. If hepatic precoma or coma is reached the mortality is 70%.

Hepatic histology may be virtually indistinguishable from acute virus hepatitis. Milder cases show spotty necrosis becoming more extensive and reaching a stage of diffuse liver injury and collapse. Bridging is frequent; inflammatory infiltration is variable. Chronic hepatitis may sometimes be a sequel. The drugs causing this type of reaction may do so by the production of toxic metabolites injurious to the liver *per se* or the metabolite may act as a hapten with cell protein, so inducing immunological liver injury.

An enormous number of drugs cause this hepatic reaction. They may emerge only after the drug has been released on the general market. Specialist textbooks should be consulted for individual drugs. Isoniazid, methyl dopa and halothane are described in detail, but any drug should be suspected. An individual drug can cause more than one reaction and there may be overlap between acute hepatic, cholestatic and hypersensitivity reactions.

The reactions tend to be severe, particularly if the drug is continued after liver damage has started. Patients with acute, fulminant drug-related liver failure must be considered for hepatic transplantation. Corticosteroids are of doubtful benefit.

Older women are at particular risk, whereas the reactions are unusual in children

Chronic Hepatitis

The picture strikingly resembles 'autoimmune' chronic hepatitis in clinical, biochemical, serological and his logical features. The patients recover when the drug is withdrawn. Anti-organelle antibodies have been found a number of patients.

Chronic hepatitis was first described following the laxative oxyphenisatin and this has now been withdrawn from most parts of the world. Chronic active hepatitis can develop insidiously after many years of methyl dopa therapy and without an acute episode. Improvement follows withdrawal of the drug.

Nitrofurantion may be related to chronic hepatitis, usually in women, 4 weeks to 11 years after starting.

Other causes include *clometacin, fenofibrate, isoniazid, papaverine, minocyclin* and *dantrolene.* Minocyclin can cause a picture resembling autoimmune chronic hepatitis.

General Hypersenstivity

A large number of drugs cause hepatic reactions of 'hypersensitivity' type of variable severity and with or without jaundice, rash, arthritis, hemolytic anemia and eosinophilia. Sometimes the picture resembles infectious mononucleosis. The reaction usually appears within 4 weeks of starting therapy and is most frequent with multiple exposures. Challenge is usually positive. There is considerable overlap with the acute hepatitis and hepatocanalicular groups. Liver histology shows focal, spotty necrosis of liver cells, with a mononuclear and sometimes eosinophilic reaction in the portal zones. Granulomas are sometimes found.

Canalicular Cholestasis

Various *androgens* and *estrogen* steroids can cause canalicular cholestasis. Estrogens contained in contraceptive pills are good examples but cholestasis is decreasing with reduction in the content of active ingredients. The estrogen is the important agent, although the progestin may augment the effect. Bile salt independent bile flow is reduced probably through suppression of N a+K-ATPase activity. Sinusoidal membranes become less fluid. Peri-cellulalar permeability (tight junctions) may be increased cytoskeleton is affected with failure of the peri-canalicular micro-filaments to contract.

The cause is usually, but not always, a C17-alkylated testosterone. The reaction is dose-dependent and reversible even if large doses have been taken over many years. This type of cholestasis is also seen with nor-ethandrolone, methyl testosterone, norandrostenolone, stanozolol, megesterol and danazol.

The patient suffers from itching with variable bilirubinaemia. Serum transaminases values are variable but in about one-third may exceed five times normal. Serum alkaline phosphatase may be disproportionately low.

Liver biopsy shows normal architecture and zone 3 cholestasis with surrounding reaction. *Electron microscopy* shows cholestasis and mild hepatocellular damage.

Prognosis is excellent. Rarely jaundice is severe and prolonged but usually the patient recovers when the drug is stopped. Recurrence is liable to follow resumption.

Hepato-Canalicular Cholestasis

Here the reaction is predominantly cholestatic but, in addition, hepato-cellular features are present. In many, immunological liver injury is suggested. There is an overlap with hypersensitivity and hepatic drug reactions.

The cholestatic reaction is usually mild but can be severe and prolonged lasting many months or even years.

Acute cholangitis in the early stages is followed by the chronic phase of ductopenia defined by the absence of interlobular bile ducts in at least 50% of small portal tracts. Recovery is usual, but occasionally, hepatic transplantation is indicated.

Many drugs cause cholestasis. The penicillin derivatives (Augmentin, Flucloxacin), lphonomides (Septrin, Bactrim), the erythromycins, promazines and procarbazine are particularly important.

Ductular Cholestasis

The bile ducts and canaliculi are filled with dense, inspissated bile casts without any surrounding inflammatory reaction. The plugs contain bilirubin, probably in combination with a drug metabolite. The picture has been particularly associated with *benoxyprofen,* which has a half-life of 30 hours in the young, but 111 hours in the elderly. Generalized poisoning by the drug and its metabolites seems likely. Benoxyprofen has now been withdrawn.

Biliary Sludge

This complicates treatment with the antibiotic, *ceftriaxone*. The patient may be symptom-free or suffer reversible biliary colic. It is dose-dependent. Sludging is related to sharing a common pathway with bile acids for hepatic transport and also to add interaction with biliary lipid excretion. The sludge consists of a small amount of cholesterol and bilirubin but the major component is the calcium salt of ceftriaxone.

Sclerosing Cholangitis

Causes include hepatic arterial infusion of cytotoxic drugs such as 5-fluorouridine, thiabendazole caustics introduced into hydatid cysts and the Spanish toxic oil syndrome.

Bile duct stricture can follow 10 years after upper abdominal *radiotherapy.*

Hepatic Tumors

The association of hepatic adenoma, a hitherto very rare benign tumor, with oral contraceptives was first suggested in 1973. It is rare but the risk increases dramatically with duration of use, particularly after 48 months. The incidence is falling with the use of pills containing smaller amounts of hormone.

Familial adenomas have been described, where sufferers have never taken oral contraceptives.

Adenomas have been induced by norethisterone in patients of renal dialysis.

Table 87.3: Summary of pathological manifestations of drug-induced hepatotoxicity

- Acute hepatocellular injury
- Acute viral hepatitis-like picture - INH, halothane, diclofenac, troglitazone
- Mononucleosis like picture - Phenytoin, sulfonamides, dapsone
- Chronic hepatocellular injury - Pemoline, methyldopa
- Massive necrosis - Acetaminophen, halothane, diclofenac
- Steatosis
  - Macro vesicular steatosis - Alcohol, methotrexate, corticosteroids, minocycline, nifedipine, TPN
  - Micro vesicular steatosis - Alcohol, valproic acid, tetracycline, piroxicam
  - Steatohepatitis - Amiodarone, nifedipine, synthetic estrogens, didanosine
- Pseudo alcoholic injury - Amiodarone
- Acute cholestasis - Amoxicillin-clavulanic acid, erythromycin, sulindac
- Chronic cholestasis - Chlorpromazine, sulfamethoxazole-trimethoprim, tetracycline and ibuprofen
- Granulomatous hepatitis - Carbamazepine, allopurinol, hydralazine
- Vascular injury - Steroids
- Neoplasia - Contraceptives, anabolic steroids
- Adenoma - Steroids
- Angiosarcoma - Vinyl chloride
- Hepatocellular carcinoma - Anabolic steroids, aflatoxin, arsenic, vinyl chloride

CLINICAL AND PATHOLOGICAL MANIFESTATIONS OF DRUG-INDUCED LIVER DISEASE

Drug hepatotoxicity manifests with clinical signs and symptoms caused by an underlying pathologic injury. The clinical presentation may or may not suggest the underlying liver injury, and therefore the types of injuries are sometimes described separately. Some drugs usually can cause one clinical and pathologic injury and other drugs can cause a variety of injuries, often making the diagnosis more challenging.

Clinical Manifestations

The manifestations of drug-induced hepatotoxicity are highly variable, ranging from asymptomatic elevation of liver enzymes to fulminant hepatic failure. The injury may suggest a hepatocellular injury with elevation of aminotransferase levels as the predominant symptom, or a cholestatic injury, with elevated alkaline phosphatase levels (with or without hyperbilirubinemia) being the main feature. In addition, drugs that cause mild aminotransferase elevations with subsequent adaptation are differentiated from those that result in true toxicity that require discontinuation.

- Asymptomatic elevations in aminotransferase: Some drugs cause asymptomatic elevation of liver enzymes that do not progress despite continued use of the drug.
  - This tolerance is also observed in 25-50% of the patients taking drugs such as phenytoin, and it is especially well described with INH.
  - 5-Hydroxy-3-methylglutaryl-coenzyme A (HMG-CoA) reductase inhibitors are also associated with a mild elevation in enzyme levels in less than 5% of cases. Other drugs include sulfonamides, salicylates, sulfonylureas, and quinidine. If the clinician is not familiar with the drug or if any question remains about the safe continuing a drug, consultation with a hepatologist should be considered.
- Elevated aminotransferase levels with acute hepatocellular injury: Drug-induced liver injury is designated hepatocellular if the ALT levels are increased to more than twice the upper limit of reference range, with alkaline phosphatase levels that are within the reference range or minimally elevated. Elevation of aspartate aminotransferase (AST) greater than ALT, especially more than 2 times greater, suggests alcoholic hepatitis. Elevation of AST less than ALT is observed in persons with viral hepatitis. In viral and drug-induced hepatitis, the AST and ALT levels steadily increase and peak in the low thousands range within 7-14 days. Many drugs can cause increases in AST, such as acetaminophen, NSAIDs, ACE inhibitors, nicotinic acid, INH, sulfonamides, erythromycin, and antifungal agents such as griseofulvin and fluconazole, acetaminophen overdose, transaminases levels greater than 10,000 IUIL are also noted.
- Elevated aminotransferase and bilirubin levels suggestive of subfulminant or fulminant necrosis.

  With increasing hepatocellular injury, bilirubin levels are invariably increased, suggest worse prognosis. Normally, the total bilirubin level is less than 1.1 mg/dL and approximately 70% is indirect (unconjugated) bilirubin. Unconjugated hyperbilirubinemia (>80% of the total bilirubin is indirect) suggests hemolysis or Gilbert syndrome. Conjugated hyperbilirubinemia (>50% of the total bilirubin is direct) suggests hepatocellular injury or cholestasis. When the bilirubin level is above 25-30 mg/dL, extrahepatic cholestasis an unlikely diagnosis; because the predominantly conjugated bilirubin is water soluble easily excreted by the kidney in extrahepatic cholestasis. Subfulminant hepatic failure most commonly results from acetaminophen, halothane methoxyflurane, enflurane, trovafloxacin, troglitazone, Ketoconazole, dihydralazine: mushroom poisoning, ferrous sulfate poisoning, phosphorus poisoning, and cocaine toxicity. Drugs that result in massive necrosis are propylthiouracil, INH, phenytoin, phenelzine, sertraline, naproxen, diclofenac, kava kava, and ecstasy.
- Elevated alkaline phosphatase (acute cholestatic injury) levels: Acute intrahepatic cholestatic injury divisible into 2 broad categories, (1) cholestasis without hepatocellular injury (pure cholestasis) and (2) cholestasis with variable hepatocyte injury.
  - The most common biochemical abnormality is elevation of the alkaline phosphate the usually without hyperbilirubinemia. Men and older patients are more prone to these adverse effects. The interval of developments is usually less than 4 weeks and may long as 8 weeks. Fever, rash, and eosinophilia may be observed in as many as 30% individuals, but these findings do not define the disorder.
  - Some common drugs associated with cholestatic injury include chlorpromazine, ciprofloxacin, ofloxacin, cimetidine, phenytoin, naproxen, captopril, erythromycin, azithromycin, and dicloxacillin. Amoxicillin-clavulanic acid is also an important cause cholestatic jaundice. Extrahepatic cholestasis secondary to biliary sludge or calculi caused by sulindac or octreotide.
- Extrahepatic manifestations: Some drugs cause systemic reactions. Extrahepatic manifestations of drug-induced hepatotoxicity are as follows:
  - Chlorpromazine, phenylbutazone, halogenated anesthetic agents, sulindac - Fever eosinophilia.
  - Dapsone - Sulfone syndrome (i.e., fever, rash, anemia, jaundice).
  - INH, halothane - Acute viral hepatitis.
- Chlorpromazine, erythromycin, amoxicillin-clavulanic acid - Obstructive jaundice.
- Phenytoin, carbamazepine, phenobarbital, primidone - Anticonvulsant hypersensitivity syndrome (i.e., triad of fever, rash and liver injury).
  - Para-amino salicylates, phenytoin, sulfonamides - Serum sickness syndrome.

– Clofibrate - Muscular syndrome (i.e., myalgia, stiffness, weakness, elevated creation level).
– Procainamide - Antinuclear antibodies (ANAs).
– Gold salts, propylthiouracil, chlorpromazine, chloramphenicol - Marrow injury.
– Amiodarone, Nitrofurantion - Associated pulmonary injury.
– Gold salts, methoxyflurane, penicillamine, paraquat - Associated renal injury.
– Tetracycline - Fatty liver of pregnancy.
– Contraceptive and anabolic steroids, rifampin - Bland jaundice.
– Aspirin - Reye syndrome.

• Sodium valproate - Reye like syndrome.

Diagnosis

When a single agent is involved, the diagnosis may be relatively simple. But, with multiple agents, arriving at the the cause is difficult. In order to facilitate the diagnosis of drug-induced hepatic injury, several clinical tools have been developed to assist the clinician.

- *History:* History must include dose, route of administration, duration, previous administration concomitant drugs, including over-the-counter medications and herbs. Knowing whether the same drug before may be helpful. The latent period of idiosyncratic drug reactions is higher. The history of every drug ingested in the past 3 months is essential.
  – Onset: The onset is usually within 5-90 days of starting the drug.
  – Exclusion of other causes of liver injury/cholestasis: Excluding other causes of liver damage.
- *Dechallenge:* A positive dechallenge is a 50% fall in serum transaminases levels within 8 days. The positive dechallenge is very helpful in cases of use of multiple medications.
- *Track record of the drug:* Previously documented reactions to a drug aid in diagnosis.
- *Rechallenge:* Deliberate rechallenge in clinical situations is unethical and should not be allowed the rechallenge in the past has provided valuable evidence that the drug was indeed hepatotoxic.

Table 87.4: Differential diagnosis

Acute viral hepatitis	Autoimmune hepatitis
Shock liver	Cholecystisis
Cholangitis	Budd-Chiari syndrome
Alcoholic liver disease	Cholestatic liver disease
Pregnancy-related conditions of liver	Malignancy
Wilson's disease	Hemochromatosis
Coagulation disorders	

WORKUP

Laboratory Studies

Performing laboratory tests to assess and diagnose the effects of the suspected medication is essential. The complete blood cell count, basic metabolic profile, and urinalysis. Patients with a hepatocellular injury have disproportionate elevation in serum aminotransferase levels compared with alkaline phosphatase while cholestasis has the opposite findings. Hepatitis B serology (hepatitis B surface antigen, anti-hepatitis B, anti-hepatitis B core antibody, hepatitis C serology) and hepatitis A serology (anti-hepatitis A) are performed to exclude an infectious etiology. ANA testing may help in cases of possible autoimmune hepatitis.

Hepatic function tests and their interpretations are as follows:

- Bilirubin (total) - To diagnose jaundice and assess severity.
- Bilirubin (unconjugated) - To assess for hemolysis.
- Alkaline phosphatase - To diagnose cholestasis and infiltrative disease.
- AST/serum glutamic oxaloacetic transaminase (SGOT).
- To diagnose hepatocellular disease. ALT/serum glutamate pyruvate transaminase (SGPT) - Albumin - To assess severity of liver injury (HIV infection and malnutrition may confound) Gamma globulin - Large elevations suggestive of autoimmune hepatitis.
- Prothrombin time after vitamin K - To assess severity of liver disease. Antimitochondrial antibody - To diagnose primary biliary cirrhosis.
- ASMA - To diagnose primary sclerosing cholangitis.

Imaging Studies

Imaging studies are used to exclude causes of liver pathology, after which a diagnosis can be made.

- *Ultrasonography:* Ultrasonography is inexpensive compared with CT scanning and MRI. Ultrasonography is effective to evaluate the gall bladder, bile ducts, and hepatic lesions.
- *CT scanning:* CT scanning can help to detect focal hepatic lesions 1 cm or larger and sometimes can be used to visualize adjacent structures in the abdomen.
- *MRI:* MRI provides excellent contrast resolution. It can be used to detect cysts, hemangiomas and secondary tumors. The portal vein, hepatic veins, and biliary tract can be visualized.

Procedures

- *Liver biopsy:* Histopathologic evaluation remains an important tool in diagnosis.

Treatment

Treatment of toxic and drug induced-hepatic disease is largely supportive, except in acetaminophen hepatoxi-city. Acute poisoning is treated by a high calorie, high carbohydrate diet and along the usual lines for acute hepatorenal failure including dialysis. In patients with fulminant hepatitis resulting from drug hepatoxicity, liver transplantation may be live saving. Withdrawal of the suspected agent is indicated at the first sign of an adverse reaction. In the case of the direct toxins, liver involvement should not divert attention from renal or other organ involvement, which may also threaten survival. Corticosteroids may have a role in immune mediated disease. Glucocorticoids for drug hepatotoxicity with allergic features, silibinin for hepatotoxic mushroom poisoning, urodeoxycholic acid for cholestatic drug hepatotoxicity have never been shown to be effective and are not recommended.

Acetaminophen Hepatotoxicity

Acetaminophen is the most widely used analgesic and antipyretic, in part because of the finding of relationship between Reye syndrome and salicylates. Consequently, acetaminophen is commonly ingested by young children or taken in an intentional overdose by adolescents.

Pathophysiology

Acetaminophen toxicity results from the formation of highly reactive intermediate metabolite, N-acetyl-p-benzoquinoneimine (NAPQ1). When therapeutic doses are administered, only a small amount (4%) of a dose is metabolized by hepatic cytochrome P-450 enzymes to NAPQ1,which is immediately conjugated with glutathione to form a harmless mercapturic acid conjugate. When hepatic stores of glutathione are depleted to less than 70% of normal, the NAPQI metabolite can combine with hepatic macromolecules to produce hepatocellular damage. The acute toxic dose of acetaminophen is generally considered to be more than 200 mg/kg in children younger than 12 years. A single ingestion of more than 7.5 g is considered a minimum toxic dose in adolescents and adults. Repeated administration of acetaminophen at doses exceeding those recommended may lead to hepatic injury or failure in some children. Parents should be advised to follow closely the manufacturer's dosing guidelines and be aware of its presence in combination products.

Children younger than 6 years are unlikely to develop significant toxicity after a single ingestion of even relatively large doses of acetaminophen. Nevertheless, at this time, children with a significant ingestion should have their plasma acetaminophen level measured and receive treatment with N-acetylcysteine (NAC) if the level falls within the toxic range on the nomogram. Adolescents have a higher incidence of toxic plasma levels after ingestion than do children. Even if a serous case of hepatotoxicity develops, the mortality rate is less than 0.5%. Patients who recover have no sequelae when observed 3-12 months after the acute toxicity. Severely affected patients may require liver transplantation.

Clinical and Laboratory Manifestations

If untreated, patients who have acutely overdosed pass through four stages of toxicity (Table 87.5). Because early symptoms are nonspecific, physicians may fail to diagnose the ingestion without a good history or high index of suspicion. If a toxic ingestion is suspected, a plasma acetaminophen level should be measured 4 hours or more may be used to determine if ingestion has occurred, but cannot be used to determine the severity of an overdose. Liver function studies including enzymes, bilirubin, and prothrombin time should be followed daily in all patients with acetaminophen levels falling within the toxic range on the nomogram.

Table 87.5: Stages in the clinical course of acetaminophen toxicity

Stage	*Time After Ingestion*	*Characteristics*
I.	½- 24 hours	Anorexia, nausea, vomiting, malaise, pallor, diaphoresis.
II.	24 – 48 hours	Resolution of above, right upper quadrant abdominal pain and tenderness, elevated bilirubin, prothrombin time, hepatic enzymes, oliguria.
III.	72 – 96 hours	Peak liver function abnormalities, anorexia, nausea, vomiting, malaise may reappear.
IV.	4 days - 2 weeks	Resolution of hepatic dysfunction or complete liver failure.

Treatment

After large acute overdose, when the need for antidotal treatment is anticipated and when treatment can be started within 1-2 hours of the ingestion, activated charcoal administration should be considered. The antidote for acetaminophen poisoning is N-acetylcysteine (NAC or Mucomyst). NAC serves as a precursor for glutathione synthesis, thus replenishing glutathione stores and preventing the reaction of NAPQI with hepatocytes. NAC therapy should be initiated as soon as possible after ingestion but may have value even started 24-36 hours after the ingestion in severe cases. The dose of NAC is 140 mg/kg loading followed by 70 mg/kg qid for 17 doses. The route is oral. The common side effects of this drug are nausea and vomiting. NAC is unpalatable and irritating to the gastrointestinal tract and should be diluted to a 5% solution with soda or fruit juice to minimize vomiting. Antiemetics may be used to control vomiting or NAC may be given directly into the stomach or upper intestine by tube. An intravenous preparation of NAC should soon be available.

Prognosis

The prognosis of drug or toxin induced liver injury depends on its type and severity. Injury is usually completely reversible when the hepatoxic factor is withdrawn. The mortality of sub massive hepatic necrosis with fulminant liver failure may, however exceed 50%. With continued use of certain drugs, such as methotrexate, effects of hepatoxicity may proceed insidiously to cirrhosis. Neoplasia may follow long-term androgen therapy. Rechallenge with a drug suspected of having caused previous liver injury is rarely justified and may result in fatal hepatic hepatic necrosis.

Drugs Withdrawn from the Market Secondary to Hepatotoxicity

In the last few years, the US Food and Drug Administration (FDA) have withdrawn 2 drugs from the market for causing severe liver injury: bromfenac and troglitazone. Bromfenac (Duract), a nonsteroidal anti-inflammatory drug (NSAID), was introduced in 1997 as a short-term analgesic for orthopedic patients. Although approved for a dosing period of less than 10 days, patients used it for longer period. This resulted in more than 50 cases of severe hepatic injury, and the drug had to be withdrawn in USA. Troglitazone (Rezulin) is a thiazolidinedione and was approved in 1997 as an antidiabetic agent. In 5 years, more than 90 cases of hepatotoxicity were reported, which resulted in withdrawal of this drug.

Recently, kava kava, a herb used for anxiety, was reported as being hepatotoxic and was withdrawn from the German market. The FDA has also issued a warning in this country. This demonstrates importance of post marketing surveillance to identify reactions that are not reported or are under drug trials.

Pemoline (Cylert), used for attention deficit disorder and narcolepsy is no longer available in the States. The Food and Drug Administration (FDA) concluded that the overall risk of liver toxicity from pemoline outweighs the benefits. In May 2005, Abbott chose to stop sales and marketing of their of pemoline (Cylert) in the U.S. In October 2005, all companies that produced generic versions of pemoline also agreed to stop sales and marketing of pemoline.

Other drugs that have significant limitations of use because of their hepatotoxic effects are felbamate (Felbatol), an antiepileptic used for complex partial seizures; zileuton (Zyflo) [indicated for asthma] tolcapone (Tasmar), used for Parkinson disease; trovafloxacin (Trovan), an antibiotic and tienlic acid, a diuretic.

CONCLUSIONS

Before marketing a new drug, testing must be done on both an acute and chronic basis and on more than one species or strain. Both the drug and its known metabolites must be used. The albumin-binding properties of the drug must be noted. The role of the drug as a hepatic enzyme-inducer must be studied. Clinical trials must include regular pre- and post-treatment estimations of serum bilirubin and transaminases levels. A needle liver biopsy, after informed consent, is particularly helpful in establishing the relation between a drug and liver injury and in determining the type of injury.

The serum transaminases may rise during the first 4 weeks of therapy only to subside despite the drug being continued. When a hepatic reaction is possible, as with isoniazid, it is wise to check serum transaminases 3 and 4 weeks after commencing treatment. If more than three times increased, the drug should be stopped. If less, a further value is taken 1 week later when an increase is an indication for stopping the drug. Continuance of therapy once a hepatic reaction has commenced is the most common cause of a fatal outcome.

The safety of a drug which causes transient rises in transaminases and apparently no other hepatic effect remains obscure. Many valuable drugs in widespread use fall into this category. In many instances, challenge is the only method of linking a drug with a hepatic reaction, but if its consequence is likely to be serious, this is ethically impossible. However, reporting agencies and drug manufacturers should pay particular attention to the results of inadvertent challenge and to the effects of withdrawing the drug (de-challenge).

Intake of a drug, such as paracetamol, within the therapeutic range, may cause liver injury if the patient is ingesting another drug such as alcohol which by enzyme induction increases the production of hepatotoxic metabolites.

An iatrogenic cause must be considered in any patient presenting with any clinical pattern of hepato-biliary disease. This is particularly so with a picture suggesting viral hepatitis in a middle aged or elderly patient, especially a woman. In the absence of evidence supporting genuine viral hepatitis, the cause is very frequently drug related.

KEY LEARNING POINTS

- Drugs are capable of causing toxic effects mimicking almost every naturally-occurring liver disease.
- Liver metabolizes virtually every drug, biochemical processes in the hepatocytes render drugs hydrophilic (water soluble) to enable inactivation and easy excretion.
- Drug metabolism and production of toxic metabolites are performed by P_{450} system of hemoproteins situated in the endoplasmic reticulum of the hepatocytes.
- Manifestations of drug-induced hepatotoxicity are

highly variable, ranging from asymptomatic elevation of liver enzymes to fulminant hepatic failure.
- Prognosis of drug-induced liver injury depends on its type and severity.

FURTHER READINGS

1. Aithal PG, Day CP. The natural history of histologically proved drug-induced liver disease. *Gut* 1999; 44:731-735.
2. Alisan MR, Sarraf CE. Liver cell death: Patterns and mechanics. *Gut*1994; 35:577-581
3. Benichou C. Criteria for drug induced liver disorder. Report of an international consensus meeting. *Hepatology* 1990; 11:272-276.
4. Bissell DM *et al.:* Drug induced liver injury: Mechanisms and test systems. *Hepatology* 2001; 33:1009-1014.
5. Clark JA, Zimmermann, Tanner LA. Labelatol hepatoxicity. *Ann Intern Med* 1990; 113:210-214.
6. Dalton TA, Perry RS. Hepatoxicity associated with sustained released niacin. *Am J Med* 1992; 93:102-107.
7. Ernst E. Safety concerns about kava. *Lancet* 2002; 359:1865-1867.
8. Gupte S, Anderson RA. Pediatric hepatology. In: Gupte S (ed): *The Short Textbook of Pediatrics,* 10th edn. New Delhi: Jaypee 2004: 422- 426.
9. Heubi JE, Baracci MB, Zimmermann. Therapeutic misadventures with acetaminophen. Hepatotoxicity after multiple doses in children. *J Pediat* 1998; 132:22-25.
10. James LP, Wells E, Beard RH, *et al.:* Predictors of outcome after acetaminophen poisoning in children and adolescents. *Pediatr* 2002; 140:522-526.
11. Lee WM. Drug-induced hepatoxicity. *N Eng J Med* 1995; 333:1118-1121.
12. Leeder J S. Pharmacokinetics and pharmacogenomics. *Pediatr Clin North Am* 2001; 48:765-781.
13. Lewis JH, Zimmermann. Drug-induced liver disease. *Med Clin North Am* 1989; 73:775-792.
14. Nehra A, Mullick F, Ishak KG, *et al.:* Pemoline associated hepatic injury. *Gastroenterology* 1984; 87:1185-1190.
15. Nolan CM *et al.:* Hepatoxicity associated with isoniazid: Preventive therapy. *JAMA* 1999; 281:1014-1018.
16. Nolan CM. Hepatoxicity associated with isoniazid: Preventive therapy. *JAMA* 1999; 281:1014-1018.
17. Perry HE, Shannon W: Efficacy of oral versus intravenous N-acetylcystiene in acetaminophen overdose: Result of an open label, clinical trial. *Pediatrics* 1998; 132:149-152.
18. Pillans PI. Drug associated hepatic reactions in New Zealand: 21 years experience. *NZ Med J* 1996; 09:315-319.
19. Roberts EA. Drug induced liver injury in children. In: Suchy FJ, Sokol RJ, Balistreri WF (eds): *Liver Disease in Children*, 2nd edn. Philadelphia: Saunders 2001: 463-492.
20. Rollins B J. Hepatic veno-occlusive disease. *Am J Med* 1986; 81; 297-299.
21. Sherlock S, Dooley J. Drugs and liver. In: Sherlock S, Dooley J (eds): *Diseases of the Liver and Biliary System,* 10th edn. London: Blackwell 1996: 337-369.
22. Suchy F J. Drug and toxin-induced liver injury. In: Behrman RE, Kliegman RM, Jenson HB (eds): *Nelson Textbook of Pediatrics*,17th edn. Philadelphia: Saunders 2004: 1339-1341.

88 Acute Liver Failure

John Matthai • Sarah Paul

INTRODUCTION

Acute liver failure (ALF) is a complex multisystem disorder that follows an acute, severe insult to the liver. It is the consequence of severe hepatocyte dysfunction and results in severe coagulopathy, increased intracranial tension, metabolic derangements, renal dysfunction and susceptibility to infections. Early diagnosis and prompt management improve the outcome. The dramatic, unpredictable and often fatal course of the disease is responsible for the confusion regarding definitions and the many treatment protocols available.

DEFINITIONS

Acute Liver Failure

A multisystem disorder with severe impairment of liver cell function, with or without encephalopathy, occurring in association with hepatocellular necrosis in a patient with no recognizable underlying chronic liver disease.

Fulminant Hepatic Failure

A potentially reversible condition, the consequence of severe liver injury, in which the onset of hepatic encephalopathy occurs within 8 weeks of the first symptom of illness, in the absence of pre-existing liver disease.

Late Onset Hepatic Failure

Development of hepatic encephalopathy between 8 and 24 weeks from the onset of jaundice.

CLASSIFICATION

This is based on the time interval between jaundice and onset of encephalopathy. The absence of pre-existing liver disease is also not mandatory for making a diagnosis of fulminant hepatic failure. Three forms of liver cell failure are recognized:

1. Hyperacute Liver Failure

Encephalopathy develops in less than 7 days. Despite the high incidence of cerebral edema, the chances of survival are the highest.

2. Acute Liver Failure

Encephalopathy occurs between 1 and 4 weeks. The incidence of cerebral edema is high and the prognosis is poor without liver transplantation.

3. Subacute Liver Failure

Encephalopathy occurs between 5 and 12 weeks. The incidence of cerebral edema is low and the child recovers from the encephalopathy, but the long-term prognosis for liver function is not good.

According to the International Association for the Study of Liver (IASL) 1999:

Hyperacute hepatic failure: Encephalopathy occurring within 10 days of onset of jaundice.

Acute hepatic failure: Encephalopathy developing from 11 to 28 days of onset of jaundice.

Subacute hepatic failure: Encephalopathy and/or progressive ascites beyond 4 weeks but within 24 weeks of onset of jaundice.

ETIOLOGY

Acute liver failure is the end-result of a variety of insults to the liver. The cause varies with the age of the child. Congenital infections and inborn errors of metabolism are common in neonates. Viral hepatitis and other metabolic causes are more common in older children.

In India, acute viral hepatitis is the most common cause and hepatitis A predominates the scenario. Hepatitis E is also being increasingly recognized as an important cause. Hepatitis B infection is an important cause in some regions of high prevalence. The sudden reactivation of latent HBV infection may result in fulminant hepatitis. Co-infection or superinfection with hepatitis D virus increases the risk of fulminant disease in patients with HBV infection. Drugs are an important cause, but are often overlooked. Valproate,

Paracetamol, phenytoin and INH are known to cause fulminant hepatitis. In children with pre-existing liver disease many drugs can precipitate acute liver failure. Wilson's disease is important in children above 8 years of age. In India a large number of cases have no identifiable etiology and this probably reflects non-availability of diagnostic tests. Factors that precipitate acute liver failure in children include intercurrent infections, persistent high fever, hypovolemia, and concomitant zinc deficiency.

Galactosemia, tyrosinemia, perinatal hemochromatosis and hereditary fructose intolerance can cause fulminant hepatitis in infants. Septic shock can also cause liver cell failure in neonates. Common causes of acute liver failure are given in Table 88.1.

Table 88.1: Etiology of acute liver failure

Children	*Neonates / Infants*
Hepatitis viruses: Hepatitis A, E , B, A and E,	Perinatal hemochromatosis
Other viruses: Herpes, EB virus, Parvo B_{19}, CMV	Tyrosinemia type I
Drugs: Paracetamol, INAH, Valproate, Phenytoin	Galactosemia
Wilson's disease	Hereditary fructose intolerance
Glycogen storage disease type IV	Congenital infection-CMV, ECHO, Herpes
Alpha 1 antitrypsin deficiency Autoimmune hepatitis Unknown	Sepsis

PATHOLOGY

Pathological features of acute liver failure depend upon the etiology. However, there are three basic features:

1. Hepatic Necrosis

Extensive hepatocyte necrosis results in loss of lobular architecture and collapse of the reticulin framework. Viral hepatitis and idiosyncratic drug reactions have extensive hepatocyte necrosis. The distribution is pan-acinar in viral hepatitis and zonal in toxic hepatitis.

Fulminant hepatic failure is associated with massive confluent necrosis. The type and distribution of the inflammatory infiltrate may help establish the etiology. In some cases there is no evidence of regeneration, while attempted regeneration results in proliferation of duct like structures. The extent of hepatic necrosis does not correlate with the development of encephalopathy or the chances of recovery.

2. Hepatocellular Degeneration

In metabolic diseases, the characteristic lesion is hepatocellular degeneration associated with diffuse fatty infiltration of hepatocytes. Inflammatory infiltrates and hepatocyte necrosis are minimal. In children with Reye's syndrome the intracellular fat is micro vesicular and does not displace the nuclei. The histology returns to normal on recovery. Fulminant hepatic failure due to hereditary fructose intolerance, acute-onset tyrosinaemia and galactosaemia show diffuse swelling of hepatocytes with condensation of organelles and cytoplasmic elements. There is scattered hepatocyte necrosis and many show macrovesicular fat with displacement of nuclei.

3. Hepatocellular Regeneration

Recovery from fulminant hepatic failure is characterized by hepatocellular regeneration. In most patients who survive, there is complete histological recovery. Some patients with massive confluent necrosis survive but later develop post-necrotic cirrhosis.

BIOCHEMICAL EVALUATION

Serum alanine aminotransferase (ALT) and asparate aminotransferase (AST) are usually significantly elevated in children with fulminant hepatic failure. Serum aminotransferases may be 1,000 to 10,000 IU/L. Aminotransferase level at admission is not useful in predicting the outcome. A rapidly falling aminotransferase value in a deteriorating patient signifies 'exhaustion' of the hepatocyte mass and terminal hepatic failure.

The serum bilirubin levels usually increase rapidly. Hemolysis and catabolism of hepatic hem proteins result in increased production of bilirubin. Early in the illness much of the bilirubin is conjugated and this is due to excretory dysfunction. Later it becomes predominantly unconjugated, reflecting massive destruction of hepatocytes. Prothrombin time is always prolonged and represents loss of synthetic function of the hepatocytes. Renal function needs careful monitoring. Blood urea levels may not always reflect the deteriorating renal function, since the diseased liver cannot synthesize urea from ammonia. Presence of significant amounts of fibrin degradation products in the blood also indicates poor liver cell function. Nonspecific markers of sepsis and multiple cultures are always important in management. After initial stabilization of the patient, tests to determine the etiology need to be done.

MANIFESTATIONS

1. Encephalopathy

Encephalopathy is an essential prerequisite for diagnosis of acute liver failure. The pathogenesis is not well understood, but is probably multi factorial. The onset is acute and usually progresses over a few days through stages of drowsiness, hypersomnia and unresponsiveness to coma. Several substances have been implicated in encephalopathy—Ammonia, Amino-acids and their metabolic products and neurotransmitters (serotonin) catecholamine, glutamate (aspartate) fatty acids and substances that act on the GABA receptor complex. Unlike chronic liver failure, hyperammonemia is a consistent feature of acute hepatic failure. Ammonia produced by intestinal bacteria and from breakdown of dietary protein is normally cleared from the circulation by urea cycle enzymes in the liver. Rising ammonia levels are detrimental to brain function. It causes post synaptic inhibition and also increases blood brain barrier permeability.

Early encephalopathy is difficult to recognize in children. EEG changes (slowing of alpha rhythm down to the delta range) may precede psychological changes early in the course of the disease. In established encephalopathy, EEG monitoring does not offer any advantage over clinical assessment.

2. Cerebral Edema

Cerebral edema is uncommon in stages I and II but seen in all patients with stage IV encephalopathy. Cerebral edema raises intracranial pressure and decreases cerebral perfusion. It may be cytotoxic or vasogenic edema. Changes in the vascular integrity of the cerebral circulation result in the transfer of solute and water into the brain parenchyma. Hypotension, hypoxia, hypoglycemia, sepsis, hyperkalemia and GI bleeding worsen intracranial hypertension. Pupillary abnormalities, muscular rigidity, decerebrate posturing, focal seizures and loss of brain stem reflexes are clinical indicators. CT or MRI imaging of the brain are diagnostic. Cerebral edema is the most important cause of death in acute liver failure.

3. Coagulopathy and Bleeding

Failure of hepatic synthesis of clotting factors and fibrinolytic factors, platelet dysfunction and intravascular coagulation are responsible for the coagulopathy. Thrombocytopenia develops rapidly and is due to immune mediated platelet destruction as well as decreased synthesis of hepatic factors necessary for platelet maturation in the bone marrow. It commonly manifests as gastrointestinal bleeding. The incidence of GI hemorrhage has decreased since the use of H 2 blockers in management. Prothrombin time expressed as INR is a good assessment of hepatic synthesis of clotting factors. While FDP levels are mildly elevated in acute liver failure, very high levels indicate sepsis.

4. Hypoglycemia

Hypoglycemia is common and the blood glucose levels may be less than 40 mg/dl. This is due to two reasons:

1. Defective gluconeogenesis.
2. Increased plasma insulin levels as a result of deranged hepatic metabolism of insulin.

The resulting hypoglycemia is therefore difficult to correct. It is important to administer a steady infusion of dextrose and monitor blood glucose levels regularly, as the classic signs and symptoms of hypoglycemia are often masked.

5. Renal Dysfunction

A majority of children with fulminant hepatic failure have functional renal failure (Hepatorenal syndrome). There is acute sodium retention (urinary spot Na^+<20 mEq/L), normal urinary sediment and oliguria (<1ml/kg/hr). However, acute tubular necrosis can sometimes occur. In hepatorenal syndrome there is hyperdynamic circulation and decrease in renal perfusion pressure. Activation of the sympathetic nervous system results in the increased synthesis of several vasoactive mediators such as rennin, angiotensin, adrenaline, ecosanoids and endothelins. This results in vasoconstriction with a rise in renal vascular resistance and decreased glomerular filtration. Gastrointestinal hemorrhage may produce a disproportionate increase in blood urea. Serum creatinine is therefore a more reliable marker of renal dysfunction in acute liver failure.

6. Hemodynamic Instability

Children with ALF may have hyperdynamic circulation with decreased systemic peripheral vascular resistance and increased cardiac output—"Warm Shock". Severe vasodilatation can lead to hypovolemia and hypotension. This is mediated by prostaglandins or nitric oxide. Invasive pressure monitoring is therefore ideal to determine the volume of fluid to be infused. Progression of the disease results in circulatory failure from falling cardiac output and depressed brain stem function due to cerebral edema. Electrolyte disturbances (hypo or hyperkalemia, acidosis and cardiac irritation due to the central venous catheter) may result in cardiac arrhythmias.

7. Electrolyte Disturbances

All children with ALF have disturbed sodium homeostasis, either hypo or hypernatremia. Hyponatremia is more common despite sodium retention by the kidney. This is due to SIADH or excess administration of hypotonic saline. Hypernatremia occurs from intravenous fluids containing high sodium levels or the administration of lactulose or mannitol. Hypokalemia may be secondary to hyperaldosteronism, vigorous diuretic use or continuous nasogastric suction. Hyperkalemia may be observed in patients with massive hepatic necrosis and / or hemolysis.

Acid-base abnormalities are common. This may be secondary to liver failure or the underlying metabolic disease, especially in infants. Respiratory alkalosis due to central hyperventilation may be seen early. Metabolic alkalosis may be due to hypokalemia or excessive diuretic therapy. Metabolic acidosis may be due to anaerobic metabolism, renal failure as well as excessive administration of citrate-preserved blood. Deepening coma may result in respiratory failure and respiratory acidosis.

8. Infections

There is increased risk of bacterial infections in patients with acute liver failure. Alteration in the immune system in the form of impaired Kupffer cell/polymorphonuclear function and reduction in many components of the complement system predisposes to infection. Sick children with poor respiratory effort and weak cough reflex are at high risk for serious infection while in the intensive care unit. Infection can cause sudden deterioration in children with acute liver failure. Fever and polymorphonuclear leukocyte response may not always be present. *Staph aureus*, *Coliforms* and *Candida* are often responsible.

MANAGEMENT

Acute liver failure is a medical emergency since it may be rapidly fatal. Sick children must be transferred to specialized centers at the earliest for best outcome. Intensive care monitoring and early recognition of complications can help avoid transplantation or death. Management is aimed at life support as well as prevention and treatment of complications, to facilitate recovery of the liver.

Assessment: History should be carefully taken and should include a good family history, consanguinity and history of exposure to drugs and toxins. A careful clinical examination should be done to look for signs of underlying chronic liver disease and the presence of K.F. ring.

General measures: A quiet environment with minimal stimulation reduces acute changes in the intracranial pressure. Intensive care and continuous monitoring is necessary in all children. Patients with encephalopathy are aggressive and may require restraint and sedation. Benzodiazepines are recommended only in ventilated patients.

Monitoring: All patients should be carefully monitored for the following:

- Oxygen saturation.
- Urine output.
- Central venous pressure.
- Blood pressure.
- Blood gas analysis.
- Electrolytes.
- Blood sugar.
- Prothrombin time.
- Blood counts.

Blood and urine cultures should be done as required. Coma scale and neurologic evaluation should be done twice daily.

1. Management of Encephalopathy

A hypertonic enema should be given soon after admission to evacuate the colonic contents. Subsequently the large bowel should be washed out twice daily. Lactulose may be given orally or with the help of a nasogastric tube in doses of 0.5 ml/kg/dose (max 30 ml/dose) four times a day to produce 2-4 loose stools/day. Lactulose decreases urea producing gut organisms and also traps ammonia in the gut. Oral neomycin or ampicillin will sterilize the gut and prevent ammonia production. Branched chain amino acids, flumazenil and extracorporeal circuits can improve encephalopathy, but results have not consistent to recommend their routine use. Anti-convulsants like phenytoin or phenobarbitone are required if there are seizures.

2. Diet and Nutrition

A constant intravenous infusion of 10% dextrose should be administered to maintain blood sugar above 80 mg%. Total fluid intake should be restricted to two thirds of normal maintenance to decrease cerebral edema. Protein restriction is not necessary in Grade I and Grade II encephalopathy. Vegetable proteins are usually preferred. Micronutrients, Vitamin C, Vitamin E and Zinc must be given. Parenteral nutrition reduces ammonia production. Enteral feeds should be started as early as possible.

3. Electrolyte Balance

Maintenance fluid is usually 10% Dextrose with 1 mEq/kg/day of sodium. Fluid volume is adjusted to the CVP and urine output. Dilutional hyponatremia need not be corrected unless the serum sodium is below 117 mEq/L. Hypokalemia may be associated with metabolic alkalosis and must be corrected. Severe metabolic acidosis may require intravenous sodium bicarbonate (8.4%), elective ventilation or bicarbonate dialysis.

4. Increased Intracranial Pressure

Cerebral edema is the most frequent cause of death in fulminant hepatic failure. The head end of the bed should be raised 20-30 degrees and the head should be in the neutral position. An osmotic agent like mannitol in doses of 0.5 gm/kg every 4 to 6 hours is useful to reduce intracranial pressure. It should be used with caution in patients with renal failure. Frusemide acts synergistically with mannitol. For optimal benefit, mannitol should be started before the ICT becomes very high. Hypoxia and hypercapnea should be corrected to reduce vasodilatation. Short term hyperventilation may be useful to reduce ICP. High dose barbiturates and controlled hypothermia may decrease cerebral edema by reducing cerebral blood flow. Steroids have not been shown to be beneficial.

CT or MRI brain scan will show flattening of the gyri and reduction in ventricular size. Loss of the definition of grey/white matter is a poor prognostic sign. Fixed, dilated pupils indicate irreversible brain damage.

5. Coagulopathy

Bleeding and coagulopathy is a major complication associated with acute liver failure. The Vit K dependent factors II, V, VII, IX and X are significantly reduced and result in the prolongation of prothrombin and partial thromboplastin time. Prolongation of prothrombin time indicates the severity of liver failure. Coagulation defects require administration of fresh frozen plasma or blood for immediate correction. Massive infusion of F.F.P can lead to fluid overload and hypernatremia. Severe thrombocytopenia requires platelet transfusions.

Gastrointestinal hemorrhage can be massive and life threatening. Cold saline washes every 4 hours along with injection ranitidine and oral antacids can help control gastric bleeding. Exchange plasmapheresis causes a rapid improvement in coagulation parameters.

6. Hypoxia and Respiratory Complications

Though the patient may be breathing spontaneously, ventilation is often inadequate. Elective mechanical ventilation should be initiated at the first sign of respiratory failure. Patients with stage II-III encephalopathy often hyperventilate leading to respiratory alkalosis. Patients in stage IV coma develop hypoventilation, hypoxia and hypercapnia. Positive pressure ventilation may reduce hepatic perfusion and exacerbate metabolic acidosis.

Pulmonary edema can occur due to vasodilatation and loss of vascular integrity in the lung. Diuretics are useful in treatment. Secondary lung infections are usually due to Staph aureus, Pseudomonas and Candida. Aspiration pneumonia and pleural effusion may also complicate the clinical course. Pulmonary hemorrhage is often terminal.

7. Renal Insufficiency

Around 75% of children develop renal insufficiency. This may be due to functional renal failure, pre-renal uremia or acute tubular necrosis. Dehydration and gastrointestinal bleeding contribute to the prerenal uremia. Increased muscle breakdown produces a marked increase in blood creatinine concentration. Acute tubular necrosis may be due to hypovolemia or dehydration. Electrolyte imbalance, sepsis, hypovolaemia and endotoxaemia all contribute to renal injury.

Pre-renal failure may be managed initially with a fluid challenge followed by adequate fluid administration to maintain the CVP. Frusemide can be used in mild renal failure. Dopamine helps maintain renal perfusion. Dialysis should be considered if there is azotemia and urine output is persistently less than 1 ml/kg/hr.

8. Infections

Bacterial and fungal infections are always seen in sick children with acute liver failure. Signs of sepsis may be very subtle. Broad spectrum antibiotics are usually recommended. Amino glycosides are best avoided as it may contribute to renal failure. All infected indwelling catheters must be removed.

9. Antidote

N. Acetyl cysteine (140 mg/kg initially followed by 70 mg/kg 4 hourly) is the specific antidote for paracetamol poisoning. It replenishes the depleted glutathione stores in the liver. It should be given within 12-15 hours after the ingestion of the drug and continued until the liver failure resolves. There is little evidence of its efficacy in other causes of acute liver failure.

Temporary Hepatic Support

This helps to support the patient and prevent neurological impairment while awaiting hepatic regeneration or liver transplantation. Pharmapheresis, exchange transfusions, Extracorporal blood cleansing, liver assisted devices containing cultured hepatocytes and cross circulation with animals have been tried. Molecular adsorbant-recirculating system (MARS) has shown promising results in adults but is very expensive. Experience in children is limited.

Liver Transplantation

Liver transplantation remains the only definitive treatment that has improved the outcome in acute liver failure. It should be considered in all children with stage III or stage IV hepatic coma. Contraindications for transplantation include irreversible brain damage, uncontrolled sepsis and severe respiratory distress syndrome. Success rates in liver transplantation for acute liver failure are lower than that done for other indications.

Auxiliary liver transplantation, where the recipient's liver is left in situ to regenerate, while grafting the new liver, can be tried if there are chances of recovery of the diseased liver. The donor liver atrophies if the native liver recovers and becomes functional again. If that happens, immunosuppressant drugs can then be withdrawn.

PROGNOSIS

The prognosis is generally poor in children under 10 years of age. The cause of liver failure is an important factor that determines the outcome. Hepatitis A infection and paracetamol poisoning have the best prognosis. Absence of an obvious etiology in child with acute liver failure and encephalopathy indicates a poor prognosis.

The severity of the encephalopathy determines survival. Only 18% of children with grade IV hepatic coma survive. Cerebral edema and significant renal failure are usually associated with a bad prognosis. Prothrombin time is the best indicator of prognosis. Alpha-feto protein level has no prognostic value. Recovery is usually complete in most patients who survive acute fulminant liver failure.

KEY LEARNING POINTS

- Acute liver failure is a complex multisystem disorder with an unpredictable course and high mortality in children.
- Time interval from onset of jaundice to encephalopathy is currently used to classify acute liver failure.
- Congenital infections and metabolic diseases are the most common causes in infants. Viral hepatitis predominates in older children. No cause is identified in many cases in India, reflecting the lack of facilities for investigations.
- Encephalopathy is an essential prerequisite for diagnosis. Cerebral edema is the most important reason for death in acute liver failure.
- Rapidly falling ALT values along with increasing prothrombin time in a clinically deteriorating patient indicates poor prognosis.
- Management is aimed at life support and prevention of complications while facilitating regeneration of the liver.
- Liver transplantation is the only definitive treatment that improves outcome.

ACKNOWLEDGEMENT

The authors wish to thank Mrs. Dhanabagyam for secretarial assistance.

FURTHER READINGS

1. Aw MM, Dhawan A. Acute liver failure. *Indian J Pediatr* 2002; 69:87-91.
2. Arora NK, Mathur P, Ahuja A, Oberoi A. Acute liver failure. *Indian J Pediatr* 2003;70:73-79.
3. Bendre SV, Bavdekar AR, Bhave SA, Pandit AN, Chitambar SD, Arankale VA. Fulminant hepatic failure. Etiology, viral marker and outcome. *Indian Pediatr* 1999;36:1107-1112.
4. Blei AT, Larsen FS. Pathophysiology of cerebral edema in fulminant hepatic failure. *J Hepatol* 1999;31:771-776.
5. Bernuau J, Benhamou JP. Classifying acute liver failure. *Lancet* 1993;342:252-254.
6. Bansal S, Dhawan A. Acute Liver Failure in Walker AW, Goulet O, *et al.* (eds): *Pediatric Gastrointestinal Disease*. New York: B C Dekker Inc 2004;1491-1507.
7. Caranci P, Van Thiel DH. Acute liver failure. *Lancet* 1995; 345;163-169.
8. Durend P, Debray D, Mandel R, *et al.* Acute liver failure in infancy: A 14-year experience of a pediatric liver transplantation. *J Pediatr* 2001;139:871-876.
9. Devictor D, Taheri C, Rousset A *et al.* Management of fulminant hepatic failure in children—An analysis of 56 cases. *Crit Care Med* 1993; 21: S 348-349.
10. Fackler JC, Liver failure in Pediatric intensive care unit. *In* : Rogers MC, Nichols DG (eds): *Textbook of Pediatric Intensive Care*, 3rd edn. Baltimore: Williams and Wilkins 1996: 1178-1191.
11. Keays R, Harrison PM, Wendon JA *et al.* Intravenous acetylcysteine in paracetamol induced fulminant hepatic failure: A prospective randomized controlled trial. *Br Med J* 1991;303: 1026-1029.
12. Kay MH, McDiarmid SV, Liver failure and transplantation *In:* Wyllie R, Hyams J.S. (eds*): Pediatric Gastrointestinal Disease*, 2nd edn. Philadelphia: WB Saunders 1999: 635-650.
13. Lee WM. Acute liver failure. *N Engl J Med* 1993;230:1862-1872.
14. Munoz SJ Difficult management problems in fulminant hepatic failure. *Semin Liver Dis* 1993;13:395-413.
15. O'Grady JG, Schlm SW, William R. Acute liver failure redefining the syndromes. *Lancet* 1993;342:273-275.
16. Poddar V, Thapa BR, Prasad A, Sharma AK, Singh K. Natural History and risk factor in fulminant hepatic failure. *Arch Dis Child* 2002; 87:54-56.
17. Prasad A, Thapa BR. Recent advances in the management of fulminant hepatic failure. In: Thapa BR (ed) *Recent Advances in Pediatric Clinical Gastroenterology.* Chandigarh. Relume Press 2001;308-319.
18. Russel G.J, Fitzgerlad JF, clark J.H. Fulminant hepatic failure. *J Pediatr* 1987; 111:313-319.
19. Shah U, Habib Z, Kleinman RE. Liver failure attributable to hepatitis A virus infection in a developing country. *Pediatrics* 2000;105:436-438.
20. Sherlock S, Dooley J. Acute Liver Failure. *In: Diseases of the Liver and Biliary System,* 11th edn. London: Blackwell 2002: 111 -126.
21. Tandon BN, Bernuau J, O'Grady J, *et al.* Recommendations of the International Association for the study of the liver: Sub-committee on nomenclature of acute and subacute hepatic failure. *J Gastroenterol Hepatol* 1999;14:403-404.
22. Thapa B R, Walia A. Acute liver failure. *In* Gupte S (ed) *Recent Advances in Pediatrics–15*. New Delhi: Jaypee 2005:76-88.
23. Vinholt SF, Davern TJ, Obaid SA, *et al.* Viral hepatitis-related acute liver failure. *Am J Gastroenterol* 2003;98:448-53.
24. Whitington PF, Soriano HE, Alonso EM. Fulminant hepatic failure in children. *In*: Suchy FJ, Sokol RJ, Balistreri WF (eds): *Liver Disease is Children*, 3rd edn. Philadelphia: Lippincott Williams and Wilkinson 2001: 63-88.

89 Portal Hypertension

Rajeev Redkar

INTRODUCTION

The portal vein transports blood from the gastrointestinal tract and the spleen to the liver. It is the only venous system in our body, which begins with capillaries and ends with capillaries. The intrahepatic branches of the portal vein terminate in small vessels that supply the hepatic sinusoids.

Embryologically, the systemic veins of our body develop from the intra-embryonic anterior and posterior cardinal veins while the portal system develops from the extra-embryonic vitelline and umbilical veins, which drain from the yolk sac and the placenta.

DEFINITION

Portal hypertension could be defined as a direct measurement of pressure in the portal system of over 11 mm of mercury or a splenic pulp pressure of over 16 mm of mercury. A rise in the portal pressure leads to splenomegaly and the development of natural porto-systemic shunts at the following sites:

- Lower end of the oesophagus and cardia through the gastro-oesophageal veins.
- The anal canal via the haemorrhoidal veins.
- In the falciform ligament via the umbilical veins.
- In the abdominal wall and retroperitoneum.

The diagnosis of portal hypertension should be suspected in a child after the occurrence of any large gastrointestinal bleed. In this age group, esophageal varices are the most likely cause for such an event. Variceal bleeding is associated with a mortality rate of 5-9 percent in children with portal vein obstruction but there is a higher risk of death of those with cirrhosis.

CLASSIFICATION

The etiology of portal hypertension in children is classified as:

I. Cirrhotic—e.g. biliary atresia, cystic fibrosis.
II. Non-cirrhotic
   a. Prehepatic e.g. portal vein thrombosis.
   b. Intrahepatic:
      i. Presinusoidal–e.g. congenital hepatic fibrosis.
      ii. Parasinusoidal–e.g. fatty liver, nodular hyperplasia.
      iii. Postsinusoidal–e.g. veno-occlusive disease of liver.
   c. Suprahepatic–e.g. Budd-Chiari syndrome.

The most frequent causes of cirrhosis in childhood include biliary atresia, alpha-1- antitrypsin deficiency and metabolic liver diseases. Many of these patients have the stigmata of their underlying disease and the diagnosis of portal hypertension is not difficult.

Diagnosis may not be so obvious in children with non-cirrhotic portal hypertension. Portal vein thrombosis (extra-hepatic portal hypertension), for example, may present within the first five years of life as a major haematemesis with only splenomegaly and a reduced platelet count as clues to the diagnosis. Many affected patients have no documented cause for their portal hypertension, although a history of umbilical vein canulation, abdominal infection, trauma or pancreatitis may be responsible for the portal thrombosis. The liver function tests in such patients are essentially normal. A confirmation of portal vein occlusion may be obtained by ultrasound demonstration of collateral venous channels in the porta hepatis replacing the portal vein. Approximately 40% of these patients have a history of umbilical vein catheterization or abdominal sepsis in the neonatal period but the venous occlusion in the majority appears to be congenital in origin.

Congenital hepatic fibrosis may also present with an acute haematemesis and normal liver function tests but the clinical features include hepatomegaly. A liver biopsy shows bands of fibrous tissue joining the portal tracts and this condition may be associated with polycystic disease and other renal disorders.

There are several reports of portal hypertension in children presenting with haematemesis and splenomegaly in whom the liver histology is normal and in whom the portal vein is patent.

Further studies have shown a subendothelial thickening of intrahepatic branches of the portal vein causing presinusoidal obstruction to portal blood flow within the liver leading to the formation of collateral venous channels in the porta hepatis. The condition has been known under a variety of names such as non-cirrhotic portal hypertension but the best is perhaps 'hepato-portal sclerosis'. The aetiology is unknown.

Suprahepatic obstruction caused by either a web in the inferior vena cava above the entrance of the hepatic veins or thrombotic occlusion of the hepatic veins (Budd-Chiari syndrome) is extremely rare in childhood. The clinical features may be mimicked by constrictive pericarditis but echocardiography and venography should make the diagnosis clear.

CLINICAL FEATURE

In portal venous occlusion, the presentation is usually in younger children (5 years) with acute episode of upper or lower gastrointestinal bleeding or splenic enlargement. Anorectal varices and haemorrhoids are identified in almost two-thirds of patients with portal venous occlusion.

However, in chronic liver disease, the presentation of portal hypertension is due to splenomegaly, which is usually noted in slightly older children (8 years). Encephalopathy and abdominal distension due to ascitis may complicate the haematemesis in patients with cirrhosis. Growth retardation is a well-recognized complication of cirrhosis and portal hypertension is a contributory factor to it due to mucosal oedema and lymphatic congestion leading to malabsorption and protein losing enteropathy.

In patients with Budd-Chiari syndrome, intractable ascitis with hepatomegaly is the usual initial presentation. Jaundice is variable.

INVESTIGATIONS

Blood Investigations

Hypersplenism may result in anaemia and reduced WBC and platelet count. Plasma concentrations of procoagulant and anticoagulant proteins may be reduced in portal venous thrombosis or Budd-Chiari syndrome. Biochemical liver function tests are abnormal in cirrhosis, but are rarely deranged in portal venous occlusion. Serum albumin levels are depleted in acute variceal bleed.

Ultrasound Scan of Abdomen

Large collateral veins, portal cavernoma and splenomegaly, which are the features of portal hypertension, may be identified on sonography of abdomen. Doppler studies provide the information about the direction, velocity and waveform characteristics of portal blood flow. In cirrhosis of liver, the maximum velocity of the blood flow in the main portal trunk is inversely correlated with the severity of the liver disease. In Budd-Chiari syndrome, Doppler sonography of the hepatic veins and the inferior vena cava can be conclusive.

Upper and Lower Gastrointestinal Endoscopy

This modality is useful in the diagnosis and treatment of varices of the esophagus, stomach and the ano-rectal area. Various grading systems are used in the assessment of oesophageal varices (Fig. 89.1). Smaller varices are bluish with a relatively thick mucosal covering while the larger ones may have signs of recent or impending bleed like 'cherry red spots' or 'varices on varices'. Portal congestive gastropathy is characterized by mucosal hyperaemia with dilated submucosal veins.

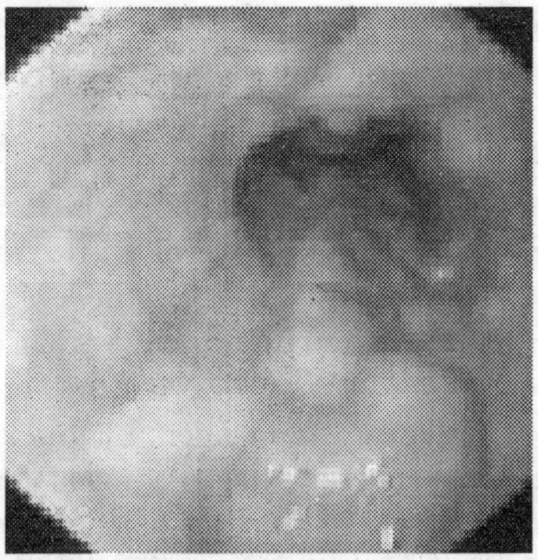

Fig. 89.1: Endoscopic appearance of esophageal varices (See for colour figure Plate 9)

CT Angiography and MRI Scan

The above modalities are increasingly used in the diagnosis of Budd-Chiari syndrome and to identify liver lesions associated with portal hypertension like focal nodular regenerative hyperplasia. MR angiography is recently used as a non-invasive alternative to conventional angiography to delineate porto-mesenteric venous anatomy.

Angiography

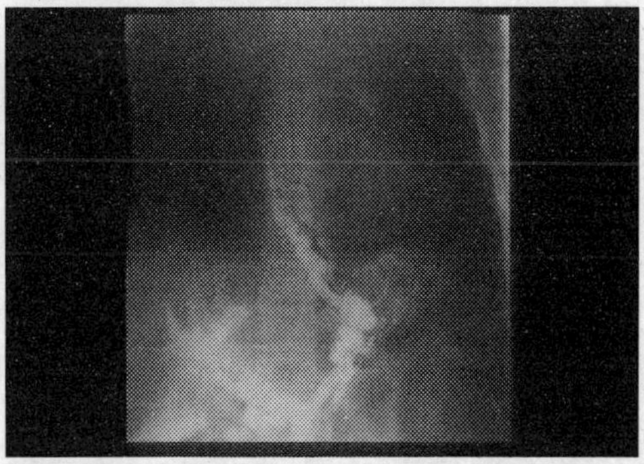

Fig. 89.2: Portal venography demonstrating oesophageal varices

MANAGEMENT

A. Treatment of the Acute Bleed

Acute variceal bleeding, particularly in young infants, can pose problems in management. Medical measures include blood transfusion and the intravenous infusion of vasopressin (0.2-0.4 units/1.73 m/min) which may arrest the bleeding. Vasopressin or its precursor, glypressin, may be used alone or in combination with nitrates to reduce the portal venous pressure. Unfortunately, these agents have side-effects related to systemic vaso constriction like headache, nausea and abdominal cramps. Somatostatin reduces splanchnic blood flow and portal pressure with minimal side-effects, but it has a short half life of less than 3 minutes. Octreotide, a long acting analog of somatostatin, has a plasma half-life of more than 1 hour. Although the effectiveness of octreotide has been studied in a small number of children, its safety and side-effect profile have encouraged its use in cases of acute variceal bleeding.

Continued bleeding may be controlled with injection sclerotherapy but the small size of the pediatric endoscope channels can limit the clearance of blood from within the esophagus. The Sangstaken-Blackmore (S-B tube) compression balloon may be life-saving when there is a failure of visualization of the varices due to overwhelming haemorrhage. However, the dangers of this instrument cannot be overemphasized. Correct placement of the gastric balloon must be checked with X-ray control in order to avoid the inflation within the lumen of the esophagus. This accidental inflation with the esophagus may result in esophageal rupture or suffocation from airway obstruction. Inflation of the gastric balloon and moderate prolonged traction achieved by securing the S-B tube to the side of the face with an adhesive tape is usually sufficient to stop the bleeding. It is rarely necessary to inflate the esophageal balloon present on the standard instrument. Balloon deflation is performed 18 to 24 hours later and this is followed immediately with endoscopic variceal injection.

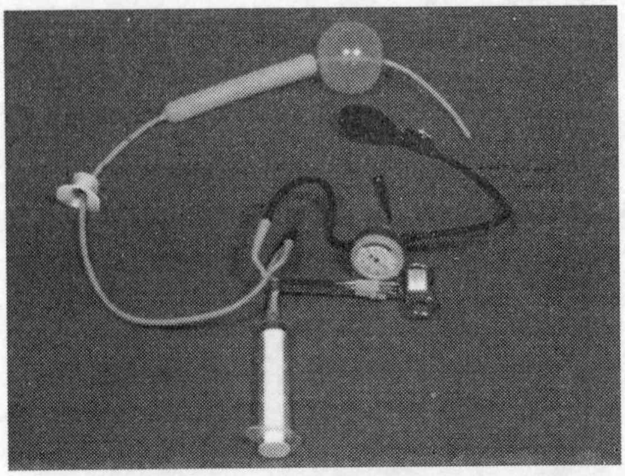

Fig. 89.3: Sangstaken-Blackmore (S-B) tube

B. Injection Sclerotherapy for Long-term Treatment

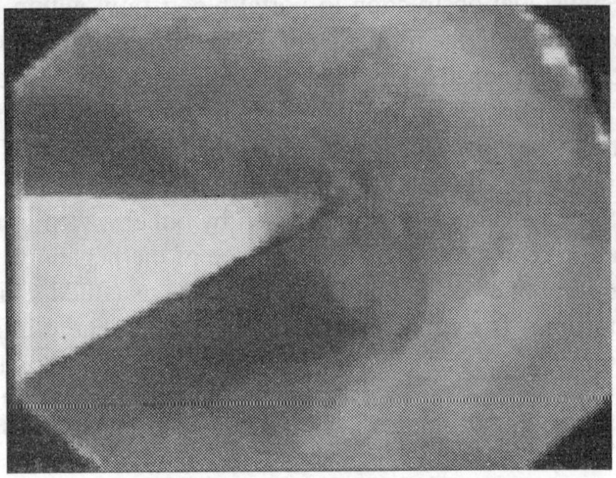

Fig. 89.4: Injection sclerotherapy
(See for colour figure Plate 9)

Injection sclerotherapy was suggested for the treatment of esophageal varices in children because of failures and complications of primary surgery. Portosystemic shunt thrombosis and rebleeding, the hazards of splenectomy in children and long-term risks of encephalopathy all encouraged an alternative therapy. Controlled trials in adult patients confirmed that early endoscopic sclerotherapy after the onset of bleeding significantly reduced the risk of rebleeding and may prolong survival in the cirrhotic. Injections are performed through a flexible upper GI endoscope under general anaesthesia with an endotracheal tube in place. Intravenous sedation has been used occasionally in older children. A variety of sclerosants are available including ethanolamine oleate, sodium tetradecyl sulphate, sodium morrhuate and polidocanol. The injections are given either intra or para-variceal and are mostly given into the cardia and lower 3 cm of the oesophagus. A maximum of 3 ml is injected into each varix to a maximum of 5 to 20 ml per session depending on the age and the size of the patient. A nasogastric tube is inserted in small infants to control the degree of gastric distension. The initial 3 injections are given at weekly intervals and subsequent treatments on a monthly basis until the varices are obliterated.

Mild symptoms of retrosternal discomfort and a transient fever are common after endoscopic sclerotherapy. The variceal hemorrhage may recur, particularly between the first 2 or 3 treatments and esophageal ulceration may be followed by stricture formation and dysphagia. Rare serious complications have included broncho-esophageal fistula, chylothorax and pericarditis. One case of paraplegia has been reported from injection of segmental spinal vessels.

An analysis of seven reports (published since 1984) of the results of sclerotherapy in 248 children shows a mortality rate of 3 percent and a rebleed rate of 12 percent. The rebleed rate in a series of 7 reports of surgery for portal hypertension (1980-86) was 14 percent.

C. Variceal Banding

This technique, which involves application of an elastic band to a variceal column, is done through flexible upper gastrointestinal endoscopes. The strangulated varix, subsequently, thromboses and sloughs. Usually upto three bands are applied at each session. Multi-band devices allow the application of several bands without the need for reloading. Treatment is performed initially at 1 to 2 weekly intervals, extending to monthly intervals once the larger varices are treated. The incidence of oesophageal stricture and systemic side-effects is lower with this treatment modality. At present, equipment limitations make this technique difficult to use in small children less than 2 years of age.

D. Transjugular Intrahepatic Porto-systemic Shunt (TIPS)

The indications of TIPS in children include uncontrolled variceal bleeding especially the ones who are awaiting liver transplantation. Some patients of Budd-Chiari syndrome or intractable ascitis may also benefit by this procedure. Portal vein thrombosis, bacterial sepsis and coagulopathy are contraindications to TIPS.

This intervention involves insertion of an expandable metallic stent from the hepatic to the portal vein through the percutaneous tranjugular route under radiological guidance. Under fluoroscopic control, a guidewire is passed into a hepatic vein. A needle is then advanced over a guidewire into the hepatic vein and thence to the portal vein. A balloon catheter is subsequently used to dilate the intrahepatic tract and the stent is deployed.

E. Surgery—Porto-systemic Shunts

Endoscopic sclerotherapy with banding is an effective primary treatment modality of bleeding oesophageal varices in majority of children with reasonable liver function. However, surgical intervention is indicated for the following cases:

- Uncontrolled bleeding from the oesophageal varices not responding to at least 2 sessions of banding or sclerotherapy.
- Bleeding gastric or ectopic varices not responding to endoscopic treatment.
- Hypersplenism or massive symptomatic splenomegaly.
- Lack of access to endoscopic treatment.
- Symptomatic biliary obstruction due to choledochal varices.
- Selected patients with Budd-Chiari syndrome.

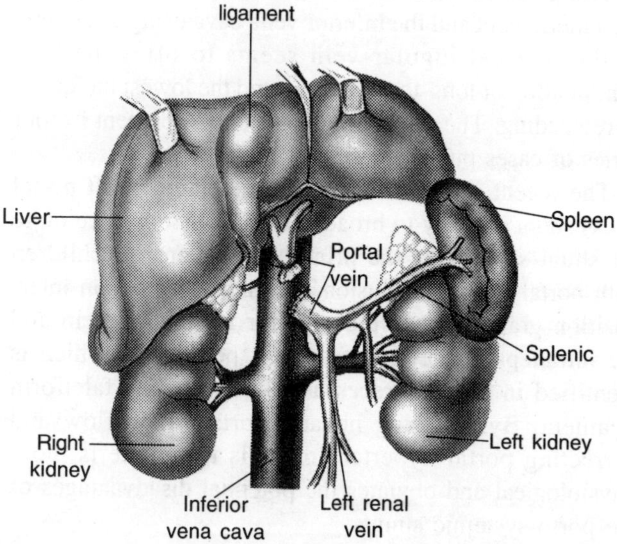

Fig. 89.5: Porto–caval shunt (See for colour figure Plate 9)

The great variety of surgical procedures advocated for the management of portal hypertension was reflected in a French multi-centre study of children treated both in European countries and North Africa. Thirty different operations, which included a range of porto-systemic shunts and various devascularization techniques (Fig. 89.6), were reported from the treatment of 109 children. The variety of surgical techniques can be explained by both the varied pathology of the portal venous system and the preferences and experience of individual surgeons. Occlusion of the portal system in the extrahepatic portal hypertension, for example, may affect the portal vein alone or may involve either the splenic or the superior.

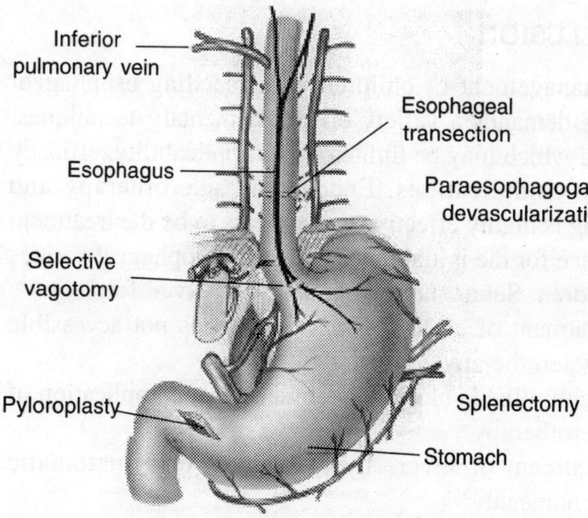

Fig. 89.6: Devascularization procedure (See for colour figure Plate 9)

The construction of a shunt between the superior mesenteric vein and the inferior vena cava using a segment of the internal jugular vein seems to offer the best combination of long-term patency and the lowest incidence of rebleeding. The rebleed rate was only 6 percent in four series of cases published since 1981.

The recent introduction of the mesenterico-left portal (Rex) shunt is likely to broaden the indications once more for shunt surgery as the primary treatment for children with portal venous occlusion.This shunt utilizes an interposition graft between the superior mesenteric vein and the intrahepatic portion of the left portal vein which is identified in the Rex recessus adjacent to the falciform ligament. By restoring hepatic portal blood flow and correcting portal hypertension, this technique is more physiological and obviates the potential disadvantages of the porto-systemic shunts.

The complications of porto-systemic shunting are not only concerned with rebleeding. Deterioration of liver function and hepatic encephalopathy are further hazards, particularly in children with cirrhosis. In a recent series of 37 children, 1 died in the early postoperative period with encephalopathy and 9 out of 31 with a patent shunt showed deterioration of mental function during a mean follow-up period of 5 years.

Porto-systemic shunt surgery should be regarded as a complementary therapy to endoscopic treatment. Porto-mesenteric venous anatomy does not permit successful shunt surgery in every child, and shunt thrombosis has been recorded with all types of shunts especially in smaller children.

Liver transplantation is the treatment of choice for children with variceal bleeding complicating end-stage chronic liver disease.

CONCLUSION

The management of children with bleeding esophageal varices demands a variety of complementary techniques, each of which may be limited by its applicability, efficacy and its complications. Endoscopic sclerotherapy and banding is highly effective and appears to be the treatment of choice for the initial management of esophageal varices in children. Shunt surgery should be reserved for:

a. Treatment of gastric or ectopic varices not accessible to sclerotherapy.
b. Uncontrollable bleeding secondary to a complication of sclerotherapy.
c. Treatment of severe hypersplenism or symptomatic splenomegaly.
d. Treatment of children living in communities far away from adequate medical care and blood transfusion facilities.

Liver transplantation is the procedure of choice for patients with complications of portal hypertension associated with end-stage liver disease. The role of newer modalities like the TIPS and Rex shunt has yet to be conclusively proven.

KEY LEARNING POINTS

- Portal hypertension is defined as direct measurement of pressure in the portal system > 11mm Hg or a splenic pulp pressure > 16 mmHg.
- Any child presenting with a large gastrointestinal bleed should be suspected to have portal hypertension.
- Special investigations include ultrasound scan of abdomen, endoscopy, CT angiograph and MRI scan, angiography, etc.
- Of the various management modalities, endoscopic sclerotherapy and banding appear to be the treatment of choice for initial management of esophageal varices.
- Shunt surgery should be reserved for certain situations such as varices not accessible to sclerotherapy.
- Portal hypertension with end-stage liver disease is the procedure of choice.
- Newer modalities like TIPS and Rex shunt remain to be evaluated.

FURTHER READINGS

1. Bismuth H, Franco D, Alagille D. Portal diversion for portal hypertension in children. *Ann Surgery* 1980; 192: 18-24.
2. De Ville de Goyet J, Alberti D, Clapuyt P *et al.* Direct bypassing of extrahepatic portal venous obstruction in children: A new technique for combined hepatic portal.
3. Fonkalsrud EW, Myers NA, Robinson MJ. Management of extrahepatic portal hypertension in children. *Ann Surg* 1974;180: 487-491.
4. Fonkalsrud EW. Surgical management of portal hypertension in childhood. *Archiv Surgery* 1980;115: 1042-1045.
5. Howard ER, Stringer MD, Colombani PM. *Surgery of the Liver, Bile Ducts and Pancreas in Children.* London: Arnold 2002, 2nd edn.
6. Howard ER, Stringer MD, Mowat AP. Assessment of injection sclerotherapy in the management of 152 children with oesophageal varices. *B Surgery* 1988; 75:404-408.
7. Poddar U, Thapa BR, Puri P, *et al.* Non-cirrhotic portal fibrosis in children *Indian J Gastroenterology* 2000; 19: 12-13.
8. Stringer MD, Howard ER, Mowat AP. Endoscopic sclerotherapy in the management of oesophageal varices in 61 children with biliary atresia. *J Pediat Surg* 1989; 24: 438-442.

90 Indian Childhood Cirrhosis

Suraj Gupte

INTRODUCTION

Occurrence of cirrhosis from various diseases such as atresia of bile duct, neonatal hepatitis, cystic fibrosis, hepatolenticular degeneration, galactosemia, glycogen-storage disease, syphilis or schistosomiasis is well-known. Nevertheless, until a decade or two back, In India and West Indies, a large chunk of cirrhosis in pediatric age group was accounted by the so-called the *Indian childhood cirrhosis* and *Jamaican cirrhosis* or *veno-occlusive disease (VOD) of liver*.

Indian childhood cirrhosis (ICC), now infrequently seen, is a fatal familial disease peculiar to the Indian infants and children, usually 6 months to 4 years of age and coming predominantly from low or middle-income Hindu families of rural origin. No age is exempt, however. We have infrequently seen ICC in early months of life too. It was first described by Sen in 1887 from Calcutta. Occasionally cases have been seen in Indonesia, Sri Lanka, Nepal, Pakistan, Burma, Israel, Bangladesh, Afghanistan, Egypt, Western Africa, UK, USA and Canada.

This designation was suggested by Professor DB Jelliffe in early 1950s and appears most appropriate. Infantile cirrhosis, infantile biliary cirrhosis, hypertrophic biliary cirrhosis, subacute toxic cirrhosis, etc. are the other names by which this condition has been referred to in the literature. Logically, however, these are misleading and obsolete now.

EPIDEMIOLOGY

- ICC is prevalent all over India.
- The following communities are predominantly affected:
  - South India—Brahmins
  - Central India—Banias
  - North India—Banias and Jats
  - North Indian Hills—Rajputs.
- Rarely, ICC has been encountered in Muslims and Christians as well.
- Males suffer 4 times more than females; the first-born is at greater risk.
- A large majority of the cases belong to low middle-class families (rural).
- Majority of the patients have vegetarian dietetic background.
- A definite family predisposition is the hallmark of ICC. Siblings and twins are frequently affected. Though blood group incompatibilities and chromosomal defects have not been encountered, same workers have found abnormal dermatoglyphics. An increased prevalence of peptic ulcer, asthma, diabetes and migraine in the pedigrees affected by ICC has been observed.

According to an estimate by Pune researchers, incidence of ICC in 1980 was 1:4100 to 1:9400. Over the last more than two decades, we have noticed a steady decline in its incidence in Jammu region so much so that it has become infrequent to see a case now. Similar is the experience from Pune and Chandigarh and, perhaps, from other parts of the country. The remarkable decline in ICC incidence appears to be related to declining practice of employing copper/brass utensils for boiling milk.

ETIOLOGIC CONSIDERATIONS

ICC continues to be a disease of obscure etiology. The various hypotheses are as follows:

A. *Nutritional*

Until recently, it was believed that malnutrition was an important cause of cirrhosis. This view is no longer held.

The objections to this hypothesis are:

- Cirrhosis is rare in children suffering from kwashiorkor. This observation is based on cross-sectional as well as longitudinal follow-up studies.
- Cirrhosis is rare in Africa, the home of kwashiorkor.
- Cirrhosis is uncommon in the poor in whom malnutrition is common. On the contrary, the incidence of ICC is high in the middle-class families.
- Fatty change that is so characteristic of liver in kwashiorkor is either absent or very insignificant in ICC.

Nutrition does not seem to play a clear role in its pathogenesis, except that marked malnutrition perhaps prevents the occurrence of this disease.

B. *Viral*

Since there is fever, leukocytosis, jaundice and splenomegaly and superficial morphologic resemblance to hepatitis, ICC has been thought to be a consequence of neonatal or infective hepatitis. The viral etiology is generally favored by workers from south India. The demonstration of Australia antigen in some cases of ICC is often quoted in support of this speculation. This observation may assume considerable significance if it can be demonstrated that the antigen continues to persist in cases of ICC. The objections to this hypothesis include:

- Natural history of ICC, unlike the experience reported from south India, differs from that of hepatitis. In most of the cases, there is no definite history of preceding jaundice.
- Epidemics of infective hepatitis have not been followed by high incidence of ICC.
- No definite virus has so far been isolated from ICC cases.
- Viral hepatitis is universal but ICC is almost exclusively seen in India.
- The histologic picture of liver in ICC does not bear close resemblance to the known features of hepatitis. In fact, at a certain stage, it attains such distinctive character as to become almost pathognomonic for ICC.

C. *Hepatotoxic*

Since infantile cirrhosis seen in West Indies, i.e. Jamaican cirrhosis (VOD), is known to result from the hepatotoxic effect of harmful pyrrolidizine alkaloids contained in the bushtea, it has been postulated that ICC may well be due to some such agent. The morphologic pattern of ICC liver has much in common with the changes produced by alcohol and other hepatotoxic substances, both in man and animals. This hypothesis regarding the etiopathogenesis of ICC is being seriously investigated now. Many workers believe that the so-called *guttis* fed to the infants may contain agents possessing hepatotoxic properties. *Aflatoxin*, a hepatoxic agent produced by *Aspergillus flavus* that grows on ground nuts, maize and rice, has also been blamed but so far the cause-effect relationship is not established.

D. *Genetic*

The reported familial predisposition points to the possibility of some underlying genetic factor. It has, however, been pointed out that this familial occurrence of ICC may well be the operation of an environmental factor.

E. *Metabolic*

The reported occurrence of defects like amino aciduria, aminoacidemia, mellituria and disturbed lactose, zinc, copper and magnesium metabolism in ICC has raised the possibility of a metabolic basis. These observations, however, need to be substantiated. Further, these defects may well be the result of ICC *per se*.

It has been claimed to be *an inborn error of tryptophan metabolism*. It has been demonstrated that both ICC patients and their asymptomatic relatives have altered tryptophan metabolism.

Sur and Bhatti, the advocates of the theory "incriminating tryptophan metabolic defect" in its etiology have made an interesting recommendation. They feel that "given a positive history, children excreting abnormal amounts of metabolities (3-HAA) can be considered at risk". Adults in such families who excrete abnormal amounts of 3-HAA could be carriers. A child at risk should be put on a low tryptophan diet and massive doses of vitamin B_6. This should be done at the first warning sign of liver disease to arrest ICC.

More recently, resurgence of interest in the copper as the possible etiologic factor has resulted. It is now felt by several workers that the many-fold increase in liver copper in ICC may be related to early introduction of feeds contaminated with copper from copper and/or brass utensils. The high hepatic copper may well be due to:

- Increased absorption.
- Reduced excretion in bile.
- Increased amount of metallothionin, an enzyme known for high binding capacity for copper.
- Some unknown metabolic factors.

Detailed analysis of feeding histories of ICC cases has established that the source of copper in them is top milk (started quite early in infancy), boiled or stored in brass vessels.

F. *Autoimmune*

Antibodies against liver tissue in great majority of the cases of ICC have been reported by some centers. High serum immunoglobulins, reduced serum complement, depressed or delayed hypersensitivity reaction and abnormal cellular immune response have also been observed. A more recent investigation reveals 52% incidence of alpha-fetoprotein (AFP) as against 9% in controls. These interesting observations have led to the postulation that ICC may well be an autoimmune disease.

Table 90.1: Common immunologic disturbances in ICC

- Impaired CMI
- High serum immunoglobulins
- High alpha-fetoproteins (AFP)
- Low serum complement C_3 level
- Presence of immunocomplexes

Whether the immunologic defects in ICC are responsible for the disease or result from it as epiphenomena is purely speculative. Further work may provide the right answer.

To conclude, no single factor seems to be the cause of ICC. It is possible that a genetically-prone child suffers from one or more of the superadded factors (viral, toxic, metabolic and/or autoimmune), leading to the overt picture of ICC.

PATHOLOGY

The basic pathologic change is the diffuse liver cell damage by way of degeneration going on to necrosis and replacement fibrosis. In an established case, there is combination of:

a. Complete disorganization of liver architecture, resulting in the formation of macronodules and micronodules.
b. Absence of regenerative activity indicated by regenerating nodules which are encircled by bands of fibrous tissue.
c. Gross pericellular (creeping) fibrosis in the hepatic lobules.
d. Predominant neutrophilic exudate in lobules.
e. Intracellular hyaline that is identical to the so-called *Mallory hyaline* seen in the alcoholic cirrhosis of adults. There is no primary disease of intrahepatic biliary system. Fatty change is either absent or as at its minimal.
f. Gross excess of copper and/or copper associated protein (*orcein*).

Electronmicroscopy (EM) shows degenerative changes in hepatocytes, scattered fibrosis, electronulecent cytoplasmic areas with loose arrangements or ganelles, indistinct outline of mitochondria, fine fibrillar Mallory hyaline and irregular dense bodies (cuprosomes).

Similar histopathology is seen in a newly-identified disorder, *hepatic copper overload syndrome*, in American children. This form of cirrhosis has a genetic disturbance in copper metabolism as in Wilson's is disease. However, onset is early and the affected children die before the age of 6 years or so.

CLINICAL FEATURES

Two modes of presentation are known:

1. Insidious which occurs in a large majority of the cases.
2. Acute which is less common and some time mimics VOD.

I. *Insidious onset*: There are three arbitrary stages which tend to merge with each other.

A. *First Stage*

It is the stage of vague manifestations. Liver is enlarged by 3 to 5 cm and has a firm feel with sharp, leafy border. Abdominal distention, anorexia or voracious appetite, lassitude, irritability, slight fever, constipation or diarrhea with clay-colored, sticky, formed stools, and growth failure may accompany.

B. *Second Stage*

This stage is characterized by further exaggeration of the manifestations of first stage. Liver size increases and it is more firm. Definite jaundice is evident. In addition, manifestations of portal hypertension dominate the picture. These include splenomegaly, ascites, hematemesis, anemia, prominent superficial abdominal veins and thrombocytopenia. There may be high incidence of intravascular hemolysis.

C. *Third Stage*

This is the terminal stage. The clinical picture is that of an apathetic and emaciated child having deep jaundice, protuberant abdomen with prominent superficial veins and ascites. Liver may be grossly enlarged (sometimes below the umbilicus) or shrunk. Spleen is usually considerably enlarged and hard. In addition, manifestations of hepatocellular failure usually supervene. Restlessness and confusion may ultimately pass on to hepatic coma in which case flapping tremors of the arms may be observed. The child generally dies at this stage either from hepatic failure *per se* or intercurrent infections.

The total duration of illness in this type of onset varies between 6 months and 3 years. It has been convincingly demonstrated that significant retardation in growth occurs in these patients. It is probably due to alteration in ratio of collagen synthesis involving skeletal tissue as indicated by low hydroxyproline index which is an accepted measure of active growth.

II. *Acute onset:* ICC may occasionally have sudden onset with jaundice, fever, clay-colored stools and hepatomegaly. All this may have rapid downhill course, the child finally dying in hepatic coma. This is called fulminant or malignant hepatitis. Some cases belonging to the category of "acute onset" may become symptomatic for a variable period and then again have reappearance of the manifestations which behave like ICC of insidious onset.

DIAGNOSIS

Diagnosis is clear in a full-blown case and no investigations may, in fact, be needed. Nevertheless, high index of suspicion plays a vital role in detecting cases of ICC. At times, thalassemia major, tuberculous hepatosplenomegaly, kwashiorkor, malaria and kala-azar require to be considered in the differential diagnosis.

Liver biopsy is the only reliable method of arriving at a foolproof diagnosis. However, it may not be feasible in an advanced ICC when prothrombin time is prolonged. In such a situation, *cupriuresis* test may be employed. In this test, following oral administration of d-penicillamine, a two-fold hike in urinary copper has a sensitivity of 86% and specificity 60%. Using urinary copper/creatinine ratio as the index parameter, sensitivity of 73% and specificity of 95% with positive and negative values of 83% and 91%, respectively, is obtained.

Table 90.2: Clinical scoring scale in ICC

Criteria	*Score*
1. **Age**	
9 to 24 months	2
25 to 36 months	1
Under 9 and over 36 months	0
2. **Sex**	
First born male	2
Boy	1
Girl	0
3. **Caste**	
Jain/Brahmin/Agarwal/Marwari	2
Maheshwari/Sindhi/Jat/Rajput	1
Muslim/Christian/Tribal	0
4. **Socio-economic status**	
Middle	2
Upper middle	1
Lower and high	0
5. **Feeding details**	
No breast milk	2
Animal milk from 2 to 4 months age	1
Only breastfeeding up to 12 months	0
6. **Utensils for milk boiling and storing**	
Brass (peetal)	2
Occasional brass or brass with inadequate tin (kali) coating	1
Steel or aluminum	0
7. **Examination of liver**	
Under 5 cm, hard with sharp or leafy margin	2
3 to 5 cm, firm with sharp margin	1
Soft with round margin	0
8. **Clinical signs of portal hypertension**	
Splenomegaly*/ascites/edema/prominent abdominal veins/hematemesis/fetor* hepaticus	
All present	3
Any 4 or more present	2
Any 2 or 3 present	1
Maximal score	22

Interpretation of the score obtained

17 and above	Strong possibility of ICC
12 to 16	Fair possibility of ICC
Under 12	ICC unlikely

It has been suggested that hair copper, reflecting the change in liver copper, may be employed as a noninvasive technique for the diagnosis of ICC.

Treatment

Until recently, ICC was dubbed as a "frustrating situation" for which no specific treatment was available. Today, if a diagnosis is made at an early stage (before the development of jaundice or ascites), ICC is potentially treatable.

Table 90.3: Indian childhood cirrhosis (ICC) vs veno-occlusive disease (VOD)

Factor	*ICC*	*VOD*	
Onset	Generally insidious	Always acute	
Etiology	Not known	Hepatotoxic	Component of bushtea
Presence of veno-occlusive element	Not seen in most cases	Outstanding feature	

In the initial stage, an adequate diet with enough of good quality proteins, vitamins and minerals is desirable. Intercurrent infections/infestations should be adequately treated. Administration of corticosteroids, gamma globulins, d-penicillamine or levamisole is advocated by some workers. The best outcome has been obtained in cases treated with d-penicillamine. The drug, administered in a dose of 20 to 40 mg/kg/day for 12 to 18 months, leads to marked improvement and even total reversal in the histopathologic picture.

In the terminal stage when the patient has entered precoma or coma, protein intake should be reduced. Administration of neomycin by gavage and 20% IV glucose drip are helpful. Oxygen may be given as and when warranted. Exchange transfusion to remove the circulating toxins gives gratifying results in some instances.

In case of portal hypertension causing hematemesis, *Sengstaken tube* may be of help in controlling an esophageal bleed. A portocaval anastomosis may be done to relieve the portal hypertension and complications of hypersplenism.

PROGNOSIS

Despite the best of efforts, ICC invariably had a fatal outcome in the past. Recent claims regarding survival of some cases require to be critically examined.

PREVENTION

Those favoring the etiologic role of copper suggest a trial of excluding use of brass and copper utensils for handling infant foods in the susceptible areas. According to them, "children with ICC always give history of being fed large

Table 90.4: Strategy of preventing ICC through lowering of the copper intake

Source of high dietary copper	*Action plan to lower it*
• Brass and copper vessels for	Use of aluminum and steel transportation, storage and for tin-coating on brass boiling of milk
• Copper and brass pots for	Change-over to earthenware or storing drinking water steel and aluminum
• Food cooked and stored in brass	Encourage use of aluminum and copper utensils and steel
• Introduction of animal milk	Promotion of breast-feeding before 2 to 3 months of age
• Copper content of drinking water	Demineralize water under 0.1 mg/L
• Foods rich in copper content	Avoid them or minimize their (liver, nuts, chocolates) consumptions

quantities of top milk boiled or stored in brass utensils since early infancy". If brass and copper vessels are scrupulously avoided for infant feeding with prolonged breastfeeding and cereal supplementation, ICC should not occur. An aggressive education campaign to switch the rural population from using brass feeding vessels/utensils to aluminum or stainless steel ones is advocated.

KEY LEARNING POINTS

- A peculiar disease seen almost exclusively in Indian infants and children is now infrequently encountered.
- Etiologically, it appears that a genetically prone child suffers from one or more of the triggering factors (copper overload, viral, toxic, metabolic, autoimmune) leading to the overt picture of the disease.
- Basic pathologic change is diffuse liver cell degeneration progressing to necrosis, and replacement fibrosis.
- Characterized by either insidious onset (common) in which liver is usually greatly enlarged and the disease progresses in three stages, the last stage ending up in fatality, or acute onset with rapid course and death.
- Despite best of efforts, prognosis remains grave.
- Prevention lies in avoiding use of brass feeding vessels/utensils.

FURTHER READINGS

1. Sharda B. Indian childhood cirrhosis. In: Gupte S (ed): *Recent Advances in Pediatrics* - 6. New Delhi: Jaypee 1992:119.
2. Sur AM, Bhatti A. Indian childhood cirrhosis. *Br Med J* 1978;2:650-654.
3. Tanner MS. Indian childhood cirrhosis: Copper ingestion, pencillamine treatment and prevention. *Indian J Pediatr* 1987;54:467-472.

91 Diseases of the Gallbladder

Renu Kumar • Ragavan M

INTRODUCTION

In recent years, gallbladder (GB) diseases have become increasingly common in children. Whether this increase in incidence is due to actual rise in diseases *per se* or simply increased detection by routine use of ultrasonography is not known. Other diseases of the gallbladder are hidden by the extreme prevalence of cholelithiasis. In children 30% of the diseases are due to acalculous causes.

Gallbladder diseases are classified as congenital anomalies, infection of gallbladder, systemic diseases involving gallbladder, gallbladder trauma and gallstone disease. Hydrops of the gallbladder, acalculous cholecystitis, biliary dyskinesia and gallbladder polyps are not uncommon in children nowadays.

ANOMALIES OF THE GALLBLADDER

These include rudimentary gallbladder, absent galladder, duplication or triplication of gallbladder.

Absent gallbladder predisposes to increased bile duct stones and bile ductal malignancy.

Intrahepatic gallbladder of the fetal position may persist into adulthood also. A pseudodiverticulum from the fundus of the gallbladder "**Phrygian cap**" is the most common anomaly of shape.

Giant cystic malformation of the GB has been described and it could be a variant of choledochal cyst.

Heterotropic tissue are found in GB include hepatic, pancreatic, intestinal or gastric. Occasionally gastric tissue can give rise to peptic ulcer of GB.

Floating gallbladder occurs due to long mesentery or short mesentery only consisting of cystic duct and cystic artery. It is more prone to torsion of GB which presents like acute cholecystitis.

Gallbladder can be **traumatized** in penetrating abdominal injury, percutaneous liver biopsy or percutaneous transhepatic cholangiography.The incidence has increased as more and more interventions are being performed under radiological guidance.

INFECTIONS OF THE GALLBLADDER

Acalculous Cholecystitis

It occurs in severe illness like sepsis, burns, or systemic trauma that results in dehydration, hypotension and ileus. The addition of TPN in this setting may decrease the gallbladder contractility with progressive distention, stasis, and predisposition to infection. It usually occurs in patients in intensive care units. Occasionally, children may worm, infestation like Ascariasis and *Giardia lamblia.* Repeated doses of opiates in postoperative or traumatized patients cause increased sphincter spasm and increase the luminal pressure above systolic blood pressure that results in ischemia and cascade of cholecystitic events.

There are no specific clinical or histological differences between calculous and acalculous cholecystitis, but for obvious reasons the morbidity and mortality remains high in acalculous form.

Diagnosis needs high index of clinical suspicion. Ultrasonography shows increasing mural thickening, gallbladder sludge and increasing distention with evidence of pericholecystic fluid which are indications for cholecystectomy. Cholescintigraphy using technetium labeled iminodiacetic acids is more sensitive test which shows nonvisualization of the gallbladder with good hepatic uptake and good drainage into the duodenum. Moreover, the rim sign that is increased pericholecystic activity indicates gangrene of the GB. Free peritoneal spill of radiotracer indicates GB perforation that mandates emergency laparotomy.

Acalculous cholecystitis needs to be followed by USG, resolving findings and improvement in symptoms usually precedes uneventful recovery. In case clinical deterioration, best treatment is emergency laparotomy and cholecystectomy. However, cholecystostomy (tube drainage of gallbladder) which is not otherwise recommended in presence of gangrenous gallbladder could be life-saving in critically ill patient. Cholecystostomy may be appropriate in children as gangrenous changes are uncommon.

Rare Types of Cholecystitis

Typhoid fever can cause either acute or chronic cholecystitis. Children can harbour salmonella typhi for rest of their life and are more prone to develop gallbladder carcinoma.

Staphylococci can rarely cause acute cholecystitis, bacteria reaching GB through blood stream.

Acute emphysematous cholecystitis results from infection with gas-forming organisms like clostridia or coliforms. Typically, it occurs in diabetics when they present with right hypochondriac pain, fever, right subcostal tenderness and toxemia. Plain X-ray abdomen shows gas filled gallbladder. The primary pathology here is obstruction of cystic duct or cystic artery and secondary infection with gas forming organisms.

Chronic gallbladder inflammation may occur in systemic sclerosis.

Xanthogranulomatous cholecystitis is a rare type of cholecystitis where gallbladder is shrunken, nodular, chronically inflamed with foci of necrosis and hemorrhage. Abundant histiocytes packed with lipids impart the yellow color to its wall as the name suggests. Gallstones are usually present. Similar condition xanthogranulomatous pyelonephritis occurs in kidney, in association with chronic infection and nephrolithiasis. On gross pathology they resemble malignancy (pseudotumor). Gallbladder is quite often affected in polyarteritis nodosa (PAN), but acute cholecystitis is rare.

Cholecystosis

Cholesterolosis is condition where triglycerides and cholesterol are deposited in the macrophages of lamina propria and also in the epithelial cells. These deposits project from the mucosa as small polyps. Diffuse cholesterosis produces "**strawberry gallbladder**" with yellow flecks of cholesterol extensively studded on a red inflamed red mucosa. These polyps can break of and form a nidus for cholesterol stones which are seen in 10-15% of cases of cholesterolosis. The etiology is obscure but increased absorption of cholesterol and its esterification by the gallbladder wall could be the possible mechanism.

Adenomyomatosis (Adenomyosis)

This condition is characterized by hyperplasia of the mucosa, specially the muscularis and by presence of intraluminal diverticula or crypts (Rokitansky-Aschoffs sinuses).

The localized form is adenomyoma, which is a pseudoneoplasm, appears as sessile mass in the fundus, which bulges into the lumen and is often umbilicated. The segmental form is marked by a constricting ring or septum in the fundus or body that separates the gallbladder into two compartments.

Diffuse form causes generalized thickening of the wall with structures resembling the glands and cysts hence the **cholecystitis glandularis proliferance** and diverticulosis. Pigment stones are frequently trapped in these diverticula.

Etiology is unknown but increased luminal pressure seems a plausible mechanism as in colonic diverticulosis. **Porcelain gallbladder** is form of **hyalocalcinosis** of gallbladder wall to hard and bluish white texture resembling porcelain ceramic. Gallstones cause chronic irritation of the gallbladder; it becomes irritated, and precipitates calcification that might necessitate surgery.

HYDROPS

Hydrops is a massive distention of the gallbladder in the absence of stones, infections or congenital anomalies. It is most often reported in typhoid fever, leptospirosis, systemic infections like streptococcal or staphylococcal, hemolytic diseases like sickle cell crisis, thalassemia, TPN with or without prolonged fasting, NNEC, Henoch-Schöenlein purpura and viral hepatitis. It is often seen in Kawasaki's (mucocutaneous lymph node) disease and is due to transient obstruction of the cystic duct or to increased mucus secretion by gallbladder resulting in poor emptying. Hydrops is also seen in Sjogren's syndrome. Further distention causes more angulation of the cystic duct further increasing the distention. Usual symptoms are right hypochondriac pain with or without vomiting. Tender gallbladder may be palpable.

Management is conservative with antibiotics and early initiation of enteral feeding to stimulate gallbladder emptying. If it does not resolve and serial USG shows progressive distention with increasing pain or in presence of toxemia indicating gangrene of the gallbladder immediate cholecystectomy should be considered.

Biliary Dyskinesia

Of late, biliary dyskinesia is being increasingly diagnosed in children. It is characterized by poor gallbladder contractility and presence of cholesterol crystals in the bile. Diagnosis is made when typical biliary pain is not associated with gall stones on ultrasound. Gallbladder contractility can be assessed by cholescintigraphy after cholecystokinin (CCK) injection. The ejection fraction (EF) of gallbladder in these patients is usually less than 35%. Changes of chronic cholecystitis are seen on histology. The management is laparoscopic cholecystectomy, which resolves the symptoms in 80% of children. Pain, nausea, vomiting in the absence of gallstones on USG and gallbladder ejection fraction less than 15% on CCK-cholescintigraphy are the predictors of benefit from cholecystectomy. Children with EF more than 15% did show predictable response to cholecystectomy. Typical histological changes of Crohn's disease have been seen in patients with granulomatous enteritis. Sclerosing cholangititis almost always involves the cystic duct and gallbladder.

NEOPLASMS

Pseudotumors include inflammatory polyps, cholesterol polyps, heterotropic nests and adenomyoma, the localized form of adenomyomatosis. Adenoma is the most common type true benign neoplasm. It can be either sessile or papillary and is usually solitary. Adenomatous polyps have been seen in Peutz-Jeghers syndrome. Ten percent of polyps are multiple. Gallbladder polyps also have become more frequent in children. Presence of biliary symptoms or size greater than equal to 1 cm is an indication for cholecystectomy.

GALLSTONE DISEASE

Children of all ages may develop gallstones; prevalence varies with age and geography. There is bimodal distribution with peaks in infancy and early adolescence. In early childhood the incidence is more in boys than girls whereas during adolescence there is female preponderance. The rising incidence of gallstones in children is probably due to increased detection by USG rather than genuine increase in incidence. Gallstone disease could be hemolytic or non-hemolytic.

There are five types of gallstones found in children compared to only four types in adults.

1. **Mixed cholesterol stones** are composed of cholesterol plus calcium, they are rounded or faceted in shape. Yellowish white in color with brown ring /specks, usually multiple, are sterile stones. Female sex and obesity are the risk factors, and more common in adults and adolescents.
2. **Pure cholesterol stones:** Contain only cholesterol, round and smooth, yellow or white color, often single, sterile in nature, risk factors are female sex and obesity.
3. **Bilirubin pigment stones** are composed of bilirubin pigment and calcium bilirubinate, are smooth or faceted, exclusively black in color, often multiple and sterile, hemolysis is the only risk factors. In young children (prepubertal), most common stones are black pigment ones due to haemolysis and total peripheral nutrition.
4. **Brown pigment stones:** Calcium bilirubinatenate +Calcium salts of fatty acids, oval and irregular in shape, brown in color and soft BR/soft single or multiple, exclusively found in infected system, cholangits /stricture are the main predisposing factors. Brown pigment stones are the result of stasis and infection, are most common in ducts.
5. **Calcium carbonate stones** are irregular, round or faceted, brown or white often single, sterile in nature, seen in children with gallbladder obstruction. Lately calcium carbonate stones are commonly reported in children.

Overall gallstones associated with hemolytic disease form the significant proportion of gallstone disease in children. Fifty percent of children with sickle cell anemia will develop gallstones by 20 years of age. In hereditary sherocytosis the incidence of cholelithiasis range from 43% to 63%, hence ultrasonography is required to look for gallstones before contemplating elective splenectomy so that cholecystectomy can be performed at the same setting. With the advent of hypertransfusion therapy for thalassemia major the incidence of cholelithiasis in this disease has decreased. Hypertransfusion suppresses bone marrow so that fragile RBC's are not available for hemolysis.

Biliary sludge is a complex mixture of mucin matrix, calcium bilirubinate and cholesterol crystals. Total parenteral nutrition, fasting, pregnancy, sickle cell disease ceftriaxone (pseudolithiasis) or octreotide administration and bone marrow transplantation are the proven risk factors. Biliary sludge usually regresses once inciting factor is eliminated; otherwise it progresses to gallstone disease. It itself can cause biliary complications. On USG it is echogenic without an acoustic shadowing (stones always have a posterior acoustic shadow). Biliary sludge is frequently documented in sickle cell anemia, so few authors recommend elective cholecystectomy in presence of sludge with or without gallstones.

Etiology

Biliary stasis, excess bilirubin production as in sickle cell anemia, hereditary spherocytosis and thalassemia major, lithogenic bile (supersaturated bile), prevalence of pigment stones increases with age, hemolytic uremic syndrome (HUS), ABO or Rh incompatibility, cardiac valve replacement, premature babies particularly susceptible to TPN induced GSD, Ileal resection or ileal diseases those especially on TPN and cyclosporine therapy.

Gallstone diseases in newborns are seen in polycythemia, phototherapy, and following multiple transfusions. Symptomatic GSD occur in 10-20% of short bowel syndrome. Ileal Crohn's has increased risk of cholelithiasis. In adolescents, risk factors like adults–female, fatty, fertile, family history. Choledochal cyst, biliary ductal anomalies and biliary dyskinesias are the other risk factors.

Clinical Features

Signs and symptoms are age dependent, fetal gallstones are also reported and found to resolve spontaneously. Premature babies are at a greatest risk for GSD due to poor contractility of gallbladder to enteral feed, furesemide therapy, Rptd BT, immature bile excretion system, systemic sepsis and biliary infection. In newborns usually remain asymptomatic and complications are uncommon.

Older children will have abdominal pain, associated with nausea or vomiting, clinical features of obstruct jaundice and pancreatitis may also be seen. Fatty food intolerance, biliary colic, acute cholecystitis–Fever, RHC tend palpable mass. Many children remain asymptomatic and are detected incidentally on USG.

Complications of untreated gallstones include acute cholecystitis, cholangitis and gallstone pancreatitis.

Diagnosis

Ultrasound on a fasted patient is the investigation of choice. Mobile, solitary/multiple echogenic structures with a characteristic posterior acoustic shadow is the classical finding. Stone size, number, GB wall thickness, and CBD diameter, liver status can also be inferred easily. In children 20-50% of Gallstones are radio-opaque, compared to only 10% in adults. DISIDA (Di-Isopropyl Imino-Diacetic Acid hepatobiliary scintigraphy) is very useful in the diagnosis of acute cholecystitis. DISIDA can be used even in the presence of poor liver function. MRCP is done in case of CBD stones or complicated stone disease. ERCP has therapeutic role only in older children due to technical problem.

Management

Occasionally gallstones resolve spontaneously either by dissolution or passage into the gut. Management of asymptomatic GSD in older children is controversial, but cholecystectomy is beneficial. Elective cholecystectomy should be considered in hemolytic gallstones. GB sludge resolves spontaneously after resumption of enteral feeds after TPN. Cholecystokinin or UDCA are used to clear biliary sludge. Dissolution therapy has little valve. ESWL is rarely used in children.

Standard of therapy for symptomatic or complicated GSD is cholecystectomy. In a severely ill child initial cholecystostomy is a safe option. In non-hemolytic incidental gallstones expectant treatment may be considered. Presence of gallstones whether symptomatic or asymptomatic in any hemolytic disorder is an indication for cholecystectomy and preferably by laparoscopic technique. In hereditary spherocytosis and thalassemia major even with asymptomatic gallstones cholecystectomy should be done at the time of splenectomy. Prophylactic cholecystectomy is not indicated in hereditary spherocytosis without gallstones. Laparoscopic cholecystectomy (LC) is the preferred technique in children. Infants can also be successfully treated with LC.

CBD STONES IN CHILDREN

CBD stones are less frequent in children than adults, but pancreatitis is not uncommon. Incidence of CBD stones varies between 15-20% of all biliary stone diseases. History suggestive of obstructive jaundice and cholangitis may indicate the presence of CBD stones.

KEY LEARNING POINTS

- Gallstone disease is uncommon in children though the incidence appears to be increasing over the recent past.
- Hemolytic disorders are the major cause.
- Early surgical intervention is needed to prevent complications.
- Laparoscopic cholecystectomy is the preferred technique even in children and infants.

FURTHER READINGS

1. Holcomb GW III, Morgan WM III, Neblett WW III, *et al.* Laparoscopic cholecystectomy in children: Lessons learned from the first 100 patients. *J Pediatr Surg* 1999; 34:1236-1240.
2. Holcomb GW III, Andrews WS. Gallbladder disease and hepatic infection. In:Grosfeld JL, O'Neill JA Jr, Fonkalsurd EW, *et al.* (eds): *Pediatric Surgery*, 6th edn. St. Louis: Mosby–Year Book 2006: 1635-1649.
3. Stringer MD. Disorders of the gallbladder and biliary tract. In Oldham KT, Colombanii PM, Foglia RP *et al.* (eds): *Pediatric Principles and Practice of Pediatric Surgery,* 2nd edn. Philadelphia: Lipincott Williams and Wilkins–Year Book 2004:1495-1507.
4. Suchy FJ. Diseases of gallbladder. In: Behrman RE, Kiegman RM, Jenson HB (eds): *Nelson Textbook of Pediatrics.*17th edn. Philadelphia: Saunders–Year Book 2004: 1345-1346.
5. Walker TM,Hambleton IR, Serjeant GR. Gallstones in sickle cll disease: Observations from the Jamaican cohort study. *J Pediatr* 2000;136:80-83.
6. Williamson RC. Acalculous disease of the gallbladder. *Gut* 1988; 29:860-872.

92 Cystic Diseases of the Liver and Biliary Tract

Renu Kumar • Ragavan M

INTRODUCTION

With widespread use of ultrasound, cystic diseases of the liver and biliary tracts are being detected more frequently nowadays.

Liver cysts have been estimated to occur in 5% of the population. They could be infective or noninfective in origin. Infective cysts are caused by an echinococcal species, or as the sequel of a treated amebic or pyogenic abscess. The noninfective cysts are simple cyst, polycystic syndromes (usually with coexisting renal disease), choledochal cyst and Caroli's disease.

Sometimes hepatic fibrosis may be associated with cystic diseases. The association of cystic disease with congenital hepatic fibrosis may be considered as "hepatobiliary fibrocystic continuum".

In addition, there are a variety of cystic neoplasm and a miscellany of unusual forms.

All cyst detected on ultrasound should be subjected to CT or MRI for accurate diagnosis and management.

SIMPLE CYSTS

Etiology of simple liver cysts is unknown, but is believed to be congenital. The cysts are lined by biliary type epithelium. Possibly they are microhamartomas that fail to develop normal connections with the biliary tree, as these cysts seldom contain bile. Typically, cyst fluid has an electrolyte composition that mimics plasma. Bile, amylase, and white blood cells are absent. These are generally benign. They can be solitary or multiple. Typically they are small and often asymptomatic.

Asymptomatic cysts do not require any treatment. Large cysts can cause pain, or get into complications like bleeding, rupture, infection or obstructive jaundice. These can be unroofed either by laparoscopic or open approaches. Infected cysts are treated as hepatic abscesses. In presence of cystobiliary communication, biliary opening should be repaired or drained by a cysto-jejunostomy. Simple needle aspiration of the cyst is not curative as epithelial lining of the cyst continually secretes fluid.

POLYCYSTIC LIVER DISEASE

Polycystic kidney disease, autosomal dominant form (AD-PLD), is occasionally associated with, adult polycystic liver disease (AD-PCLD) Occasionally; PCLD has been reported in the absence of polycystic kidney disease. The kidney cysts usually precede the liver cysts. PKD often results in renal failure, whereas liver cysts are asymptomatic. Hepatic fibrosis and liver failure are rare. Patients may be symptomatic because of hepatomegaly. Symptomatic liver cysts are treated by surgical drainage. Liver resection of the most affected part is also effective. Rarely cystadenoma or cysteadenocarcinoma occurs in liver and are distinguished by the presence of septae or mass and are treated by resection.

NEOPLASTIC CYSTS

Hepatic tumors with central necrosis on imaging studies can be misdiagnosed as liver cysts. True intrahepatic neoplastic cysts are rare. These cystic tumors are lined with biliary-type cuboidal or columnar cells and are surrounded by ovarian-like stroma. Cystadenoma is a premalignant lesion with a tendency for malignant transformation into cystadenocarcinoma.

CHOLEDOCHAL CYST (CDC)

Choledochal cysts, more appropriately called "congenital biliary dilatations". They are isolated or combined congenital dilatations of the extrahepatic biliary tree, intrahepatic biliary radicles, or both. Two third of children with CDC have signs or symptoms before the age of 10 years. It is amongst the most common abnormalities affecting the biliary system of children. It is more prevalent in females of Asian descent. In some cases CDC may not become clinically apparent until adult age.

Classification

Todani's modification of Alonso-Lej's classification system for choledochal cysts is the most accepted one (Fig. 92.1).

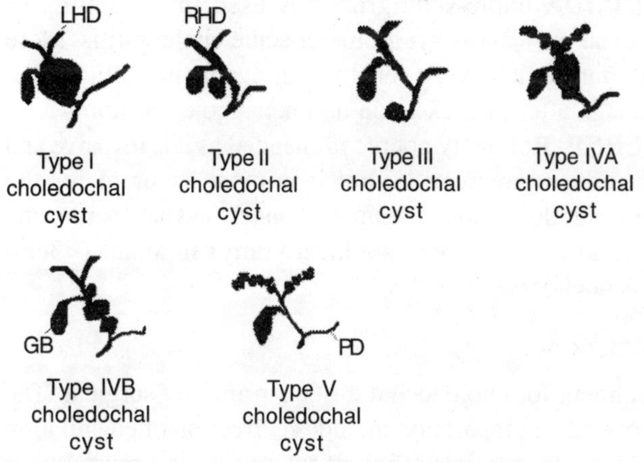

Fig. 92.1: Types of choledochal cysts
LHD: Left hepatic duct; RHD: Right hepatic duct; GB: Gall bladder; PD: Pancreatic duct

Type I - Most common (80-90%) type is dilatations of the entire common hepatic and common bile ducts or of segments of each. They can be cystic or fusiform. The gallbladder usually enters the CDC. The right and left bile ducts and the ducts within the liver are usually normal in size.

Type II is a diverticulum from common bile duct (CBD), although the CBD itself is normal. They may be sessile or connected to CBD by a narrow stalk.

Type III also called as choledochocele, is a localized area of dilation terminal CBD within the duodenum or pancreas, rest of the biliary tree is usually normal. There is almost always some degree of narrowing or blockage around the ampulla. Pain, in particular, is characteristic of this type.

Type IVA cysts - Multiple dilatations of both intra and extrahepatic biliary tree, frequently, a large, solitary cyst of the extrahepatic duct is associated with multiple intrahepatic cysts.

Type IVB cysts are multiple dilatations of only the extrahepatic bile duct.

Type V cysts - Dilatation of intrahepatic biliary ducts with periportal fibrosis (Caroli's disease). Numerous cysts are interposed with strictures that predispose to intrahepatic stone formation, obstruction, and cholangitis. Cysts are typically bilobar. Occasionally, unilobar disease frequently involves left lobe.

Types VI - Few cases of isolated dilatation of cystic duct have been reported. They may be called Type VI CDC. However, they are extremely unusual and are not included in Todani's classification.

Fruste forme (FFCC) represents 4-21% of all choledochal cysts. It is described as "minimal dilatation of CBD" which does not grow with time, almost always associated with long common channel and partial obstruction of terminal CBD. CBD dilatation is 6-10 mm, associated with fever, jaundice abdominal pain, recurrent pancreatitis and altered LFT. The histology of the excised extra hepatic biliary tree (EHBD) shows partially denuded mucosa with ulceration or sloughing, minimal fibrosis, and inflammatory cell infiltration. It is better diagnosed on by intraoperative cholangiopancreatography or MRCP or ERCP in a clinical setting of CDC. The treatment of choice for FFCC in children is EHBD excision and hepatico-jejunostomy.

There are reports on the association of choledochal cyst with biliary atresia.

Etiology and Pathophysiology

The exact etiology is not known. The pathogenesis is probably multifactorial with a congenital predisposition and an acquired damage. Majority (90%) of patients with choledochal cysts have an anomalous pancreatobiliary junction (APBJ). An APBJ is characterized by the entry of the pancreatic duct into the common bile duct 1 cm or more proximal to where the common bile duct reaches the ampulla of Vater.

APBJ → Reflux of pancreatic secretions and enzymes into the CBD→ Alkaline conditions in CBD→ Activate pancreatic proenzymes → Results in inflammation and weakening of the bile duct wall. →Complete denuding of the common bile duct mucosa→ Cystic dilatation of CBD.

Other theories are congenital weakness of CBD, abnormal canalization of CBD, obstruction at the level of duodenum, abnormalities of autonomic innervation, sex-linked defect, prenatal rupture of CBD (type II) and congenital duodenal duplication (in type III).

Clinical Features

Clinical presentation varies with the patient's age. Clinically there are two distinct forms of CDC, infantile form and adult form.

Infantile form is seen in 1-3 months of age, usually with in first month. Symptoms are overt and dramatic. Clinical picture is like that of complete bile duct blockage. The features are obstructive jaundice with yellow skin and eyes, acholic stools, hepatomegaly and low grade fever. Jaundice manifest at 1-3 weeks of age. Pain and features of cirrhosis are rare. An early workup to exclude biliary atresia is also mandatory in this setting.

Adult form can present any time after 6 months of age, usually after 2 years. Manifestations are more subtle and protean, usual symptoms are abdominal pain (stretching of the dilated duct or to cholangitis), palpable abdominal mass, intermittent jaundice, signs of cholangitis or cirrhosis and rarely pancreatitis. The diagnosis of CDC is difficult in children with pancreatitis. Indeed, a classical (Charcot's) triad of abdominal pain, jaundice, and a palpable right hypochondriac mass is seen in only 10% of cases. CDC's in older children or adults can present with a number of serious complications like cholangitis, cysts rupture with biliary peritonitis, cholelithiasis, severe pancreatitis, hepatic abscesses, hepatic cirrhosis, malignancy and portal hypertension. Toxic cholangitis presents with fever, vomiting, jaundice, abdominal pain and disorientation (known as Reynold's pentad).

In utero (Fetal CDC) – Nowadays many CDC are diagnosed by antenatal ultrasound as early as15th week of gestation. However they become evident clinically after 1 to 3 weeks of birth. Antenatal diagnosis facilitates thorough investigations and elective definitive surgical therapy, before complications settle in. The treatment is delayed primary cyst excision. The recommended age is after 2 months when the infants physiology more suitable for anesthesia unlike in neonates. Percutaneous drainage can be done in neonates with severe obstructive jaundice.

Investigations

Basic blood chemistries like liver function tests including amylase and lipase, coagulation profile, hemogram and cross match for blood are done. Diagnostic investigations include:

Ultrasonogram is the initial screening test for any patient with suspected hepatobiliary pathology. It gives an idea about the echotexture of the liver, intrahepatic biliary radicals, status of entire extrahepatic biliary and vascular structures. Pertinent findings include a cystic extrahepatic mass.

MR cholangiopancreaticography (MRCP) is used to visualize CDC and is the confirmatory study in children with choledochal cysts (Fig. 92.2) because it does not require breath holding (latest TSE technology), and is also noninvasive. It delineates the cyst and associated anomalies of the pancreatic duct junction with the CBD, and the long common channel formed by the two are usually well demonstrated.

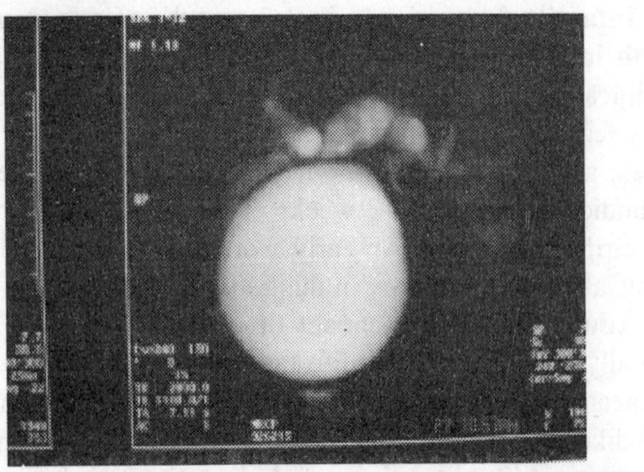

Fig. 92.2: MRCP, type I, depicting the choledochal cyst (See for colour figure Plate 10)

CECT Scan is highly accurate, helps in diagnosis and planning surgery. Recently, CT cholangiography has been used in the diagnosis of choledochal cysts.

DISIDA chole-scintigraphy is used in the setting of neonatal cholestasis syndrome or acute cholecystitis. More importantly, it is very sensitive in evaluating bilioenteric drainage after cyst excision and hepaticojejunostomy.

ERCP- Routinely not recommended as it is invasive and can induce pancreatitis, but it is most accurate for the demonstration of long common channel, and has therapeutic advantage (endoscopic sphincerotomy) in small (<3cm) choledochoceles.

Treatment

Treatment for choledochal cysts is primarily surgical. The preoperative preparation includes correction of coagulation problems by administration of vitamin K and fresh frozen plasma if required, prophylactic antibiotics, adequate hydration and preoperative carbohydrates.

The aim of surgery is to completely excise the dilated ductal system and to establish bilioenteric drainage. The procedures include excision of the cyst with hepatico-jejunostomy in type I and type IV, excision of the diverticula in type II, transduodenal sphincterotomy, sphincteroplasty, pancreatoduodenectomy for type III. In type V (Caroli disease)-Unilobar disease, usually left, can be treated with lobar resection. Bilobar diseases with biliary cirrhosis, portal hypertension, or liver failure are candidates for liver transplantation. Recently, laparoscopic techniques have been successfully applied to the management of choledochal cysts.

If untreated, complication like jaundice, recurrent cholangitis, pancreatitis, gallstones, cholecystitis, cirrhosis with portal hypertension, cyst rupture and carcinoma of CBD, gallbladder, pancreas and liver can occur. Risk of malignancy is age related, less than 10 years it is 0.7%, between 11-20 years it is 6.8% and more than 20 years it is 15%.

HYDATID DISEASE

The term, *hydatid*, literally means water vesicle or drop of water. It's a zoonotic infestation caused by larval tapeworm (platyhelminths) of the genus echinococcus. Highly endemic in Mediterranean, Middle East, Southern South America, Iceland, Australia, New Zealand, Southern Africa and especially North Indian states like Jammu and Kashmir, Himachal Pradessh, Uttaranchal, Punjab and Haryana. Incidence is quite variable. There is no sex predilection, but usually active member of family is affected. Hydatid is a disease of young adults, average age of manifestation is 30-40 years, but in endemic areas children and adults are equally affected. Peak incidence in childhood is seen between 5-15 years.

Parasitology

Four species of echinococcus are identified, of these only

three are of medical importance. *Echinococcus granulosus* causes cystic echinococcosis, *E. multilocularis* causes alveolar echinococcosis, *E.vogeli* is most rare, and usually seen in southern part of South America and *E. oligartus* whose life cycle not known. E. granulosus is the most common of the three and E. multilocularis is rare but most virulent.

Life Cycle

The definitive hosts are domestic or wild dogs those carry the adult tape worm, which measures <1cm, which is a true hermaphrodite and lives in the canine ileal villi and continuously shed eggs (30μ). The eggs are then taken by the grazers (intermediate host) where it develops into larva and hydatid cyst. Dogs get infected by ingesting viscera of intermediate animals. Intermediate hosts are sheep, cow, goat, camel, and buffalo. Humans are accidental intermediate hosts and are dead end for the parasite (**mortal combat**). Direct pet handling is the most common route of infestation in children. Indirectly children can acquire the ova by contaminated food or water and also by handing contaminated objects.

Development in Humans

In human beings, the ingested hexacanth embryo is activated by bile salts in the duodenum and the onchosphere are released. They penetrate the gut mucosa and gains access into portal circulation. In the liver, if not destroyed by Kupffer cells or filtered by sinusoids, the larval stage develops into a "Hydatid cysts". Eighty percentage develop hydatid cysts in the liver alone and right lobe is commonly affected. Rest escape and enter the lungs and other organs. First response of the tissues to the invasion by the larva is to wall it off by fibrous tissue (advential reaction). Then chitin secretion with central vacuolization is done by the parasite itself. As early as 12 hours, a small hydatid follicle is formed. By the end of 7 days the parasite is demarcated by a vascular reaction but still it is vulnerable to phagocytosis. After 15 days a microscopic hydatid cyst forms. By the end of 3 weeks the cyst is visible to the naked eye. At 3 months it can be measured 4-5 cm in diameter. They are usually spherical, but can have distorted shape that suggests compression by adjacent bile ducts or vessels. Pericyst is formed by 5 months. Cysts in the centre of the liver have slow growth due to parenchymal compression. Peritoneal cyst and superficial cysts will have rapid growth as there is room for expansion. Normal growth rate of the cyst is 1mm per month (1-2 cm/year). Sometimes the cyst becomes extensively calcified but every calcified cyst is not dead.

Hydatid Cyst Structure

It consists of three layers: pericyst, ectocyst and endocyst (Fig. 92.3). Pericyst is formed from host tissue, ectocyst and endocyst are formed by the parasite. **Pericyst** is an avascular atrophic layer of liver cells forming an adventitious capsule, which can be separated from the ectocyst. **Ectocyst** is the laminated membrane, formed by the chitin secreted by the parasite itself, which gives rigidity, and more importantly it conceals parasitic antigen so that there is no systemic reaction from the host, measures approximately 0.5 cm thick, acts as barrier for bacteria and ultra filter for proteins. **Endocyst** is the germinative membrane, has nutritional and proliferative function roughly measures 1-2 mm, it produces hydatid fluid, ectocyst, brood capsules, protoscolices and daughter cyst. It has three layers outer tegument that gives rise to laminated membrane, middle tegument cell region responsible for transport of nutrients and ions, inner layer with the reproductive function.

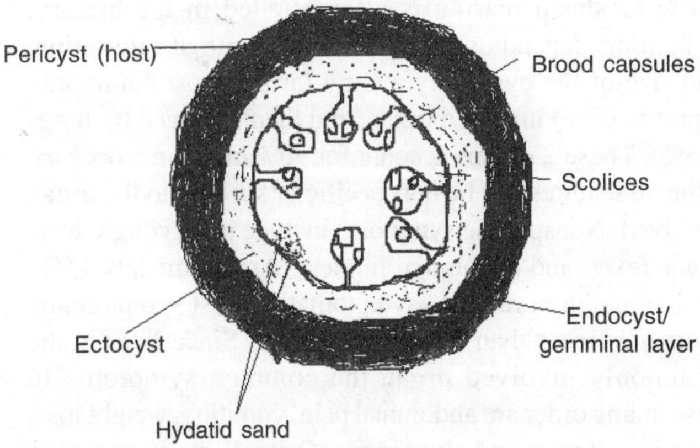

Fig. 92.3: Hydatid cyst structure. Note the three layers

Cyst Contents

A process of **endogenic vesiculation** from the germinal membrane produces brood capsules which form the future worm heads known as protoscolices. Protoscolex measure about 150 μ, they are sturdy, mobile and free floating. They implant only on serosal surfaces and not on epithelial surfaces. In definitive host like dogs they develop into an adult worm. In intermediate host like sheep or human beings (accidental host) they develop into a new hydatid cyst in the target organ. Hydatid fluid is sterile, colorless and highly antigenic. "**Hydatid sand**" is formed by free brood capsules, protoscolices, and calcareous bodies in hydatid fluid. In horses hydatid cysts are parasitologically sterile and do not produce brood capsules.

Organs affected

Virtually any organ of the human body can be involved. Apart from liver and lungs, other organs affected include Muscles (5%), Bones (3%), Kidneys (2%), Brain (1%) and Spleen (1%). Organ specific symptoms indicate a significant increase in size of the cyst with pressure effects of the organ concerned. Pressure effects are initially vague and have delayed manifestations except brain and eyes.

Types of Hydatid Cysts

Univesicular cysts are those which have intact laminated membrane and they contribute to 50% of cysts. *Multivesicular cysts* (MVC) are those which do not have an intact LM. LM is ruptured by pressure necrosis or trauma. Here the pericystic cavity is filled with degenerated fragments of LM, innumerable daughter cyst, amorphous hydatid debris, bile and often small cystobiliary communication is present. This appears as 'thin pus' which is sterile. Patients with MVC are more prone to anaphylaxis.

Clinical Features

Living in or visiting an endemic area, contact with pets and cattle or sheep rearing is often elicited in the history. Symptoms depend on the parasite load, site of infestation, and size of the cysts. Liver is by far the most commonly (approx. 63%) involved organ, and then followed by lungs (25%). These 2 organs account for 90% of echinococcosis. Clinical features can be nonspecific or specific to the organ involved. Nonspecific symptoms include pain, cough, low-grade fever, and abdominal fullness. Approximately 15%-25% of children remain asymptomatic. Most symptomatic cysts are larger than 5 cm in diameter. Since liver is the commonly involved organ the common symptoms in descending order are abdominal pain, vomiting, weight loss, jaundice, fever and dyspepsia. Overall most common symptom is right hypochondriac pain with or with hepatomegaly. Pressure effects of liver hydatid includes features of obstructive jaundice, are due to cyst-biliary fistula or extrinsic compression. Abdominal pain due to starching of Glisson's capsule. Signs include hepatomegaly, palpable mass and icterus. Spider angiomas are suggestive of portal hypertension due to biliary cirrhosis or inferior vena cava obstruction. Urticaria and erythema are due to allergic reactions. Pyrexia occur secondary to infection or allergic reaction. Hypotension is suggestive of anaphylaxis due to cyst leak or intervention. Tender hepatomegaly suggests infected cyst. Splenomegaly indicates splenic cyst or portal hypertension. Pressure effects of pulmonary hydatid are chronic cough, dyspnea, pleuritic chest pain and hemoptysis grossly decreased breath sounds over the affected area are seen in lung hydatid with or without airway obstruction. Sympathetic pleural effusion occurs on the ipsilateral side. More dangerously diaphragmatic erosion and rupture into ipsilateral hemithorax can result in shock and pyothorax. Central nervous system pressure effects are headache, dizziness, altered consciousness and site specific focal neurologic deficits. In CNS hydatid cysts nonspecific or focal neurologic deficit can be seen. Mild to full coma or cerebral herniation can also occur. Eyes are rarely affected; decreased visual acuity, blindness, and exophthalmus are the usual signs. In hydatid of extremities bone-tenderness, palpable mass arising from bone or muscle and rarely signs of peripheral nerve compression or specific sensory and/or motor deficit. Any child with these pictures especially in an endemic area should be suspected to have hydatid until proved otherwise.

Clinical Course and Complications

Fifteen percent to 25% of children remain asymptomatic and 65% to 85% become symptomatic. Rate of complication of hydatid are more in children than adults. Approx 40% give rise to complications in children suppuration (11-27%) or Rupture (1-4%) and only 5% are to undergo spontaneous abortion. Simple uncomplicated liver hydatid can remain asymptomatic till old age.

Suppuration

Due to increased intracystic pressure leakage in laminated membrane occurs that allows the entry of serum and bile into the cyst resulting in bacterial growth forming a pyogenic abscess. It is blessing in disguise as the parasite dies. Most common organism is E. coli. The abscess may erode the diaphragm and rupture into bronchus-resulting in bronchobiliary fistula. Management of suppurated hydatid is surgical drainage, antibiotics and albendazole therapy.

Rupture

Major rupture leads to fatal anaphylactic reaction, which is common in endemic areas. *Minor leaks* may produce allergic reactions like flushing and urticaria. *Obscure rupture* is endocyst rupturing into pericyst. *Communicant rupture* is cyst rupturing into the biliary/bronchial (Hydatidoptysis) tree. *Free rupture* occurs into cavities like peritoneal, pleural, pericardial, or into the intestines. Intraperitoneal rupture could be silent rupture with delayed presentation as disseminated abdominal hydatidosis or acute rupture with or without anaphylaxis and its sequalae. In endemic areas "Dumb-bell" hepatoperitoneal cysts are also seen that can rupture leading to ascites.

Intraperitoneal rupture occurs due to increase in intracystic pressure leads to pressure necrosis of superficial pericyst. It results in discharge of all cyst contents into peritoneal cavity with or without residual liver scar. It causes "Secondary echinococcosis" where multiple intraperitoneal hydatid cysts develop causing intestinal obstruction, abdominal distension and ascites. In highly endemic areas rupture presents with a variety symptoms. *Hydatid emesis* is vomiting of hydatid membranes or its contents, seen in cyst rupture into the stomach. *Hydatid enterica* is passage of hydatid cyst membranes or its contents per rectum occurs in cyst-enteric fistula. *Hydatiduria* is passing cyst membranes or its content in the urine seen in rupture of genitourinary hydatids. Hydatopyothorax (shoulder pain) rupture into thorax results in empyema or lung abcess. *Hydatidoptysis* is coughing out hydatid cyst contents; it indicates the presence of cystobronchial fistula. *Hydatid cachexia* is seen in children harboring large or multiple hydatid cyst.

Five to 10% of live cysts rupture into the biliary tract. It amounts to 60% of all complications. Rupture can be tangential or terminal and 90% are silent. Rupture can result in spontaneous cure, or cholangitis and can cause luminal obstruction manifesting as obstructive jaundice. Cyst at the porta can cause extrinsic compression of CBD/hepatic ducts and rupture into them. Rupture leads to conversion of univesicular cyst to a multivesicular cyst. Rupture could be the cause of unresolving secondary infection of pericystic cavity.

Spontaneous abortion

Spontaneous abortion is a fortunate event and the etiology is not known. Breach in pericystic layer leads to non-functioning pericyst. Subsequently fibrosis and calcareous deposition ensues resulting in total calcification and shrinkage in size. Ultimately residual asymptomatic calcified mass is left behind. Occasionally aseptic necrosis with no evidence of parasite can also occur (sterile pus).

Lab Studies

Blood tests are highly nonspecific. LFT may reveal elevated bilirubin or serum alkaline phosphatases. Leukocytosis is seen in cases of infected cyst. Eosinophilia is seen 25% of all infected persons. Hypogammaglobinemia is present in 30% of patients. All serodiagnostic techniques used for evaluation of hydatid cysts have variable results. Casoni test is of historical importance now due to its low sensitivity (only 70%).

Most common test done now is indirect hema-agglutination (IHA). Enzyme linked immunosorbent assay (ELISA) and IHA have sensitivity of 90% in liver and 40% in pulmonary hydatids. IHA and ELISA are the initial screening tests of choice. Many other immunological tests like basophil degranulation test and T lymphocyte cytokine mRNA expression test also exist. Confirmatory test is demonstration of antibody against antigen 5' (arc 5b) by immunodiffusion or immunoelectrophoresis (IEP). IEP is highly specific for active infection (cross reacts with cysticercosis). It turns negative within 6-12 months after surgery or death of the parasite. Basophil degranulation test turns negative 1 week after surgery.

Radioimaging

Plain X-rays may show thin rim or streak of calcification delineating a cyst, which is suggestive of an inactive echinococcal cyst. In alveolar eichinococcosis, plain films may be normal. In endemic areas eleveted hemidiaphragm on postero-anterior view of chest X-ray is suggestive of liver hydatid.

Ultrasound (USG) is the first line diagnostic modality. Used for screening in endemic areas as well as for monitoring treatment and follow up. Intra-operative USG is used for localization of deep cysts. However, accuracy of ultrasound is operator dependent. Effectiveness of medical therapy is determined by decrease in cyst size, development of pseudo-solid pattern and presence of transonic halo around cyst wall. World Health Organization Informal Working Group (2003) has described a new ultrasound classification based on the natural history of the disease (Table 92.1).

Table 92.1: WHO's new ultrasound classification of hydatid cyst

Type	*Status*	*USG features*	*Remarks*
CL	Active	Not pathognomonic, unilocular, no cyst wall	Consider DD
CE1	Active	Cyst wall (+), hydatid sand	Fertile
CE2	Active	Multivesicular, cyst wall, rosette pattern	Fertile
CE3	Transitional	Detached LM, Waterlily sign	Daughter cyst+/-
CE4	Inactive	Heterogenous degenerating contents, No dauht cyst	No living protoscolices DD needed
CE5	Inactive	Complete or partially calcified wall, Not pathognomonic, but highly suggestive	No proto-scolices

(+)- Present, CE-Cystic Eichinococcosis. CL-Cystic Lesion.

CT scan is the most informative investigation to know the location, dimensions and biliary and vascular relationship, presence of cyst elsewhere. Accuracy is 98%. It differ-entiates hydatid from amebic and pyogenic liver abcess. Irregular outline suggests degenerating hydatid cyst. Alveolar echinococcosis mimics hepatocellular carcinoma. Spiral CECT with 3D reconstruction is very accurate in showing the vasobiliary relationship to the cyst.

MRI has no real advantage over CT scan; however it is specifically useful in cardiac, skeletal and vertebral hydatidosis.

ERCP has both diagnostic (cystobiliary fistula) and therapeutic in intrabiliary rupture and cholangitis due to hydatid cyst, in whom sphincterotomy and extraction can be performed. Indications for endoscopic papillotomy include hydatid debris in CBD, biliary fistula persisting for more than 3 months, high output biliary fistula and jaundice with caustic sclerosing cholangitis.

Management

Management is primarily surgical. Indications for surgery are:

- Large liver cysts with multiple daughter cysts.
- Presence of cystobiliary communication.
- Superficial single liver cysts because of the risk of traumatic or spontaneous rupture.
- Presence of pressure effects on vital organs/structures.
- Infected cysts, pulmonary hydatid cysts (they are prone to cystobronchial fistula), cysts of brain, kidneys, eyes and bones.

Preoperative Preparation

- Prophylactic antibiotic at induction; septic patients should be started on appropriate antibiotics based on the culture and sensitivity of the pus or blood culture.
- Life saving drugs like adrenaline, steroids, chlorpheniramine, etc. should be available ready in the ward and operation theatre.
- Entire medical team should take universal precautions while handling the cyst material.

Operative Procedures

- *Cyst evacuation* with external drainage, capittonage, omentoplasty, introflexion.
- *More radical procedures* have lower risk of relapses but have higher risk of complications. Radical procedures include:
  - Closed cystopericystectomy.
  - Open cystopericystectomy.
  - Liver resection (either anatomic or atypical).
- *Liver transplantation* in bilobar disease may be indicated.

Medical Management

Indications for primary medical management are multiple cysts in multiple organs, inaccessible or deep (>4cm) cysts, inoperable primary liver or lung cysts due to inaccessible location calcified cysts as they are mostly inactive, very small cysts, poor medical status, disseminated cyst and intra-operative spillage of cyst contents. Chemotherapy is not the primary mode of therapy with limited role only in 30-40%. Benzimidazole carbamates like albendazole, mebendazole, flubendazole and isoquinoline derivative-praziquantel are used for the treatment and prophylaxis. They are more effective in pulmonary rather than hepatic hydatid, and are not effective in extra-hepatopulmonary disease. Contraindications to chemotherapy are bone marrow suppression, chronic hepatic disease, large cysts with the risk of rupture, bone cysts, inactive and calcified cysts.

Albendazole

It acts by decreasing the ATP production in worm, causing energy depletion and immobilization leading to death of the parasite. It acts as ovicidal, larvicidal and vermicidal also. Has poor aqueous solubility, so poorly absorbed from GI tract. However, it is metabolized to albendazole sulfoxide which is easily absorbed. Plasma level rise after fat rich meal.

Mebendazole

It irreversibly blocks the glucose uptake by the parasite. Most poorly absorbed drug so high dosage is required to be effective. Primary (only) medical therapy is 40-50 mg/kg/d per oral for 3-6 months, but in adjunctive therapy (in addition to surgery) it is started 4 days prior to surgery and continued till 1 month postoperatively. Dosage not established in children <2 years; > 2 years: 50 mg/kg/d, tolerate well. Contraindications are hypersensitivity. Adverse effects are neutropenia, hepatitis, alopecia and glomerulonephritis.

Praziquantel (PZQ)

It is absorbed well by the GI tract. It increases cell membrane permeability resulting in loss of intracellular calcium that causes massive muscle contractions and paralysis of the musculature. It is more effective as adjunct to albendazole. It is very active against protoscoleces, so after intraoperative spillage, it is used at a dose of 40 mg/kg/d X 2 weeks postop. with praziquintal pulmonary cysts become more prone to rupture.

Pediatric Dosage: Not established in <4 years; > 4 years: Like adults 40 mg/kg PO q wk.

Contraindications include hypersensitivity and ocular cysticercosis. Adverse reactions are hepatotoxicity, anemia, thrombocytopenia, alopecia embryotoxicity and teratogenicity.

Primary Therapy (without surgery)

There is no standard protocol for medical therapy. However, the commonly followed regimen is albenadazole-10-15 mg/kg/day for 28 days (3-6 cycle) separated by 14-day intervals between each (WHO).

Adjunctive Therapy (with surgery)

Peri-operative albendazole or mebendazole reduce the risk of secondary echinococcosis. To be started 4 days before surgery and continued for 1-3 months postoperatively in uncomplicated cases. For complicated cases like multivisceral cyst or intraoperative spillage drugs should be continued till 6 months. Optimal treatment can be continued for 3-6 months, with no increase in adverse effects. If mebendazole is used it has to be given for 3-6 months orally; 40-50 mg/kg/d.

KEY LEARNING POINTS

In addition to simple cysts and polycystic liver disease, choledochal cysts and hydatid cysts are important.

Choledochal Cyst (CDC)

- Congenital biliary dilatations of the extrahepatic biliary tree, intrahepatic biliary radicles or both, usually manifesting < 10 years of age, is of infantile form and adult form.

- Toni's modification of Alonso-Lej's classification is currently followed.
- Special investigations are ultrasonogram, MRCP, CECT scan, DISIDA and, infrequently, ERCP.
- Complications include: jaundice, recurrent cholangitis, pancreatitis, gallstones, choleystitis, cirrhosis with portal hypertension, rupture and malignancy.
- Treatment is primarily surgery.

Hydatid Disease

- Liver is the most common site followed by lungs though any human organ may be involved.
- Most common manifestations are abdominal pain (right hypochondriac pain with or without hepatomegaly and pressure symptoms such as obstructive jaundice), vomiting, weight loss, jaundice, fever and dyspepsia.
- Special investigation include IHA and ELISA (initially), IEP (confirmatory) and radioimaging with CT scan being the most informative.
- Treatment is surgery and/or pharmacotherapy employing albendazole, mebendazole or PZQ.

FURTHER READINGS

1. Kayaalp C. Hydatid cyst of liver. In: Blumgart LH, Belghiti G, Jarnagin WR, de Matteo RP, Chapman WC *et al.* (eds): *Surgery of the Liver, Biliary Tract and Pancreas*, 4th edn. Philadelphia: Saunders 2007: 952-970.
2. Manickam S, Ramadan K and Adams BK. A rare choledochal cyst of the cystic duct with an anomalous pancreaticobiliary union in an adult patient: A case report. *Clin Radiol Ext* 2004; 59:68-71
3. Miyano T. Choledochal cyst. In: Stringer MD, Oldham KT, Pierre D, Mouriquand E (eds): *Pediatric Surgery and Urology: Long-term Outcomes*. 2nd edn. Cambridge: Cambridge University Press 2006; 465-479.
4. O'Neill JA Jr. Choledochal cyst. In: Grosfeld JL, O'Neill JA Jr, Fonkalsurd EW, *et al.* (eds): *Pediatric Surgery*, 6th edn. St. Louis: Mosby–Year Book 2006:1620-1634.
5. Quereshi FG, Nadler EP, Ford HR. Biliary stone diseases. In: Stringer MD, Oldham KT, Pierre D, Mouriquand E (edn): *Pediatric Surgery and Urology: Long-Term Outcomes*. 2nd edn. Cambridge: Cambridge University Press 2006; 480-490.
6. Suchy FJ. Cystic diseases of liver and gallbladder. In: Behrman RE, Kiegman RM, Jenson HB (eds): *Nelson Textbook of Pediatrics*.17th edn. Philadelphia: Saunders–Year Book 2004; 1343-1345.

93 Liver Tumors

Ragavan M • Renu Kumar

INTRODUCTION

Liver tumors of infancy and childhood include a broad-spectrum of benign and malignant lesions. The liver is the third most common site for intra-abdominal malignancy in children, following adrenal neuroblastoma and Wilms' tumor. Statistically, malignant tumors are more common than the benign tumors with a ratio of 2.5:1. Liver tumors account for 1-2% of all childhood malignancies.

Hemangioendothelioma and mesenchymal hamartoma typically occur in the first year of life, accounting for 50-60% liver tumors. Hepatoblastoma typically occurs before 5 years of age. Hepatocellular carcinoma and adenoma mostly occur in the second decade of life.

CLASSIFICATION

Table 93.1 gives the classsificaton of tumors involving the liver.

INFANTILE HEMANGIOENDOTHELIOMA

Infantile hemangioendothelioma is the most common liver tumor in infancy. It occurs as a single or multicentric liver mass in early childhood. At present 80% of patients are lees than 6 months of age. The female-to-male ratio is 3:1. They are considered to be benign hamartomatous proliferation of vascular tissue and a variant of hemangioma. In adults asymptomatic hemangioma is common. The massive arterio-venous shunting within the hemangioendothelioma can cause high-output cardiac failure.

Pathology

The lesions appear as blood filled endothelial lined spaces with associated central calcification and fibrosis. Individual lesions appear circumscribed but are not capsulated. The tortuous vascular spaces can trap blood elements leading to thrombocytopenia and consumptive coagulopathy (Kasabach-Merritt syndrome) and even microangiopathic anemia. Heart failure and anemia in utero may result in nonimmune hydrops which may be seen in antenatal scan. Two types of histological patterns, type I comprises 80% of cases and are made up of variably sized vascular spaces

Table 93.1: Classification of liver tumors in children

Type	*Benign tumors*	*Malignant tumors*
Mesenchymal origin	Rhabdoid tumor Mesenchymal hamartoma Cavernous hemangioma Inflammatory pseudotumor	Undifferentiated (embryonal) sarcoma Angiosarcoma Rhabdomyosarcoma Rhabdoid tumor
Epithelial origin	Focal nodular hyperplasia Hepatocellular adenoma Nodular regenerative hyperplasia Mixed hamartoma Developmental cysts	Hepatoblastoma Hepatocellular carcinoma Fibrolamellar carcinoma
Germ cell neoplasia **Metastatic tumors**	Teratoma	Endodermal sinus tumor Neuroblastoma Malignant germ cell tumors Leukemia Lymphoma Sarcoma

lined by immature endothelial cells, separated by a supporting fibrous stroma and interspersed with scattered bile ductules. Type II histology differs from type I in the character of the endothelial cell proliferation with larger and more pleomorphic endothelial cells. Both histological variations can be present in the same liver. Immunohistochemistry show positive staining for factor VIII-related antigen and more variably with lectin and von Willebrand's factor.

Clinical Features

The common clinical manifestations are abdominal mass, respiratory distress, congestive cardiac failure, jaundice, failure to thrive, fever, Kasabach-Merritt syndrome, liver failure, rupture and death.

Investigations

Ultrasound Doppler shows blood filled spaces with high flow pattern. Contrast enhanced computerized tomogram show late enhancement, and delayed picture show retention of contrast in the blood filled spaces. MRI shows regular, less intenseT1 and hyperintense T2 images. HIDA scan reveals no uptake of radiotracer, and blood pool scan show persisting enhancement. Angiogram shows diffuse angiomatous lesion with rapid filling of hepatic veins and large feeding artery. It has value in the management as it shows the detailed anatomy of the hepatic vasculature. Preoperative percutaneous biopsy of hepatic vascular tumors is unnecessary and dangerous because of the risks of intra-peritoneal bleeding. Liver function tests are usually normal, but the alpha-fetoprotein level can be moderately elevated. Ectopic production of either TSH or a TSH-like hormone is reported.

Treatment

A variety of treatment options have been suggested. The natural history of hepatic hemangioendotheliomas, like the hemangioma located elsewhere in the body, follows a biphasic pattern of proliferation followed by spontaneous involution. Imaging studies can usually confidently enable the diagnosis, allowing for a conservative approach in many cases. When symptomatic the treatment options available are oral steroids (prednisolone 3-5 mg/Kg body weight per day), alpha-interferon, antimitotic agents, principally cyclophosphamide, external beam radiation, embolization, hepatic artery ligation, laser coagulation, and surgical resection. Steroids provide 40-50 % response rate. Surgical treatment consists of lobar resection if the lesion is confined to one area (the minority) or ligation of the hepatic artery if the lesion is bilobar. Embolization using gelfoam, polyvinyl alcohol and steel coils has apparently good results. Although the outcome for solitary and asymptomatic masses is good, mortality in the face of uncontrollable heart failure and multifocal lesions remains high (15-40%). Malignant degeneration to angiosarcoma is rare but has been documented. Cardiac failure can cause death in upto 70% of untreated infants before adequate regression of the lesion occurs. Younger the age of presentation and the more severe the cardiac symptoms poorer is the prognosis.

CAVERNOUS HEMANGIOMA

In adults cavernous hemangioma is the most common benign tumor of the liver and is present in approximately 1% population, whereas in children pure cavernous hemangiomas *per se* is rare rarely seen.The characteristic histopathology includes irregular large vascular spaces lined by flattened endothelial cells and separated by a paucicellular or myxoid stroma. They tend to be stable over time, without the proliferative and involuting phases which is characteristic of infantile hemangioendothelioma.

MESENCHYMAL HAMARTOMA OF THE LIVER

This lesion is considered as a hamartoma though there is controversy. The lesion is believed to be the result of aberrant hamartomatous development of primitive mesenchyme in the portal tracts. As it occurs late in embryogenesis the liver maintains its normal lobular architecture and biliary connection. Cytogenetic analysis revealed a specific translocation involving the long arm of chromosome 19 (19q 13.4) and also imply that it may after all be a true neoplasm rather than a developmental anomaly or hamartoma. It is the second most common benign hepatic lesion and is seen in children less than 2 years of age. It has predilection for the right lobe and in 5% of cases involve both the lobes. The male female ratio is 1.6:1.

Pathology

Grossly, the lesion is well encapsulated and the cut surface shows multiple cysts with yellowish or colorless watery or mucoid material separated by thin walled septation. Usually no bile staining is seen in the tumor. Microscopically, the lesion shows mesenchymal loose myxoid tissue with islands of hepatocytes throughout the lesion though normal hepatic architecture is not seen. The loose myxomatous tissue consists of mature collagen fibrils, fibroblast and small vessels. The hepatocytes in the lesion are arranged in groups and show normal ultra structural features of mature heaptocyte.

Clinical Features

Children with this lesion present with mass abdomen, pain, vomiting and respiratory distress etc. They can remain asymptomatic and jaundice is very rare. There are also prenatal case reports. It has been postulated that the rapid growth of the tumor may be secondary to cystic degeneration or destruction and dilatation of lymphatics.

Investigations

Ultrasonography is useful for diagnosis. The mass shows cystic spaces with intervening solid septa. The size and contents of cystic and solid components of the mass may vary. Contrast enhanced CT scans is ideal to confirm the diagnosis (Fig. 93.1). Calcification is rarely present in the lesion. A sulfur colloid liver scintigraphy reveals a large defect and can be used as an adjunctive modality. Angiographically the mass is hypovascular or vascular but is not needed for diagnosis. There is non-specific elevation of serum AFP levels. It needs to be differentiated from other masses like hemangioendothelioma, teratoma, simple cysts or the rare cystic hepatoblastoma and masses arising from adjacent organs.

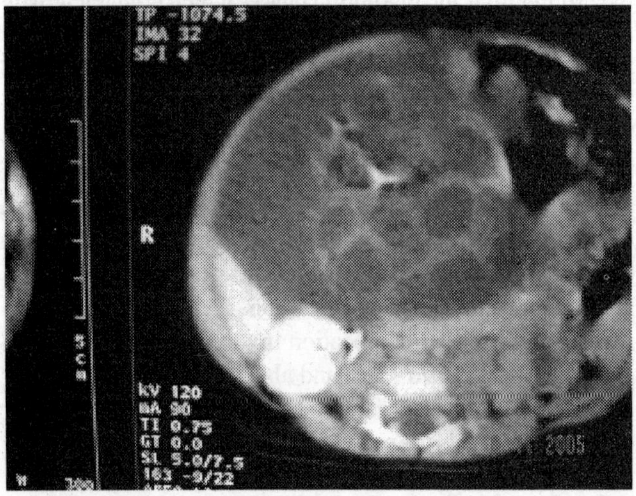

Fig. 93.1: CT scan showing liver mass with solid and cystic area suggestive of mesenchymal hamartoma

Treatment

Surgical excision is the treatment of choice. The surgical options are enucleation, wide excision or formal hepatic lobectomy. Long-term follow up is warranted due to rare risk of development of angiosarcoma.

FOCAL NODULAR HYPERPLASIA (FNH)

Focal nodular hyperplasia is a benign tumor that occurs most commonly in young adult women accounting for 4-10% of all benign liver tumors. It comprises 2% of all childhood liver tumors. The female-to-male (F/M) ratio is 3:1. Presents as an asymptomatic mass in an otherwise normal child, and is associated with a variety of clinical conditions and syndromes like hemi hypertrophy, VACTERAL syndrome, sickle cell anemia, intra and extrahepatic vascular malformations, brain tumors, congenital cardiovascular anomalies, and glycogen storage disease type I. Oral contraceptive use may induce growth or hemorrhage within a preexisting focal nodular hyperplasia.

It occurs as a single circumscribed or, less commonly, multifocal lesion. In children, 60% occur in left lobe, 30% in the right, and 10% are bilateral. Although usually subcapsular in location, deeply situated or pedunculated masses may occur. On cut surface a highly characteristic central stellate scar, present in at least 50% of cases. This feature distinguishes focal nodular hyperplasia from other liver masses. The mass has no bile staining and rarely shows hemorrhage or necrosis.

Microscopically, the central scar shows thick walled vessels with marked fibromuscular hyperplasia and myxoid change and the septa also contain vessels that may be thick walled. These septa are without a central bile duct but show prominent ductular proliferation at the interface between the fibrous tissue and hepatocytes.

A characteristic central scar on CT scan is pathognomonic for FNH. Unenhanced CT scans show a hypodense well-defined lesion. In dynamic CT scan during the arterial phase FNH appears as an early contrast-enhanced homogenous lesion that becomes isodense with the normal liver parenchyma on delayed images. A less enhanced central scar can be seen in fewer than 50% of lesions. Differentiating FNH from adenomas may require technetium sulphur colloid scan, which shows uniform uptake by FNH lesions. Open biopsy may be required for definitive diagnosis in rare circumstances. Distinguishing focal nodular hyperplasia from hepatocellular carcinoma on biopsy or fine needle aspirate material depends largely on the cytologic features of malignancy. The reported association of FNH with fibrolamellar carcinoma raises concerns of potential malignancy arising within incompletely resected lesions. However, even with incomplete excision or diagnosis by biopsy only, outcome seems to be excellent. As FNH does not carry the risk of hemorrhage associated with benign adenomas and is not known to undergo malignant degeneration, resection is not always necessary and treatment can be individualized.

HEPATOCELLULAR ADENOMA

Hepatocellular adenoma is a rare tumor, accounting for 5% of benign liver masses in childhood. It is less common than focal nodular hyperplasia. These tumors can occur in any age. There is strong association between hepatic adenoma and oral contraceptive intake. The average lag time between starting oral contraceptives and diagnosis of hepatic adenoma is about 5 years. Thus, in children the incidence is equal in male and female.

It presents as mass associated with pain and fever. In adult women taking oral contraceptives, acute hemorrhage or rupture can occur and presents as an emergency. In about 50% of childhood hepatic adenoma there is associated glycogen storage disease (GSD) I or Fanconi's anemia. Hepatic adenomas appears as a single, large (> 10 cm), circumscribed, bulging, yellow-tan mass in the right hepatic lobe with or without central hemorrhage and necrosis.

The histopathology of the tumor shows well-differentiated hepatocytes arranged in 2 to 3 cell thick cords, or in sheets. Peliosis, a recognized complication of androgen therapy, is seen in the adjacent liver parenchyma in approximately 50% of cases. The treatment is to discontinue oral pills and surgical excision. Associated conditions like Fanconi's anemia make the prognosis guarded.

RARE BENIGN TUMORS

Nodular Regenerative Hyperplasia

It consists of small but widely distributed nodules of hepatocytes without associated fibrosis. The nodules are small in size, varying from 1 to 4 cm. It occurs in association with a wide variety of disease processes, and is considered to be a result of abnormal hepatic blood flow. Portal hypertension occurs in approximately 50% of adult cases. In the largest reported series in children, hepatosplenomegaly or suspected intra-abdominal tumor was the most common clinical presentation.

Developmental Cysts

These are also relatively common and include a variety of lesions, like those associated with polycystic renal disease or extra hepatic choledochal cysts. Primary hepatic cysts occur rarely in childhood and include the solitary or simple cyst, epidermoid cyst, ciliated hepatic foregut cyst, and hepatobiliary cystadenoma.

Inflammatory Pseudo Tumor

Also called "inflammatory myofibroblastic tumor", it presents with fever, weight loss, obstructive jaundice and mass abdomen. There is hypergammaglobulinemia and leukocytosis. It can occur in other parts of the body like abdominal wall, pancreas, retroperitoneum etc. The liver lesion is poorly circumscribed mass composed of a variety of cells in varying proportions, including spindle cells or myofibroblast, lymphocytes, plasma cells, macrophages, foam cells. Venous invasion frequently occurs and may result in portal and/or hepatic vein thrombosis. They tend to recur locally and may very rarely metastasize distally.

HEPATOBLASTOMA

Hepatoblastoma is the most common primary hepatic malignancy in children. It accounts for 45% of all pediatric liver tumors. The conditions which predispose to hepatoblastoma are familial adenomatous polyposis syndrome, Beckwith-Wiedemann syndrome and hemihypertrophy. The typical presentation is a child younger than 3 years with an abdominal mass, pain, respiratory distress, vomiting, anemia and failure to thrive.

Investigations

Laboratory abnormalities include an elevated alpha feto protein (in 90%) and thrombocytosis. Abdominal ultrasonogram is done to localize the mass and estimate the extent of tumor within the liver. Doppler evaluation is used to evaluate the patency of the inferior vena cava, the hepatic veins, and the portal vein. CECT scans of the abdomen and chest are used to assess resectability and evaluate for the presence of pulmonary metastasis. Volumetric reconstruction can be done using dynamic CT. Hepatic angiography or MRI angiography is helpful to determine resectability and to delineate the vascular anatomy more precisely. Patients with hepatoblastoma with low titer of AFP have bad prognosis. Pathological diagnosis can be done by FNAC or by percutaneous or open biopsy.

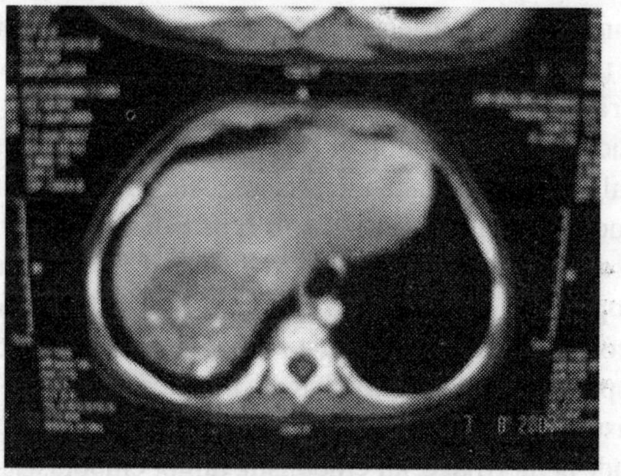

Fig. 93.2: CECT scan showing hepatoblastoma in right lobe of liver

There are many staging systems used for staging, management and outcome analysis. The Children's Oncology Group (COG) uses the extent of tumor and outcome of surgical resection as critical criteria for staging.

Table 93.2: COG staging of hepatoblastoma

Stage I:	Complete resection
Stage II:	Resection with microscopic residual disease
Stage III:	Resection with gross residual tumor
	Tumor spill and/or positive lymph nodes
	Incomplete resection of primary tumor
Stage IV:	Distant metastases.

International Society of Pediatric Oncology on Childhood Liver Tumors (SIOPEL) uses the pretreatment extent (PRETEXT) of diseases staging based on the imaging. This system divides the liver into 4 sectors; the anterior and posterior on the right side and the medial and lateral sectors on the left. Based on the tumor location, the patient is categorized as four stages:

Stage I if three adjoining sectors are free.
Stage II with two adjoining sectors free.
Stage III with one sector free; and

Stage IV when no sectors are free of tumor or large central hilar mass extending to all sectors. It is also taken into account whether portal or hepatic veins are involved or if extra hepatic spread has occurred. Both staging systems directly correlate with patient survival.

Treatment

Complete surgical resection remains the goal of current therapy for HB. Planning a major hepatic resection begins with adequate imaging studies to ensure resectability. Treatment begins with laparotomy for resection if possible or biopsy if the tumor is unresectable. About half of tumors can be resected, and postoperative chemotherapy consists of cisplatin, vincristine, and 5-fluorouracil. Monotherapy with cisplatinum or PLADO regimen consisting of cisplatinum and doxorubicin are used. Approximately 50% of tumors are unresectable at the time of diagnosis and require chemotherapy before surgical resection. Characteristics of an unresectable tumor include multicentricity, invasion of the inferior vena cava (IVC) or portal vein, or distant metastases. Adequate response to chemotherapy is observed in 70% of patients who then go on to complete resection followed by additional postoperative chemotherapy. In patients with tumors that do not adequately respond to resection, orthotopic liver transplantation is an option if there is no evidence of regional or distant metastases. Major intra-operative complications include hemorrhage, air embolism, tumor embolus, and bile duct injury. Postoperative complications include hemorrhage, bile leak, abscess formation, pulmonary complications, and wound problems. Only 20% of the normal liver is necessary to maintain hepatic function; thus, postoperative insufficiency is rare. Postoperative care consists of adequate fluid replacement, intravenous albumin supplementation, vitamin K, and clotting factors for the first 3-4 days. The liver function test results generally normalize within the first 2 weeks, and hepatic insufficiency is reasonably rare. Follow up protocol consists of US, chest radiographs, and serial AFP levels, generally at 3- to 6-month intervals. AFP is an early marker of recurrence, and elevated levels should prompt thorough investigation. The survival rate has improved in the last 3 decades, and the overall survival is currently 85%-92%. Outcomes based on the SIOP PRETEXT staging are 100%, 91%, 68%, 57% for Stage I, II, III and IV respectively.

HEPATOCELLULAR CARCINOMA

Hepatocellular carcinoma (HCC) accounts for about 20% of pediatric hepatic malignancies and has bimodal age of presentation, the first occurring at ages 0-4 years and the second between ages 10-14 years. Predisposing conditions include hepatic fibrosis and cirrhosis secondary to metabolic liver disease and viral hepatitis. Less commonly, HCC occurs in children without preexisting liver disease. Hepatocellular carcinoma is associated with hepatitis B and hepatitis C infection. The incubation period for genesis of hepatocellular carcinoma from the time hepatitis virus infection is extremely short in children with perinatally acquired virus. Several specific types of nonviral liver injury and cirrhosis in children are associated with hepatocellular carcinoma, including: tyrosinemia, biliary cirrhosis, and alpha-1-antitrypsin deficiency. Patients with HCC typically present with abdominal pain caused by the large size of the lesion. Associated weight loss, anemia, and fever may also be present. Liver function tests are routinely elevated; the AFP is elevated in half of thc cases. Metastases usually occur in the lung and lymph nodes. Workup and staging are similar to those used in HB.

More than 70% of these tumors are considered unresectable at the time of presentation and, unlike HB, they respond poorly to chemotherapy. Treatment is a combination of chemotherapy and surgery. Vincristine, cisplatin, 5-FU, and doxorubicin have had little impact on the progression of this disease. Newer therapeutic strategies have included chemoembolization, intra-arterial chemotherapy, and intraoperative cryotherapy.

The overall survival rate remains poor, with a 41% disease-free survival rate at 2 years and a 27% disease-free survival rate at a longer follow-up interval. In children with recurrent liver disease or multifocal extensive primary malignancies, hepatic transplantation is an option.

HEPATIC METASTASES

Hepatic metastases in the pediatric population arise from a variety of primary malignancies, including neuroblastoma (Fig. 93.3), Wilms tumor, rhabdomyosarcoma, rhabdoid tumor, non-Hodgkin lymphoma, adrenal cortical carcinoma, and osteogenic sarcoma. Current criteria for resection of these hepatic metastases include control of the primary tumor, a solitary or limited number of metastases, and a reasonable expectation of prolonged survival.

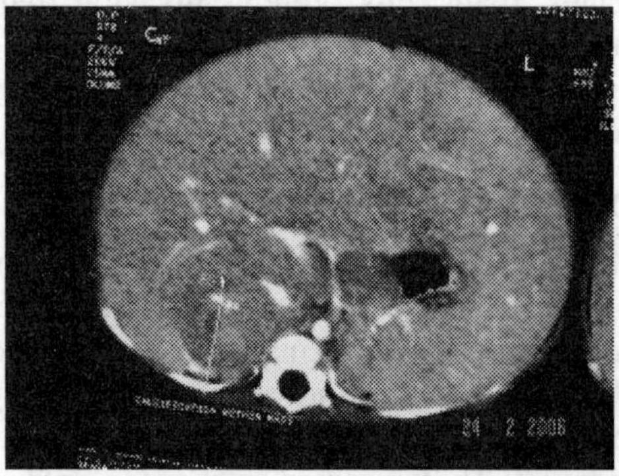

Fig. 93.3: CT scan showing diffusely enlarged liver from extensive metastasis. The child had a right adrenal mass suggestive of stage IV neuroblastoma

KEY LEARNING POINTS

- Liver is the third most common site for intra-abdominal malignancy (others being adrenal neuroblastoma and Wilm's tumor).
- Hemangioendothelioma and mesenchymal hamartoma typically occur in the first year of life.
- Hepatoblastoma typically occurs in preschool age group.
- Hepatocellular carcinoma and adenoma mostly occur in the second decade of life.
- Hepatic metastasis arise from a variety of primary malignancies, say Wilm's tumor, non-Hodgkin's lymphoma, adrenal cortical carcinoma and ostogenic sarcoma.

FURTHER READINGS

1. Atkinson JB, Deugarte DA. Liver tumors. In: Grosfeld JL, O'Neill JA Jr, Fonkalsurd EW, *et al.* (eds): *Pediatric Surgery,* 6th edn. St. Louis: Mosby 2006: 502-514.
2. Belgiti J, Viligrain V, Paradis V. Benign liver lesions. In: Blumgart LH, Belghiti G, Jarnagin WR, *et al.* (edn). *Surgery of the Liver, Biliary Tract and Pancreas*, 4th (edn). Philadelphia: Saunders 2007: 1131-1151.
3. Corbally MT, Spitz L. Malignant potential of mesenchymal hamartoma: An unrecognized risk. *Pediatr Surg Int* 1992; 7: 321-322.
4. Cohen RC, Myers NA. Diagnosis and management of massive hepatic hemangiomas in childhood. *J Pediatr Surg* 1986; 21: 6-9.
5. De Maioribus CA, Lally KP, Simik, *et al.* Mesenchymal hamartoma of the liver. A 35 years review. *Arch Surg* 1990; 125: 598-600.
6. Herzog CE. Neoplasm of the liver: In: Behrman RE, Kliegman RM, Jenson HB *Nelson Textbook of Pediatrics*, 17th edn. Philadelphia: Saunders 2007: 1725-1745.
7. Nguyen L, Shandling B, Ein S, *et al.* Hepatic hemangioma in childhood: Medical management or surgical management. *J Pediatr Surg* 1982; 17: 576-579.
8. Philip C, Guzzetta JR. Nonmalignant tumors of the liver. In:Grosfeld JL, O'Neill JA Jr, Fonkalsurd EW, *et al.* (eds): *Pediatric Surgery*, 6th edn. St. Mosby Louis 2006: 495-501.

94 Liver Transplantation

Vani Gopalareddy • Stephen Dunn

INTRODUCTION

Liver transplantation has changed the prognosis for many infants and children dying of end-stage liver failure. In this chapter we will discuss the historical aspects of liver transplantation, indications and contraindications for transplantation, preoperative care, various available surgical strategies, postoperative management, possible surgical complications, long-term survival and follow-up care.

HISTORICAL ASPECTS

The first human liver transplantation was attempted in 1963 both in USA and in Paris. There was not much success until 1967, when a child with hepatoma was successfully transplanted. The 1-year survival has increased since then from 30% to about 90% currently, mainly due to improvements in preoperative management of hepatic complications and nutritional support, postoperative immunosuppression and improved surgical techniques. In addition, the multivisceral transplantation including the small intestine, has made the survival of children with short gut a reality.

INDICATIONS

Liver transplantation is a standard therapy for fulminant liver failure, end-stage liver disease due to chronic liver disorders, hepatic-based metabolic liver disease, stable liver disease with significant morbidity and primary liver tumors (Table 94.1).

Table 94.1: Indications for pediatric liver transplantation

Chronic liver diseases

1. Biliary atresia
2. Idiopathic neonatal hepatitis
3. Alagille's syndrome
4. Progressive familial intrahepatic cholestasis (PFIC)
5. Non-syndromic paucity of bile ducts
6. α_1-Antitrypsin deficiency
7. Cystic fibrosis
8. Glycogen storage type IV
9. Tyrosinemia type I
10. Wilson's disease
11. Chronic hepatitis: Autoimmune, Idiopathic, Postviral (hepatitis B, C, other)
12. Cryptogenic cirrhosis
13. Fibropolycystic liver disease +/– Caroli syndrome

Acute liver failure

1. Autoimmune
2. Halothane exposure
3. Paracetamol poisoning
4. Viral hepatitis (A, B, C, E, or NA-G)
5. Fatty acid oxidation defects
6. Neonatal hemochromatosis
7. Tyrosinemia type I
8. Galactosemia
9. Wilson's disease

Inborn errors of metabolism

1. Crigler-Najjar type I
2. Familial hypercholesterolemia
3. Primary oxalosis
4. Organic acidaemia
5. Urea cycle defects

Liver tumors

1. Benign tumors causing hepatic dysfunction
2. Unresectable malignant tumors

LIVER TRANSPLANTATION IN CHRONIC LIVER DISEASES

- ***Biliary atresia:*** It is still the most common indication for liver transplantation in children, comprising over 50% of pediatric liver transplants in USA. Transplantation is required for children who present with cirrhosis, portal hypertension and its complications and who have an unsuccessful Kasai portoenterostomy or recurrent cholangitis.
- ***α_1-Antitrypsin deficiency:*** Most common form of inherited metabolic liver disease presenting in childhood. Only about 20% require transplantation in childhood.

- ***Tyrosinaemia type I:*** Prior to the introduction of NTBC, [2-(2-nitro-4-trifluoromethylbenzoyl)-1,3-cyclohexenedione], liver transplantation was indicated for acute or chronic liver disease, development of hepatocellular carcinoma (HCC). Liver transplantation is now only indicated for those children who have a poor quality of life, do not respond to NTBC, or in whom hepatic malignancy is thought to have developed.
- ***Wilson's disease:*** It is a rare indication for liver transplantation in childhood but is indicated for those children who present with advanced liver disease, fulminant liver failure or who have progressive hepatic disease despite therapy.
- ***Cystic fibrosis (CF):*** Liver transplantation is indicated only for those children with decompensated, severe malnutrition or complications of portal hypertension unresponsive to medical management, such as ascites or uncontrolled variceal bleeding
- ***Glycogen storage diseases (GSD):*** Type I should respond to appropriate nutritional management. Transplantation is indicated only for those children who develop multiple hepatic adenomas. GSD types III and IV may progress to cirrhosis needing transplantation.
- ***Autoimmune liver disease:*** The majority of children with autoimmune liver disease types I/II respond to immunosuppression. Liver transplantation is indicated for those children who have advanced portal hypertension or do not respond to immunosuppression or those who present with fulminant hepatic failure.
- ***Chronic hepatitis B or C:*** Most children are asymptomatic in whom the development of cirrhosis and HCC may evolve over several years. Main indication for transplantation is end-stage liver disease. Recurrence with hepatitis B or C post-transplantation is likely in 90% of patients without continued prophylactic therapy.
- Prognosis for other cholestatic disorders in infancy, such as Alagille's syndrome, non-syndromic paucity of bile ducts, familial intrahepatic cholestasis is variable. Liver transplantation is indicated for the development of cirrhosis and portal hypertension, development of malnutrition or growth failure unresponsive to nutritional support, or intractable pruritus, which is resistant to maximum medical therapy or biliary diversion.

In summary, children with chronic liver disease having any significant delay in developmental parameters, growth failure, complications such as chronic hepatic encephalopathy, hepatorenal syndrome, hepatopulmonary syndrome, small hepatocellular carcinoma, refractory ascites, intractable pruritus or recurrent variceal bleeding despite optimum management need transplantation.

INDICATIONS OF LIVER TRANSPLANTATION IN ACUTE LIVER FAILURE

Poor prognostic factors for children with fulminant hepatitis requiring listing for liver transplantation are as follows:

1. Non-A to G hepatitis.
2. Rapid onset of coma with progression to grade III or IV hepatic coma.
3. Diminishing liver size.
4. Falling transaminases.
5. Increasing bilirubin (>17.5 mg/dl).
6. Persistent coagulopathy (INR >4).
7. Acute renal failure.

PRETRANSPLANT EVALUATION (Table 94.2)

Evaluation should:

1. Assess the severity of the liver disease and the presence or absence of hepatic complications.
2. Establish the urgency for transplantation.
3. Assess whether the operation is technically feasible.
4. Consider any significant contraindications to successful transplantation.
5. Establish whether the transplant operation is appropriate for the child and family.
6. Prepare the child and family psychologically.

CONTRAINDICATIONS FOR TRANSPLANTATION

1. Severe systemic sepsis, particularly fungal sepsis, at the time of operation.
2. Malignant hepatic tumors with extrahepatic spread (pulmonary metastasis responsive to treatment is not a contraindication) and primary extrahepatic unresectable malignancy.
3. Irreversible neurologic injury.
4. Severe systemic oxalosis with cardiac involvement.
5. Mitochondrial cytopathies with multisystem involvement.
6. Giant-cell hepatitis with autoimmune haemolytic syndrome because of disease recurrence.

HIV-positive status alone without AIDS, hepatitis B and C are no longer considered absolute contraindications for OLT in many centers.

PREPARATION FOR TRANSPLANTATION

It is important to correct the abnormalities noted during the pre-transplant evaluation. Live vaccines are usually contraindicated in the immunosuppressed child, and so it is

Table 94.2: Pre-transplant evaluation

1.	*Nutritional status:* Height, weight, triceps skinfold, mid-arm muscle area
2.	*Identification of hepatic complications:* Ascites, hepatosplenomegaly, varices on endoscopy
3.	*Hematology:* Full blood count, platelets, blood group. HLA matching is not required
4.	*Cardiac assessment:* ECG, echo, chest X-ray
5.	*Respiratory function:* Oxygen saturation*, ventilation perfusion scan*, lung function tests†
6.	*Neurological and developmental assessment:* EEG, developmental scales, intelligence scales
7.	*Renal function:* Urea, creatinine, electrolytes,urinary protein/creatinine ratio
8.	Dental assessment
9.	*Radiology:* Ultrasound of liver and spleen for vascular anatomy Wrist X-ray for bone age and rickets, MRI/angiography‡
10.	*Serology:* Cytomegalovirus, Epstein-Barr virus, Varicella Zoster, Herpes simplex, HIV, Measels, Hepatitis A,B, C

*If cyanosed.
†In cystic fibrosis.
‡If portal vein anatomy equivocal.
ECG, Electrocardiogram; EEG, Electroencephalogram; HIV, Human immunodeficiency virus; MRI, Magnetic resonance imaging.

important to ensure that routine immunizations are complete including hepatitis A and B vaccination. Correct malnutrition and treat any complications of portal hypertension. Psychological preparation in children older than 2 years is essential. Parents and appropriate relatives must be fully informed of the necessity for liver transplantation in their child and of the risks, complications and the long-term implications of the operation.

ORTHOTOPIC LIVER TRANSPLANT SURGERY (OLT)

The majority of donor organs are retrieved from heart-beating cadavers, but can be obtained from live donors (Living related transplants). Liver transplantation involves three operations—the donor operation, the back table operation which may include liver reduction or liver splitting and the recipient operation.

The Liver Graft (Donor Operation)

The recipient is selected on the basis of a compatible blood group, size matching, medical urgency and time on the waiting list. Occasionally, blood group O may be given to blood groups A or B, if medically necessary. Cadaver livers are retrieved from heart beating donors that have fulfilled the criteria of brain death. Malignancy (except brain tumors) and uncontrolled bacterial sepsis or viral infections such as HIV remain absolute contraindications to donation. A hard fibrotic or a grossly fatty liver is unusable. When in doubt, histological examination of a frozen section of the liver is essential.

Back Table Operation

Most hepatic reduction or splitting is performed in-situ in the cadaver donor. The back table operation may be selected for hepatic splitting or reduction. It is performed at the recipient hospital and is synchronized with the recipient operation. Whole liver graft back table operation is relatively straightforward; however, the majority of pediatric liver transplants require a liver reduction operation to be performed, to generate either a single reduced-size graft or a pair of split liver grafts.

The principles of liver reduction are based upon the work of Couinaud, who described the segmental anatomy of the liver (Fig. 94.1). The liver is composed of eight segments including the caudate lobe (segment I), three segments (II-IV) of the anatomical left lobe and four segments (V-VIII) of the right lobe. The liver is usually divided along the plane of the falciform ligament to provide a left lateral segmental graft (segments II and III) drained by the left hepatic vein. In the reduced graft, the common bile duct, portal vein and hepatic artery are all preserved with the left lateral segment. In contrast, when the liver is split, usually the main trunks of these structures, together with the inferior vena cava are left with the right graft. At implantation, microvascular techniques and biliary re-construction using a Roux loop of jejunum are required for the left split graft (Fig. 94.2) The technique of liver reduction was modified to enable split-liver grafting, so that a single liver could be used for two recipients. The organ is preserved in the cold preservation liquid (Wisconsin solution) until ready to be

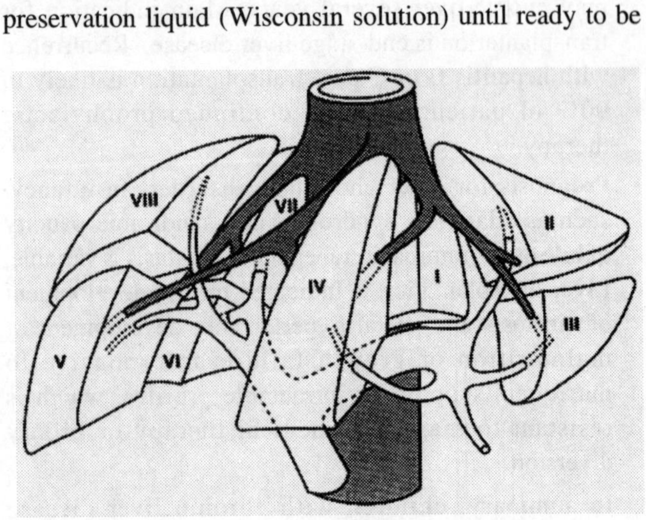

Fig. 94.1: Couinaud segments of liver

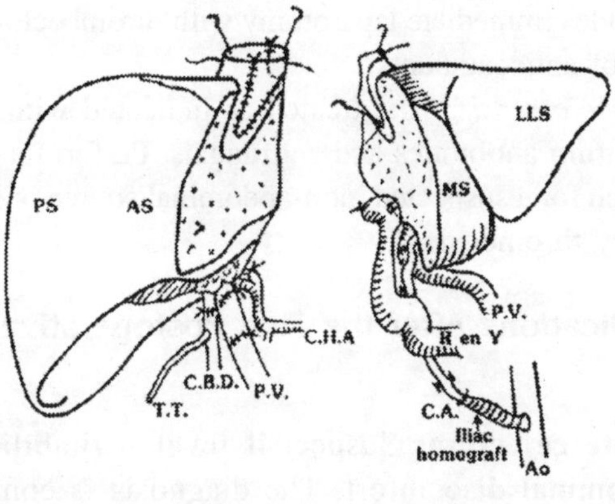

Fig. 94.2: Split liver graft with roux loop of jejunum

implanted into the recipient. The optimal "*cold ischemic time*" is less than 6-8 hours.

The Recipient Operation

The recipient liver transplant operation is carried out through a bilateral subcostal incision, often with an upper midline extension. The operation can be divided into two phases: total hepatectomy, in which the old liver is dissected and removed; and liver graft implantation.

Once the liver graft is removed from the cold preservation fluid it starts to warm. The vascular anastomoses are performed quickly in order to minimize warm ischemic injury. It is optimal to keep "*warm ischemia time*" to less than 60 minutes. Following completion of the venous anastomoses the liver is flushed with a rinsing solution to remove preservation fluid which has a high potassium concentration, and the venous clamps removed. Following reperfusion of the liver from the portal vein, the arterial anastomosis is carried out. The final anastomosis is to the graft bile duct. In adults and children without previous biliary pathology the donor and recipient common bile ducts are joined together.

Children with biliary atresia require a choledocho-jejunostomy using a Roux-en-Y loop of recipient jejunum. During the first hour after reperfusion there is usually evidence that the liver is working with spontaneous correction of acidosis and clotting factors, and production of bile.

LIVING RELATED ORTHOTOPIC LIVER TRANSPLANTATION (LRLT)

LRLT has improved the supply of liver grafts for small children who might otherwise die whilst waiting for a suitable cadaveric organ. LRLT also allows optimal timing of the transplant as an elective procedure. There have been reports of several donor deaths; risk of donor mortality is estimated at between 1:100 and 1:1000 depending upon whether a larger right liver graft or a smaller left graft is taken. Preoperative investigations include liver function tests, serology and imaging to assess the size of the intended segmental graft as well as its vascular and biliary anatomy.

For a child less than 25 kg the graft from a live donor is usually a left lateral graft (liver segments II+III). The size of the graft must be between 0.8 and 6% of recipient body weight for optimal results. In the USA approximately one-third of pediatric liver transplants are now performed from living donors.

AUXILIARY LIVER TRANSPLANTATION

Auxiliary liver transplantation involves transplantation of a donor liver graft without removal of the entire native liver. Its purpose is to retain the native liver in case of spontaneous recovery such as fulminant or subfulminant hepatic failure when there is potential for the original liver to recover. Once the native liver has recovered, immunosuppression is gradually withdrawn and the liver graft atrophies due to chronic rejection. This is done in very few centers in the world.

POSTOPERATIVE MANAGEMENT

1. **Ventilation:** Although it is possible to extubate some patients in the operating room, it is generally advisable to stabilize the patient in the intensive care unit (ICU) to ensure that liver function is satisfactory with good hepatic artery and portal vein flow on Doppler ultrasound before discontinuing ventilation.
2. **Fluid management:** Maintain urine output > 1 ml/kg/h. Provide 2/3 of fluids as crystalloids and replace wound drainage with albumin.
3. **Prophylactic antibiotics:** Broad spectrum intravenous antibiotics are prescribed for 48 hrs or until peritoneal drains are removed. Oral nystatin to prevent oral and esophageal candidiasis for 6-12 months. Bacterium prophylaxis against PCP pneumonia for 6 months. CMV prophylaxis with weekly immunoglobulin for 7 doses and if CMV positive donor, also treat with gancyclovir for 6 weeks. There is no satisfactory prophylaxis for EBV.
4. **Antiplatelet therapy:** Aspirin 3 mg/kg/day PR or NG (maximum 81mg) for 3 months.
5. **Anticoagulation (if necessary):** Heparin (60-120 units/kg/day) to maintain PT 20-30s.

6. **Antacid therapy**: Ranitidine 3 mg/kg/dose TID, Proton pump inhibitor 1mg/kg/dose BID.
7. **Antihypertensives:** Calcium channel blockers, ACE inhibitors.
8. **Immunosuppression:** Post-transplantation immunosuppression consists of induction and maintenance medication regimens as well as treatment protocols for acute cellular rejection. The highest risk of acute cellular rejection occurs early in the posttransplant period, so intravenous corticosteroids are used initially and tapered rapidly over several days and oral corticosteroids are used in the long-term.

   There have been many recent advances in immunosuppressive drugs, but current protocols consist of the calcineurin inhibitors:

   - Tacrolimus combined with prednisolone.
   - Cyclosporin microemulsion (Neoral), prednisolone.
   - Others: Sirolimus, Azathioprine, Mycophenolate mophetil (MMF) may be used as an adjuvant agent to permit lower doses of the calcineurin inhibitors in an effort to reduce toxicity. Sirolimus should not be used in the early post operative period due to concerns of thrombosis.

Steroids are reduced over the first 2 weeks and withdrawn after 3 months to improve growth. Cyclosporin or tacrolimus are continued for life. Although most immunosuppressant drug monitoring is with trough levels, peak cyclosporin levels may be more effective in preventing rejection and reducing side-effects. Anti-interleukin-2 receptor antibodies (IL-2 antibodies) are monoclonal antibodies, which selectively target the IL-2 receptors on activated T-cells, which is a key step in the development of cell-mediated immunity. Two anti-bodies are available, Basiliximab and Daclizumab, both of which are renal sparing and provide effective induction immunosuppression post-transplant in combination with a calcineurin inhibitor in adults.

POSTOPERATIVE COMPLICATIONS

Early Postoperative Complications

1. *Primary non-function:* It is a serious complication which requires immediate retransplantation. It may be suspected if there is persistent coagulopathy, acidosis, a high potassium and high transaminases and renal failure. Treatment consists of retransplantation or an increase in immunosuppression.
2. *Hepatic artery and portal vein thrombosis:* Treatment includes immediate laparotomy with thrombectomy and use of anticoagulants.
3. *Systemic sepsis:* It is treated as indicated with broad-spectrum antibiotics and antifungals. Perform a careful search for a suspected intra-abdominal source or hepatic artery thrombosis.

Complications After the First Postoperative Week

1. **Acute rejection:** Suspect if fever, irritability and abdominal discomfort. The diagnosis is confirmed by detecting a rise in bilirubin, GGTP and transaminases. Liver biopsy shows mixed inflammatory infiltrate in portal tracts with sub-endothelial lymphoid infiltration (endothelialitis) and inflammatory infiltration of bile ducts. Treatment is with pulse methylprednisolone (20-40 mg/kg/day) intravenously over 2 or 3 days. If there is inadequate response, may require higher levels of tacrolimus or the addition of other agents, including mycophenolate mofetil and muromonab-CD3 (Orthoclone OKT3), which is a monoclonal preparation of antibodies directed against CD3 cells.
2. **Chronic rejection:** It occurs in <10% of children at any time post transplant. The diagnosis is suggested by the gradual onset of jaundice, pruritus and pale stools which indicate biliary obstruction. Biochemical changes include a higher rise in bilirubin, alkaline phosphatase and GGT than in transaminases. Histology may demonstrate extensive damage and loss of bile ducts (vanishing bile duct syndrome) with arterial obliteration and fibrosis. Most children respond to an increase in immunosuppression, but some require retransplantation.
3. **Biliary complications:** Such as biliary strictures and leaks.
4. Sepsis.
5. Immunosuppression side effects (Table 94.3).
6. CMV or EBV infection.
7. Post-transplant lymphoproliferative disease (PTLD). There is a close relationship between primary EBV infection and the development of lymphoproliferative disease (PTLD). The clinical features may represent infectious mononucleosis, isolated lymphoid involvement or malignant lymphoma. EBV-PCR is usually positive, but is not diagnostic of PLTD. The diagnosis is based histology from the affected tissue, which may demonstrate polymorphic B-cell proliferation or lymphoma. EBER staining for EBV is

Table 94.3: Side effects of immunosuppressive treatment

Tacrolimus	*Cyclosporine*	*Prednisone*
Nephrotoxicity	Nephrotoxicity	Osteoporosis
Tremor	Tremor	Osteonecrosis
Hypertension	Hypertension	Diabetes
Headache	Hyperlipidemia	Hyperlipidemia
Cardiomyopathy	Hirsutism	Hirsutism
Alopecia	Gingival hyperplasia	Hypertension
Hyperglycemia	PTLD	Cushingoid habitus
PTLD		

positive. Almost any organ in the body may be affected, although the liver and gut are most commonly involved. Treatment includes: reduction of immunosuppression, intravenous acyclovir (3mg/m^2) or ganciclovir (10 mg/kg/day) and anti CD20 antibody (Rituximab). Chemotherapy is required if the PTLD becomes overtly malignant.

SURVIVAL FOLLOWING LIVER TRANSPLANTATION

1-year survival after paediatric liver transplantation may be as high as 90%. Long-term survival (5-8 years) ranges from 60 to 80%. Survival may be affected by the recurrence of the original diseases such as hepatitis B, hepatitis C, autoimmune hepatitis, including de novo autoimmune hepatitis.

QUALITY OF LIFE FOLLOWING TRANSPLANT

It is essential to encourage both child and family to return to a normal life. Children who survive the initial 3 months post-transplant without major complications should achieve a normal lifestyle despite the necessity for continuous monitoring of immunosuppressive treatment. Majority of children who have had a successful liver transplant will have normal growth pattern, puberty.

OUTPATIENT MONITORING

Initial post-transplant management includes frequent follow-up by the transplant centre, usually at weekly intervals, extending with time to monthly, 3-monthly, and then 6-monthly intervals.

Monitoring should include assessment of nutritional status, liver function tests, annual abdominal ultrasound examinations, immunosuppression monitoring to prevent rejection and reduce toxicity. Monitoring for PTLD by EBV PCR 3-6 monthly.

KEY LEARNING POINTS

- OLT has evolved from an experimental therapy to state-of-the-art therapy.
- OLT is a standard therapy for most fulminant liver failure, and end-stage liver disease with complications.
- Early referral of potential recipients allows timely evaluation of potential living donors or time for acquisition of a cadaveric donor organ.
- Improved surgical techniques and immunosuppressive therapy have improved survival rate to over 90% in pediatric patients.

FURTHER READINGS

1. Al-Hussiani A, Tredger MJ, Dhawan A. Immunosuppression in pediatric liver and intestinal transplantation: A closer look at the arsenal. *J Pediatric Gastroenterol Nutr* 2005; 41: 152-165.
2. Andrews WS, Shimaoka S, Sommerauer J *et al.* Steroid withdrawal after pediatric liver transplantation. *Transpl Proc* 1994; 26:159-160.
3. Andrews W, Sommerauer J, Roden J *et al.* Ten years of pediatric liver transplantation. *J Pediatr Surg* 1996; 31:619-624.
4. Arora N, Bunn S, McKiernan P, Beath S, *et al.*: Long term evaluation of renal function after paediatric liver transplantation. *Hepatology* 2000; 32, 341A.
5. Bismuth H. Surgical anatomy and anatomical surgery of the liver. *World J Surg* 1982; 6:3-9.
6. Bismuth H, Houssain D. Reduced size orthotopic liver grafts in hepatic transplantation in children. *Surgery* 1984; 95: 367-370.
7. Codoner-Franch P, Bernard O & Alvarez F. Long-term follow-up of growth in height after successful liver transplantation. *J Pediatr* 1994;124, 368-373.
8. Gregorio GV, Portmann B, Reid F *et al.* Autoimmune hepatitis in childhood: A 20-year experience. *Hepatology* 1997; 25;541-547.
9. Kelly D, Mayer D. Liver transplantation. In: Kelly D (ed) *Diseases of the Liver and Biliary System in Children*, 2nd edn Oxford: Blackwell 2004: 378-401.
10. Malatack JJ, Schald DJ, Urbach AH *et al.* Choosing a paediatric recipient of orthotopic liver transplantation. *J Pediatr* 1987; 112:479-489.
11. McDiarmid SV, Anand R, Lindblad AS. The Principal Investigators and Institutions of the Studies of Pediatric Liver Transplantation (SPLIT) Research Group. Development of a pediatric end-stage liver disease score to predict poor outcome in children awaiting liver transplantation. *Transplantation* 2002;74:173-181.
12. McDiarmid, S Current status of liver transplantation in children. *Pediatric Clin North Am* 2003;50:1335-1374.

13. Newell KA, Alonso EM, Whitington PF, *et al.*: Post-transplant lymphoproliferative disease in paediatric liver transplantation. Interplay between primary Epstein-Barr virus infection and immunosuppression. *Transplantation* 1996;62:370-375.
14. Zitelli BJ, Gartner B, Malatack JJ, *et al.* Pediatric liver transplantation: Patient evaluation and selection, infectious complications, and life-style after transplantation. *Transplant Proc* 1987; 19:3309-3316.

Part C
Pediatric Nutrition

95 Nutritional Requirements

Suraj Gupte • EM Gomez

INTRODUCTION

No doubt, adequate nutrition is of paramount importance during childhood, especially in the first 3 years of life, when growth is most rapid and the child is, by and large, totally dependent on his caretaker(s), usually the parents. Over and above these increased needs for rapid growth, there are high maintenance needs on account of higher metabolic and nutrient turnover rates in infants and children.

Since an important factor responsible for adequate growth is balanced nutrition, erroneous nutrition leads to inadequate growth in addition to undernutrition and poor weight gain. Naturally, a basic knowledge of nutritional requirements at various ages as also sources of such vital nutrients as vitamin A and micronutrients as iron and zinc is mandatory.

Macronutrients are protein, carbohydrates and fat. Micronutrients are vitamins, trace elements and electrolytes. Failure to obtain any of the nutrients may cause harm. At times, it may prove catastrophic.

The term, *energy requirement,* denotes the amount of dietary energy required to balance energy expended and deposited in new tissues (growth). Table 95.1 gives the breakup of energy expenditure.

Table 95.1: Breakup of energy expenditure

Growth	12%
Physical activity	25%
Basal metabolism	50%
Fecal loss	8%

In order to meet the growth needs in first 3 years and during adolescence, a higher energy dense diet (less complex carbohydrates and larger quantity of fat) is needed.

Water, proteins, carbohydrates, fats, vitamins and minerals are the chief constituents of food. These six factors form the human body in the following way:

Water	63%
Proteins	17%
Fats	12%
Carbohydrates	1%
Vitamins and minerals	7%

WATER

It is second only to oxygen as a "must" for survival. Compared to adults, infants require much larger amount of water per unit of body weight. Its requirements at different ages are given in Table 95.2.

Table 95.2: Water requirements at different ages

Age range	*Water requirement (ml/kg)*
First 3 days	80 to 100
3 to 10 days	125 to 150
15 days to 3 months	140 to 160
3 to 12 months	150
1 to 3 years	125
4 to 6 years	100
7 to 9 years	75
10 to 12 years (and thereafter)	50

ENERGY

Calorie or energy requirement varies from age to age as is shown in Tables 95.3 and 95.4. On an average, 50% of calories should come from carbohydrates, 35% from fats and 15% from protein.

It is worth remembering that daily requirement is 100 to 120 k calories per kg for the first year of life. During the following period, it decreases by around 10 k calories per kg for each succeeding 3-year duration. succeeding 3-year duration.

Table 95.5 presents the total daily calorie requirement during the first year of life. It is apparent that an infant of 1 year of age needs about 1,000 k calories. A rough rule is to add 100 calories per each year of age upto a maximum of

1,500 k calories. About adolescence; when the growth spurt occurs, calorie needs are much higher. According to this rule a child of 5 years of age needs 1,000 + 400 = 1,400 k calories.

Second popular method of calculating energy requirements is by employing the Holiday and Segar formula (Box 95.1).

Box 95.1: Calculation of energy (calorie) requirement

I. Beside Method

1 year	1000 kCal

Subsequently100 kCal for every year in addition to 1000 kCal until adolescence.

Thus, for 1 child of:

1 year	1000 kCal
2 years	1000+100=1100 kCal
3 years	1000+200=1200 kCal
4 years	1000+300=1300 kCal
5 years	1000+400=1400 kCal
6 years	1000+500=1500 kCal
7 years	1000+600=1600 kCal
8 years	1000+700=1700 kCal
9 years	1000+800=1800 kCal
10 years	1000+900=1900 kCal
11 years	1000+1000=2000 kCal
12 years	1000+1100=2100 kCal

II. Holiday and Segar Method

Expected Weight	upto10 kg	100 kCal/kg
	10 to 20 kg	1000+50 kCal/kg
	over 20 kg	1500+20 kCal/kg

Thus, for a child of:

1 year (10 kg)	1000 kCal
2 years (12 kg)	1000+100=1100 kCal
3 years (14 kg)	1000+200=1200 kCal
4 years (16 kg)	1000+300=1300 kCal
5 years (18 kg)	1000+400=1400 kCal
6 years (21 kg)	1500+20=1520 kCal
7 years (24 kg)	1500+80=1580 kCal
8 years (27 kg)	1500+140=1640 kCal
9 years (30 kg)	1500+200=1700 kCal
10 years (33 kg)	1500+260=1760 kCal
11 years (36 kg)	1500+320=1820 kCal
12 years (39 kg)	1500+380=1880 kCal

Backup of energy is as follows:

- Maintenance of basal metabolism 50%
- Specific dynamic action 5%
- Growth 12%
- Physical activity 25%
- Losses in stools etc. 8%

Table 95.3: Daily calorie requirement of infants

Age range (months)	*Requirement calorie per kg*
0 to 3 months	120
3 to 6 months	115
6 to 9 months	110
9 to 12 months	105

Table 95.4: Daily requirement of calories

Age range (years)	*Requirement k calorie per kg*
Under 1 (average)	110
1 to 3	100
4 to 6	90
7 to 9	80
10 to 12	70
13 to 15	60
16 to 19	50
Adult	40

Table 95.5: Absolute daily requirement for calories during first year

Age (months)	*Calorie requirement*
1	500
2	600
4	700
5	800
9	900
10	1,000

Tables 95.3, 95.4 and 95.5 give approximate requirements for calories.

PROTEINS

Proteins of animal origin are termed "biologically complete proteins" since these provide good deal of essential amino acids, namely lysine, leucine, isoleucine, tryptophan, valine, methionine, phenylalanine, threonine and histidine. On the contrary, proteins of vegetable origin are usually "biologically incomplete" since they lack one or more of the essential amino acids. However, when different vegetable sources of protein are combined, result is a product that is likely to provide all the essential amino acids. Higher amounts of vegetable proteins are needed to make allowance for low biological value.

Table 95.6: Daily requirement for proteins

Age range (years)	*Protein requirement (g/kg)*
Under 1	3.5 to 2.6
1 to 3	2.5 to 2.0
4 to 6	3.0
7 to 9	2.8
10 to 12	2.0
13 to 15	1.7
16 to 19	1.5
Adult	1.0

Biologic value is defined as the fraction of absorbed nitrogen retained in the body for growth or maintenance. It is of 100 for egg protein which is regarded as the "reference protein", 75 for milk and fish and 67 for rice.

There are 10 essential amino acids, 7 conditionally essental amino acids and 4 non-essential amino acids (Table 95.7).

Table 95.7: Various amino acids

Essential	*Conditionally essential*	*Non-essential*
Leucine	Taurine	Alanine
Isoleucine	Tyrosine	Glutamate
Valine	Cysteine	Asparagine
Lysine	Glycine	Aspartate
Tyrosine (Phenylalanine)	Serine	
Methionine (Cysteine)	Proline	
Threonine	Glutamine	
Tryptophan		
Histidine		
Arfinine		

CARBOHYDRATES

Maximum bulk (55-60%) of calories (energy) needs to be obtained from carbohydrates. In fact, the balance of the calories needed, after meeting the needs of proteins and fats, is provided by this constituent.

Carbohydrates are of two types:

1. Simple which may be monosaccharides (glucose, fructose, galactose, ribose, deoxyribose) and disaccharides (sucrose, lactose, maltose).
2. Complex (polysaccharides): Starch, glycogen, fiber. With the exception of fiber, all carbohydrates are converted to glucose which is either employed as a fuel by the brain and muscles or stored in liver and muscles as glycogen. Carbohydrates consumed in excess are converted to fat.

Fiber (polysaccharides like cellulose, hemicellulose, pectin, gums, mucilages; nonpolysaccharides like lignins), a constituent of plant cell walls, mainly remains unabsorbed since it is resistant to digestion by enzymes of the human small intestine. It usually enhances the bulk of the diet. Dietary fiber is a complex mixture of both water-soluble (pectin, gums, mucilages, hemicelluloses) and water-insoluble (cellulose, lignin, hemicellulose) fiber. Its food value is negligible.

It is important for normal functioning of the GIT, preventing and even curing chronic constipation. Important fiber-containing foods include cereals, fruits, vegetables and dried beans.

Very high fiber intake containing phytate (inositol hexaphosphate) may interfere with bioavailabilty of calcium (e.g. calcium-deficiency rickets). Similarly excess of dietary oxalates in fiber may cause iron-deficiency anemia (IDA).

Recommended intake in children is age plus 5 g per day.

FATS

Whereas carbohydrates are readily available source of energy, fats constitute concentrated energy-giving element, thereby enhancing the calories without much increase in bulk. The minimal requirement are not accurately defined. Usually upto 30 % of total energy should be from fats (3.5 % of calories should be supplied by linoleic acid and 0.3 % from linolenic acid). Since human body is incapable of synthesizing this acid, it has got to be supplied in diet. Its deficiency in infants causes dryness and thickening of the skin with desquamation and intertrigo.

Important lipids are: Triglycerides (fats and oils), phosphilopids (lecithin) and steroids (cholesterol).

Depending on the length of the carbon, fatty acid may be:

- Short-chained
- Medium-chained
- Long-chained.

Depending on the saturation, triyglycerides may be:

- Saturated
- Unsaturated: Monounsaturated and polyunsaturated.

Saturated fatty acids are obtained from meat and coconut oil. Human body can also produce it from carbohydrates and proteins.

Unsaturated fatty acids are obtained from vegetables, nuts and seeds. Whereas monounsaturated fatty acids (MUFA) such as oleic acid may also be produced by the body, polyunsaturated fatty acids (PUFA), also called essential fatty acids (EFA), must be provided by the dietary sources. PUFA consists of omega-6 fatty acids (linoleic acid, arachiodinic acid) present in normal balanced diet and omega-3 fatty acids e.g. linolenic acid, eicosapentanoic acid (EPA) and docaosahexaenoic acid (DHA) which are present in fish and seafoods.

Lecithin is a major component of cell membrane. It is synthesized by the liver.

Though cholesterol, an important component of cell membrane, may be produced by the human liver, its dietary sources include animal fats (egg, meat especially kidney and liver, cheese, desi ghee). It may be transformed to hormones, vitamin D and bile. The daily intake of cholesterol should not exceed 250-300 mg/day.

VITAMINS

(Table 95.8)

MINERALS AND TRACE ELEMENTS

Cations like calcium, magnesium, sodium and potassium and anions like phosphorus, sulfur and chloride which are

Table 95.8: summarizes the requirements of vitamins which are essential for the maintenance of good health

Vitamins	*Requirement*
A	1,500 to 5,000 IU
B_1 (thiamine)	0.5 to 1.5 mg
B_2 (riboflavin)	0.5 to 2.5 mg
Niacin (niacinamide, nicotinamide, nicotinic acid)	0 to 20 mg
B_6 (pyridoxine)	0.4 to 1.4 mg
B_{12} (cyanocobalamine)	1 to 1.5 mcg
Folic acid	25 to 1000 mcg
C	30 to 50 mg
D	400 IU
E	4 to 5 IU

needed in amounts exceeding 100 mg/day are called "macrominerals". Elements like iron, zinc, copper, cobalt, iodine, selenium, molybdenum and chromium which are needed in very small amounts (upto 100-200 mcg/g matrix) are called *microminerals.*

The recommended intake of important minerals is given in (Table 95.9).

Table 95.9: Daily requirement for minerals

Mineral	*Requirement*
Iron	Infants: 1 mg/kg (6 to 10 mg)
	1 to 3 years: 15 mg
	3 to 12 years: 10 mg
	12 to 18 years: 18 mg
Calcium	Infants: 400 to 600 mg
	1 to 10 years: 0.7 to 1.0 g
	Over 10 years: 1.2 to 1.5 g
Potassium	1.5 mEq/kg (1 to 2 g)
Sodium	2.0 mEq/kg
Zinc	0.3 or more mg/kg
Magnesium	Infants: 40 to 70 mg
	1 to 3 years: 100 to 150 mg
	3 to 12 years: 200 to 300 mg
	12 to 18 years: 300 to 350 mg
Iodine	0.2 mg
Copper	0.05 to 0.1 mg/kg
Fluorine	0.5 to 1 mg

Iron, available from food, is of two types, namely heme and nonheme. Heme iron is found in nonveg foods, say meat, liver, chicken and fish. Around 15-35% heme iron gets absorbed from the gut. Nonheme iron is present in plants, legumes, eggs, milk and cereals. Its absorption is much less, i.e. hardly 1%. Several factors influence its absorption (Table 95.10). During adolescence, iron needs enhance. This is especially true in case of menstruating teenagers.

Zinc is normally present in our body in sufficient amount. No supplementation is, therefore, required by the healthy individuals. In certain situations, say persistent diarrhea, malnutrition, ITS, and acrodermatitis enteropathica, zinc deficiency occurs and, therefore, zinc supplementation is strongly recommended to hasten recovery. Normal daily requirement of zinc is 4-6 mg/day. Excess of zinc intake may be complicated by copper deficiency.

Table 95.10: Foods affecting absorption of iron from the gut iron from the gut

Absorption enhanced	*Absorption reduced*
Vitamin C-rich foods	Tea
Guava	Coffee
Lemon	Maize
Orange	Phytates (whole meal bread)
Tomatoes	
Indian gooseberry	
Foods cointaining heme iron	
Liver	
Meat	
Chicken	
Fish	
Fermented/germinated foods	

Table 95.11 lists salient features of important minerals.

FREE OXYGEN RADICALS AND ANTIOXIDANTS

The term, *free radicals,* refers to atoms or molecules that contain one or more unpaired electrons that are capable of altering (usually enhancing) their chemical reactivity and cause tissue damage. These are produced in large amounts during all tissue activities (infection, phagocytosis, tissue injury, ischemia-perfusion). Examples of free radicals are superoxide anions, singlet oxygen, peroxide anion, hydroxyl radical and hydrogen peroxide.

To counter the free radicals, defenses are provided in the form of *antioxidants* which are defined as substances in food that significantly decrease the adverse effects of free radicals. Examples of antioxidants are superoxide dismutase, transferrin, glutothionine peroxidase, vitamin C (ascorbic acid), vitamin E (tocopherol), beta-carotene, selenium, zinc, iron, manganese, nicotinamide, riboflavin and lycopene.

Excess of free radicals results either from their higher production or from inadequate antioxidant defense. Disorders in which free radicals appear to play a significant role include retinopathy of prematurity, Rh hemolytic disease, hemolytic anemia of the newborn, hypoxic-ischemic encephalopathy, septicemia, intraventricular hemorrhage, bronchopulmonary dysplasia, ARDS, necrotizing enterocolitis, inflammatory bowel disease, advanced PEM (kwashiorkor), cholestatic liver disease, pancreatitis, iron-overload (hemochromatosis) and copper-overload (Wilson's disease, ICC).

Recently, a number of synthetic antioxidants N-acetyl

Table 95.11: Salient features of important minerals/trace elements

Mineral/ Trace element	*Source*	*Deficiency*	*Excess*
Iron	Green vegetables, meat, yolk, whole grains, nuts, legumes. Milk, especially breastmilk, is a poor source.	Microcytic-hypochromicanemia	Hemosiderosis; poisoning
Zinc	Cheese, nuts, grains, meat, fish	Dwarfism with iron-deficiency anemia, hyperpigmentation, hepatosplenomegaly, hypogonadism; acrodermatitis enteropathica: poor wound healing; depressed immunocompetence, ITS, LBW	Gastrointestinal upset, copper deficiency, reduced high density lipoprotein
Copper	Legumes, nuts, whole grains, meat, liver, oyster (shell-fish)	Refractory anemia, osteoporosis, neutropenia, depigmentation, ataxia, raised serum cholesterol	Indian childhood cirrhosis (ICC)
Magnesium	Cereals, legumes, nuts, meat, milk	Tetany	None
Calcium	Milk and its products, fish, green leafy vegetables	Tetany rickets	Renal stones, heart block
Phosphorus	Milk and its products, fish, green leafy vegetables	Rickets	Tetany
Iodine	Sea-foods, vegetables from iodine-rich soil, iodized salt	Goiter, cretinism	Goiter
Fluoride	Sea-food, tea	Dental caries	Fluorosis
Chromium	Drinking water, animal foods, yeast	Impaired glucose tolerance; diabetes mellitus in animals	None

cysteine. Glutathione, glutathione peroxidase analogue (ebselen), coenzyme Q derivatives and superoxide dismutase are available. These are yet to be successfully tried in humans.

INDIAN SCENARIO

Survey conducted by the National Nutrition Monitoring Bureau (NNMB) indicate that diet of the Indian preschoolerst is grossly deficient in each and every category of food (Table 95.12). Overall, it is the deficiency of calories (energy) whereas protein intake is, by and large, satisfactory. A noteworthy observation is that diet of children belonging to the higher strata of society show intake of protein that is in excess. It is, therefore, important to lay stress on total intake of food rather than just protein as is often done in practice.

Table 95.12 presents the recommended balanced diets for children.

Table 95.13 gives nutritive value of some commonly used foods in India as per the ICMR with minor modifications.

> **KEY LEARNING POINTS**
>
> - Adequate nutrition, particularly enhanced during periods of rapid growth, including maintenance needs, is of paramount importance.

Table 95.12: Balanced diet for children

	Preschool children						*School children*	
	1 to 3 years Veg. (g)	*4 to 6 years Nonveg. (g)*	*7 to 9 years Veg. (g)*	*10 to 12 years Nonveg. (g)*	*Veg. (g)*	*Nonveg. (g)*	*Veg. (g)*	*Nonveg. (g)*
Cereals	150	150	200	200	250	250	320	320
Pulses	50	40	60	50	70	60	70	60
Green leafy vegetables	50	50	75	75	75	75	100	100
Other vegetables/roots and tubers	30	30	50	50	50	50	75	75
Fruits	50	50	50	50	50	50	50	50
Milk	300	200	250	200	250	200	250	200
Fats and oils	20	20	25	25	30	30	35	35
Meat fish and eggs	-	30	-	30	-	30	-	30
Sugar and jaggery	30	30	40	40	50	50	50	50

Table 95.13: National Nutrition Monitoring Bureau (NNMB) survey data on actual vis-à-vis recommended dietary consumption by Indian preschoolers as per Indian Council of Medical Research document

Dietary item	*Actual intake*	*Recommended intake*
Cereals (g)	147	150-200
Pulses (g)	16	40-50
Leafy vegetables (g)	4	50-75
Other vegetables (g)	14	30-50
Fruits (g)	7	40-50
Milk and milk products (g)	80	200
Fats and oils (g)	4	20-25
Flesh foods (g)	4	30
Sugar and jaggery (g)	5	30-40
Calories (kcal)	758	1200-1700
Protein (g)	22-30	22-30
Iron (mg)	6.9	11.5-18.4
Calcium (mg)	193	400
Vitamin A (mcg)	220	400
Riboflavin (mg)		0.7-1.0

- Erroneous nutrition leads to inadequate growth, undernutrition and poor weight gain.
- In order to meet the growth needs in first 3 years and adolescence, a higher energy dense diet (less carbohydrates and larger quantity of fat) is needed.
- Water, proteins, carbohydrates, fats, vitamins and minerals are the chief constituents of food.
- On an average, 50 percent of calories should come from carbohydrates, 35 percent from fats and 50 percent from protein.
- Antioxidants are needed to counter the free radicals.
- *Macronutrients* are protein, carbohydrates and fats whereas *micronutrients* are vitamins, trace elements and electrolytes; *antioxidants* (superoxide dismutase, transferring, glutathione peroxidase, vitamin C vitamin E) are substances in food that significantly decrease the adverse effects of free radicals.
- Any imbalance in nutrition leads to undernutrition, poor weight gain and growth faltering.

FURTHER READINGS

1. Anderson JW, Smith BM, Gustafson NJ. Health benefits and practical aspects of high fiber diets. *Am J Clin Nutr* 1994;5 (Suppl 5): 1242S-1247.
2. Beird WC. Nutritional requirements during infancy. In: Browman BA, Russel RM (eds): Present Knowledge in Nutrition, 8th edn. Washington: International Science Institute Press 20001:416-425.
3. Gupte S. Marasmus and kwashiorkor. *Pediatrics* 1975; 56: 152-153.
4. Gupte S. Perspectives in infant nutrition. In: Gupte S (ed) *Newer Horizons in Tropical Pediatrics* 2nd edn., New Delhi: Jaypee 1986: 206-243.
5. Ghosh S. Nutritional needs of children. In: Ghosh S (ed) *Nutrition and Child Care: A Practical Guide*. New Delhi: Jaypee 2000:1-12.
6. Indian Council of Medical Research: *Dietary Allowances for Indians*. Supp Rep Ser No. 60, 1968.
7. Park K. Nutrition and health. In: *Park's Textbook of Preventive and Social Medicine*, 18th edn., Jabalpur: Banarsidas Bhanot 2005:392-425.
8. Williams CL, Bollella M. Is a high-fiber diet for children. *Pediatrics* 1995;96:1012-1019.

96 Breastfeeding

Bratati Banerjee

INTRODUCTION

"The essential characteristic of a mammal is not the capacity for gestation, but the further manifestation of maternal care, the possession of mammal to secrete milk for the young."

Lactation in its simplest form is an extremely ancient physiological function, probably dating back about 200 million years. The offspring of the most evolved of the mammalian class—the placental mammals—are entirely dependent in early life on nourishment in the form of milk secreted by exocrine glands—the mammal. It has been suggested that primitive mammary glands may have developed originally from modified apocrine sweat glands in reptiles. Such highly developed mammals have certain universal characteristics. They are warm-blooded and carry their young in utero, nourished by placental nutrient exchange. Their offsprings are all immature in varying degrees, so that they are usually unable to search for food and all are in need of warmth, contact and maternal protection. Lastly, and in contrast with all other classes, the mammal mother is the sole supplier of food in the form of milk produced directly from her body. Infant survival depends on the mother's presence, her ability to secrete milk, and on the partly reflex, partly learnt interaction by the mother-contact that leads to the initiation and successful continuation of lactation.

Among placental mammals, those who have to be able to run or swim almost immediately after birth have a relatively long gestation period and are born mature. Man is unique in this respect, as there is both a long gestation period and an immature newborn, incapable of unaided locomotion and completely dependent on the mother. The newborn is even unable to reach the breast unaided.

The hypothesis of Bostock suggests that the human fetal period must be considered as of 18 months duration. Labour occurs after 9 months to permit the large head to pass the relatively narrow birth canal. Thus the termination of uterine gestation takes place when the limit of brain and head size compatible with birth has been reached, long before the offspring is mature. Human newborn can therefore be considered to be an 'extero-gestate' or external fetus for about the first 9 months after birth. During this time he is completely dependent on the mother for protection and warmth, and her breasts function nutritionally as an external placenta. Following this, in traditional circumstances, the baby passes slowly through the 'weaning period', when he is gradually accustomed to new foods and moves from breast milk to the adult diet. During this phase, the human infant has been termed as a 'transitional'.

PHYSIOLOGY OF LACTATION

The breast consists partly of glandular tissue and partly of supporting tissue and fat. The gland tissue makes the milk, which moves along the nipple along small ducts. Before the ducts reach the nipple, they become wider and form lactiferous sinuses beneath the areola.

Stages of Lactation

Lactation, or the process of breastfeeding, results from the interplay of hormones and of instinctive, reflex and learned behaviour by mother and newborn. In this process four overlapping stages may be recognized:

1. *Milk initiation (Lactogenesis):* This process commences in the latter part of pregnancy, when colostrum secretion occurs as a result of stimulation of the breast alveolar cells by placental lactogen, and is continued after birth as an automatic process.
2. *Milk secretion (Galactopoiesis):* The continuing secretion of milk is mainly related to sufficient production of anterior pituitary hormone prolactin and to maternal nutrition.
3. *Milk ejection:* Movement of milk from the alveoli, where it is secreted, to the mouth of the infant is an active process within the breast, brought about by the let-down or milk ejection reflex.
4. *Milk ingestion:* The last stage of lactation is the ingestion of breast milk by the sucking baby. This is dependent on

the interactions between the mother and the newborn, and especially on the functioning of the letdown reflex and the neonatal feeding reflexes.

However, recent studies have provided evidence for the existence of appetite control in human newborn. Ultimately it is the infant's demand for breast milk which regulates milk supply and lactation capacity is not the controlling factor.

Breastfeeding Reflexes

Neonatal: The full term healthy newborn baby possesses three instinctive reflexes needed for successful breastfeeding.

1. The rooting reflex, in which tactile pressure on the cheek or circumoral area, and possibly the smell of the mother's breast, leads to turning of the head and opening and closing the mouth as the baby seeks for the nipple.
2. The sucking reflex, in which the tactile 'sign stimulus' of the nipple and the areola of the breast filling the mouth sufficiently and adequately leads to a milking action by the tongue against the hard palate.
3. The swallowing reflex, in which when the baby's mouth is full of milk he swallows it.

The suckling reflex begins to develop by the seventeenth week of fetal life and matures by the thirty second to thirty sixth week of pregnancy. In healthy full term babies, the rooting and sucking reflexes are strongest shortly (20-30 min) after birth, so that the vigorous nipple stimulation at that time can assist in initiating a letdown reflex. Also early nursing after birth avoids mammary congestion which can interfere with breastfeeding mechanically, as the swollen oedematous breast may make it difficult for the baby to grasp the nipple. These neonatal feeding reflexes are feeble or absent in smaller premature or low-birth-weight babies, or in a variety of general illnesses of the newborn.

Maternal: There are three main maternal reflexes involved in breastfeeding:

1. Prolactin reflex, in which every time the baby sucks at the breast the nerve endings of the nipple are stimulated, resulting in production of the hormone prolactin from the anterior pituitary, which leads to secretion of milk from the breast.
2. Nipple erection reflex, where stimulation of the mother's nipple by the baby's mouth leads to nipple erection, which makes the nipple protractile thereby assisting in the milking of the breast by the suckling reflex.
3. Let-down reflex (draught, milk-ejection or oxytocin reflex), which is a psychosomatic reflex, where oxytocin is produced by the posterior pituitary as a result of the baby's suckling. Oxytocin makes the muscle cells around the alveoli contract and the milk is pushed down towards the nipple.

TYPES OF HUMAN MILK

Colostrum

It is the thick yellowish fluid that is secreted in the first few days after delivery. It is very rich in proteins and protective antibodies and therefore, along with the excess white blood cells present in it, provides the 'first immunisation' against infections likely to be acquired by the baby after birth. The antibodies also probably help to prevent allergies. Colostrum contains Epidermal Growth Factor (EGF), which results in a mild purgative effect, which helps to clear the newborn's gut of meconium, thereby clearing bilirubin and also helps baby's immature intestine to develop after birth. It is richer than mature milk in vitamins A and K, thus preventing infections and hemorrhage in the newborn.

Transitional Milk

This comes during the following two weeks when the milk increases in quantity and changes in appearance and composition as per the baby's needs. Fat and sugar content of this milk is high, while immunoglobulin and protein content are low.

Mature Milk

Mature milk starts from the third or fourth day. The quantity increases gradually and the milk changes from a whitish to a yellowish colour. The composition of mature milk changes from the beginning to the end of a feed, the milks of these two stages being termed as fore and hind milk.

Fore milk is produced at the beginning of a feed, and looks grey and watery. It contains plenty of protein, lactose, vitamins and minerals, but not much fat. It satisfies the baby's thirst.

Hind milk is produced towards the end of a feed and looks much whiter. It is rich in fat and provides about half of the energy of a feed and satisfies the baby's hunger.

Preterm Milk

This is secreted following birth of a premature baby. This milk contains more protein, Na+, iron, IgG and calories.

COMPOSITION OF HUMAN MILK

Indian mothers secrete 450-600 ml of milk daily with 1.1 g protein per 100 ml. The energy value of human milk is 70 kcal per 100 ml. The composition and output of human milk varies with many factors including the stage of lactation, maternal nutrition, ethnic groups and individual variation. Diurnal variation in breast milk has also been reported.

The composition of breast milk is ideally suited to the needs of the baby and has all the nutrients that he needs for the first 6 months of life. The nutrients of breast milk can be more easily digested and absorbed than artificial milk. A baby needs less breast milk than artificial milk to grow well.

Biologically, human milk is a highly complex and unique secretion with many marked differences from milk of other species, which have successfully been used to rear babies in different cultures. However, cow's milk has been the most commonly used one and therefore deserves comparison with human milk.

Lactose

Almost all the carbohydrate in milk is lactose, but small quantities of other substances are also present, including galactose, fructose, and numerous nitrogen-containing carbohydrates, as well as 'bifidus factor'. Breast milk contains more lactose than any other milk and this is essential for human body. It provides energy and helps in the absorption of calcium. The enzyme lactase helps to digest lactose. Lactose is metabolized in the infant's body to galactose, a constituent of galactolipids, needed for the development of the central nervous system. Together with the bifidus factor, lactose promotes the growth of lactobacilli in the intestine.

Fats

Breast milk contains more polyunsaturated and essential fatty acids. There may be slightly less fat if the mother is severely malnourished. The fat content varies with the time of suckling. There is a three-fold increase in fat content in the last milk of the feed 'hind milk'. Diurnally the fat rises from early morning to a plateau at about midday. Fat content is lower in the later months of lactation. Levels of essential polyunsaturated fatty acids, particularly linoleic acid and oleic acid, are greater in breast milk. The cholesterol levels in human milk are higher than in cow's milk.

Triglycerides, the main constituents of milk fat, are broken down to diglycerides and monoglycerides by the enzyme lipase present in the intestine. However, in contrast to cow's milk, human milk is itself rich in lipase, thus making free fatty acids easily available, even before the digestive phase in the intestine. Fat in human milk is thus more efficiently digested and absorbed than cow's milk.

Proteins

Cow's milk contains about three times more protein than human milk, largely in the form of casein. However, the protein in breast milk forms soft curds, due to precipitation of caseins, which are easily digestible, while the protein in artificial milk forms thick curd in the baby's stomach which is difficult to digest. Breast milk contains enough essential amino acids, which artificial milks do not. Taurine, which is plentiful in breast milk, has been seen to enhance growth of baby's brain. Breast milk is much richer in lactoferrin, lysozyme and IgA, with no β lactoglobulin.

The amino acid composition of the two milks also differs in a variety of ways. The cystine content of human milk is higher than that of cow's milk, while tyrosine and phenyl alanine are greater in cow's milk. These differences are important as newborns, especially premature babies, fed on cow's milk develop 'transient tyrosinaemia', with potential late sequelae.

Vitamins

All vitamins, except vitamin K are present in human milk. Breast milk contains water soluble vitamin D, besides the fat soluble fraction which protects against rickets. It also contains more vitamins A, C and E than cow's milk. In addition, vitamin E is present in the appropriate ratio with the polyunsaturated fatty acids present. The breastfed baby does not require any vitamin supplements or fruit juice. However, dark-skinned infants are at increased risk of developing rickets, particularly if they are primarily breast-fed, and, therefore, require vitamin D supplementation. The levels of most vitamins in milk are increased by maternal dietary supplementation.

Minerals and Water

Milk contains almost all known minerals needed by the body such as calcium, phosphorous, sodium, potassium, magnesium, cobalt, copper, iodine etc. Breast milk contains the correct amount of calcium and phosphate. The concentration of minerals is over three times greater in cow's milk than in human milk. Iron content of both bovine and human milk is extremely low. But iron in human milk is better absorbed than iron in cow's milk. Fluoride content of human milk depends on the level of the mineral in drinking water. Cow's milk contains more fluoride than human milk. Mammary gland, like the thyroid gland concentrates iodine, which appears in milk.

Milk contains enough of water for the baby, even in hot climate, as a result of which the baby does not need to drink any extra water. The renal solute load of cow's milk is much greater than that of breast milk. By contrast, human milk is a low solute fluid, which is designed as a 'supply and demand' source of nutrients and water, in response to both hunger and thirst.

Composition of Breast Milk of Mothers with Premature Babies

The composition of milk in mothers with premature babies is different from that in case of term babies. It contains more energy, fat, protein, sodium, zinc, anti-infective factors and cells (polymorphs and lymphocytes) and has lower concentration of lactose, calcium and phosphorous.

Table 96.1: Comparison between breast milk during the first month of lactation and unprocessed cow's milk

Constituent	*Breast milk (g/L)*	*Cow's milk (g/L)*
Proteins	11	33
Casein	4	28
Soluble proteins	7	5
Lactalbumin	3.5	1.5-1.8
Beta-lactglobulin	0	3.7
Lactotransferrin	1-2	0.2-0.5
Immunoglobulin	1-2	0.5
Lysozyme	0.5	Traces
Non-protein Nitrogeneous substances		
Lipids	35	35
Linoleic acid	3.5	1
Carbohydrates	70	50
Lactose	62	50
Nitrogenous oligosaccharides	8	0
Minerals	2	8
Calcium	0.33	
Phosphorous	0.15	
Iron	0.4-1.5 mg	0.3-0.5 mg
Vitamins		
C	60 mg	20 mg
D	50 IU	25 IU
Energy	640-720 kcal 2670-3000 kJ	650 kcal 2717 kJ

TERMS FOR INFANT FEEDING

- *Exclusive breastfeeding:* When a baby has no other food or drink except breastmilk, including milk expressed or from wet-nurse. The baby should not even have a pacifier or dummy. Drops, syrups (vitamins, minerals, medicines) may be given.
- *Predominant breastfeeding:* When a baby has small amounts of another food or drink, such as small drinks of water or water based products as tea, fruit juice etc. and drops or syrup, it is almost exclusive breastfeeding or predominant breastfeeding.
- *Partial breastfeeding:* When a baby has some breast feeds and some artificial feeds or other drinks, or has started weaning foods but continues to breast feed.
- *Token breastfeeding:* When a child mostly has other food, but still breast feeds sometimes.
- *Artificial feeding:* When a baby has artificial milk feeds and no breast milk at all.
- *Bottle feeding:* This means the baby is fed from a bottle, whatever is in the bottle, including expressed breast milk.
- *Timely complementary feeding:* This means giving a baby other food in addition to breastfeeding, when it is appropriate, after the age of 6 months.

ADVANTAGES OF BREASTFEEDING

It has been established that breast feeding is the ideal form of feeding the newborn. Global efforts to protect human and child rights have been initiated and among them is the right to a healthy start of life by the best nourishment a mother can provide. Breastfeeding has many advantages:

To the baby:

1. It is safe, clean, hygienic and available to the infant at the correct temperature.
2. It fully meets the nutritional requirements of the infant in the first 4-6 months of life. It is easily digested and utilized by both normal and premature babies.
3. It contains anti-microbial factors such as macrophages, lymphocytes, secretary IgA, anti-streptococcal factor, bifidus factor, antiviral factor, lysozyme and lactoferrin, lactoperoxidase, complements, interferon, which provide considerable protection not only against diarrheal diseases and necrotizing enterocolitis, but also against respiratory infections in the first months of life.
4. Sucking is good for the baby, helping in the development of jaws and teeth and prevents caries teeth.
5. It protects the baby from the tendency to obesity and also prevents under nutrition, and is good for a low-birthweight baby.
6. It provides several biochemical advantages such as prevention of neonatal hypocalcaemia and hypomagnesaemia.
7. Babies on breast milk are less likely to get colic, infantile allergies and eczema than artificially fed babies.
8. Presence of growth factors in breast milk helps the baby's intestines to grow and develop, so that he is able to digest and absorb other foods.
9. Breastfeeding has sometimes been associated with a positive effect on intelligence and cognitive scores of the child and also better visual development and visual acuity, leading to reading and learning readiness.
10. Risk of infantile diarrhea, asthma, cot or sudden infant death and also lymphoma is probably reduced in breast fed babies.
11. Breastfeeding helps in prevention of adulthood diseases, such as hypertension, diabetes and coronary artery diseases.
12. Breastfed babies are less likely to become smokers and alcoholics in later life.

To the mother

1. It is the simplest way to feed the baby and available at any time and any place, without requiring any preparation.
2. The mother has a feeling of satisfaction and achievement and psychologically it makes her happier.
3. Lactating mothers are likely to return to pre-pregnancy figure earlier than non-lactating mothers due to utilization

of fat reserve laid down during pregnancy and due to involution of the uterus.

4. Lactating mothers experience easier expulsion of placenta and earlier termination of post partum bleeding.
5. Breastfeeding increases the period of lactation amenorrhoea after child birth, which helps to conserve iron store of the mother, thus preventing anaemia.
6. Breastfeeding lowers the risk of breast and ovarian cancer.
7. Breastfeeding allows for daily rest periods for the mother.

To the family

1. Breastfeeding is less expensive. The cost of extra food that a lactating mother requires is much less than the cost of milk substitutes.
2. Breastfeeding protects the baby against many diseases, thus reducing the cost of treatment.
3. It promotes bonding between the mother and the baby, resulting in a healthy family.
4. Lactation amenorrhoea prevents more births than all the family planning methods put together.

To the society

1. It contributes to child survival.
2. It leads to decreased health care costs due to reduced morbidity in breastfed infants.
3. Government spending on subsidized infant formula feeding programme is decreased.

To the employer

1. It leads to increased productivity as the mother is more satisfied.
2. Decreased absenteeism as the baby falls sick less often.

To the environment

1. Breastfeeding does not cause environmental degradation as artificial feeding does, i.e. in the manufacturing of Infant Milk Substitutes (IMS), bottles, nipples; heating of IMS, bottles, nipples; disposal of bottles, nipple.
2. Sanitary material used by non-lactating, menstruating women also leads to pollution by their disposal.
3. Manufacturing promotion material for formula feeding, paper used in sanitary material etc. causes depletion of natural resources.

IMMUNOLOGIC CONSEQUENCES OF BREASTFEEDING

The predominant immunoglobulin is secretory IgA, which acts locally within the infant's gastrointestinal tract. Human breast milk contains IgA antibodies against E. coli, and it is known that breast fed babies are less prone to enteric infections than are bottle fed babies. Human milk also contains both T and B lymphocytes from the mother. The amounts of protective factors in human milk appear to vary between individuals, being much richer in the milk of young women compared to that of older women.

Table 96.2: Prevention of diseases by human milk

Disease	*Ameliorating property of human milk*
Infectious diseases	
Acute respiratory infections	Immunoglobulin, especially IgA, IgM, IgG
Diarrhea	Macrophages, lymphocytes, polymorphs
Necrotizing enterocolitis	Lactoferrin, lysozyme, lactoperoxidase, complement factor, bifidus factor etc.
Otitis media	Antibody protection and/or lack of irritation from cow's milk
Other diseases	
Sudden infant death	Anti-infectious, anti-allergic
Neonatal hypocalcemia	Ideal calcium/phosphorous ratio, better calcium resorption
Iron deficiency anaemia	Better iron absorption, no blood loss from intestines
Gastrointestinal infections	Humoral and cellular anti-infectious factor
Necrotizing enterocolitis	Immunologic factors, macrophages, osmolarity of human milk
Infantile eczema	No species-non-specific proteins
Acrodermatitis enteropathica	More efficient zinc absorption
Vitamin E deficiency anaemia	Sufficient vitamin E in human milk
Chronic constipation	Stools soft
Hypernatremic dehydration	Low mineral and sodium content
Childhood lymphoma	Increases resistance and immunity
Hypertrophic pyloric stenosis	Uncertain; speculated that breast feeding prevents pyloric spasm and oedema
Liver disease	Protease inhibitors, including anti-trypsin
Atopic disease (allergies, asthma)	Inhibits potential antigen molecules from entering neonate by providing passive barrier
Celiac disease	Protects against development of villous atrophy in intestinal mucosa
Crohn's disease	Uncertain

CONTRAINDICATIONS TO BREASTFEEDING

In Mother

1. Chronic diseases such as active tuberculosis, leprosy, malignancy, beri beri etc. Many authorities advocate continuing breastfeeding in the first two, provided chemotherapeutic coverage is being given.
2. Mothers stubbornly addicted to alcohol or heavy doses of some drugs like heavy metals, phenobarbitone, hydantoin, steroids etc.
3. Psychosis.
4. Local conditions like breast abscess, cracked nipple etc.

In Infant

1. Gross prematurity of baby and other conditions in which newborn cannot suck.
2. Inborn errors such as phenylketonuria, galactosemia and lactose intolerance.
3. Breast milk jaundice, provided serum bilirubin approaches critical level.
4. Biological mother may avoid breastfeeding an infant who is to be passed to another couple.

However, the only true contraindications for stopping breast milk are galactosemia and phenylketonuria. Maternal illness should not result in interruption of breastfeeding. If need arises, expressed breast milk (EBM) may also be given.

PREPARATION DURING PREGNANCY

The expectant mothers, particularly primiparas and those experiencing difficulties with lactation management earlier, should be motivated and prepared to exclusively breast feed. This should be achieved by educating, through a personal approach, about the benefits and management of breastfeeding. In the last trimester of pregnancy, breast and nipples should be examined and relevant advice given. Expectant mothers should be counselled to eat extra green vegetables. Additional rest of half to one hour and, wherever possible, switching to relatively lighter work during the last trimester should be propagated. For delivery, it is important to choose a hospital where breastfeeding is supported. Indiscriminate use of sedatives, analgesics and anaesthetics should be avoided as it prevents the mother establishing a close contact with her infant immediately after the delivery and also diminish the newborn infant's sucking capability. Breastfed infants whose mothers smoke have a 5 times higher level of cotinine, a nicotine by-product, in their urine than infants of smokers who do not breastfeed. Nursing mothers should, therefore, stop smoking.

STARTING BREASTFEEDS

Practically all mothers, including those with mild to moderate chronic malnutrition, can successfully breastfeed. Soon after delivery, the mother should be allowed to keep the newborn with her (rooming-in). After a normal delivery, babies should receive the first breastfeed as soon as possible, and preferably within half hour of birth. During this period and later, the normal newborn should not be given any other fluid or food, known as prelacteal feeds, like honey, "ghutti", animal or powdered milk, tea, water, glucose water etc. since these are potentially harmful. It is essential that the baby gets the first breast milk called colostrum, which is all the food and fluid needed at this time—no supplements are necessary, not even water. The mother, especially with the first birth, may need help in the proper positioning for breastfeeding. Breastfeeds should be given as often as the baby desires and each feed should continue for as long as the infant wants to suckle. After a caesarean section, breastfeeding should be started as soon as possible and preferably within 4 hours of delivery. The mother will need help to put the baby to the breast for a day or two.

In order to 'kick out' the swallowed air, the act of nursing should be followed by burping. It should be done by holding the baby erect over the mother's shoulder or making him sit in mother's lap and then patting or rubbing his back, so that he eructates the swallowed air. Failure to do so may cause regurgitation, vomiting and even abdominal pain.

POSITIONING A BABY AT THE BREAST

Correct positioning of the baby at the breast is important for effective milk transfer from the mother to the baby. The mother and the baby need to be comfortable during breastfeeding. An incorrect sucking position may lead to sore nipples, refusal to feed, and the feeling that there is not enough milk. This may lead to engorged breasts.

- The mother should sit or find a comfortable position for herself.
- She should hold her baby in her arms so that he faces the breast and his abdomen is against the mother's. The baby's entire body should face towards the breast.
- The mother should hold and offer her whole breast and not just the nipple or areola.
- She should then touch the baby's cheek or the side of his mouth with the nipple to stimulate the rooting reflex.
- Baby should be in good attachment, that is close to the mother and chin touches breast, has mouth wide open and cheeks are full, lower lip has turned out and tongue can be seen, takes slow deep sucks which causes no pain to the mother.
- Many mothers prefer to breast feed while lying down. As long the baby has access to the breast, he can be fed satisfactorily in any position.
- She should start the child on a different breast each time to help both breasts produce the maximum amount of milk.

DRUGS SECRETED IN MILK

Most drugs given to the mother are secreted in the milk. Many factors influence this, including the concentration of drugs in the plasma, the degree of protein binding of the drug, plasma and milk pH, degree of ionization, lipid solubility, and molecular weight. Drugs are secreted in milk usually in concentrations no higher than in maternal plasma. Consequently the amount of drug ingested by the infant is small.

Drug therapy should be avoided in lactating mothers and when necessary, a safer alternative should be prescribed. Drug intake should preferably be timed during or immediately after breastfeeding. Majority of the commonly used preparations are compatible with safe breastfeeding. Only a few drugs necessitate discontinuation of breastfeeding.

Table 96.3: Medication for breastfeeding mothers

Breastfeeding contraindicated
- Cytotoxic drugs
- Anticancer drugs (antimetabolites)
- Radioactive substances—stop breastfeeding temporarily
- Lithium

Breastfeeding should continue, monitor the baby for drowsiness:
- Psychiatric drugs and anticonvulsants
- Barbiturates and diazepam – problems sometimes occur. Change the drug, but if there is no alternative continue breastfeeding and observe the baby

Use alternative drugs if possible
- Sulphonamides
- Chloramphenicol, tetracycline
- Oestrogen—may decrease breast milk supply
- Thiazide diuretics—may decrease breast milk supply

Use with caution
- Ephedrine
- Ergot
- Aspirin
- Indomethacin
- Nitrofurantoin
- Nalidixic acid

Safe in usual doses
- Antibiotics
- Analgesics
- Antihistamines
- Antacids
- Insulin
- Digoxin
- Bronchodilator
- Corticosteroids
- Chloroquin
- Anthelmintics
- Antituberculars
- Nutritional supplements of iron, iodine, vitamins

BREASTFEEDING IN THE MALNOURISHED MOTHER

Breast milk is fairly well protected from the influence of malnutrition in the lactating mother. A review of available literature reveals that even among malnourished mothers, breast milk is sufficient to sustain the growth and development of the infant upto 4-6 months of age. Maternal undernutrition has been shown to have no effect on vitamin A, vitamin E, iron, calcium, magnesium, copper and zinc content of colostrum. Among anti-infective factors, IgA content is lower but there is no difference in lactoferrin, lysozyme, IgG and IgM content of colostrums. Protein and lipid content has also been found to be lower in malnourished mothers.

In mature milk, among mothers receiving upto 60 percent of Recommended Daily Allowance no significant decrease in protein concentration of breast milk has been observed. Some amino acids, such as lysine and methionine, have been reported to be lower in the milk of malnourished mothers. The concentration of lactose and fat is not affected by mother's nutrition.

The nutrients in human milk are affected only when the nutritional status of the mother is considerably affected. Nutrients affected may be considered on a 'sliding scale' with water soluble vitamins most easily affected, fat, protein and calcium to a minor degree and lactose the least. An Expert Committee of Indian Academy of Pediatrics, in 1988, has recommended that even inadequately nourished mothers can provide milk in sufficient quantity during the first 4-6 months of the baby's life. The quantity and quality of human milk is severely affected only in severe malnutrition states. However, studies have not yet established the threshold for the level.

DIET OF LACTATING MOTHER

A lactating woman should be advised to eat an extra helping of the family food and regular consumption of green leafy vegetables. There is no need to avoid any specific food. However, use of excessive caffeine, tobacco, and alcohol etc. should be discouraged.

BREASTFEEDING BY WORKING WOMEN

In the present day most of the rural and urban mothers work, majority in the unorganized sector. This is often the reason for discontinuing breastfeeding. However, breastfeeding can well be continued, if the mother is willing, by the following ways:

1. In the organized sector there is a provision of maternity leave, which can be availed of partly before and partly after delivery. Mothers with uncomplicated pregnancy can take the major part of this leave after delivery. After maternity leave is exhausted other kinds of leave can be continued for as long as possible. During the total leave period the baby should be exclusively breast fed.
2. On resuming work, if the workplace is close to her residence, the mother can take breaks from work and come back home to breast feed her baby.
3. If the workplace is far away the mother can take the baby along with her, if facility of crèche or child care centre is available.
4. If such facilities are not available, the mother should breast feed her baby as many times as possible – early in the morning, before leaving for work, immediately after returning from work, and throughout the rest of the evening and night.
5. For the rest of the day that she is away from home the mother should express her breast milk before going for work, so that the expressed milk can be fed to the baby during her absence. This milk can be stored for 6-8 hours at room temperature and upto 24 hours if refrigerated.

It is not necessary to reheat the milk before giving it to the baby. If the milk separates it can be shaken up. It remains good for use.

6. At the workplace the mother should express the milk regularly, to maintain adequate lactation.

BREASTFEEDING IN SPECIAL SITUATIONS

Sickness of the Baby

1. *Low birth weight babies:* Babies weighing more than 1200 g may safely be given expressed breast milk through nasogastric tube, cup or spoon. Bottles should not be used for feeding these babies as this poses a risk of infection and nipple confusion later. The baby can also be put to an empty breast to provide non-nutritive sucking.
2. *Twins:* If two babies are breast fed simultaneously, prolactin and oxytocin secretion increases accordingly, making more milk available to both babies. The mother needs to be reassured of this possibility.
3. *Diarrhea:* Breast fed babies normally pass 8-10, semi-formed, soft, curdy, frothy, yellowish stools, smelling like yoghurt. This is because of the high lactose content of milk. It may be wrongly interpreted as diarrhea by some mothers. However, in infective diarrhea baby passes frequent, watery stools and may become dehydrated. In invasive diarrhea, the stool contains blood and mucus. It should be ascertained if the baby has received anything other than breast milk, especially a bottle feed, which is a common cause of diarrhea. Breast feeding should not be discontinued and ORS should be given with a spoon between feeds.
4. *Jaundice:* Physiological jaundice in the newborn, which may appear on the second to the tenth day and is not above 14 mg/dl, subsides on its own. Infrequent breast feeding may lead to higher levels of bilirubin in physiological jaundice. Mothers should be counselled on the necessity and conditions of continuing breastfeeding that does not cause any complications.
5. *Cleft lip and palate:* Such babies should be held upright to prevent milk from leaking through the cleft palate. The baby should be well attached to the breast, with the whole areola in his mouth, so as to close the cleft with the breast tissue.
6. *Neurologically impaired babies:* Hypotonic babies and those with Down's syndrome may lack muscle tone in the jaw muscle, and require careful positioning so as to attach properly to the breast. The baby should be woken up every 2 to 3 hours for feeding. If necessary, the child may be fed on expressed breast milk.
7. *Surgery in breast fed baby:* When a breast fed baby needs surgery, the mother should carry on breastfeeding the baby for as long as possible prior to the surgery. For the period the baby cannot be put to the breast, the mother should express her breast milk and resume breastfeeding as soon as the baby recovers. These mothers require psychological support to allay their anxiety which inhibits oxytocin reflex.
8. *Inborn errors of metabolism:* Some metabolic disorders severely limit or render impossible the use of certain milk components. In galactosemia no kind of milk can be given. In phenylketonuria breastfeeding may be continued with monitoring of blood phenyl alanine.

Sickness of the Mother

1. *Cesarian section:* The mother should commence breast-feeding as soon as consciousness is regained, which may be within 4 hours after the surgery. Extra support is required to initiate breastfeeding for the first few days following surgery.
2. *Mental illness:* In puerperal psychosis or puerperal depression, the mother is usually capable of looking after her baby normally. Mother and baby should be together and breastfeeding continued. But she should have a helper to ensure that she doesn't neglect or injure the baby.
3. *Breast problems:* In mastitis or breast abscess, breast-feeding should be continued.
4. *Tuberculosis:* Breastfeeding can be continued, but the mother should be treated and the baby given BCG vaccination. If she is sputum positive INH 5 mg/kg/day should be given to the baby for 3 months. After 3 months a tuberculin test should be done and if negative BCG vaccination given.
5. *Leprosy:* Breastfeeding should be continued and the mother treated for leprosy. Dapsone is passed in the breast milk in sufficient quantity to afford protection to the baby.
6. *Diabetic mother on insulin:* Breastfeeding should be initiated and continued normally. Insulin passed in milk is inactivated by the baby's digestive enzymes.
7. *Herpes simplex:* If there is no lesion on the breast, breast-feeding should be continued. She should wash her hands before handling the baby. In case of lesion in the breast, feeding should be continued from the other breast.
8. *Hepatitis B:* Babies whose mothers are hepatitis B surface antigen positive should receive hepatitis B vaccine and HBIG (0.5 ml) at birth, and second and third doses given at one and six months of age. Breastfeeding should be continued as normal.
9. *HIV positive mother:* Vertical transmission of HIV occurs during pregnancy, child birth or breastfeeding. Babies who are not breastfed are 14 times more likely to die of common childhood sicknesses than exclusively breast fed babies, especially of low income families. On the other hand, in an HIV positive mother put on AZT in pregnancy and postpartum, the risk of transmission to

baby is greatly reduced. Hence, the decision to breast feed or not should be taken by the mother and the family, after weighing the advantages and disadvantages.

PROBLEMS ENCOUNTERED BY A LACTATING MOTHER

Breast Engorgement

When the milk first comes into the breasts, they feel hard and painfully full. The best way to prevent this engorgement is to let the baby suckle as often and as soon after birth as possible. Engorgement should be treated as soon as it develops by using warm compress on the breast. The baby should be allowed to suckle, and if he cannot hold the breasts the mother should express milk and feed him. Hand expression is preferable to the pump. After expressing some milk, baby should be put to breast. Milk should be expressed as often as necessary to make the breasts comfortable.

Blocked Duct, Mastitis and Breast Abscess

If a milk duct becomes blocked, a painful lump forms. The lump should be gently massaged towards the nipple to unblock the duct. Feeding from the breast should be continued. If a blocked duct is not cleared, the breast tissue may become infected, and the breast itself becomes tender and swollen. If untreated, an abscess develops. The mother should be encouraged to continue feeding the baby. If suckling is painful milk should be expressed every 3 hours. Warm compress helps to relieve the pain. If mother develops chill, fever and bodyache, she may need a full course of antibiotics or drainage of abscess if required.

Sore Nipples, Cracked Nipples

If the baby does not take enough breast into the mouth, the mother can get sore nipples, which may even damage the nipple skin and a fissure or crack appears. This can be prevented by good positioning during suckling. If sore nipple develops, suckling should be continued. No cream should be applied and nipples should not be washed with soap before or after each feed. They should be washed only during bath, once or twice a day. The nipples should be exposed to air and a little creamy hind milk may be applied after each feed. If the baby has oral thrush it should be treated and the same cream should be applied to the nipples. If suckling is impossible for a few days, milk should be expressed and this should be fed to the baby from a cup.

Expression of Milk by Hand

- A cup or glass should first be washed, then rinsed in boiling water, or dried in strong sunlight, or preferably boiled for 2-3 minutes.
- The mother must wash her hands thoroughly and then follow these steps:
  1. Lean forward and support the breast with her hand.
  2. Place her thumb on the areola above the nipple and her first finger on the areola below the nipple.
  3. Press the thumb and finger.
  4. Press the areola behind the nipple between the finger and the thumb.
  5. Continue pressing and releasing.
  6. Milk will begin to drip and then flow in a stream.
  7. Press the areola in the same way from the sides to express milk from all segments of the breast.
  8. The nipple itself must not be squeezed, but only the areola.

DEFICIENT LACTATION AND RELACTATION

Causes

1. Poor development of breast tissue: occurs as a constitutional defect and may be genetic and familial. The large breast is often the one with the most fat and the least glandular elements and does not always function well. The nipples may be small, flat or inverted and thus impede suckling.
2. General ill health and poor nutrition: may act over a long period and during pregnancy.
3. Acute illness: may arise in connection with the delivery-shock, haemorrhage and serious infection, often leading to destruction of anterior lobe of the pituitary gland.
4. Baby not breast fed often enough: feeding less than 5-6 times per day may lead to insufficiency.
5. Introduction of other food: giving artificial milk, prelacteal feed etc. reduces the production of breast milk.
6. Incorrect positioning: proper positioning is important for effective transfer of milk from the mother to the baby.
7. Failure of the baby to suckle effectively: may result from prematurity, illness, congenital abnormalities of the mouth and laziness. There is often a vicious circle, as the baby is lazy at suckling because he realizes there is little milk for him; this in turn has an adverse effect on the supply. Cracking and soreness of the nipples may make it necessary to stop suckling for a time and this nearly always interferes with the supply of milk.
8. Failure of the baby to empty the breast: supply of milk depends on emptying the breast fairly completely at the end of each feed, failing which milk supply is decreased.
9. Psychological considerations: mother's willingness to breast feed, her determination to make it successful, bonding with the baby and absence of undue anxiety over the thriving of her baby makes lactation successful. That willingness to breast feed is so important is seen from the fact that even grandmothers, when compelled in adverse circumstances, can breast feed.

Signs that a Baby May Not be Getting Enough Milk

Reliable Signs

1. Poor weight gain.
2. Passing small amounts of urine.

Possible

1. Baby not satisfied after breast feeds.
2. Baby cries often.
3. Very frequent breast feeds.
4. Very long breast feeds.
5. Baby refuses to breast feed.
6. No milk comes when mother squeezes.

Management

1. Psychological and physical preparation during pregnancy.
2. Ensuring the mother that she is healthy in mind and body.
3. Advice on care of nipples and breasts.
4. Correct positioning of the baby during feeding.
5. Adequate fluid intake, at least 3 litres in 24 hours.
6. If the baby fails to empty the breast at a feed, any remaining milk should be removed by pump or expression.
7. Exclusive breastfeeding to be maintained.
8. If baby refuses to suckle on 'empty' breast, milk may be given with a dropper or by a tube attached to the breast and to a cup of milk at the other end.
9. Some food, drink and herbs, believed to increase the mother's milk supply, may be given. These act by increasing the woman's confidence and helping her to relax. These may also improve her nutrition.
10. Galactagogues may be used, the safest being metoclopramide, given in a dose of 10 mg orally 8 hourly for 7-10 days. Chlorpromazine may also be given in a dose of 25 mg 8 hourly.

Evidence of Successful Relactation

- Appearance of first milk secretion in 2 to 10 days.
- Partial restoration of breastfeeding with reduction of top feed to half of the initial.
- Complete restoration of breastfeeding with total withdrawal of top feed.

BOWEL PATTERN IN BREASTFED BABIES

Healthy infants maintain adequate hydration status when exclusively breast fed and therefore do not require additional water. There is a great variation in colour and consistency of stools in breast fed babies. There may be several stools per day or only one per week. Consistency may vary from soft to watery or may even be explosive. Colour may be golden yellow to greenish and contain mucus and even reducing substances. This is not diarrhea and does not necessitate use of medication. Most babies may also strain and even cry while passing motion. This should not be interpreted as constipation or difficulty in evacuation. Bowel pattern changes frequently over the first 6 months of exclusive breastfeeding.

When a nursing mother starts menstruating her breast milk contains higher concentration of prostaglandins which increase gut motility in her infant. So an increase in frequency of stools, increase in fluidity and sometimes green colour with mucus may be seen. It does not require medication, water or ORS.

GROWTH MONITORING OF A BREASTFED INFANT

Growth references in common use, such as the NCHS and Tanner data sets, do not describe accurately the natural trajectory, and the breastfeeding infant, in both industrialized and developing countries, grows rapidly in the first two months, slowing thereafter. This deceleration in weight velocity was once described as 'growth faltering' and speculatively attributed to shortfall in energy intake from breast milk.

Part of the normal ongoing monitoring of the newborn and infant development is the measurement of weight, length, height and simple motor skills compared to large data sets of clinically normal infants. The 20-year-old charts of WHO were based on growth patterns of babies fed formula-milk, not taking into account the fact that breast-fed babies tend to grow slower. As a result millions of healthy infants were assessed as growing too slowly because of inadequate international child-growth standards. Consequently, many infants were taken off breast milk and given solid foods before they needed them, with potentially life-threatening consequences.

The original standards differed between countries and in the time when the control data was collected (some based on data from 1970s or earlier). This has recently changed with the release of WHO international child growth standards using entirely new data sets. These standards were developed using data collected in the WHO Multicentre Growth Reference Study (MGRS), which is a community-based, multi-country project involving more than eight thousand children from Brazil, Ghana, India, Norway, Oman, and USA. On 27 April 2006 World Health Organization (WHO) released a New International Child Growth Standards for Infants and Young Children, to provide evidence and guidance for the first time about how every child in the world should grow.

The new standards are based on the breastfed child as the norm for growth and development. This brings coherence for the first time between the tools used to assess growth, and national and international infant feeding guidelines which recommend breastfeeding as the optimal source of nutrition during infancy. This will now allow accurate assessment, measurement and evaluation of breastfeeding and complementary feeding.

The first of this set of new growth charts released includes growth indicators such as weight-for-age, length/height-for-age, and weight-for-length/height. For the first time, there now exists a Body Mass Index (BMI) standard for children upto age five, as well as the Windows of Achievement standard for six key motor development milestones such as sitting, standing and walking.

FACTORS INFLUENCING PRACTICE OF BREAST-FEEDING

The patterns of breastfeeding are influenced by a variety of socio-demographic characteristics. Of these, the most consistent effect observed has been that of urban-rural residence. But with urbanization and development of rural areas even this difference is on the decline. The other factors noted to have a negative effect on breastfeeding, namely maternal education and increasing socio-economic status, use of modern methods of contraception and exposure to mass media, are all effects of modernity. The significance of most other influences varies from one cultural milieu to another. The western countries have gone through the whole cycle of changes in infant feeding practices induced by these factors and are returning to the old-fashioned tradition of prolonged breastfeeding. The developing world is unfortunately in mid-cycle.

GLOBAL TRENDS IN BREASTFEEDING

The practice of lactation by humans dates back to 100 million years. Wet nursing appeared as the first alternative in about 2000 BC, followed by animal milk as substitute. Use of artificial milk started in the present century. Following the Second World War, there was a rapid decline of breastfeeding in the western world. A lot of propaganda and marketing technology made patented food extremely popular, even in low income families, consequently leading to a tremendous rise in the prevalence of malnutrition among children, with its sequelae of increased morbidity and mortality. The picture was the same in the non-industrialized countries also. From the 1970's, the scientific communities started realizing the unique properties of breastfeeding, and efforts for protecting and promoting breastfeeding was initiated.

The global efforts for protection of breastfeeding started at a joint WHO/UNICEF meeting held in October 1979, where recommendations were made in Infant and Young Child Feeding. International code on marketing of breast milk substitutes was brought by WHO in 1981, followed by other declarations and policies. Finally in 1992 the Baby Friendly Hospital Initiative (BFHI) was initiated, to be adopted worldwide.

BREASTFEEDING PRACTICES IN INDIA

The prevalence of breastfeeding is almost universal in India, in both rural and urban areas. The urban women from high socio-economic societies, who used to prefer formula feeding, are now beginning to realize the advantages of breastfeeding. For most of the rural mothers, this is a natural method of feeding, and they do not consider any other alternative method. A review of Indian studies showed 96-100 percent of infants being breast fed.

Newborns are generally breast fed for the first time only 48-72 hours after birth. In a small proportion of cases, initiation of breastfeeding is reported after 24 hours or between 13 and 24 hours. However, in some tribal areas breastfeeding is initiated within 6-12 hours of birth. A Rapid Household survey reported the proportion of women who started breastfeeding within 2 hours of delivery (26.3 percent) to be higher in urban women and increased with the women's education and economic status, but same between SC/ST and non-SC/ST women (R). In many areas colostrum is discarded because of the general belief that it is not good for the child. This view occurs from the fact that as the colour of the initial breast milk is not white, it is considered to be impure and therefore can harm the child. As a result prelacteal feeds are often given, like beverages such as tea, boiled water, honey, sugar, jaggery or glucose with plain water or diluted animal milk. The most common ones are water sweetened with honey, sugar or jaggery. In some cases ghee, castor oil and some herbal preparations are also used as pre-lactation foods for infants.

It has been observed that in India, particularly in rural areas, due to ignorance and poverty, women continue to breastfeed their children exclusively for upto 8 months and in some cases for even upto 12 months. This delay in introducing supplementary foods is one of the major causes of malnutrition among infants. In India, when babies are very young (0-3 months), generally they are fed on demand. Breastfeeding during sleep is also quite common.

According to NFHS-2, only 37 percent of newborn children were put to the breast within one day of birth and even fewer were breastfed within one hour of birth. Most mothers squeezed out the 'first milk' before breastfeeding. These practices are widespread across all subgroups of women, although the more educated women are somewhat more likely than most other women to initiate breastfeeding within a day of childbirth. Initiation of breastfeeding is earlier for children born in a health facility, particularly a public health facility, than children born at home. Only 55 percent of children under four months of age are exclusively breastfed. Ninety-two percent of children are still being breastfed at 12 months of age and 59 percent are still being breastfed at 24 months of age. Children are breastfed for 25 months and exclusively breastfed for 4 months, on average. The median duration of exclusive breastfeeding is only 2 months. However the median duration of breastfeeding is two months shorter for girls than for boys. In general, urban women, more educated women, Sikh and Jain women, richer women, and women who gave birth in health facilities breastfeed for a shorter length of time than most other women.

Table 96.4: Undesirable practices associated with infant feeding in the Indian context

Undesirable practice	*Recommended practice*
Discarding first milk (colostrum)	Initiate breastfeeding as soon as possible after birth (within ½ hr after normal delivery and within 4 hrs after caesarian section).
Late initiation of breast feeding	No feed should be given to the baby before initiation and giving prelacteal feeds of breastfeeding. These introduce the first infection, may be aspirated into the lungs and reduce baby's need to suckle on the breast thereby reducing the production of breast milk.
Giving top feeds before 4-6 months of age	In the first 4-6 months of life the baby should be given only breast milk and nothing else. It meets all the needs of the baby.
Bottle feeding for milk/ water	Bottle should never be used to feed the baby, as it is a source of infection. If required, a cup and spoon may be used.
Delay in starting complementary	Start giving complementary feeds (3-4 feeds) to a feeding baby, when he is 4-6 months old, and increase to 4-6 feeds in a day to a child after 9 months of age, in addition to breastfeeding.
Complementary feeding is inadequate	Give 4-6 feeds of semi-solids to the baby in a day.

BOTTLENECKS IN SUCCESSFUL BREASTFEEDING

A lot of obstacles come in the way of successful breastfeeding. These are:

1. Mismanagement by elders in the family.
2. Erroneous role played by the electronic and print media.
3. Erroneous impression among some women that 'formula' is a status symbol.
4. Lack of interest on the part of health personnel to promote breastfeeding.
5. Non-availability of reasonable place for breastfeeding in the working places.
6. Inadequate breastfeeding or nursing leave for mothers.
7. Inadequate preparation for breastfeeding during antenatal check-ups.
8. Lack of 'will' for breastfeeding on the part of the mother.

EFFORTS MADE TO PROTECT, PROMOTE AND SUPPORT APPROPRIATE INFANT FEEDING PRACTICES IN INDIA

The Indian Government is a signatory to the 'Innocenti Declaration on the protection, promotion and support of breastfeeding'. The five pronged strategy given below includes the recommendations of the declaration, as well as resolution passed unanimously by World Health Assembly in May 1994. The strategies are:

1. Setting up a National Breastfeeding Committee.
2. Human Lactation Management Training (HLMT) and promotion of breastfeeding by supporting the concept of Baby Friendly Hospital Initiative (BFHI).
3. Extension of maternity leave and other support for a breastfeeding mother, and improving nutrition of pregnant and lactating women.
4. Enactment of Infant Milk Substitutes, Feeding Bottles and Infant Foods (Regulation of Production, Supply and Distribution) Act (1992).
5. Information, Education and Communication in support of breastfeeding.

The Department of Women and Child Development of the Government of India has set up a National Committee. A few state governments have also set up such committees.

THE INTERNATIONAL CODE OF MARKETING OF BREAST MILK SUBSTITUTES (1981)

Breast milk and breastfeeding need to be protected from formula promotion activities. This requires regulation of the promotion of sale of the formula. For this purpose, in 1981, the World Health Assembly adopted The International Code of Marketing of Breast Milk Substitutes, based on which every country should make its own specific rules.

Table 96.5: Main points of the international Code

1. No advertising of breast milk substitutes and other products to the public.
2. No free sample to mothers.
3. No promotion in the health service.
4. No company personnel to advise mothers.
5. No gifts or personal samples to health workers.
6. No pictures of infants or other pictures idealizing artificial feeding, on the labels of the products.
7. Information to health workers should be scientific and factual.
8. Information on artificial feeding, including that on labels, should explain the benefits of breastfeeding, and the costs and dangers associated with artificial feeding.
9. Unsuitable products, such as sweetened condensed milk, should not be promoted for babies.

INFANT MILK SUBSTITUTES, FEEDING BOTTLES AND INFANT FOODS (REGULATION OF PRODUCTION, SUPPLY AND DISTRIBUTION) ACT (1992)

Protection and promotion of breastfeeding needs special attention in India, so as to reduce mortality, morbidity and malnutrition among children. There has recently been an unprecedented fall in the number of breastfeeding mothers due to various reasons. Government of India has therefore actively promoted breastfeeding and is providing the necessary support for this, by passing a law entitled 'The Infant Milk Substitutes, Feeding Bottles and Infant Foods (Regulation of Production, Supply and Distribution) Act, 1992'. This law is based on the guidelines provided under The International Code of Marketing of Breast Milk Substitutes.

Table 96.6: Salient features of the infant milk substitutes, feeding bottles and infant foods (Regulation of Production, Supply and Distribution) Act, 1992

Promotion to public

- No person shall advertise any kind of infant milk substitute (IMS) or feeding bottles (FB).
- No person shall take part in the promotion of IMS, FB or infant foods (IF).
- No person shall give free samples or gifts of IMS or FB or gifts of utensil or other articles.
- No person shall offer inducement of any other kind for the purpose of promotion of sales of IMS or FB.
- No donation of IMS or FB to any person except to an orphanage.
- Not to use educational material on prenatal, postnatal care or infant feeding, for the purpose of promoting sale of IMS or FB.

Promotion to health care system

- No display of posters or placards on IMS, FB or IF in the hospitals.
- Information or education material relating to IMS and FB can only be distributed by medical practitioners and should have minimum prescribed information as per rules.
- No payment of any kind to a person working in health care system by any person producing, distributing or selling IMS, FB or IF.
- No direct or indirect financial inducements or gifts to health workers.

Company employees

- No commission to employees on the basis of sales volume by the producer, distributor, supplier or seller of IMS, FB or IF.

Labelling

- Containers of IMS, FB and IF or a label on it should carry certain information prescribed in the Act and Rules.
- No picture of an infant or woman is allowed on the label or tins of IMS.
- No use of words like 'humanised' or 'maternalised' on the label, container or advertisement of IMS.
- No use of words like 'recommended' or 'approved' by medical profession.
- No use of words like 'full protein', 'complete food' or 'energy food' on labels of IF.

Penalty

- Violation of the Act can lead to some fine and/or imprisonment up to 3 years.

BABY FRIENDLY HOSPITAL INITIATIVE (BFHI)

UNICEF and WHO launched BFHI as a part of the global effort to protect, promote and support breastfeeding. The word 'friendly' implies cordiality and warmth indicating an environment amenable to the baby. The global BFHI has listed ten steps, which the hospitals must fulfill to achieve the 'Baby Friendly' status. Hospitals should also keep this displayed for generating awareness among all concerned.

The BFHI was initiated in India with focus on the metropolitan cities initially and then spread to the whole country. The National Task Force comprising representatives from GOI, UNICEF, WHO, and professional bodies like IMA, IAPA, TNAI etc., with a secretariat located in IMA headquarters in New Delhi, provides the policy guidelines and technical support. Each state has a State Task Force, with representatives of all the agencies constituting the National Task Force. The 'Baby Friendly' hospitals in India are also expected to adopt and practice guidelines on other interventions critical for child survival including antenatal care, clean delivery practices, essential newborn care, immunization and oral rehydration therapy.

If a hospital wishes to invite assessment in order to be designated as 'Baby Friendly' by National Task Force (NTF) criteria, a complete self-assessment form provided by the NTF may be submitted. The assessment is conducted by an external team. If the health care facility meets the criteria, it receives a Baby Friendly Hospital designation and a plaque.

Table 96.7: Breastfeeding policy: Ten steps to successful breastfeeding

1. Have a written breastfeeding policy that is routinely communicated to all health care staff.
2. Train all health care staff with skills necessary to implement this policy.
3. Inform all pregnant women about the benefits of management of breastfeeding.
4. Help mothers initiate breastfeeding within half an hour of birth.
5. Show mothers how to breast feed, and how to maintain lactation even if they should be separated from their infants.
6. Give newborn infants no food or drink other than breast milk, unless medically indicated.
7. Practise rooming-in. Allow mothers and infants to remain together 24 hours a day.
8. Encourage breastfeeding on demand.
9. Give no artificial teats or pacifiers (also called dummies or soothers) to breastfeeding infants.
10. Foster the establishment of breastfeeding support groups and refer mothers to them on discharge from hospital or clinic.

FEEDING PRACTICE INDICATORS

To study feeding practices it is essential to have a common set of indicators. WHO has developed a common set of breastfeeding indicators, which are as follows:

1. Exclusive breastfeeding rate.
2. Predominant breastfeeding rate.
3. Timely complementary feeding rate.
4. Continued breastfeeding rate.
5. Bottle feeding rate.

Other indicators to monitor progress in connection with Baby Friendly Hospital Initiative

6. Breast milk substitutes and supplies receipt rate.
7. Rooming-in rate.
8. Timely first suckling rate.

BANKING OF HUMAN MILK

According to a joint statement of WHO and UNICEF "The best food for a baby who cannot be breastfed is milk expressed from the mother's breast or from another healthy mother....The best food for any baby whose own mother's milk is not available is the breast milk of another healthy mother". "Where it is not possible for the biological mother to breast feed, the first alternative, if available, should be the use of human milk from other sources. Human milk banks should be made available in appropriate situations." A human milk bank is "a service which collects, screens, processes, and dispenses by prescription human milk donated by nursing mothers who are not biologically related to the recipient infant".

Prior to the advent of commercial formulas, wet nursing was frequently the only way for an infant to survive. As wet nurses became harder to find, physicians interested in the survival of infants and children looked for other ways to provide human milk to sick children. Thus the concept of donor human milk banking was born. In the US the first donor milk bank was founded in Boston in 1911. During the late 1920s there were numerous donor milk banks in the USA. The American Academy of Pediatrics first published guidelines for milk-banking operations in 1943.

In India, the neonatology department of Lokmanya Tilak Municipal General Hospital (Mumbai) has established the one of its kind milk-bank in the country, which offers breast milk to around 25 babies daily. The milk bank was founded on November 27, 1989. Success of this unique concept in Mumbai, has encouraged other cities like Hyderabad and Vadodara to come up with their own milk-bank.

Two concerns are often raised by donors, milk recipients and health care providers regarding potential risks of using banked human milk:

1. Viruses, including HIV, have been shown to transmit through breast milk, for prevention of which breast milk donors should be screened very carefully.
2. Some of the worthwhile components of breast milk are compromised in the pasteurization process, but most are not. Though the enzymes in breast milk appear to be most affected by the heat, immune factors are less sensitive to heat and growth factors and fatty acids are stable at pasteurization temperatures. Therefore, safe processing should be done at lowest possible temperature.

CONCLUSION

Feeding is a critical aspect of caring for infants and young children. Breast milk is the ideal food for a human infant and is sufficient to meet his requirements for the first 6 months of life. Appropriate breastfeeding practices stimulate bonding with the mother and psycho-social development. It leads to improved nutrition and physical growth, reduced susceptibility to common childhood infections and better resistance to cope with them. Improved health outcomes in young children have long-lasting health effects throughout the life-span, including increased performance and productivity, and reduced risk of certain non-communicable diseases. However, this ideal practice is currently being threatened due to lack of awareness among mothers and also amongst the health providers. So every effort must be made to propagate the message among all concerned.

KEY LEARNING POINTS

- Educate and prepare the mother and the family for correct infant feeding during antenatal period.
- Initiate breastfeeding immediately after birth (on the labour table itself), and positively within half an hour after normal delivery and within four hours after cesarean section.
- Babies should be kept with the mother all the time.
- Give breast feeds on demand (i.e. whenever baby feels hungry) from both the breasts.
- The mother can feed the baby in any position she finds comfortable – lying down, sitting, reclining etc.
- The baby should be attached properly to the breast. The whole nipple and most of the areola should be in the baby's mouth. The head of the baby should also be at a slightly higher level than the rest of the body.
- The baby should be exclusively breast fed for the first 6 months, i.e. nothing other than breast milk, not even water, is to be given to the baby.
- Complementary feeding should be started at 6 months of age.
- Breastfeeding should be continued for as long as possible.

FURTHER READINGS

1. Anand RK. Feeding practices in infants and young children. In Anand RK, Kumta NB, Kushwaha KP, Gupta A (eds): *The Science of Infant Feeding*. New Delhi: Jaypee 2002: 3-20.
2. Banapurmath CR, Banapurmayh S, Kesaree N. Breastfeeding Problems. In: Anand RK, Kumta NB, Kushwaha KP, Gupta A (eds): *The Science of Infant Feeding*, New Delhi: Jaypee 2002: 138-154.
3. Bokare U, Dandge V, Meenakshi, Mujawar N, Vincent A, Dua H. Breastfeeding: Right policy, wrong target. Indian Progress in Reproductive and Child Health 2004. *Proceedings of 6th World NARCHI RCH Congress and XIV India Conference on Reproductive and Child Health,* New Delhi 2002.
4. Breast Feeding Management—Training of Trainers course Trainer's Manual. National Task Force, Baby Friendly Hospital Initiative, New Delhi.
5. CDC, "Human milk banks", www.cdc.gov/breastfeeding/compend-milkbanks.htm

6. Chetan R, Indira Bai K. Breastfeeding promotion: Practical guidelines. In Gupte S (ed): *Recent Advances in Pediatrics,* Special vol. Nutrition, Growth and Development: New Delhi: Jaypee 1993: 51-62.
7. Child growth and development available at http://www.who.int/nutrition/topics/childgrowth/en/index.html
8. Cornell experts help call for new international child-growth references By Susan Lang/Cornell Chronicle | | Cornell News Service Home Page |http://www.news.cornell.edu/Chronicle/97/8.21.97/child-growth.html
9. Fernandez A, Mondkar J, Nanavati R. The establishment of a human milk bank in India. *J Hum Lact* 1993; 9: 189-190.
10. Fernandez A, Mondkar J, Vaz C. Experiences with milk banking in Bombay. *Indian J Pediatr* 1990: 57:375-379.
11. Ghosh S. *Nutrition and Child Care—A Practical Guide*. New Delhi: Jaypee 1997.
12. Gupta A, Kushwaha KP, Sobti JC, Jindal T. Breastfeeding and complimentary feeding. In:*Guidelines for Doctors*. New Delhi: Breastfeeding Promotion Network of India 2000.
13. Gupte S, Anderson RA. Pediatric Gastroenterology. In Gupte S (ed): *The Short Textbook of Pediatrics*, 10th edn. New Delhi: Jaypee 2004: 365-402.
14. Gupte S, Gomez EM. Growth and Development. In Gupte S (ed): *The Short Textbook of Pediatrics,* 10th edn. New Delhi: Jaypee 2004: 30-54.
15. Gupte S, Gomez EM. Pediatric nutrition and nutritional deficiency states. In Gupte S (edn): *The Short Textbook of Pediatrics,* 10th edn. New Delhi: Jaypee Brothers 2004: 125-166.
16. Gupte S, Singh K. Pediatric Bacterial Infections. In Gupte S (ed): *The Short Textbook of Pediatrics,* 10th edn. New Delhi: Jaypee 2004: 197-221.
17. Gupte S. Infant Feeding. In Gupte S (ed): *The Short Textbook of Pediatrics*, 10th edn. New Delhi: Jaypee 2004; 113-124.
18. Heird WC: The feeding of infants and children. In Behrman RE, Kliegman RM, Jenson HB (eds): *Nelson Textbook of Pediatrics*, 17th edn Pennsylvania: Saunders 2004;157-166.
19. IAP Policy on Infant Feeding available at Http://www.Iapindia.Org/Policyinfant.Cfm
20. Jindal T, Chatterjee S. Anatomy and Physiology of Lactation. In Anand RK, Kumta NB, Kushwaha KP, Gupta A (eds): *The Science of Infant Feeding*. New Delhi: Jaypee 2002: 23-35.
21. Kulkarni ML. Breastfeeding and lactation management. In: *Manual of Neonatology*. New Delhi: Jaypee 2000: 188-221.
22. Kumta NB, Gupta S. The ecological aspects of infant feeding. In Anand RK, Kumta NB, Kushwaha KP, Gupta A (eds): *The Science of Infant Feeding*. New Delhi: Jaypee 2002: 48-58.
23. New News on Breast Feeding available at http://www.rehydrate.org/breastfeed/news.htm
24. Patnaik S, Sharma S, Sinha S, Roy K. Case study of a lactating grandmother. *Indian J Public Health* 1999; 43: 10, 25.
25. Sengupta P. Breastfeeding and working women. In Anand RK, Kumta NB, Kushwaha KP, Gupta A (eds): *The Science of Infant Feeding*. New Delhi: Jaypee 2002: 210-216.
26. Singh KC, Gupte S. Pediatric viral Infections. In: Gupte S (ed): *The Short Textbook of Pediatrics*, 10th edn. New Delhi: Jaypee 2004: 177-196.
27. Singh T, Gupte S. Community pediatrics. In Gupte S (ed): *The Short Textbook of Pediatrics*, 10th edn. New Delhi: Jaypee 2004: 71-96.
28. The WHO Child Growth Standards. World Health Organisation, Geneva. Available at http://www.who.int/childgrowth/standards/en/
29. United Nations Children's Fund (UNICEF), Facts for Life, New York, 2002 available at: http://www.unicef.org/ffl/text.htm
30. WHO Updates Outdated Pediatric Growth Charts available at http://www.medindia.net/news/view_news_main.
31. Wright, Nancy E. Donor human milk in preterm infants. *J Perinatology* 2001, 21:249-254.
32. World Health Organization releases New Child Growth Standards available at https://www.who.int/mediacentre/news/releases/2006/pr21/en/index.html
33. World Health Organization releases new Child Growth Standards available at http://www.who.int/mediacentre/news/releases/2006/pr21/en/index.html
34. World Health Organization Releases New Child Growth Standards. WHO Child Growth Standards. Available at http://www.who.inthttp://www.medicalnewstoday.com/medicalnews.

97 Complementary Feeding

Suraj Gupte

INTRODUCTION

The now obsolete term *weaning* means "to be taken off the breasts" or "introduction of foods other than breast milk". The latter meaning is more relevant in infant nutrition. Though in vogue for several decades, the "weaning" is an inappropriate terminology. The better terminology is *complementary feeding*.

DEFINITION

By current definition, complementary feeding means introduction of nutritious foods over and above breastfeeding. These energy-dense foods should be cost-effective, affordable, easily available and well-tolerated.

RECOMMENDED AGE

Six months is the most appropriate time for introducing complementary feeding. *The whole process should be gradually completed by 9 months to 1 year of age* when the child should be taking almost the adult diet.

Whereas delayed introduction of complimentary foods is known to cause malnutrition and growth retardation, premature introduction of such foods exposes to the risk of infections and the resultant morbidity and mortality.

Besides infections, too early introduction of complimentary feeds, including cow milk, or buffalo milk has other problems (Table 97.1) and is not recommended except under special circumstances such as when the mother is not able to produce sufficient milk despite the best of efforts.

Table 97.1: Problems associated with too early initiation of complementary feeds

Short-term
- Decreased suckling frequency and intensity, leading to decreased milk production.
- Iron deficiency unless cereal preparations used are rich in iron.
- Hypernatremia
- Weaning diarrhea

Contd.

Contd.

Long-term
- Malnutrition in the poor
- Obesity in the affluent
- Hypertension
- Arteriosclerosis

ATTRIBUTES OF AN IDEAL COMPLEMENTARY FOOD

Home-made
Indigenous
Hygienic
Fresh
Calorie dense.

TYPES OF COMPLEMENTARY FOODS

The complementary foods can be divided into different groups (3 "A"s) based on their availability and nutritional advantages (Box 97.1)

Box 97.1: Types of Complementary Foods

Appropriate (First Line) Weaning Food

These includes fresh home-made, locally available, culturally acceptable, hygienically prepared, energy dense and cost-effective foods like:

a. Combination of cereals and pulses (khichadi, dal-rice etc.), porridge, suji, dalia, kheer, khaman, dhokla, idli, dosa, ragi, rice preparations etc. in any form fortified with sugar and oil or fried.
b. Mashed banana, sweet potato and potato.
c. Milk added to cereals preparations.
d. Sprouted legumes, nuts, dry fruits etc. depending upon the affordability.

Acceptable (Second Line) Weaning Foods

These include home available foods like (a) breads, cakes, pastry, biscuits, cheese, ice cream etc. (b) caloric dense fruits etc.

Avoidable (Third Line) Weaning Foods

a. Commercially available artificial foods or tinned foods.
b. Fast food or junk food.
c. Low caloric fruits juices, soups.
d. Repeatedly fried foods containing trans fatty acids (which predispose to obesity, atherosclerosis, cardiac and neurological problems in future life).

SCHEDULE FOR COMPLEMENTARY FEEDING

It is initiated in the form of some liquids like fruit juices and soups and semisolid and solids like gruel, biscuits and mashed fruits and vegetables. Remember, grape juice is preferable to other juices since it is low in sorbitol and fructose/glucose ratio, a potential cause of carbohydrate malabsorption (often without clinical symptoms).

To begin, with one of the foods like a cereal, mashed ripe banana, mashed potato, curd, pulses, *khichri*, etc. should be introduced when the child is about 4 to 6 months of age. The food should be given in small amounts which can be built up slowly. Every 1 or 2 weeks, a new food may be added. If the child does not like a particular food, this may be omitted.

Germinated cereal flour or pulse flour is an amylase-rich food (ARF) and is able to dramatically reduce the viscosity of high dietary porridges. It makes an excellent weaning food.

Fish, egg, meat, etc. should be introduced later, in view of the possible risk of allergy to proteins. In case of egg, begin with the "yolk".

Box 97.2: Age-related guidelines for complementary feeding

6-9 months

- Start with cereal-based porridge that is enriched with oil or mashed fruit.
- Start with small amounts and gradually go up on increasing the amount and frequency so that by 9 months he is taking around ½ cup of foodstuff daily.

Contd.

Contd.

- Eventually, he should be taking his share from the family food i.e. rice, pulses, khichri, fish, egg, meat, chapatti (softened), fruits, vegetables, as 4 to 5 meals a day.

9 - 12 months

- Give a variety of soft foods (chopped/pounded) rather than mashed foods (since the child can chew now) out of the family/household foods with increasing amount of serving.
- Give swerving 4 to 5 times daily.

KEY LEARNING POINTS

- Strictly speaking, it denotes introduction of nutritious foods over and above the breastfeeding.
- Complementary foods should be fresh, hygienic, energy-dense, cost-effective, easily-available, affordable, and well-tolerated.
- Six months is the most appropriate time for starting complemnary feeding; it should be gradually completed by 9 months to 1 year of age when child should be taking almost the adult diet.
- Amylase-rich foods (ARFs) reduce the viscosity of high dietary porridges, making excellent complementary foods.
- Fish, egg white and meat should be introduced later.

FURTHER READINGS

1. Brown KH, Sharma S. Editorial: Complementary feeding of infants and young children. *Indian Pediatrics* 1999;36:547-550.
2. Ghosh S. *Nutrition and Child Care*. New Delhi: Jaypee 1997.
3. Gupte S, EM Gomez. Infant feeding. In: Gupte S (ed): *The Short Textbook of Pediatrics,* 11th edn. New Delhi: Jaypee 2008.

98 Amylase-Rich Foods

Meenakshi N Mehta • Romeen Lalvani • Nitin J Mehta

INTRODUCTION

Germination and fermentation are two widely-used traditional technologies in Asia and Africa which hold great promise to improve young child nutrition. The addition of a small quantity of germinated cereal flour, rich in alpha-amylase is able to dramatically reduce the viscosity of high dietary bulk porridges, thereby making it easy for an infant toddler to consume. Germination of a variety of pulses, especially mung (beans sprouts) is widely practised in S-E Asia and of a variety of pulses and to a lesser degree wheat, in India. "Kimea" (germinated sorghum flour) is routinely used in brewing beer in Africa and has been promoted in East Africa for reducing the viscosity of additional sorghum gruels. Nonalcoholic fermentation and souring of cereal porridges by lactic acid producing bacteria is widely practised in Africa and is traditionally used as a weaning food. Advantages of sour porridge are that it enhances bioavailability of proteins/vitamins/minerals the low pH makes it resistant to pathogenic bacterial contamination and is palatable.

The autofermentation which occurs when cereal or pulse flours are steeped in water overnight reduces the viscosity of the subsequently cooked gruel to some extent. Fermented batters subsequently steamed (*Idli, Dhokla*) or fried (*Dosa*) are household food processing technologies in India. Another fermentation technology most popular and widely practised in India is the preparation *Dahi* (curd, yoghurt). The therapeutic properties of yoghurt and butter milk are well appreciated and these products are used for feeding of young children on a daily basis and particularly when they suffer from diarrhea and fever. The fermented food such as tempech, Tofu of SE Asia are some well-known home foods that are relished by young weaning age children of that region and should be promoted for these children by that specific community and culture for their enhanced nutritional and health properties.

CONCEPT OF AMYLASE-RICH FOOD

Alpha amylase is the liquefying enzyme that breaks down long chain carbohydrates present in all cereals into shorter chain dextrins. Hence, any food abundantly rich in alpha-amylase ought to reduce the viscosity or 'dietary bulk' of a traditional gruel. Germinated cereal flours are extermely rich in alpha-amylase and in catalytic amounts are able to thin cooked (70°C) paste cereal flour slurries (upto even 30% solid concentration) instantly. Amylase-rich foods can also liquify cooked slurries made from habitual diet of cereal/pulse or os soya-fortified-bulgar etc. Preparation of the ARF consists of steeping the grains overnight, germinating for 48 to 96 hours, sundrying for 5 to 8 hours, toasting on a flat skillet, devegetating, and milling the grains. ARF preparation from as little as 100 to 200 g of any cereal grain for a cost of 20 to 40p (fraction of one US cent) would be sufficient to thin one child's gruel daily for one whole month. ARF can be prepared from germinated pulses also (mung, chickpea, cowpea, soyabean etc.) but would have substantially less amylotytic power.

Among wheat, sorghum, maize or other millets, wheat was found to have the shortest germination period (48 hours) and had the highest amlyase activity (4500 maltose units/g ARF). A 20 g percent cooked paste gruel of any cereal powder would require hardly 1 g wheat ARF for its thinning. As far as possible it is best to avoid germinated sorghum which elaborates dangerous levels of hydrocyanic acid (HCN). Moisture in the ARF can destroy the enzyme. Hence the ARF must be rendered bone dry and should be stored in a cool dry place.

Germination is biochemically a rather straight-forward process in which amylase hydrolyses starch, producing several effects. Firstly, the viscosity is reduced. This is important if efforts to decrease dietary intake are to be successful. An average gruel contains 10 percent of solid or less by weight. It is estimated that the infant can only take 200 to 300 ml per meal. Considering this, an infant can comfortably take about 600 to 900 ml per day, if fed three times a day. This would thus provide 60 to 90 g solids per day. Any cereal when taken in this quantity would give about 240 to 360 kcal which is less than even one third the daily requirements of an infant. The hypothesis is that ARF is able to reduce viscosity and bulk so that greater volume of food is eaten. The benefits are via effects on swallowing, especially during illness. Gastric emptying time may be reduced, thereby increasing the number of feeds. In addition, there may be reduction in the phytic acid content of cereal foods such as minerals including iron.

GERMINATION—THE STATE OF THE ART

Germination of cereals is a household technology, common in Asia and Africa, often for making local beer. The technology has been described and scientifically evaluated and germinated flour termed "power flour" used to reduce dietary bulk and raise nutrient density of weaning foods.

Which Cereal to Germinate?

Various cereals like wheat, sorghum, maize and pearl millet can be used. Wheat was found to have the shortest germination period, i.e. 48 hours and had the highest amylase activity, i.e. 4500 maltose units/g ARF. Germination periods of other cereals are; sorghum – 72 hours, pearl millet–72 hours, maize – 96 hours. A potential problem with sorghum is the high cyanide content of certain strains.

Food Intake

Food intake by young children is dependent on many factors, including the state of the child's health, number of meals (feeding frequency) per day and consistency of food.

During the crucial weaning age between 12 to 24 months, viscosity of the food is crucial as the child cannot easily eat stiff food. Reduction of dietary bulk using 'power flour' therefore has a useful application here to raise nutrient intake.

Positive Effects of Germination on Nutrient Content

Significant increments occur in thiamine (20%), riboflavin (175%), niacin (30%) and pantothenic acid (190%). Lysine, the most limiting amino acid increases significantly in sorghum averaging 10 percent. Antinutritional factors such as tannin decrease significantly (40%) while phytic acid decreases marginally.

Nutrient Availability In Vitro

Protein digestibility is variety dependent and increased by an average of 20 percent during germination. Ionizable iron increases significantly by 100 percent. In vivo, rat bioassay showed increased protein digestability in germinated high tannin sorghm of 26 percent. Increment in iorn availability also occurred 2 to 6 times compared to undergerminated white sorghum when germination was followed by 2 to 3 days autofermentation.

Cost

If one takes 100 g whole cereal grain to make ARF powder, this small amount will cost about 0.8 to 1.5 rupees (e.g. 1 kg wheat costs approximately 8 to 15 rupees). This amount will suffice for one child's gruel for one month.

Storage

ARFs have a shelf-life of a year when stored in well stoppered bottles at ambient temperatures (35 to 42°C) and fairly high relative humidity.

How to use ARF?

In African regions, high nutrient weaning foods with low bulk are prepared by thinning with 'power flour', then reheated to pasteurise it or the ingredients are mixed, made to stand overnight, then cooked and the children fed.

Alternatively, the dry method developed in India could be used. Here the cereal is germinated, dried or roasted and ground into flour which can then by prepared into porridge and rich supplements such as groundnut flour, pulse flour or milk added. This approach has the advantage that a large amount of flour can be prepared and used over a time within adequate shelf-life. It reduces the work-load and the frequency of having to go through the germination, drying and milling proceeses. It also provides the chance to exercise good quality control for a good and safe product, though storage might pose a problem.

Technological Considerations

- In a cereal-based weaning food, starch is the cheapest source of calorie.
- Higher levels of solids in weaning formula can increase energy density (so that a smaller volume of intake can satisfy the energy need of infants).
- But higher solid levels also build up viscosity of food (resulting in thick gruel, difficult to swallow in large amounts by the child).
- Reducing viscosity of weaning foods:
  - Results in an increased intake, i.e. the infant 'drinks' more formula.
  - Reduces dietary bulk, i.e. the formula can have a higher solids level without viscosity build up.
- Viscosity reduction is achieved by the liquefying action of alpha-amylase: large starch molecules are attacked at several places, randomly breaking them down (many smaller polymers). The most immediate effect is observed in reduction of viscosity.
- Requirements for viscosity reduction by alpha-amylase activity are:

1. A substrate, weaning food mixture.
2. A source of alpha-amylase enzyme.
3. A suitable set of conditions for enzyme action:

i. Constituting a slurry of weaning food mix in water.
ii. Heating the slurry to promote GELATINIZATION of starch.
iii. Maintenance of temperature (50 to 70 °C) and agitation of viscous mass containing enzyme to promote THINNING.

Enzyme activity is most effective on gelatinized starch.

Option 1:

Enzyme can be added after slurry has been gelatinized into a viscous mass.

Option 2:

Enzyme can also be present (added) in pregelatinized slurry, if desired viscosity reduction can be achieved during the course of heating and cooling the slurry.

The principle of viscosity reduction by alpha-amylase can be used in several processing options. The choice of a particular option depends on the scale of operation, and the extent of processing applied to the weaning food.

Constraints

Despite extensive promotion, difficulties have been encountered in using the amylase-rich flour correctly, possibly because it has been specifically promoted as a "power flour", giving rise to the mistaken perception that the amylase-rich flour itself is the energy source.

The concept of making a thick porridge and then thinning it may be difficult and puzzling for those who traditionally make their porridge thin.

Concern has also been expressed about the safety of amylase-rich flours with regard to the risk of aflatoxin contamination and, for sorghum, the risk of cyanide poisoning.

Advantages

The advantage of ARF are:

- Cheap cost.
- Widely known and practised household technology.
- Small amounts to be made only intermittently; and
- Adaptability of making at the household, the community level or even at the scaled-up commercial level. The single and unique contribution of ARF is that it can permit the mother to mix in much more flour into the gruel and consequently make it high in energy density, yet low in viscosity and dietary bulk.

PREPARATION OF WHEAT ARF

Although various cereals wheat, sorghum maize and pearl millet can be used, wheat selected is known to have the shortest germination period, i.e. 48 hours and has the highest amylase activity, i.e. 45 maltose units/g ARF. Several varieties of wheat were tried for germination of which 'Lokwan' variety of wheat yielded best germination and hence 'Lokwan' variety of wheat was used for the preparation of ARF at the LTMG Hospital, Mumbai.

Following steps are involved in preparation of wheat ARF:

Preparation of ARF begins with the germination of wheat, which forms part and parcel of the Culinary culture of Asia. For its use as a viscosity reducer of infant foods, additional care is required to ensure sanitation and safety. ARF production starts with the selection of grains with good germination quality and ends with an appropriate storage of the powder of dried grains for an extended shelf-life.

Major steps:

1. *Selection of grains*
   - Select whole, unbroken grains free from infestation.
   - Broken grains do not germinate well.
   - Pick out the debris from the grains and wash.
2. *Steeping*
   About 100 g of wheat is steeped overnight in 2 to 3 times its volume of water.
   Precautions: Water level should be sufficient to cover the swelling grains during steeping. Steeping for too long hampers germination.
3. *Germination*
   - Drain excess water.
   - Wrap it in a clean wet cloth.
   - Cover it by inverting with a utensil and ensure a cool, dark place.
   - Sprinkle water every 6 to 8 hours to keep the cloth moist.
   - Open after 48 hours. Most of the wheat will have sprouted by then.
4. *Drying and milling*
   This is done in two stages:
   a. Preliminary drying:
   Dry in the sun/air for 1 to 2 hours with occasional stirring.
   b. Final drying:
      - Can be either sun drying in bright sunshine for 6 hours or light roasting on a low flame using a thick bottomed *kadhai.*
      - Alternatively, roasting can be carried out on a mud *'tava'.*
5. *Devegetating*
   Manually remove roots and shoots on a sieve.
6. *Milling*
   The germinated, dried-toasted, devegetated wheat is now milled either by hand pounding or in an electric grinder. The ARF powder is now ready.
7. *Storing*
   Fill in polythene bags, keep the polythene bag in a wide mouthed screw cap bottle.

8. *How to use ARF with gruel/porridge*
   - Heat the gruel.
   - Take pan off the fire.
   - Add ARF.
   - Stir well for 10 min for ARF to act.
   - Bring the contents to boil on the fire.
   - Cool to serve.
   - Alternatively, ARF can also be added as the boiled gruel is cooled.

KEY LEARNING POINTS

- ARF should be used in child nutrition in health for the weaning foods as well as during sickness, i.e. for the dietary management of malnutrition and diarrhea.
- ARF is cheap, easy to prepare and store.
- ARF can be used even by mothers from the lower socioeconomic strata, where malnutrition poses a major problem.

FURTHER READINGS

1. Gopaldas T, Mehta P, Patil A, Gandhi H. Studies on viscosity of thick gruels with small quantities of an Amylase Rich Cereal Malt. *Food Nutr Bull* 1986;8:42-47.
2. Gopaldas T, Mehta P, John C. Bulk reduction of traditional Indian Weaning Gruels. *In:* Alnwick D, Moses S, Schimdt OG (eds). *Improving Young Child Feeding in Eastern and Southern Africa: Household Level Food Technology.* Ottawa: IDRC 1987:330-339.
3. Gopaldas T. Concept of amylase-rich food (ARF) and its role:Infant feeding and growth. In: Gopaldas T, Deshpande S (eds). *The Miracle of Germinated Cereal Grain Powders.* Proceeding International Workshop/ Publication Department of Food and Nutrition, MS University, Baroda/ International Development Research Centre, Canada. Baroda: Daya Publishing House 1992:29-34.
4. Gopaldas T. Technolgies to improve weaning foods in developing countries *Indian Pediatr* 1991:28:217-221.
5. Gopaldas T, John C. Evaluation of a controlled 6 months feeding trial on intake by infants and toddlers fed a high energy-low bulk gruel versus a high energy high bylk gruel in addition to their habital home diet. *J Trop Pedatr* 1992; 38: 278-283.
6. Marquis GS, Lopez T, Peerson JM, Brown KH. Effect of dietary viscosity on energy intake by breastfed and non-breastfed children during and after acute diarrhea. *Am J Clin Nutr* 1993;57;218-223.
7. Mehta MN. Dietary management of protein-energy malnutrition and diarrhea. *Bulletin Subspeciality Chapter on Nutrition, Indian Academy of Pediatrics* 1995; 3:2-8.

99 Protein-Energy Malnutrition

Suraj Gupte • EM Gomez • EE Gomez

INTRODUCTION

Today, nutritional deficiencies constitute a major public health problem in India and other developing countries. Not all cases of PEM are from primary dietary deficiency. Many are secondary to deficiency states resulting from other diseases such as tuberculosis, severe malabsorption or metabolic illnesses.

The incidence of severe forms, *kwashiorkor* and *marasmus*, as also low birthweight infants (LBW) has gradually fallen though only to an unsatisfactory level Nevertheless, mild to moderate malnutrition which eventually ends up in stunted growth continues to exist in around 60% of the pediatric population. These substandard survivors are likely to suffer from consequences as poor quality of life, low cognitive development and learning skills on top of other handicaps continues to exist in around 50 percent of the pediatric population. Considerable morbidity (and, at times mortality) accompanies nutritional anemias and other micronutrient and vitamin deficiencies that invariable accompany the clinical spectrum of PEM, directly or indirectly.

PROTEIN-ENERGY MALNUTRITION (PEM): A SPECTRUM

The term, protein-energy malnutrition, refers to a class of clinical conditions that may result from varying degree of protein lack and energy (calorie) inadequacy. This nomenclature replaces the relatively older designation, i.e. protein-calorie malnutrition, on the recommendation of the World Health Organization (WHO) and Food and Agriculture Organization (FAO).

The term has been adopted because it is now widely agreed that the major limiting factors in the diet of children, particularly in the countries of the Third World, are energy and proteins, usually more of the former. Deficiency of proteins is usually not primary and isolated. Almost always it appears to be due to poor intake of food (energy) as such. There is evidence that if child's energy is taken care of, it will be difficult for him to have significant protein deficiency. Else, if his energy consumption is poor, whatever proteins he takes are likely to be consumed to provide energy rather than to build the tissues.

Among the various factors that influence the clinical manifestations of protein-energy malnutrition (PEM) figure magnitude of deprivation, its duration, relative inadequacy of different principles of food and the accompanying infection or some other disease.

Broadly speaking, two major clinical syndromes, *kwashiorkor* and *nutritional marasmus*, are widely recognized. Kwashiorkor is said to result from gross deficiency of proteins though energy deficiency is also present. Nutritional marasmus, on the other hand, results from gross deficiency of energy though protein deficiency also accompanies. Thus, it is clear that there is deficiency of both, proteins and energy, in both the states. The predominance of the deficiency determines whether it is going to be kwashiorkor or nutritional marasmus.

Many malnourished children show overlap in the clinical picture, demonstrating features of both the deficiency states at a time. It is often quite appropriate to label them as *marasmic-kwashiorkor*.

But, the aforesaid severe form of PEM constitute only a tip of the widespread problem of malnutrition. A vast majority of the children suffering from mild to moderate forms of it remain hidden in the community for one or another reason. The two types of this subclinical malnutrition are: nutritional dwarfing (stunting) and prekwashiorkor.

All these form of PEM, in actuality, constitute a continuous spectrum of the manifestations of malnutrition. Growth failure and poor tissue repair (due to protein lack) and energy shortage (due to calorie deficiency) are common to all the forms.

ETIOLOGY OF PEM

A multitude of factors, often in nexus, contribute to development of PEM (Fig. 99.1).

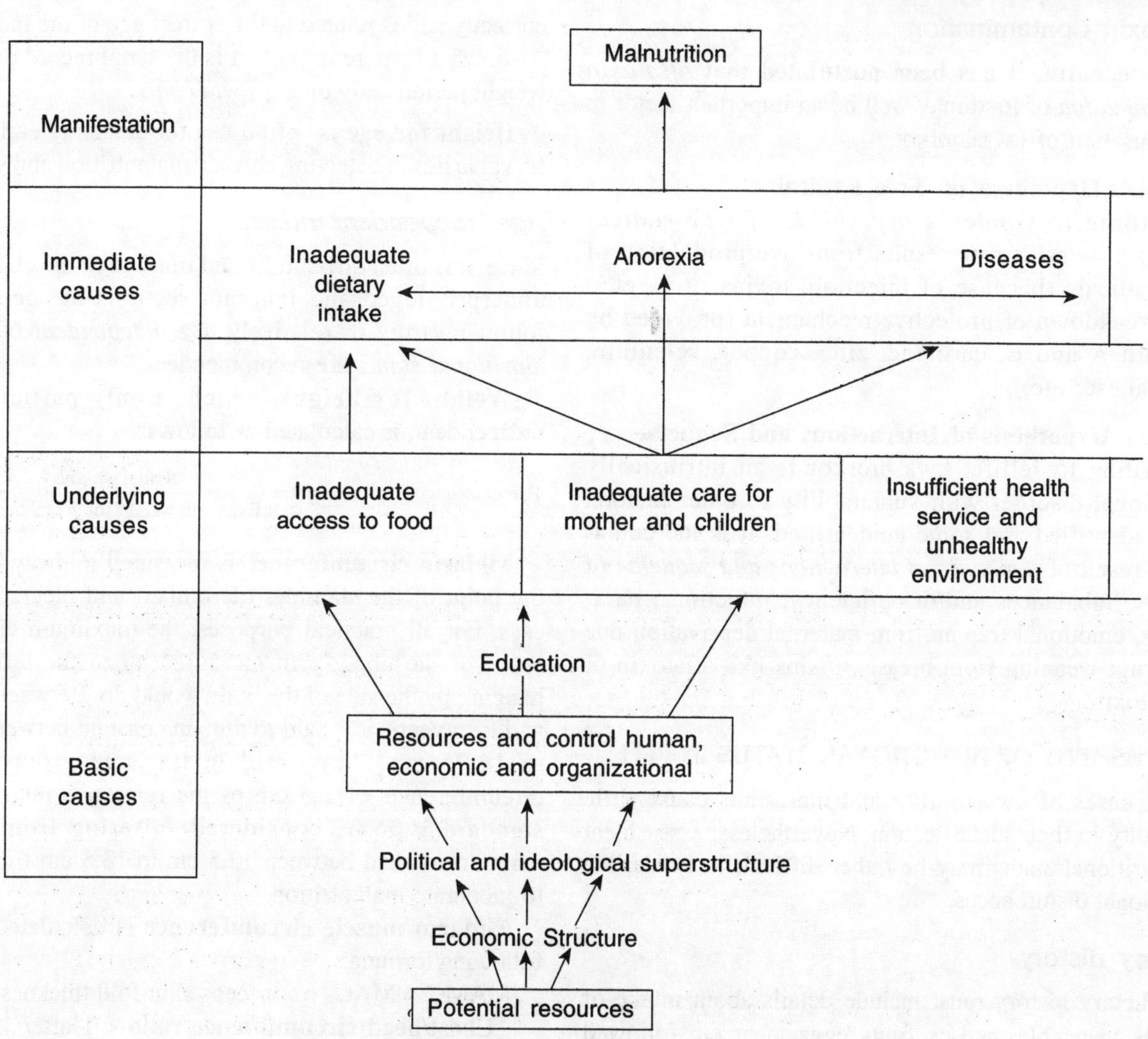

Fig. 99.1: Etiology of PEM in nutshell

EVOLUTION OF PEM (Fig. 99.1)

Why does one child develop marasmus while the other kwashiorkor under similar conditions? The answer to this oft-asked question remains elusive. The available hypotheses are briefly described here.

Dietary Hypothesis

According to the widely-accepted *dietetic hypothesis*. Kwashiorkor is predominantly a protein deficiency and marasmus an energy deficiency. Of course, both proteins and energy lack-exist in both the syndromes. This hypothesis has a good deal of support from studies in the laboratory animals as well as work on human beings.

Adaptation Hypothesis

The noted nutritionist, Gopalan, has claimed that dietary background of children suffering from kwashiorkor and marasmus may well be the same. According to his postulation, the so-called *adaptation hypothesis*, marasmus is an extreme degree of adaptation to prolonged inadequacy of proteins and energy in the diet. Kwashiorkor is a stage of adaptation failure or dysadaptation which may follow two situations. First: Continued prolongation of the stress of malnutrition. Second: Sudden precipitation or aggravation by a fulminant infection such as measles, pertussis, bronchopneumonia or acute diarrheal episode.

Gopalan feels that whereas nutritional marasmus may be the result of extreme degree of adaptation and the kwashiorkor the result of dysadaptation, relatively mild effect of adaptation may be responsible for nutritional dwarfing. Since, according to Gopalan's hypothesis, kwashiorkor follows occurrence of dysadaptation in a marasmic child, most of the cases are likely to show features of both, i.e. marasmic kwashiorkor.

Aflatoxin Contamination

More recently, it has been postulated that *aflatoxin contamination* of food may well be an important factor in the causation of kwashiorkor.

Golden's Hypothesis of Free Radicals

According to Golden's *hypothesis of free radical damage*, kwashiorkor results from overproduction of free radicals (because of infection, toxins, iron, etc.) and breakdown of protective mechanism (provided by vitamin A and E, carotene, zinc, copper, selenium, manganese, etc.).

Jellife's Hypothesis of Interactions and Sequelae

According to Jellife, kwashiorkor is an intrinsically nutritional disorder with vulnerability to other factors, some identified and some unidentified. It is the cumulative result of a *mixture of interactions and sequelae* of dietary imbalances and/or deficiency, infections, parasitosis, emotional trauma from maternal deprivation due to abrupt weaning from breasts, toxins like aflatoxin or ochratoxin.

ASSESSMENT OF NUTRITIONAL STATUS IN PEM

Frank cases of kwashiorkor and marasmus cause little difficulty in their identification. Nevertheless, assessment of nutritional status may be rather difficult in borderline nutritional disturbances.

Dietary History

The dietary history must include details about intake of cereals, vegetables, pulses, fruits, eggs, meat, etc. followed by calculations to obtain average daily consumption of proteins and calories. A rough idea about the adequacy of vitamins and minerals in the diet should also be formed.

Clinical Signs

Deficiency signs such as hair changes, anemia, xerosis, cheilosis, angular stomatitis, rachitic rosary, bleeding spongy gums, dental caries, etc. should be actively looked for.

The observations on the deficiency signs should, however, be interpreted very cautiously. As for instance, phrynoderma (toad skin), though traditionally thought to be due to vitamin A deficiency, may also be a feature of scurvy and deficiency of linoleic acid.

Anthropometry

Anthropometry is a very valuable index for evaluation of nutritional status.

Age-Dependent Indices

Weight for age is by far the simplest, the most widely used and the most reliable index, provided that it is recorded correctly and is related to the correct age of the individual. Also, what is more important is the serial record of child's weight periodically on a *growth chart*.

Height for age is of no use for detecting early PEM. Its value lies in detecting chronic malnutrition and stunting.

Age-Independent Indices

Since, it is often difficult to find true age of the child in the underprivileged and ignorant sections of society, the following truly or relatively *age-independent indices of nutritional status* are recommended.

Weight for height, which is only partially age-independent, is calculated as follows:

$$\text{Percentage weight for height} = \frac{\text{Actual weight}}{\text{Expected weight for actual height}} \times 100$$

Midarm circumference is measured midway between the point of the shoulder (acromian) and olecranon process. For all practical purposes, the maximum circumference of the upper arm measured when the left arm is hanging by the side of the body would do. Between second and fifth years, it is said to remain constant between 16.25 to 16.75 cm. Any child in this age group with a circumference < 12.5 cm of the reference international standard is to be considered suffering from severe malnutrition and between 12.5 cm to 13.5 cm from mild-to-moderate malnutrition.

Midarm muscle circumference is calculated by the following formula:

MAMC = MAC- p × triceps skin-fold thickness.

Chest/head circumference ratio < 1 after 1-2 years points to PEM.

Triceps skin-fold thickness is measured by a standard caliper (Lange, Herpenden or Best). Tanner chart gives the normal values at different ages. On an average it exceeds 10 mm in 1 to 6 years age group. A measurement between 6 to 10 mm points to mild-moderate malnutrition and under 6 mm severe malnutrition.

Mid-upper-arm/height ratio of less than 0.29 indicates gross malnutrition, the normal being 0.32 to 0.33.

Quac-stick method is a simple, easy, inexpensive and yet reliable method of detecting early malnutrition of acute onset. Quac-stick is an abbreviation of Quacker arm circumference measuring stick. The instrument consists of a stick graduated with figures for midarm circumference in relation to height. For this test, maximum left arm circumference (the arm hanging by the side of the body) is recorded. Then, the child is made to stand in front of the Quac-stick. From the graduations in the stick, his nutritional status in terms of 50, 60, 70 or 80% of the standard can be easily read.

Shakir tape method is a simple and age-independent tool for assessing malnutrition. This special tape has colored zones: red, yellow and green, corresponding to less than 12.5 cm (wasted), 12.5 to 13.5 cm (borderline) and over 13.5 cm (normal) midarm circumference.

Bangle method, another method not needing age and useful in preschool children, consists in slipping a bangle with a diameter of 4 cm up the forearm. An attempt is made to move it over to the upper arm. In case it can slip over the elbow, malnutrition is present. The method, though simple and easy, is not quite reliable.

Quetlet index based on relationship between weight and height is expressed as weight (kg) ×100/height $(cm)^2$. Normal value varies between 0.14 to 0.16. In gross malnutrition, it is less than 0.14. It is quite reliable. It is similar to BMI, except that here we take height in centimeters rather than meters.

Dugdale index too is based on relationship between weight and height. It is expressed as:

$$\frac{\text{Weight (kg)}}{\text{Height (cm)}} \times 1.6$$

Normal value varies between 0.88 to 0.97. An index of less than 0.79 suggests malnutrition.

***Rao's weight/height ratio* is expressed as:**

$$\frac{\text{Weight (kg)}}{\text{Height}^2\text{ (cm)}} \times 100$$

Normal value is above 0.15.

Investigations

Laboratory investigations include hemoglobin, serum proteins, blood levels of nutrients like vitamins, iron, etc. and amino acid level in blood and urine.

The real value of biochemical tests is to detect subclinical malnutrition that could not be revealed by anthropometry. How far these tests are of concrete value in practice remains to be convincingly substantiated.

Radiology may reveal some retardation of bone age, osteoporosis or classical signs of scurvy or rickets. Some workers have described transverse lines of arrested growth at the growing ends of long bones months prior to onset of frank PEM.

Associated Disorders

While assessing the nutritional status, one must look for signs pertaining to malabsorption, intestinal parasitic infestations, tuberculosis, etc.

Vital Statistics

For evaluation of the nutritional status of a community, the above measures should be supported by vital statistics such as infant mortality, neonatal mortality, perinatal mortality, stillbirth rate, 1 to 4 years mortality and life expectancy as also the ecological background.

EFFECTS OF PEM ON OTHER SYSTEMS/DISEASE ENTITIES

1. PEM and Disturbances of Metabolism

PEM is characterized by profound disturbances of water and electrolytes, minerals, protein, fat, carbohydrate and energy metabolism and, hence, rightly designated as a "metabolic disorder".

Water, Electrolytes and Minerals

Total body water: Total body water is increased in PEM, irrespective whether it is of kwashiorkor or marasmic type. A positive correlation exists between the magnitude of rise in body water and the extent of weight loss. Thus, lowest values are found in kwashiorkor and the highest in marasmus.

Whether the alteration is secondary to increased cellular mass which constitutes the active protoplasm of the body and reduction in the adipose tissue is not clearly understood.

A noteworthy point is that despite increased body water, a malnourished child is thirsty. This paradoxical observation is ascribed to the defective thirst mechanism in PEM.

Potassium: There is a definite reduction in the total body potassium by as much as 25%. Though all organs are depleted of potassium, the musculature suffers the most followed by the brain. Potassium depletion is more marked in cases of PEM with diarrheal disease. In kwashiorkor, it is significant even in the absence of diarrhea. Whether potassium depletion results from gastrointestinal losses through the gut or from defects in specific enzymes (that have a role in carbohydrate metabolism), or both, is not clear. Potassium deficiency may be existing despite absence of any clinical manifestations of dehydration and/or hypokalemia.

A very high frequency of pyelonephritis and acute renal failure is encountered in cases of severe malnutrition whose potassium depletion has not been attended to. Of course, the contributory role of concomitant dehydration and infection cannot be denied.

Sodium: Unlike potassium depletion, sodium is retained by the body. Sodium retention is primarily extracellular though muscle, skin, brain and viscera, too, are affected.

Intracellular sodium retention and potassium deficit may change the function of important enzymes in carbohydrate metabolism and oxidative phosphorylation.

Magnesium: Magnesium depletion in PEM is now well established. This deficiency may cause grave disturbances, including neurologic signs such as twitching, tremors and convulsions.

Phosphorus: Both forms of phosphorus (organic as well as inorganic) are decreased in the muscles of malnourished children. Adequate nutritional correction leads to increase in both the forms. The exact significance of this observation, particularly from a clinical angle, remains obscure.

Calcium: Calcium depletion is a common feature of PEM, more so when the assessment is based on blood levels. However, clinical evidence of tetany is infrequent.

Iron: Iron deficiency anemia is a common feature of PEM. It is, however, complicated by other deficiencies involving folic acid, vitamin B_{12} vitamin E and probably some other vitamins.

Copper: Low levels of copper in serum, hair and liver of subjects suffering from PEM have been documented. There may also be low levels of ceruloplasmin which plays the role of a "link" in copper and iron metabolism.

Chromium: Chromium deficiency has been blamed for the impaired glucose tolerance in malnourished children. There is evidence that it may contribute to poor growth of the child during the earlier stage of nutritional rehabilitation. Chromium therapy may accelerate growth in marasmic infants.

Zinc: Low serum as well as muscle and liver zinc values exist in PEM. Zinc deficiency may play an important role in the etiology of the *syndrome of growth retardation with short stature, hypogonadism, hepatosplenomegaly and anemia* in boys. The supplementation of zinc to such boys results in a dramatic improvement. Some time, within three weeks of initiating treatment, significant gain in weight and acceleration of sexual maturity are achieved. Zinc deficiency is also associated with infantile tremor syndrome and diarrheal disease.

Protein and Amino Acids

Total serum protein level is always reduced, principally due to hypoalbuminemia which is remarkable in kwashiorkor. The level of beta-globulins is also reduced. Alpha and gamma-globulin level is variable in absolute terms; it is invariably high in relation to other serum protein fractions.

There is a remarkable reduction in the total body protein. Its turnover, unlike that of albumin, may be high rather than low.

Significant reduction in plasma amino acids occurs in kwashiorkor. Valine, leucine, isoleucine and tyrosine are the ones most affected. There is a rise in amino acid recycling in kwashiorkor. This mechanism, together with low urea synthesis, increased ammonia and urea nitrogen utilization for protein synthesis, contributes to increased nitrogen economy in protein deficiency.

Lipids

There is a reduction in fat absorption from the gut. Also, there is increase in fecal fat (steatorrhea) even when diet is free from fat. Free bile acids are increased whereas there is a decrease in the concentration of conjugated bile acids. The latter are supposed to be essential for dissolution of lipids in the lumen of the gut and their eventual absorption.

The transport of fat from liver to tissues as low density lipoproteins is considerably reduced though transport from gut to liver is not much altered.

Various factors that may contribute to the fatty liver of kwashiorkor are increased fat transport from tissues to liver, reduced synthesis of beta-lipoproteins, increased liver lipogenesis, and probably reduced level of essential fatty acids.

Carbohydrates and Energy

Hypoglycemia occurs frequently and may prove fatal in a proportion of cases. Glucose absorption is impaired due to deficiency of disaccharidase enzymes in the intestinal mucosa. Handling of intravenously administered glucose and galactose is abnormal. Circulating insulin levels are low. The levels fail to respond to stimulation with glucose or arginine.

Disaccharide intolerance is a common transient phenomenon. Hence, it is advisable to avoid large loads of lactose containing foodstuffs during early part of management of PEM.

Levels of growth hormone are high but of somatostatin low. Basal metabolic rate (BMR) is reduced. Thyroid function, too, is low.

2. PEM and Infection

The interaction between infection and nutrition has been a subject of countless studies over the past few decades. Today it is widely recognized that there is a definite association between malnutrition and infection.

Malnutrition is the most common immunodeficiency in pediatric practice and breaks down the host resistance in by and large all segments. The most consistent abnormality detected in various studies has been the impairment in cell-mediated immunity (CMI). That explains why bacterial infections, which count on CMI for host's defence against them, are very severe in children suffering from PEM. Secondly, children with PEM are difficult to sensitize by repeated antigens. Thirdly, even the delayed hypersensitivity reactions that recall previous sensitization are also delayed.

There is evidence that iron-deficiency anemia has an adverse effect on the cellular immune response.

The underlying mechanisms include lymphopenia, reduced number of T-lymphocytes in the peripheral blood, impaired response to mitogen and antigens, decreased lymphokine production and serum inhibition.

It has been demonstrated that levamisole improves the ability of lymphocytes to proliferate *in vitro* in response to phytomitogens and increases the number of rosetting T-lymphocytes. However, the effect on lymphocyte stimulation response is less than that achieved by nutritional supplementation both at 2 and 4-week intervals after initiation of therapy. When given together with nutritional rehabilitation, levamisole administration is associated with an increase in cell-mediated response *in vivo* and *in vitro*, the change being observed earlier than a significant gain in weight. The clinical significance of these observations is not yet clear.

Interrelationship between PEM and infection is summarized in Box 1.

Box 99.1: Interrelationship between PEM and infection

Causes of Malnutrition leading to Infection

- Micronutrient deficiency: Iron, zinc, copper, selenium.
- Vitamin deficiency: Vitamin A, C, E, B_6, folate.
- Impaired cell-mediated immunity (CMI), phagocytic function and complement system.
- Reduced cytokine production.
- Reduced concentration of IgA, IgM and IgG.

Cause of Infection leading to Malnutrition

- Reduced intake of food, especially micronutrients.
- Enhanced catabolic losses.
- Reduced absorption of nutrients.
- Metabolic inefficiency because of micronutrient deficiency.

3. PEM and Family Planning

In developing countries, women (often malnourished) begin to produce children at a much younger age. They continue doing so quite frequently with poor spacing. Result: too many births. What is still more disturbing is that they continue doing so as long as they are not old enough.

This phenomenon leads to impaired nutritional status of both the mother and her babies, many of whom may be born after intrauterine growth retardation has already affected their bodies and perhaps brains. Such infants start life with a distinct disadvantage. They are also candidates for high morbidity and mortality.

Undoubtedly many of such deaths could be prevented. The biostatisticians call such deaths as excessive "reproductive wastage".

The question arises: Why do women reproduce at such a high pace in developing world? The reason is simple. Unless parents can be assured that the children they have are going to survive into adulthood, they will be unwilling to consider limiting their reproductive activities. It has, therefore, been argued that nutrition and general health activities should be coordinated to provide major support for maintaining health and promoting survival of infants and children.

A strong plea is made for promoting the traditional breastfeeding with suckling done throughout the 24 hours each day. This practice is not only a safeguard against malnutrition but it also has an effect on ovulation and birth spacing.

4. PEM and Endocrinal Status

Cortisol: Contrary to earlier studies, now it has been convincingly shown that serum cortisol levels in gross PEM are high, suggesting hyperfunction of the adrenal cortex. Such factors as infection and hypoglycemia are said to contribute to this observation.

High cortisol levels mediate the following useful functions:

- Augmentation of lipolysis.
- Enhancement of muscle protein catabolism.
- Promotion of liver protein synthesis.

Somatomedins: Serum levels of insulin like growth factor (IGF-1 and 2) are low due to one or more of the following factors:

- Low protein and/or energy supply in diet.
- Lack of essential amino acids.
- Low insulin/cortisol ratio.
- Low somatomedins levels mediate the useful function of reducing energy and oxygen utilization by retarding growth.

Insulin: Impaired serum insulin levels are found in kwashiorkor and marasmic kwashiorkor but not in marasmus due to:

- High energy low protein ratio in diet.
- Low body potassium.
- Deficient insulinotropic factors and insulin transport by the damaged pancreas.

Growth hormone: Growth hormone levels are high in PEM, reflecting increased secretion rather than impaired clearance. The causative factors include:

- Low somatomedin levels.
- Hypoalbuminemia and low amino acid levels.
- Low serum tyrosine level.

The useful functions mediated by this observation include:

- Facilitation of the process of lipolysis.
- Boosting of glucogenesis.
- Decrease in catabolism of albumin.

Glucagon: Glucagon levels are high whereas insulin levels are low in PEM, leading to low insulin/glucagon ratio. The following useful functions may be mediated:

- Reduction in glucose uptake by muscles and adipose tissue, sparing heart and brain.
- Increased muscle protein catabolism.
- Increased lipolysis and fatty acid supply to peripheral tissues.

Thyroxine: Contrary to earlier observations, thyroid hormone production is either normal or high in kwashiorkor but normal or low in marasmus.

5. PEM and Diarrhea

Diarrhea is a common accompaniment of the clinical picture of overt PEM. Its prevalence is 5 to 7 times more and its severity 3 to 4 times greater in malnourished children as compared to normal children. In the not-so-distant past, recurrent diarrhea in malnourished children was generally ascribed to superimposed infections and infestations. No doubt, malnourished patients are particularly susceptible to infection because of the impaired cellular immunity which is an important adverse sequel of malnutrition *per se*.

It was earlier suggested that, besides bacterial and parasitic contamination of the gut, gastrointestinal candidiasis may contribute to the common occurrence of diarrhea in malnutrition. The investigations from Indonesia and Australia lent support to this hypothesis.

Recently, it has been convincingly demonstrated that PEM may *per se* cause striking morphological as well as functional damage to the small intestinal mucosa, leading to malabsorption. Transitory secondary disaccharidase deficiency, causing lactose intolerance and osmotic diarrhea, has also been observed in significant proportion of the cases. The earlier reports suggesting existence of some monosaccharide malabsorption have now been substantiated. Moreover, it is to be noted that iron deficiency is a common occurrence in PEM. Since there is evidence that iron deficiency may itself contribute to an exudative enteropathy in childhood, the role of such anemia in etiology of diarrhea of malnutrition seems to be convincingly established.

A recent study has documented significant decline in histamine augmented maximum acid output as also presence of chronic gastritis and gastric mucosal atrophy in per oral gastric biopsies in marasmic children.

Finally, there is evidence that PEM may give rise to pancreatic atrophy and decreased enzyme secretion. Digestive disturbance and diarrhea may result.

Thus, it becomes obvious that diarrhea in malnutrition is of multifactorial etiology. An absolutely clear picture of the whole problem may emerge in the near future. The information as it stands today, however, does highlight some salient aspects which definitely have bearing on the line of management.

6. PEM and Anemia

Anemia is a common accompaniment of PEM. Generally, it is mild to moderate. But some of the children suffering from kwashiorkor have even severe anemia. It may be of variable morphology: hypochromic microcytic, macrocytic/megaloblastic or dimorphic—reflecting vitamin, mineral and protein deficiency.

Whereas protein lack *per se* can cause anemia, in clinical practice anemia associated with PEM is seemingly *multifactorial in origin*. Besides, dietetic inadequacy of the nutrients needed for synthesis of hemoglobin, factors such as infections and infestations and coexisting absorptive dysfunction play significant role in its etiopathogenesis. These factors need to be tackled if prompt response is the goal. Just providing nutrients does little good.

As regards the blood transfusion in treatment of such anemia, it is only infrequently required. Overenthusiasm in this behalf may mean losing the patient. The risk of CCF is particularly high. Resort to transfusion (unless anemia is very severe i.e. 2 or 3 g/dl hemoglobin) is seldom needed. It is given very slowly, preferably after administering a fast-acting diuretic like frusemide (IV) to minimize chance of precipitating CCF.

7. PEM and Cardiac Function

Gross malnutrition is known to considerably reduce the weight and the size of the heart. This is ascribed to atrophy of the cardiac muscle.

On the functional front, cardiac output is reduced in keeping with the severity of weight loss. There is prolongation of the systemic recirculation time, appearance time, bradycardia and reduced peripheral blood flow. Congestive cardiac failure may occur. ECG shows nonspecific changes. Radiology shows reduction in heart size. Not only does malnutrition *per se* affect cardiac function, but other factors such as accompanying severe anemia, reduced oxygen consumption and hypothyroid state too contribute to it.

8. PEM and Renal Function

PEM causes reversible impairment of renal function as manifested by:

- Reduction in glomerular filtration and renal plasma flow, especially when there is accompany gastroenteritis.
- Aminoaciduria, phosphaturia and inefficient excretion of an acid load from disturbed tubular function.
- Urine is acidic due to increased excretion of hydrogen ions to conserve potassium.

9. PEM and Drug Disposition

It is now well established that nutritional status of a child has significant effect on the bioprocesses involved in disposition of various drugs in the body. As a result, bioavailability of the drug(s) for therapeutic purposes is influenced, often warranting alteration in dose and frequency of administration.

The exact observations concerning different drugs in various studies are, however, far from uniform.

VARIOUS CLASSIFICATION OF PEM

I. Syndromal Classification

- Kwashiorkor
- Nutritional marasmus
- Marasmic kwashiorkor

- Prekwashiorkor
- Nutritional dwarfing (Stunting).

II. Gomez Classification

According to this classification, PEM is graded with reference to the weight for age as percentage of the expected weight (Harward standard):

First degree	Weight between 90 and 75% of expected for age
Second degree	Weight between 75 and 60% of expected for age
Third degree	Weight below 60% of expected.

III. Wellcome or International Classification

Weight between 80 and 60% of expected for age

With edema	kwashiorkor
Without edema	undernutrition

Weight below 60% of expected

With edema	marasmic kwashiorkor
Without edema	nutritional marasmus

IV. Classification of the Indian Academy of Pediatrics (IAP)

First degree	Weight between 80 and 70% of expected for age
Second degree	Weight between 70 and 60% of expected for age
Third degree	Weight between 60 and 50% of expected for age
Fourth degree	Weight below 50% of expected

In case the child has demonstrable pitting edema, the letter "*K*" is placed in front of the evaluated grade.

V. Jellife Classification

First degree	Weight between 90 and 80% of expected
Second degree	Weight between 80 and 70% of expected
Third degree	Weight between 70 and 60% of expected
Fourth degree	Weight below 60% of expected

VI. McLaren Classification

Mild	Weight between 90 and 80% of expected
Moderate	Weight between 80 and 70% of expected
Severe	Weight below 70% of expected

All these classifications recommended Harvard standard as the reference standard (now obsolete). CDC reference standards are the current recommendation.

VII. Waterlow Classification

Acute (wasted but not stunted)	Weight for height low, height for age normal
Acute/chronic (wasted and stunted)	Weight for height low, height for age low
Nutritional dwarfing (stunted but not wasted)	Weight for height normal, height for age low

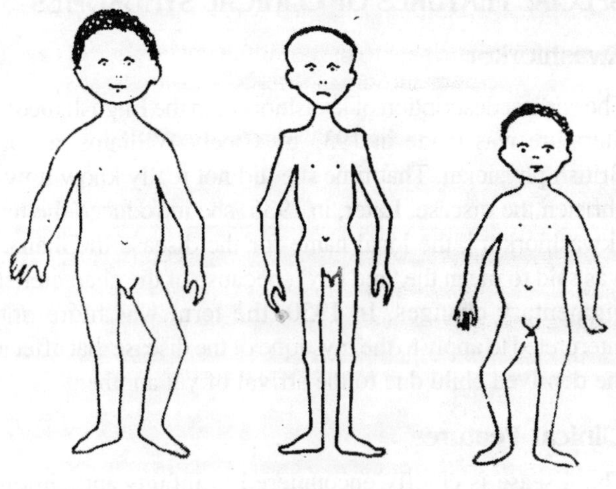

Fig 99.2: Shows a wasted child and a stunted child in comparison to a normal child. Application of sheer "weight for age" criterian shall be of no use in differentiating wasted child for stunted child. Weight for height and height for age are needed for this

VIII. WHO Classification

Table 99.1: WHO Classification of PEM

Criteria	*Moderate PEM*	*Severe PEM*
Symmetrical edema	No	Yes
Weight for height	70 - 79% of expected	< 70% of expected
(Index of wasting)	(wasting)	(severe wasting)
Height for age	85 - 89% of expected	< 85% of expected
(Index of stunting)	(stunting)	(severe stunting)

IX. Arnold Classification

It is based on midarm circumference (MAC):

Mild to moderate	MAC between 12.5 - 13.5 cm
Severe	MAC under 12.5 cm

X. Classification Based on Skinfold Thickness

Mild	80-90 % of expected for age (8-9 mm)
Moderate	60-80 % of expected for age (6-8 mm)

Severe Under 60 % of expected for age (>6 mm)

Note:

1. $$\text{Weight for height} = \frac{\text{Actual weight} \times 100}{\text{Weight of normal child of the same age}}$$

$$\text{Height for age} = \frac{\text{Actual height} \times 100}{\text{Height of normal child of the same age}}$$

2. Reference norms for comparison are CDC standards.

SPECIAL FEATURES OF CLINICAL SYNDROMES

Kwashiorkor

The earliest description of kwashiorkor in the English medical literature was made in 1933 by Cicely Williams, a noted British physician. That time she did not really know how to christen the disease. Later, in 1935, she introduced the term "kwashiorkor", the local name for the disease in Ghana. It was said to mean the "red boy", because of the characteristic pigmentary changes. In 1950, the term was more aptly interpreted to apply to the mystique of the disease that affected the deprived child due to the arrival of yet another.

Clinical Features

The disease is chiefly encountered in infants and children in the preschool age group. A vast majority of the cases are in 1 to 4 years age group. No age is, however, exempt. Occasionally, it may be seen in infants aged few months, in adolescents and even in adults.

A classical case of kwashiorkor is dull, apathetic and miserable, evincing hardly any interest in the surroundings. His growth is stunted and there is marked muscle wasting with some retention of subcutaneous fat. He has pitting edema over the legs and feet and perhaps over certain other parts of the body. There may be diarrhea, skin and hair changes, anemia and vitamin deficiency signs. Liver is, as a rule, enlarged due to fatty change.

Though this is the picture of full-blown kwashiorkor, it may be noted that only four signs growth failure, muscle wasting with retention of some subcutaneous fat, mental apathy and hypoalbuminemic edema (not of cardiac, renal or hepatic origin) taken together are sufficient by themselves to label a case as "kwashiorkor". The remaining elements may individually or collectively accompany the essential features, depending on the severity of the disease, dietary pattern and regional variations.

Biochemical Changes

These are striking. Serum proteins are always low, the maximum reduction being that of the albumin fraction; the globulins may often be found relatively elevated.

Anemia is usually moderate to severe and may be of variable morphology though iron-deficiency is a common denominator in most cases.

Low serum enzymes (esterase, amylase, lipase, cholinesterase and alkaline phosphatase), serum cholesterol, glucose, urea, certain vitamins, potassium and magnesium occur. The activity of pancreatic enzymes is considerably reduced. Total body potassium is diminished.

Imbalance of plasma amino acids and amines aciduria are common findings. Impaired cellular immunity is present.

Diagnosis

Dietetic enquiry reveals deficient intake of both proteins and calories, the protein lack being more predominant, over a prolonged period. Occurrence of an added stress like measles, whooping cough, diarrhea or bronchopneumonia often precipitates the overt picture, leading to development of pitting edema.

Diagnostic criteria may be divided into two major subdivisions: essential and nonessential.

A. Essential Features

(Minimal Diagnostic Criteria)

i. Growth retardation as evidenced by low weight and low height.
ii. Muscle wasting with retention of some subcutaneous fat.
iii. Psychomotor change as evidenced by mental apathy in the form of silent listless inertness, lack of interest in the surroundings.
iv. Hypoalbuminemic pitting edema, at least over the pretibial region. Serum albumin should be less than 2.5 g/dL and cardiac, hepatic, renal and angioneurotic causes of edema should be ruled out. These essential features are to be considered the minimal diagnostic criteria for kwashiorkor.

B. Nonessential Features

These are variable features and may or may not be present in each and every case:

i. *Hair changes* in the form of hypochromotrichia (light-colored hair), sparseness (areas of alopecia), change in texture (coarseness, silkiness) and easy pluckability. Alternate bands of light and dark color have earned the name "flag sign" which signifies periods of inadequate, adequate and inadequate nutrition over a prolonged period. This fascinating sign is only occasionally encountered.
ii. *Skin changes* include light-colored skin but the most classical dermatosis consists of areas of hyperpigmentation intervened by areas of raw red skin caused by shedding of the superficial skin flakes. This has been called *flaky-paint dermatosis*. Another similarly characteristic skin lesions of kwashiorkor is *crazy-pavement dermatosis*. Reticular pigmentation, mosaic dermatosis and pellagra-like lesions over the exposed

parts (usually dorsal surfaces) may also be encountered.

Besides the aforesaid dermatosis, kwashiorkor children may suffer from indolent sores and ulcers besides superadded skin infections like pyodermas and scabies.

iii. *Gastrointestinal manifestations* include diarrhea, vomiting and anorexia. In spite of edema, the child may develop dehydration. Diarrhea may be due to:
   a. Euperadded intestinal infections and parasitic infestations like Giardia lamblia.
   b. Effect of malnutrition *per se* on intestinal mucosa, causing reversible villous atrophy and malabsorption, inhibition of the activity of the enzyme disaccharidase (mainly lactase), causing disaccharide (mainly lactose) intolerance and damage to the pancreas, and
   c. Iron-deficiency anemia which can, on its own, lead to enteropathy by damaging the intestinal epithelium. Thus, it is obvious that diarrhea in children suffering from kwashiorkor has multifactorial etiology.

iv. *Mineral and vitamin deficiencies* are common. Anemia is usually present and is moderate to severe in intensity. It is frequently iron-deficiency type though dimorphic and even pure megaloblastic morphology may be encountered. There is evidence that PEM may *per se* cause anemia. Accompanying factors such as intestinal parasitic infestations and systemic infections may also play a contributory role.

   Other mineral deficiencies are those of potassium and magnesium.

   Deficiency of vitamin A is frequent and may lead to serious problem of keratomalacia and irreversible blindness.

   Deficiencies of vitamin B-complex, C, D and E may also complicate the picture.

v. *Hepatomegaly*, quite often fairly remarkable (liver may touch the umbilicus), is invariably present. The consistency is usually soft, the edge rounded and the surface smooth.

vi. *Superadded infections* (say, tuberculosis, bronchopneumonia, enteritis, measles, pyodermas, etc.) and intestinal parasitic infestations (*L. giardia, Ent. histolytica*, roundworm, hookworm, threadworm, *H. nana*, etc.) are common. Infection by gram-negative organisms (usually enteritis and septicemia and occasionally urinary tract infection) are most troublesome to manage in such patients.

vii. *Clubbing* may be encountered in a proportion of the children with kwashiorkor as a result of the accompanying steatorrhea.

viii. *Nonspecific ECG changes* may be found in a small proportion of the cases. A significant cardiac involvement is seldom seen.

NUTRITIONAL MARASMUS

Though kwashiorkor has received far greater attention from the researchers, nutritional marasmus is encountered more frequently in several parts of the world, particularly in north India. At times, the condition is referred to as *athrepsia or infantile atrophy*.

Clinical Features

Nutritional marasmus occurs usually in subjects less than 3 years of age; the peak incidence is seen during the first year of life. The disease may be encountered in later childhood.

A characteristic feature of the clinical picture is remarkable wasting of both muscles and subcutaneous fat. The face is wizened and shrivelled—just as in the case of a monkey. In the early stages, the child is irritable, hungry and craves for food. But, in the later stages, he may become miserable and apathetic, refusing to take anything. Edema is conspicuous by its absence. Significant hair changes, dermatosis and marked fatty liver are also absent. As in kwashiorkor, diarrhea, mineral and vitamin deficiencies, superadded infections and parasitic infestation are commonly seen (Table 99.2) provides further grading of marasmus.

Table 99.2: Grading of nutritional marasmus

Grade	*Characteristic(s)*
1.	Loss of fat from axilla
2.	Loss of fat from abdominal wall and gluteal region
3.	Loss of fat from chest and back
4.	Loss of buccal pad of fat (which consists of fatty acids); it takes longer time to disappear

Biochemical Changes

These are slight until marasmus is of very advanced degree. The reason is that the amino acids liberated from child's own tissues make possible a continuing synthesis of serum enzymes, albumin and other essential metabolites.

Anemia is mild to moderate and may be of any morphologic type though iron-deficiency anemia undoubtedly dominates the picture.

Electrolyte disturbances may occur in the presence of diarrhea and vomiting. Blood urea is usually normal and blood sugar slightly raised. Duodenal enzymes show little or no reduction.

Diagnosis

Dietetic history suggests inadequacy of both proteins and calories (carbohydrates) in child's intake in the recent past. The predominant lack is of calories. Diagnostic criteria may be essential and nonessential as outlined below:

A. Essential Feature

(Minimal Diagnostic Criteria)

1. *Growth retardation* as evidenced by marked loss of weight and subnormal height/length.
2. Gross muscle as well as subcutaneous fat wasting.
3. Absence of edema.

B. Nonessential Features

1. Hair changes are usually not present.
2. Classical dermatosis of kwashiorkor is not seen. However, indolent sores and ulcers as also superadded skin infections occurs very frequently.
3. Gastrointestinal manifestations like diarrhea and vomiting occur as in kwashiorkor. A marasmic child is, however, hungry rather than anorexic though he may develop anorexia once marasmus has advanced to extreme degree.
4. Mineral and vitamin deficiencies occur fairly commonly. Anemia is usually mild to moderate and may be of varied morphology. Potassium and magnesium deficiencies occur in patients with diarrhea and vomiting. Vitamin deficiencies occur relatively less often compared to kwashiorkor.
5. Liver is rather shrunk which is in sharp contrast to the fatty, enlarged liver of kwashiorkor.
6. Superadded infections and infestations are nearly as common as in kwashiorkor.
7. Psychomotor change is usually in the form of irritability rather than listlessness. Advanced cases may, however, become apathetic as is seen in kwashiorkor.
8. Clubbing may be seen in a proportion of marasmic children. It seems to be related to the accompanying steatorrhea.

Marasmic Kwashiorkor

Marasmic kwashiorkor refers to cases demonstrating a combination of features of kwashiorkor and marasmus. Presence of edema is essential for this diagnosis. For instance, an established case of nutritional marasmus may be mistakenly initiated on a diet consisting of lots of calories but very little proteins. Such a child is a candidate for developing hypoproteinemia and clinical edema. Remaining features of kwashiorkor may or may not be present.

Prekwashiorkor

Prekwashiorkor refers to a child who has quite poor nutritional status and certain other features of kwashiorkor such as hair changes minus edema. Such a child, unless taken care of at this very stage, may develop edema and other features of full-blown kwashiorkor.

Nutritional Dwarfing (Stunting)

If PEM starts fairly early in life and goes on and on over a number of years without causing overt picture of kwashiorkor or marasmus, child's height as well as weight may be significantly low for his age. This is what has been termed *nutritional dwarfing*.

Let us illustrate it through a specific example. An apparently healthy-looking child, appearing aged 4 years, is brought to a physician for a trivial medical problem. His height is 99 cm and weight 18.5 kg. Naturally, the physician forms an impression that the nutritional status of the child, including height and weight, is good enough for the age of 4 years. Right at this stage, the mother reveals that the actual age of the child is 8 years which indeed surprises the physician. The fact is that this child is quite stunted and underweight for his actual age.

Nutritional dwarfing is a common problem in developing countries but cases are not as frequently detected. It seems to be a kind of "adaptation" to poor diet (not as grave as to cause frank kwashiorkor or nutritional marasmus) over a prolonged period. These children are generally less active and less lively. They are more prone to diarrhea, pneumonia, tuberculosis or other infections prevalent in the region.

COMPLICATIONS OF PEM

These are given in Table 99.3.

Table 99.3: Serious complications of advanced PEM

Complication	*Remarks*
Superadded infection	Both overt and hidden: Septicemia, pneumonia, diarrhea, pyoderma, scabies, UTI, tuberculosis infections.
Dehydration and dyselectrolytemia	Usually complicating accompanying diarrhea, dyslectrolytemia often with lactose intolerance.
Hypothermia	An unattended rectal temperature of < 35 degree Celsius may prove fatal, causing sudden infant death syndrome (SIDS).
Hypoglycemia	It contributes to poor response to nutritional therapy and carries a poor prognosis.
CCF	It is usually precipitated by excessive intake of sodium and fluid or severe anemia. Since cardiac size is invariably small in PEM, even a normal sized heart in X-ray should arouse suspicion of CCF.
Anemia	Moderate to severe anemia may result from malnutrition as such or such factors as superadded infection(s), contributing to development of CCF.
Bleeding	DIC may complicate the clinical picture.
Suddent infant death syndrome (SIDS)	Sudden death 4-7 days after admission. Usually, the cause remains unclear.

MANAGEMENT OF PEM

Domiciliary (Home) Management

A. Mild-Moderate Malnutrition

Children with mild to moderate malnutrition are best managed in their own homes and kept under surveillance so as to find out improvement or deterioration in their nutritional status. The parents of such children are educated about the inadequacy in child's intake and guided how to correct it. The stress should be on the locally available economic foods rather than on expensive tinned protein preparations which should be reserved for special situations only. The parents must be apprised of the value of carbohydrates and the rationale of giving liberal amounts of semisolids and solids. They must understand why only milk will not be enough for the growing child. There is evidence that domiciliary treatment brings about gratifying results. It also reduces the unnecessary hospital load, is much less expensive, and, in addition, takes nutritional education to the family and the community.

Ours as well as many other workers' experience indicates that malnutrition relapse only infrequently when moderate PEM is treated at home. On the contrary, incidence of recurrences in hospital-treated cases is fairly high.

The management at home has got to be supervised and monitored by weekly visits of paramedicals (say an anganwadi worker), visits to a nearby nutrition rehabilitation center or OPD of a health centre/hospital.

A prerequisite to domiciliary treatment is absence of severe infection(s), fulminant gastroenteritis and electrolyte imbalance.

Good weight gain, as judged from the growth chart, is by and large the best yardstick of adequacy of response to nutritional rehabilitation.

B. *Uncomplicated Severe Acute Malnutrition (SAMN)*

Though WHO has categorically recommended hospitalization in case of SAMN, the IAP has recently advocated home treatment for this category since it is not at present feasible to offer them hospital treatment (Box 99.2).

Box 99.2: Domiciliary (Home) Treatment of Uncomplicated Severe Acute Malnutrition (SAMN) as per the Indian Academy of Pediatrics (IAP)

Diet:	Energy – Dense therapeutic diet with low bulk in the initial phase which should be home-based (prepared/modified from the family pot; indigenous ready-to-use therapeutic foods (RUTF) – Cost-effective, easily available and acceptable – Fed frequently (6-8 times/24 hours)
Supplements:	Micronutrient and minerals
Oral Antibiotics:	Usually cotrimoxazole or ampicillin for 7 days
Deworming:	Single dose
Warming Up:	Hypothermia prevented by maintaining environmental temperature and covering the child well, especially during night
Immunization:	Routine
Health Education	
Others:	Family and community participation, nutrition counselling, household food security, etc.

Management in Nutrition Rehabilitation Center (NRC)

This concept, originally started in southern America, aims at offering nutritional rehabilitation for mild to moderate PEM as a compromize between domiciliary and hospital managements. It offers a meeting point between classical treatment and prevention, embracing the positive points of both hospital and home management.

Two types of NRCs are: Day care center and residential center.

Day Care NRC: It consists of a room for children, a kitchen, an examination room and a teaching space.

At least one good meal is provided to children. Around 20 to 40 malnourished children along with their mothers who are expected to involve themselves in various activities are taken care of. The center remains open from 8 AM to 6 PM daily.

Residential NRC: This is a larger and more organized NRC with a "housemother" as the fulltime head with responsibilities that include daily work schedule of the mothers, purchase of food, issuing the correct amount of food as decided by the nutritionist, and keeping stock and maintenance of cleanliness of the center. The supervisory staff is part time and includes a doctor, a medical assistant/nurse, a home economist/nutritionist, and an agriculture teacher/extension worker. The center is attached to a health center or the pediatric department of a teaching hospital, or an under-5-clinic. The criteria for admission to the NRC are:

- Children especially at risk.
- Children who fail to gain weight over a period of 3 months.
- Children who do not catch up in growth after serious illness (measles, whooping cough, diarrhea).
- Failure to breastfeeding.
- Mothers and children who find it difficult to cope with their problems in spite of the health teaching they receive at the under-5-clinic.
- Twins and triplets.

The stress in the NRC is on nutrition and health education, household budget teaching, homecraft teaching and actual feeding, using locally available foodstuffs and local methods of cooking and preparation.

The successful rehabilitation at the NRC must be followed up at home so that the knowledge acquired during stay at the center continues to be applied at home.

Hospital Management

Complicated severe acute malnutrition (SAMN) needs to be managed in hospital in three phases:

I. Resuscitation Phase

(admission to 6-24 or even 48 hours):

Here resuscitation (stabilization) of the seriously sick child with complications is achieved through:

- Rehydration by employing WHO-recommended special rehydration solution for malnutrition (ReSoMAl) which provides high glucose and low sodium and has a low osmolarity (300 mmol/L) compared to 311 in standard WHO ORS. Alternatively, IV half-strength Darrow, half-strength Ringer lactate or even half normal saline with 5% dextrose may be used. See also Chapter (Fluid, Electrolyte….).
- Thermoregulation by keeping the child warm.
- Treatment of shock by IV fluids.
- Treatment of severe anemia by blood transfusion; and
- Treatment of superimposed infection(s) (both overt and strongly suspected) by broad-spectrum antibiotics.

II. Acute (Nutritional correction) Phase

(2nd to 7th day):

It comprises actual nutritional correction, particularly with emphasis on such components as **b**eginning of feeding, energy-dense feeding, stimulation, and **t**ransfer to home-based diet (**BEST**).

Beginning of Feeding

It should preferably be with milk-based diet, starting with low volume and then gradually building up the quantity and frequency. In many cases, it may become necessary to initiate dietary therapy with tube feeding. As soon as the child begins oral acceptance, he should be fed orally.

Calculation of Diet: The nutritional correction, the cornerstone of treatment, is carried by providing high protein and high energy diet. A daily intake of 100 kcal/kg/day of expected weight (150 - 200 kcal/kg/day of actual weight) and 3 g/kg of proteins calculated with reference to the actual weight should be achieved in very first week. This target is reached slowly, beginning with just 100 kcal/kg/day at the start. This is vital for the much-needed catch-up growth. It is advisable to provide at least 10 percent of total calories from proteins of higher biological value. The choice of foodstuffs should be based on local resources. It is good to feed small amounts of food at more frequent intervals

Transient lactose intolerance: Causing persistent watery diarrhea, may cause difficulties in initial management. In such situations, one may use one of the lactose-free milks, soyabean milk or a vegetable-protein mixture. Subjects fed on soya-based preparations are better supplemented with zinc, 1 mg/kg/day. Zinc deficiency is as such also common in severe PEM. Zinc supplementation quickly improves the dermatosis as well. In our experience, highly concentrated milk with mashed banana and/or cereal syrup makes an excellent alternative to lactose-free preparations which are either very expensive or poorly tolerated, often inducing vomiting. Such a mixture should contain 25% milk and 75% banana and/or cereals. Addition of sugar and vegetable oil (high-energy milk formula) further improves its taste and nutritional value.

Potassium Supplements: As a rule, each and every child with kwashiorkor and that of nutritional marasmus with diarrhea must receive oral potassium 5 mEq/kg/day (1 g=14 mEq) as potassium chloride solution.

Magnesium Supplements: It is helpful to give magnesium sulfate, 0.5 to 1.5 ml/day (0.3 ml/kg/day with a maximum of 2 ml) intramuscularly in 2 divided doses during the first one week or two. Thereafter, magnesium supplements should come from natural sources like milk, groundnut, peas and grains.

Treatment of Anemia and Micronutrient Deficiencies: The associated anemia and vitamin deficiencies should be treated. However, it is a good policy to give supplements of medicinal zinc, especially to patients who are fed with soya-based preparations. Since zinc-supplemented malnourished children are likely to develop plasma copper deficiency, enough copper intake in diet should be ensured. Bleeding diathesis is an indication for vitamin K (IM) and/or platelet transfusion.

Energy-Dense Feeding

After initial feeding, the child shows signs of recovery with return of appetite. This is the time to further build up his diet, employing energy-dense foods such as a mixture of cereals, pulses, jaggery and oil (preferably coconut oil).

Stimulation

Holistic approach, tender loving and emotional support contribute to recovery and catch-up growth in weight.

Transfer to Home-based Diet

The child should be gradually shifted to the home-based diet i.e. diet that is easily available, acceptable, affordable by the family.

III. Rehabilitation Phase

(7th day to 2-6 weeks):

After dietary correction spread over a week, the child accepts more and more food to make up for the deficiency. He should be encouraged to eat at libitum 10.5).

Results of Nutritional Rehabilitation

- Resumption of alertness and activity, manifested as "first smile", followed by return of appetite within first few days are good signs of recovery.
- Weight gain, after edema has disappeared, is 10 to 15 g/kg/day which is 5 times that of normal child of

same height and 10 times that of normal child of same age.

- Some infants and children with marasmus may develop edema following some correction in their nutrition. The so-called "refeeding edema" results from hyper-insulinemia causing decrease in sodium excretion. It may also follow nutritional rehabilitation with a diet that is predominant in calories (energy) with relative inadequacy of proteins.
- Disappearance of hepatomegaly and enteropathy and rise in serum albumin, though steady, are somewhat slow.
- In 1 to 3 months period, the patient attains normal weight for height and can be considered as "clinically recovered".

Discharge

Ideally, the child should be discharged from the hospital when he attains normal weight for height. It is, however, difficult to keep him in the hospital for so long because of the pressure on hospital beds. It has been suggested that discharge may be made when the child has achieved a weight that is 85% of the normal weight for height. In our experience, it takes about 2 to 4 weeks.

The hospital stay should be utilized to educate the mother about the value of high protein and high energy diet of the "family type" so that she knows how to achieve "consolidation of cure" at home. Complete recovery usually takes another 2 to 4 months after the child is back home.

Poor Response to Nutritional Rehabilitation

Primary Failure is indicated by failure of:

- Resumption of appetite by 4th day.
- Beginning of loss of edema by 4th day, and its disappearance by 10th day.
- Weight gain (a minimum of 5 g/kg/day) by 10th day.

Secondary Failure is indicated by failure to gain weight over 5g/kg/day for 3 successive days during rehabilitation phase.

There are quite a few factors that may be responsible for poor response to nutritional rehabilitation (Table 99.4).

Table 99.4: Factors contributing to poor response to nutritional rehabilitation

- Feeding Inadequacy: Faulty, inadequate
- Failure to adequately treat the accompanying infection(s) (pneumonia, diarrhea, UTI, AOM, intestinal parasitosis, malaria, tuberculosis, HIV
- Failure to properly treat accompanying dehydration and dyselectrolytemia
- Failure to attend to accompanying deficiencies (say anemia)
- Poor Facilities: Untrained and poorly motivated staff, inadequate environment
- Serious Underlying Diseases: Malabsorption, immunodeficiency, inborn errors of metabolism, malignancy.

PHENOMENA ENCOUNTERED DURING NUTRITIONAL REHABILITATION

Favorable

1. Resumption of alertness as shown by a smile and interaction with mother.
2. Initiation of weight gain.
3. Disappearance of edema (by 7-10 postherapy day).
4. Disappearance of enteropathy and hepatomegaly.
5. Elevation of serum protein.
6. Attainment of normal weight and height in 1-3 months ("clinical recovery").

Unfavorable

1. *Pseudotumor Cerebri*
   Overenergetic nutritional correction in malnourished infants may be accompanied by a transient rise of intracranial tension. The phenomenon is benign and self-limiting.
2. *Nutritional Recovery Syndrome (Gomez Syndrome)*
   The term refers to an interesting sequelae of events seen in children who are being treated with very high quantity of proteins during the course of rehabilitation from gross malnutrition. The syndrome is characterized by increasing hepatomegaly, abdominal distention, ascites, prominent thoraco-abdominal venous network, hypertrichosis, parotid swelling, gynecomastia and eosinophilia. In some instances, splenomegaly also occurs. Though the syndrome was initially described in kwashiorkor from Africa, we have recorded its occurrence in both kwashiorkor and marasmus in north India.

   Etiopathogenesis of this syndrome remains speculative. Our surmise is that its development may well be related to endocrinal disturbances. That in PEM the function of the pituitary and its target glands is set at a lower ebb is well-known. This response of the pituitary to the state of poor dietary intake appears to be an adaptive mechanism that permits survival of the patient by reducing body activity and metabolic rate, and by retarding growth. During nutritional rehabilitation, the greater utilization of the hormone by the body stimulates the pituitary to produce its trophic hormones. This results in a response by the target glands. Thus, it appears that the nutritional recovery syndrome is caused by an increase in estrogen level and by a variety of trophic hormones produced by the recovering pituitary gland.
3. *Encephalitis-like Syndrome*
   About one-fifth children with kwashiorkor become drowsy within 3 to 4 days after initiation of dietary therapy. Most often, the condition is self-limiting. Occasionally, it may be accompanied by progressive unconsciousness with fatal outcome. Even more rarely, a transient syndrome marked by coarse tremors, parkinsonian rigidity, bradykinesia and myoclonus (Kahn

syndrome) may appear 6 to several days after starting the dietary rehabilitation. Sometimes, tremors (the so-called "kwashi-shakes") may occur during the recovery phase and may take even months to resolve.

These encephalitis-like states are considered to be the result of far too much of proteins in the diet.

4. *Rickets*

   During nutritional recovery, as a result of rapid growth, vitamin D, calcium and phosphate consumption may fall short of the body needs, causing rickets. In some children, the pre-existing but hidden rickets become manifest following restoration of bone growth during nutritional rehabilitation.

5. *Anemia/Micronutrient Deficiency*

   In addition to the pre-existing anemia as a part of malnutrition, the child may manifest further worsening in hemoglobin status if iron and folic acid supplements are not provided during nutritional rehabilitation. Likewise, deficiencies of other micronutrients may too become manifest.

PROGNOSIS IN PEM

With good hospital care, mortality rate in gross PEM has today considerably fallen. Against the alarmingly high figures of 20 to 50% in the older series, the recent reports indicate 5 to 20% mortality. In our experience, it is around 5-10%, kwashiorkor children dying more often than those suffering from nutritional marasmus.

Bad prognostic signs include severe dehydration, hypoglycemia, hypothermia, CCF, superimposed infections, xerophthalmia, bleeding diathesis, hepatic dysfunction, seizures, significant change in sensorium and cachexia (extreme weight loss).

The causes of mortality include dehydration and electrolyte imbalance (dyselectrolytemia), hypoglycemia, hypothermia, fulminant systemic infections and congestive cardiac failure. In our experience, dehydration and electrolyte imbalance due to diarrheal disease and fulminant systemic infections are the chief killers of malnourished children. Congestive cardiac failure, though uncommon, carries a very bad prognosis. In some cases hypoglycemia and hypothermia may prove fatal.

LONG-TERM SEQUELAE OF PEM

Growth Retardation

Infants who suffer from significant malnutrition fairly early in life and over a prolonged period develop a permanent, irreversible stunting of growth.

Mental Impairment

Now a sort of consensus seems to have emerged concluding that IUGR and malnutrition in the first year of life, if severe enough to retard physical growth and to warrant hospitalization, may cause retardation in mental performance, eventually leading to low intelligence and impaired learning skills.

Malnutrition and Liver

It is no longer believed that PEM causes cirrhosis in the long run. The concept is based on longitudinal follow-up studies of children suffering from severe PEM and the observation that incidence of cirrhosis in Africa, the home of kwashiorkor, is fairly low.

Prevention of Malnutrition

WHO has described malnutrition as a "global problem", having adverse effects on the survival, health performance and progress of population groups. The effects are of the highest order in the developing countries.

Prevention at Family Level

The most significant in the preventive measures at family level is what is called "nutrition education". Nutrition education consists of:

i. Good antenatal care so that mother's own nutrition remains upto the mark and she does not develop malnutrition and anemia. This will be of much help in reducing the incidence of intrauterine growth retardation and LBW, the predecessors of malnourished children in very many instances.

ii. Encouragement to the mothers to breastfeed the infants for as long as they can. Even if the mother is not in a position to breastfeed the infant for some reason, it is of advantage to express her milk and feed it to him. Of course, she must take good diet and adequate amounts of fluids to maintain her lactation. In case of prolonged breastfeeding, it is to be confirmed that the lactation performance of the mother is adequate. Else, adequate supplementation of feeding becomes imperative.

iii. At the age of 6 months, the infant should start receiving nutritional supplements, in addition to breastfeeding. The supplements should be combination of cereals, protein-rich foods and fruits such as mashed banana.

iv. The practice of shifting to artificial feeding in the form of bottle feeding with diluted cow milk or tinned milk should be discouraged, particulalry in the poor in whose families it is virtually impossible to prevent occurrence of contamination of the bottle and the formula.

Prevention at Community Level

Here again nutritional education is of vital importance. Its delivery may be either through mass media such as radio, television, posters, documentary, flms, etc. or imparting knowledge to the mothers at group meetings or at the doorstep of the family by the health auxiliary.

Secondly, surveys to detect cases of mild to moderate malnutrition, using preferably age-independent criteria, should be conducted. Such children may be kept under surveillance and, if required, given nutritional supplements.

The supplementary feeding programs in India include applied nutrition program, midday meal program for school children, special nutritional program, vitamin A prophylaxis program, anemia prophylaxis program, integrated child development services (ICDS), food for work program, etc. The principal beneficiaries of such programs are the nutritionally vulnerable preschoolers, school-going children and pregnant and lactating mothers. Ample evidence is now available to support the contention that adequate supplementation through the feeding programs results in improvement of nutritional status of the target population, provided that operational efficiency is ensured.

Prevention at National Level

This consists of measures to improve food production, control price-rise, make available cheap supplementary foods, fortify and enrich foods, prevent adulteration and irradiate certain foods such as wheat, potato and onion. Also, nutrition education and containment of population explosion are of paramount importance.

Prevention at World Level

Efforts to intensify various international food programs like those of WHO, FAO, UNICEF, CARE, OXFAM, SIDO, DANIDA, Indo-Dutch, etc.

KEY LEARNING POINTS

- Over the years, spectrum of PEM has changed from dominance by severe syndromes (kwashiorkor and marasmus) to dominance by mild to moderate PEM ending up with stunting.
- Evolution of different syndromal states is still an issue of hypotheses.
- Anthropometry (especially employing the criteria weight for height) remains the most important tool for assessment of nutritional status.
- Serious complications include fulminant infections, dehydration and dyselectrotemia, hypothermia, hypoglycemia, CCF, severe anemia, bleeding and SIDS.
- Treatment depends on whether PEM is mild-moderate, uncomplicated severe or complicated severe.
- Complicated severe acute malnutrition needs to be managed in hospital in three phases, namely resuscitation phase, nutritional correction phase and rehabilitation phase.
- During treatment, favorable and unfavorable phenomenon (say, nutritional recovery syndrome) may be encountered.
- Prevention is at family level, community level, national level and world level.

FURTHER READINGS

1. Alleyne GAO, Hay RW, Picou DI, Stanfield JP, Whitehead RJ. *Protein-Energy Malnutrition*. London: Edward Arnold 1989.
2. Bhan MK, Bhandari N, Bahl R. Management of the severely malnourished child: Perspectives from developing countries. *BMJ* 2003;326:146-151.
3. Gupta P, Shah, D, Sachdev HPS, Kapil U. National workshop on "Development of guidelines for effective home-based care and treatment of children suffering from severe acute malnutrition". *Indian Pediatr* 2006;43:125-13.
4. Gupte S: Nutritional recovery syndrome. *N Engl J Med* 1972; 291:501.
5. Gupte S: Nutritional rehabilitation. *Indian J Pediatr* 1983;50:97.
6. Gupte S. *Textbook of Pediatric Nutrition*. New Delhi: Peepee 2006.
7. Jelliffe DB, Jelliffe EEP: Causation of kwashiorkor: Towards a multifactorial consensus. *Pediatrics* 1992; 4: 502.
8. Sachdev HPS, Choudhury P. *Nutrition in Children. Developing Country Concerns*. New Delhi: BI 1994.
9. WHO: Guidelines for the inpatient treatment of severely malnourished children (Part II). *Nutrisearch* 2000;7:3.

100 Micronutrients/Minerals and Other Deficiencies

Suraj Gupte • EM Gomez

INTRODUCTION

The human body minerals may be categorized into two major groups. First group includes electrolytes (sodium, potassium, etc), those with structural role (calcium, posphorus, etc), those as component of hemoglobin (iron) and minor minerals (copper, zinc, cobalt, iodine, etc). The second group conists of those whose precise functions are not yet known, e.g. nickel, tin, silicon and vanadium.

IRON DEFICIENCY DISORDERS

Iron deficiency exists in two forms:

1. Iron deficiency anemia (IDA) with overt manifestations such as anemia, poor growth and development, reduced learning capacity, cognitive function and work capacity.
2. Iron-deficient stores which sooner or later end up as IDA.

Iron-Deficiency Anemia (IDA)

As emphasized earlier, iron-deficiency is the most common etiologic factor in anemias. It is especially common in infancy because both breast as well as cow milk do not provide the baby's needs for iron. Secondly, poor iron stores in premature babies predispose to further deficiency so that, at about third month (the time for maximal physiologic reduction of hemoglobin), there may be marked iron-deficiency anemia. Twins commonly become iron deficient. At times, only one of them may suffer. Preschool age and adolescence are particularly more vulnerable for IDA because of rapid somatic growth.

In older children, the causes include inadequate intake, malabsorption, infection, chronic blood loss (ancylostomiasis) and cow milk-protein (CMP) hypersensitivity. Recently, convincing evidence has accumulated to the effect that iron-deficiency may *per se* cause an absorptive defect by damaging the small intestinal epithelium.

Rarely, in such errors of iron metabolism as sideroblastic anemia, idiopathic pulmonary hemosiderosis and congenital transferrin deficiency, iron gets stored in the body rather than being utilized for erythropoiesis.

Clinical Features

These include progressive pallor, irritability, anorexia, tiredness, weakness, failure to thrive, atrophy of tongue papillae, pica and koilonychia. Diarrhea is often present. At times, pseudotumor cerebri may occur. Occasionally, especially in severe anemia, spleen is enlarged. Hemic murmur (soft systolic, having maximal intensity over the base and changing with position) is common. When anemia is severe, cardiomegaly may be present.

Though most children learn to adapt to anemia of prolonged duration, some may suffer from CCF, particularly in the presence of an added stress.

Recently, it has been demonstrated that frank iron-deficiency anemia causes low infant behavior record (IBR) as manifested by unhappiness, lack of cooperation and shorter attention span, as also lower mental development index (MDI). Even subclinical iron-deficiency causes low MDI. Both IBR and MDI revert to normal following correction of iron-deficiency.

Diagnosis

Diagnosis of IDA rests upon demonstration of microcytic hypochronic anemia along with reduced body/serum iron. Peripheral smear examination shows aniso-poikilocytosis and polychromasia. MCV, MCH and MCHC are reduced. RDW (Red cell distribution width, a measure of variation of red cell size) is increased. There is mild reticulocytosis, leukocytosis and thrombocytosis. Serum iron is reduced (<30 mg/dL is considered diagnostic), so is serum ferritin (<10 ng/ml). Total iron binding capacity (TIBC) over 400 mg/dL strongly suggests IDA. Transferrin saturation is reduced (<12-14% in children and <16% in adolescents). Bone marrow is hypercellulor with reduced iron stores but examination of bone marrow for diagnosis is not required.

On the basis of biochemical and hematological changes iron deficiency is graded into 3 stages – Stage I – Depletion of iron stores (ferritin is decreased, transferrin saturation, serum iron and hemoglobin are normal; Stage II – Depletion of transport iron (transferrin saturation and serum iron also reduced, Hb is normal); and Stage III – State of IDA (frank features of IDA).

Differential Diagnosis

Iron dificiency anemia needs to be differentiated from anemia showing hypochromic microcytic picture, say lead poisoning, beta-thalassemia trait, thalassemia major, HB H disease (a type of alpha-thalassemia), and anemia accompanying chronic inflammations and infections.

Treatment

1. Specific treatment consists in replacing the iron deficiency with iron which may be administered orally or parenterally.

   A. **Oral therapy:** The dose of elemental iron is 3-6 mg/kg/day in 3 divided doses. Any iron can be given. But the most economic and most easily available one is the simple ferrous sulfate, containing 20% iron (Table 100.1) and available as 200 mg tablets. Oral iron, in any form, causes gastric irritation if given in excess dose. The side-effects of oral iron include nausea, vomiting, diarrhea, constipation, abdominal cramps, staining of teeth and tongue and discoloration of stools.

   Even recommended dose may cause GIT disturbance in which case readjustment of the dose becomes essential. For optimal absorption, iron dose should be administered in between meals. Concurrent administration of vitamin C enhances its absorption whereas foods rich in phytates (cereals) and phosphates (milk) reduce it. The total duration of treatment varies from 3 to 6 months. Therapy must continue in the same dose for another 6 weeks after attainment of normal hemoglobin.

   Hemoglobin rise following oral iron therapy is around 0.4 g/dl day.

   Factors contributing to poor response to oral iron include:

   - Poor tolerance.
   - Subtherapeutic dose (< 3-6 mg/kg/day).
   - Insufficient length of treatment.
   - Accompanying illness: Malabsorptive state, infection(s).
   - Persistent bleeding (occult or frank).
   - Poor compliance.
   - Iron administration soon after intake of milk (phosphates) or cereals (phytates).
   - Incorrect diagnosis of IDA in thalassemia, lead poisoning or sideroblastic anemia.

Table 100.1: Elemental iron content of various oral iron salts

Salt	*Elemental iron (%)*
Ferrous sulfate	20
Anhydrous ferrous sulfate	37
Ferrous sulfate (exsicated)	30
Ferrous fumarate	33
Ferrous fructose	25
Ferrous succinate	23
Ferrous lactate	19
Ferrous carbonate	16
Ferric ammonium citrate	15
Ferrous gluconate	12
Colloidal iron	50

   B. **Parenteral therapy:** It is indicated when one desires to cut down hospital stay, if oral medication is not feasible because of intolerance or presence of diarrheal disease, when gastrointestinal bleeding is likely to be worsened by oral iron therapy, and when there is a sufficient reason to believe that the patient is unlikely to regularly take his "pills". A small group of pediatricians prefers to initiate treatment with parenteral iron (a few injections only) and then put the patient on oral medication. They believe that such a schedule helps in tiding over the initial "difficulties" in management.

   Total dose is calculated by one of the formulas:

   Dose of parenteral iron (intravenous infusion or intramuscular) is calculated as follows:

   Iron required = 2.5 × body weight (kg) × Hb deficit (Hb deficit is the difference between measured and desired values of Hb).

   An additional 20-30% of the calculated dose is included to replenish the stores.

   Parenteral iron may be given intramuscularly or intravenously.

   Intramuscular Administration: For this purpose iron-dextran complex (Imferon) and iron-sorbitol (Jectofer) are available. Daily dose of intramuscular injection should not exceed 5 mg/kg i.e. 50 mg in infants and 100 mg in adolescents. The best site is upper and outer quadrant of thigh. To avoid repeat injection at the earlier prick, it should be given in Z fashion. The injection is given deep IM making sure that staining of skin doesn't occur. Adverse effects include local pain, fever, arthralgia, and lymphadenopathy.

   Intravenous Administration: Only iron-dextran complex (Imferon) can be given by this route. After testing sensitivity with a small dose, the total dose infusion (TDI) is given in 250-500 ml of saline slowly over 6-8 hours. It is now only infrequently employed in view of the risk of shock and anaphylaxis.

   Blood transfusion should be reserved for life-threatening situations when anemia is very severe and has associated symptoms warranting a rapid rise in hemoglobin level. If a decision to give blood has been taken, transfusion must be given slowly. Danger of CCF in such patients is really high (Table 100.2). A partial exchange transfusion is advisable in case of IDA accompanying CCF.

Table 100.2: High-risk factors in blood transfusion in severe anemia

- Age under 2 years: Poor cardiac tolerance may lead to cardiac complications especially with the presence of added stress in the form of pre-existing CCF, bronchopneumonia, congenital heart disease, edematous malnutrition, etc.
- Malnutrition: Myocardial weakness because of degenerative changes as in beriberi and circulatory overload as in kwashiorkor may lead to CCF.
- Impending CCF
- Acidosis
- Hypoglycemia
- Stored blood

Other measures include *digitalization* if the patient has CCF, adequate nutritional rehabilitation and adequate management of the underlying cause of anemia and associated illness. In our country, the worm infestations are invariably present and should be eradicated. Otherwise response to iron may be poor. Likewise, besides malnutrition, deficiencies of other hemopoietic factors such as folic acid and vitamin B_{12} (which may introduce an element of macrocytosis/megaloblastosis in children with iron-deficiency anemia) should also receive attention.

Control Measures

- Neonates born preterm and LBW should receive oral iron by 2 weeks of age, provided that they are infection-free.
- Exclusive breastfeeding should be given for first 6 months.
- Complimentary foods rich in iron, say green-leafy vegetables, beans, pulses) should be initiated at 6 months of age since only milk diet is likely to contribute to development of IDA in the infant in the second half of first year.
- Periodic treatment of intestinal parasitic infestations, especially hookworm infection, is quite helpful. Walking barefooted should be avoided.
- Iron supplements for susceptible infants and children and at puberty, especially in girls. This is usually achieved with iron tablets, syrup or drops. Alternative strategies include:
  - Availability of iron-fortified salt (a Government of India program) and food items.
  - Availability of "Sprinkles" a novel form of microencapsulated iron which can be packaged in easy-to-use sachets for fortifying weaning foods at home. A low dose of 12.5 mg/day of elemental iron is not only quite effective but also better tolerated.

ZINC DEFICIENCY

Next to iron, it is the most abundant trace element in the human body. It is an essential component of at least 20 enzymes, including alkaline phosphatase, carbonic anhydrase and pancreatic carboxypeptidase. It plays a vital role in protein synthesis and RNA. Its concentration in hair is deemed to reflect the zinc status of a subject. It is also present in erythrocytes, prostate, eye, bone and endocrine glands. Total body zinc content of a newborn is about 60 mg and that of an adult about 1,600 mg.

The dietary sources of zinc include meat, liver, fish nuts, grains, dry beans and legumes. Daily requirement is some 200 mcg.

Etiology

Zinc deficiency may occur in protein-energy malnutrition, malabsorption states, regional ileitis, rheumatoid arthritis, sickle-cell anemia, achondroplasia, chronic blood loss, excessive sweating and hyperzincuria in catabolic states or viral hepatitis. Prolonged parenteral nutrition, if not supplemented with zinc, may also cause zinc deficiency state. Consumption of fibres and phytates in excess hampers zinc absorption.

Clinical Features

Clinical manifestation of zinc deficiency include growth retardation, hypogonadism, anemia and hepatosplenomegaly. This peculiar syndrome called, "adolescent nutritional dwarfing", has been described particularly from Iran and Egypt, though cases have been seen in India and other developing countries. In our own experience, a convincing cause and effect relationship between this syndrome and zinc deficiency remains to be established. Also, it has been said that zinc deficiency in such cases may well be due to poor absorption because of phytates, calcium and other dietary components rather than low dietary intake.

Additional features of zinc deficiency include protracted diarrhea, delayed wound healing, anorexia, failure to thrive, pica, impaired taste perception (hypogeusia), hyperkeratotic skin and, perhaps, infantile tremor syndrome.

Acrodermatitis enteropathica is an inborn error of zinc metabolism in which there are skin changes at the extremities and around the orifices, diarrhea, alopecia, atrophy of nails and failure to thrive. This autosomal recessive condition usually manifests shortly after weaning and shows dramatic and sustained response to therapy with zinc.

Diagnosis

The laboratory confirmation for zinc deficiency may be obtained from a plasma zinc level of below 70 μg/dL or a hair zinc level of below 70 μg/g dry weight.

Treatment

Treatment of zinc deficiency consist in giving zinc sulfate, 0.2 to 1 mg of elemental or 1 to 5 mg of the salt as such/kg body weight/day. In very severe deficiency states, as high a dose as 20 to 40 mg/day of elemental zinc may be administered.

COPPER DEFICIENCY

Copper, rightly called the "iron twin", plays a vital role in the utilization of iron stores and in the activity of many important enzymes, including cytochrome oxidase, monoamine oxidase, dopamine betahydroxylase, delta-aminolevulinic acid dehydrogenase, ascorbic acid dehydrase, uricase and tyrosinase. Total body copper content of a newborn is about 14 mg and that of a young adult about 100 mg. Thus, there is an average growth requirement of 10 mcg/day. It is distributed in all tissues of body, including kidney, liver, brain, heart, bone marrow and bones.

Whereas in a newborn as much as 50% of body copper is found in the liver, the corresponding figure in a young adult is only 5%. Thus, just, as is the case with iron, copper stores of an infant are sufficient for the first six months of life. In the liver, copper is incorporated into a protein complex, "ceruloplasmin".

Copper is widely distributed in foodstuffs with the exception of milk; breast milk contains 40 µg/ dL and cow milk 20 µg/dL of it.

Deficiency may be encountered in the following situations:

- Protein-energy malnutrition, including nutritional rehabilitation employing predominantly soy milk and zinc supplementation in excess.
- Malabsorption states.
- Chronic diarrheal disease.
- Prolonged parenteral feeding without copper supplements.
- Premature infants being fed low-copper milk preparations.

COBALT

It is apart of vitamin B_{12} and is required for iodine utilization. It increases iron absorption. Its deficiency causes anemia and goiter. Its excess can cause dilated cardiomyopathy which is indistinguishable from primary dilated cardiomyopathy. Its excess may also cause goitre.

SELENIUM

Selenium is an integral part of glutathione peroxidase and is linked to vitamin E and is an important antioxidant co-factor. Its deficiency leads to dilated cardiomyopathy which used to be common in certain geographical parts of China ("Endemic DCM/ Keshan disease"). It was first described in 1979 and may occur in young children and women. It is a preventable cardiomyopathy, but once DCM sets in, total reversal to normality is not possible even with selenium supplementation. Four forms of Keshan's disease are recognized: an acute variety with shock, a subacute variety with both hypotension and CHF, a chronic variety with CHF and the fourth one, which presents as asymptomatic cardiomegaly. It is virtually indistinguishable from various presentations of primary DCM. Deficiency may also cause liver necrosis, arthritis and myopathy. Its excess may cause dental caries, alopecia and garlic odor in breath.

CHROMIUM

Chromium deficiency is associated with poor glucose tolerance and neuropathy. It facilitates insulin action. Its excess can lead to dermatitis and renal failure.

MANGANESE

Manganese is an enzyme cofactor in superoxide dismutase, oxidative phosphorylation and bone mineralization. Deficiency may produce growth retardation, weight loss, red hair and hypocholesterolemia. Excess may cause cholestasis, encephalopathy, basal ganglia disorder, goiter and cardiomyopathy.

FLUORINE

Fluorine is a component of bone and teeth. Upto 1 ppm in drinking water is desirable. Deficiency leads to carries tooth and excess to fluorosis.

MOLYBDENUM

Molybdenum is important in uric acid metabolism. Deficiency may lead to tachycardia, irritability, central scotoma and upper GIT cancers. Excess may unmask gout and cause bony defects like genu valgum.

NICKEL

Nickel is a component of urease and nickel plasmin. Excess may produce dermatitis, liver necrosis and lung cancer.

VANADIUM

Vanadium deficiency is associated with nutritional edema.

SILICON

Silicon is important in cross linkage of collagen and deficiency may produce defective bone growth. Excess may cause fibrosis lung.

ARSENIC

Arsenic is important in skin and nail formation.

ENDEMIC GOITER

Enlargement, of the thyroid gland as a result of iodine deficiency is endemic in sub-Himalayan belt extending from Ladakh through Himachal Pradesh, Uttar Pradesh, Bihar, Bengal, Sikkim, Bhutan, Assam, Arunachal Pradesh, Meghalaya and Nagaland to Burma. Isolated pockets are being increasingly identified, e.g. Rajasthan, Gujarat, Maharashtra, Madhya Pradesh, Andhra and Kerala.

Since sea-water is a rich source of iodine, goiter is rare in population living along the sea coast.

Subclinical deficiency of iodine may manifest in the form of goiter only at puberty or confining to the periods of stress.

The public health importance of goiter lies in the high incidence of deafmutism, mental retardation (often accompanying frank cretinism), ataxia and spasticity in the endemic areas.

Availability of iodized salt (common salt fortified with sodium or potassium iodate in a ratio of 1 in 40,000) is the most economic, convenient and effective means of mass prophylaxis in endemic areas. An alternative to iodized salt is iodized oil given as an intramuscular injection once in 3 years as a cheap, safe and long-acting prophylactic measure.

CALCIUM DEFICIENCY

By and large 99% of body calcium is found in bones and teeth. The remaining 1% is involved in clotting cascade, nerve conduction, muscle stimulation, vitamin D metabolism and parathyroid function.

Its metabolism is regulated by vitamin D, calcitonin and parathyroid hormone.

In order that calcium performs is function well, adequate magnesium, phosphorus and vitamin A, C, D and E should be available in the body.

Whereas availability of fat facilitates its absorption from the gut, phytates (cereals) reduce its absorption.

Sources of calcium include milk and its products and millets (say, ragi).

Clinical Features

1. Tetany: Muscle cramps, numbness, tingling.
2. Impaired growth.
3. Calcium-deficiency rickets.
4. Osteoporosis.
5. Nonspecific: Arthralgia, palpitations.

MAGNESIUM DEFICIENCY

Next to potassium, it is the most abundant mineral cation in cells. It is involved in:

- Synthesis of fatty acids, proteinsyclic AMP.
- Oxidative phosphorylation.
- Autonomic control of heart.

Sources include plant foods and meat.

Requirements are:

First 6 months	40 mg/day
Second 6 months	60 mg/day
Later	200 – 300 mg/day

Causes

These include PEM, diarrheal disease, malabsorption syndrome (MAS), and chronic renal failure.

Clinical Features

1. Irritabilty
2. Tetany
3. Increased or decreased reflexes.

HYPONATREMIA

It is defined as a serum sodium of less than 130 mEq/L.

Etiology

It is caused by conditions that lead to:

1. Primary sodium deficit with sodium depletion from renal losses, extrarenal losses or nutritional deficits.
2. Primary water excess with water gain.
3. Abnormal retention of sodium and water.

For details, see Table 100.3.

Table 100.3: Etiology of hyponatremia

Primary sodium deficit with sodium depletion
Renal sodium losses: Prematurity, renal salt wasting. Adrenal insufficiency with mineralocorticoid deficiency, recovery phase of acute tubular necrosis, chronic diuretic therapy, osmotic diuresis in diabetes mellitus, renal tubular acidosis.
Extrarenal sodium losses: Vomiting, gastroenteritis/diarrhea, nasogastric drainage, excess sweating, burns, cystic fibrosis.
Nutritional deficits: Water intoxication (WIC) syndrome, IV fluids poor in sodium, CSF drainage, burns, paracentesis.
Primary water excess with water gain
Syndrome of inappropriate ADH secretion (SIADH), hypothyroidism, excess IV fluids, psychogenic polydipsia, glucocorticoid deficiency, tap-water enema.
Abnormal retention of sodium and water
Nephrotic syndrome, cirrhosis, CCF, renal failure (both acute and chronic).

Clinical Features

These include restlessness, confusion, seizures, hypotension, CCF and coma depending on the severity of hyponatremia. Most subjects with serum sodium under 130 but above 120 mEq/L are asymptomatic.

Treatment

Symptomatic hyponatremia is treated by administering 3% solution of sodium chloride (saline), 10 ml/kg (maximum 12 ml/kg) at a rate of 1 ml/ minute, intravenously. This would correct hyponatremia by approximately 5 mEq/L. Thereafter, extra sodium needed (calculated as per the formula given below) may be administered slowly spread over 24 to 48 hours. Rapid correction carries the risk of pontine myelinosis.

Na Sodium deficit (mEq/L) = [serum Na expected (135) – serum Na actual] × wt (kg) × 0.6.

In hyponatremia associated with SIADH, water-overloading and renal failure, fluid restriction is required to safeguard against pulmonary edema and CCF. In hyponatremia accompanying hypoproteinemia, fluids must not be restricted.

HYPOKALEMIA

It is defined as a serum potassium level of less than 3.5 mEq/l.

Etiology

Hypokalemia may result from reduced intake, renal losses, extrarenal losses, and fall in muscle mass (Table 100.4).

Table 100.4: Etiology of hypokalemia

Reduced potassium intake
Protein-energy malnutrition
High renal losses
Diuretics: Osmotic diuretics, carbonic anhydrase inhibitors
Tubular defects: Renal tubular acidosis
Acid-base disturbances: Diabetic ketaoacidosis, alkalosis
Endocrinopathies: Cushing syndrome, primary aldosteronism, thyrotoxicosis
High extrarenal losses
GIT: Diarrhea, vomiting, catharsis, frequent enemas, biliary drainage, enterocutaneous fistulas
Skin: Profuse sweating
Miscellaneous
Decrease in muscle mass: Myopathies
Familial hypokalemic periodic paralysis

Clinical Features

These include weakness of skeletal muscles, hypotonia, hyporeflexia, abdominal distention, poor peristalsis, paralytic ileus, frank paralysis and considerable respiratory distress.

Prolonged hypokalemia leads to inability of kidneys to concentrate urine, polyuria, polydipsia and alkalosis. Poor renal function may persist even after correction of hypokalemia.

Cardiac involvement may be in the form of arrhythmias and ECG changes which include depression of ST segment, flattening or inversion of T wave, prominent U wave and prolongation of QTc beyond 0.425 sec. Yet severer hypokalemia may further cause prolonged P-R interval, sino-atrial block and extrasystoles (ventricular). Mental apathy may also be encountered.

Treatment

It consists in administering potassium 2 to 3 mEq/kg/24 hours, over 24 hours. The IV fluid must not contain more than 40 mEq/L potassium.

Hypokalemia with massive urinary losses should be treated with oral potassium, 10 mEq/kg. Indomethacin and $MgCl_2$ are indicated in Barter syndrome and Gitelman syndrome, respectively.

HYPERKALEMIA

It is defined as a serum potassium of more than 5.5 mEq/L.

Etiology

It usually results from excessive intake (often through IV fluids), impaired excretion (acute/chronic renal failure, adrenal insufficiency, hyporeninemic hypoaldosteronism, potassium-sparing diuretics), shifting or release of potassium from tissues into ECF (acidosis, injury, hemorrhage, burns, hemolysis, insulin deficiency) and drugs (succinyl-choline, digitalis toxicity).

Clinical Features

Significant hyperkalemia may cause marked muscular weakness with flaccid paralysis, tetany, paresthesia, bradycardia, shock and cardiac arrhythmias. ECG changes include elevation and tenting of T-wave, widening of QRS complex, depression of ST segment, prolongation of PR interval and short QT interval.

Treatment

Initial therapy consists in rapid IV administration of sodium bicarbonate, 1 to 3 mEq/kg, or glucose and insulin (0.5 to 1 g of 10 to 20% glucose/kg plus 1 unit crystalline insulin/ 3 g of glucose) to lower the serum potassium level, and IV calcium gluconate, 0.3 to 0.5 ml/kg of a 10% solution, slowly to counter the cardiac toxicity. It would be under ECG monitoring.

Eventually, a negative potassium balance is attained by employing ion-exchange resins, e.g. Kayexalate, 1 g/kg/24 hr (orally or as retention enema) in 2 to 4 divided doses, by hemodialysis, or by peritoneal dialysis.

KEY LEARNING POINTS

- Iron deficiency, the most common micronutrient deficiency, produces, in addition to anemia, low infant behavioral record (IBR) and low mental development index (MDI), needs not only treatment but also preventive steps.
- Zinc deficiency, implicated in causation of growth retardation, hypogonadism, anemia, hepato-splenomegaly, protracted diarrhea, etc.
- Deficiency of copper, the so-called "iron twin", may accompany PEM, malabsorption states, chronic diarrhea, TPN, etc.
- Iodine deficiency, causing endemic goiter, may lead to deafmutism, mental retardation, ataxia and spasticity, needs universal use of iodized salt for mass prophylaxis in endemic areas.
- Precise functions of some micronutrients like nickel, tin, silicon, vanadium, etc. is still being investigated.

FURTHER READINGS

1. Bhaskaran P. Micronutrient malnutrition, infection and immunity: An overview. *Nutr Rev* 2002;60:S40-S45.
2. Diaz JR, de las Cagigas A, Rodriguez R. Micronutrient deficiencies in developoing and affluent countries. *Eur J Clin Nutr* 2003;57:S70-S72.
3. Oken E, Duggan C. Update on micronutrients: Iron and zinc. *Curr Opin Pediatr* 202;14:350-353.

101 Vitamin A Deficiency (VAD)

Suraj Gupte • Shally Sharma

INTRODUCTION

Deficiency of vitamin A, *xerophthalmia*, a leading cause of blindness among the underprivileged, continues to be a problem of public health magnitude in the developing world.

Of the 10 million children suffering every year from xerophthalmia, 5 million belong to Asia. One-fourth of them are eventually blinded. Half a million go blind in India alone every year.

BACKGROUND: OVERVIEW OF VITAMIN A

Vitamin A, a fat-soluble alcohol, is an essential micronutrient that is derived primarily from a plant pigment, provitamin A carotenoids (*beta-carotene,* for example), which plays a vital role in the photochemical basis of vision. Conversion of carotene to vitamin A occurs in the intestinal wall and its absorption into the lymphatic system is facilitated by bile. It is concerned with the maintenance of epithelial tissue in the body, especially that of eye, skin and mucous membrane.

Table 101.1 summarizes salient features of vitamin A. Overdose may cause toxic effects (hypervitaminosis A) in the form of pseudotumor cerebri and hyperostosis.

Table 101. 1: Salient features of Vitamin A

Sources
Dark green leafy vegetables (DGLV), yellow fruits, dairy products, fish liver oil, liver, egg yolk
Characteristics
Fat-soluble; heat-stable; oxidation destroys it; bile essential for absorption; stored in liver; protected by vitamin E
Biochemical Action
Essential for synthesis of visual pigment (rhodopsin) as well as iodopsin; in reproduction, embryonic and fetal development, growth, bone growth, immune and epitheloid functions; in several basic cellular processes
Deficiency Signs
Ocular and extra ocular manifestations (See text)
Toxicity
Painful swelling of long bones; bone fragility; pseudotumor cerebri; anorexia; drying and cracking of skin; hepatosplenomegaly; alopecia; carotenemia; fetal abnormalities

Etiology

Vitamin A deficiency usually occurs in association with malnutrition and chronic intestinal disorders such as malabsorption states, chronic diarrheal disease, and pancreatic disease like cystic fibrosis and hepatic insufficiency. In these situations, vitamin A absorption or metabolism is disturbed.

Diarrhea is a risk factor for vitamin A deficiency; *vice versa* also is true. Severe measles too is a risk factor for vitamin A deficiency.

Prevalence

The precise incidence of xerophthalmia in the pediatric population defies evaluation. In general, 3 to 10% of the infants and children in the Third World suffer from it. In north India, surveys conducted by the Child Health Study Group reveal incidences of 6 to 7% in preschoolers and 8.1% in school-going children. The incidence in hospitalized children in Calcutta is 9.8%. The prevalence in south India is even higher.

Clinical Features

These may be considered under the two subheadings, ocular and extraocular.

A. Ocular Features

The earliest manifestation, *night blindness* or poor dark adaptation, is due to insufficient formation of the visual purple, *rhodopsin*. Often, the mother of the infant observes that he takes considerable time to adjust to dim light or darkness.

Xerosis of conjunctiva is usually the first sign that can be seen on examination. The conjunctiva becomes dry, lusterless, wrinkled and dirty brown in color. These changes are most obvious in the interpalpebral bulbar conjunctiva. In advanced cases, significantly evident involvement of conjunctiva over the lower lid and lower fornix's may be present.

Table 101.2: WHO classification of xerophthalmia

XN	Night blindness
XIA	Conjunctival xerosis
XIB	Bitot spot
X2	Corneal xerosis
X3A	Corneal ulceration/keratomalacia <1/3rd corneal surface
X3B	Corneal ulceration/keratomalacia >1/3rd corneal surface
XS	Corneal scar
XF	Xerophthalmic fundi (white retinal lesions)

Conjunctival xerosis may lead to formation of the so-called Bitot spot which consists of an almost triangular area, usually about the lateral aspect of the limbus, covered by fine, white, foamy or greasy substance. It is basically a heaped-up dry mass of conjunctival epithelium. The appearance is like grains on chalky, pasty foam. It is noteworthy that Bitot spots are generally seen in both the eyes and are present more frequently to the lateral than the medial of the limbus.

Keratomalacia is the advanced stage of xerophthalmia. It consists of softening, necrosis and ulceration of the cornea. Unlike the preceding stage of corneal xerosis, keratomalacia is irreversible, except for the possible replacement of the grossly damaged cornea by a transplant. Once cornea gets involved, photophobia accompanies the clinical profile.

With the onset of keratomalacia, cornea melts into a dead white to dirty-yellow structure; invasion by an infection (which is quite usual) further aggravates the situation. If corneal perforation occurs (which again is quite frequent), herniation of the lens and vitreous may result.

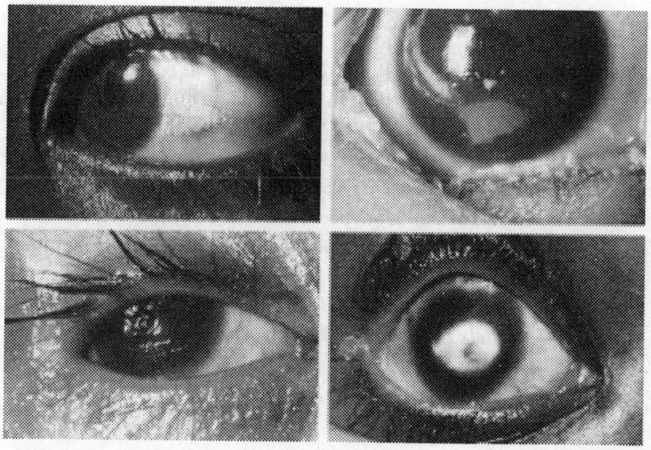

Fig. 101.1-4: Xerophthalmia (See for colour figure Plate 10)

Eventually, *panophthalmitis* leads to almost total destruction of not just the cornea but that of the whole eyeball. Irreversible blindness (which was entirely preventable) is the final outcome, the eye ending up as a shrunken globe.

During the course of destruction of the globe, retina does not lag behind in suffering. On fundoscopy, it reveals small white spots and granules, the so-called *fundus ophthalmicus*.

B. Extraocular Features

The extraocular manifestation of vitamin A deficiency include:

- Dry, scaly skin, especially lining of the hair follicles and sebaceous glands over the outer aspect of the limbs (the so-called "follicular hyperkeratosis," "toad skin" or "phrynoderma").
- Hypertrophy or even atrophy of tongue,
- Increased susceptibility to infections due to squamous metaplasia of respiratory, urinary and vaginal tract epithelium as a result of impaired immune response (both specific and nonspecific); renal and visical calculus may occur more often in such subjects.
- Growth failure.
- Anemia.
- Diarrhea.
- Cognitive deterioration.
- Pseudotumor cerebri.

Diagnosis

High index of suspicion from the clinical picture is the most important diagnostic measure. Support may be obtained from the dark adaptation test to detect early xerophthalmia.

Objective tests to detect marginal vitamin A deficiency include:

- *Conjunctival impression cytology (CIC).*
- *Vital staining of xerotic conjunctiva* (Rose Bengal, Lissamine, Kajal or other maskera) supplement clinical diagnosis of xerophthalmia.
- A relative dose response.
- Modified relative dose response.
- Determination of plasma or liver retinol (vitamin A) level is of doubtful value.
- Giving 0.2 ml/kg of cod liver oil by mouth may carry out Vitamin A absorption test. Blood samples are obtained before its administration and thereafter at 3,5,7,9 and 12 hours. Afterwards, a curve is plotted from the vitamin A values obtained on these samples. A flat curve indicates defective absorption.

Treatment

The currently recommended WHO/UNICEF schedule for

treatment of xerophthalmia is summarized in Table 101.3 It needs to be clearly noted that it is now advisable to use an oily preparation for oral and a water-miscible preparation for injection.

It is noteworthy that abuse of vitamin A may cause toxicity (hypervitaminosis A). Manifestations may include irritability, lassitude, alopecia, anorexia, fever, benign raised intracranial pressure (pseudotumor cerebri) and hard tender swellings over the bones. Steroids may be of help if used early enough in these cases. Almost all cases recover fully without any sequelae. Rarely, deaths are, however, reported.

Table 101.3: WHO/UNICEF treatment schedule of xerophthalmia

Children 1 to 6 years and above	
Immediately on diagnosis	200,000 IU vitamin A (O)
The following day	200,000 IU vitamin A (O)
Four weeks later	200,000 IU vitamin A (O)
Children under 1 year and under 8 kg weight at any age	
Half the doses as indicated for children 1 to 6 years and above	
For night blindness or Bitot spot	
Treat with a daily dose of	10,000 IU of vitamin A (O) for 2 weeks

Note: If there is a persistent vomiting or profuse diarrhea, an intramuscular injection of 100,000 IU of water-miscible vitamin A (but not an oil-based preparation) may be substituted for the first dose.

Prevention

An intake of at least 1500 IU/day in infants and children less than 4 years and 5000 IU/day in grown-up children should be ensured. Just milk meets this requirement in infants. Older children need leafy vegetables and red palm oil in addition to milk.

According to the *National Vitamin A Prophylaxis Program*, all children in the age group 6 months to 6 years in the target areas should receive 2,000,000 IU of vitamin A (in an oily base) orally every six months. By the 5th birthday, the child is expected to receive 9 oral doses of vitamin A. The agent is supplied as syrup of 100,000 units of vitamin A per ml.

For preventive purposes, use of P-carotene-rich foods, dark green leafy vegetables (DGLV), say mustard (sarson), spinach (palak), fenugreek (methi), amaranth (chaulai), drumstick (sahjan), yellow vegetables (carrot), yellow fruits (mango, orange, papaya) and vitamin A-rich foods, say fish, liver, fresh liver oil, dairy products and edible oils, should be encouraged. "Vision by vegetables" is a good slogan.

Dark green leafy vegetables are an inexpensive and superb source of P-carotene (precursor of vitamin A). Just 40 g of GLV cooked with 2 to 3 g of oil provide 1200 μg of β-carotene, which is the recommended daily allowance (RDA) as per WHO. Even in malnourished children, absorption of β-carotene is about 70 percent. Children are able to eat enough (GLV) from a single traditional meal to meet their vitamin A requirement.

Fortification of commonly eaten foods with vitamin A can be an effective prophylactic measure in a population.

Finally, adequate and timely treatment of PEM, intestinal parasitosis and diarrheal disease, especially with supplementation of the intake with dark-green leafy vegetables and edible oil, goes a long way in preventing xerophthalmia.

The pregnant and lactating mothers should get enough of retinol or carotene in their diets.

Premature babies need vitamin A since they have poor lipid absorption.

KEY LEARNING POINTS

- Vitamin A deficiency (VAD) usually occurs in association with malnutrition and chronic intestinal disorders, pancreatic disease and hepatic insufficiency.
- Clinical manifestation may be both ocular (ranging from night blindness to xerophthalmia fundi) and extraocular (ranging from dry, scaly skin to pseudotumor cerebri).
- Diagnosis needs a high index of suspicion followed, if need be, by dark adaptation test and an objective test like conjunctival impression biopsy.
- For treatment, it is advisable to follow the WHO/UNICEF schedule, employing oil-based preparation for oral and a water-miscible preparation for injection.
- Prevention lies in ensuring a minimal of 1500 IU/day and 5000 IU/day before and after 4 years of age, respectively.

FURTHER READINGS

1. Gropper SS, Smith JL, Groff JL. *Advanced Nutrition and Human Metabolism,* 4th edn. Belmount: Thomson Wadsworth 2005.
2. Morelli JG. Nutritional dermatosis. In: Klioegman RM, Behrman RE, Jenson HB , Staton BF (eds): *Nelson Textbook of Pediatrics,* 18th edn. New Delhi: Jaypee 2008: 2767:2769.
3. Oumeish OY, Oumeish I. Nutritional skin problems in children. *Clin Dermatol* 2002;19:426-431.
4. Sommer A. *Vitamin A Deficiency and its Consequences: Field Guide to their Detection and Control,* 3rd edn. Geneva: World Health Organization 1995.

102 Vitamin B-Complex Deficiency States

Suraj Gupte

INTRODUCTION

The term, *vitamin B-complex*, include several factors with varying chemical composition and function (thiamine, riboflavin, niacin, pyridoxine, biotin, vitamin B_{12} and folate). All these vitamins form important constituents of a closely-related enzyme system. Deficiency of any single constituent is usually accompanied by deficiency of other constituents. Understandably, therefore, manifestations of several vitamin B deficiencies coexist in the same child.

THIAMINE DEFICIENCY

Thiamine (vitamin B_1), a water-soluble vitamin, is an essential coenzyme for metabolism of carbohydrates, especially in oxidative decarboxylation of pyruvic acid to acetyl-coenzyme A and other alpha-ketoacids in the Kreb cycle. It is believed to play vital role in the nutrition of heart and peripheral nerves.

It is freely distributed in animal and vegetable products such as liver, egg, yolk, pork, legumes, yeast, pericarp and germ of cereals, autolysed yeast (marmite), and milk. Polishing the rice considerably destroys its thiamine content.

Etiology

Thiamine deficiency occurs either because of poor intake in the diet, malabsorption states, or prolonged illness.

Clinical Features

Thiamine deficiency leads to the disease, *beriberi* which occurs usually in infants (*wet beriberi*) though older infants and children may also suffer from its chronic form (*dry beriberi*). *Meningitic form* is also known.

The earliest symptoms, occurring in early infancy (especially if the mother is providing thiamine-deficient breast milk), include restlessness, bouts of excessive crying (as if the infant is having an abdominal colic), vomiting, abdominal distention, flatulence, constipation and insomnia.

In the acute cardiac form (wet beriberi), the infant may develop congestive cardiac failure in the form of tachycardia, gallop rhythm, dyspnea, cyanosis, hepatomegaly, cardiomegaly, edema and pulmonary edema. The possibility of thiamine deficiency should always be considered in endemic areas in subjects presenting with intractable congestive cardiac failure.

In the chronic neurologic form (dry beriberi), the manifestations may include anorexia, weight loss, weakness, diarrhea, constipation and edema. The child is usually drowsy and apathetic. Ataxia is common. There may be peripheral neuritis and various palsies, including hoarseness due to vocal cord paralysis, and nystagmus. Deep tendon reflexes are usually absent.

In the meningitic form The clinical picture is dominated by bulging anterior fontanel, dilated pupils, head retraction and coma. Convulsions may occur, leading to a mistaken diagnosis of encephalitis or meningitis. CSF reveals no abnormality.

In addition to all this, thiamine dependency has been incriminated in the etiology of:

i. Anomalies of branched chain ketoacid decarboxylase system, e.g. maple syrup urine disease, and
ii. Syndrome of optic atrophy, intermittent ataxia, lactic acidosis and hyperalaninemia due to pyruvate decarboxylase deficiency.

Differential Diagnosis

Differential diagnosis may have to be made from pyloric stenosis and other high obstruction in the presence of troublesome vomiting. Endomyocardial fibroelastosis, congenital heart disease and glycogen storage disease involving the heart (Pompe disease) may be considered in the presence of CCF. Chronic neurologic form would require differentiation from lead poisoning. Meningitic form may be confused with meningitis or encephalitis. A normal CSF may prove most helpful in such a situation.

Diagnosis

Diagnosis of beriberi is more or less clinical. In fact, a dramatic response to thiamine therapy within few hours is the best test of its deficiency. However, if facilities are available, the following investigations may be done:

1. Blood thiamine level < 4 μg/dl (normal is 10 ± 5μg/dl) is suggestive.
2. Milk thiamine level < 7 μg/dl.
3. Red cell transketolase level is low.

Treatment

As soon as the diagnosis is convincingly made, the child must receive 10 mg of thiamine intravenously. In the subsequent three days, he should be given 10 mg of the vitamin intramuscularly twice daily. Over the next six weeks, 10 mg daily should be administered orally.

The breastfeeding mother should receive thiamine (50 mg/day) therapy simultaneously.

Prognosis

Prognosis is excellent provided reasonable intake of thiamine is ensured.

Prevention

Ensuring that at least 0.4 mg of thiamine is provided in the daily diet (thrice the quantity in case of pregnant and lactating women) prevents beriberi. This requirement is met via a mixed diet containing fresh mashed fruits and vegetables plus whole grain cereals after 6 months of age (the period of exclusive breastfeeding).

RIBOFLAVIN DEFICIENCY

Riboflavin (vitamin B_2), another water-soluble vitamin, is a constituent of flavoprotein enzymes vitally concerned with the intermediary metabolism of carbohydrates. It is found in both animal and vegetable foods such as liver, fish, egg, kidney, meat, beans, yeast, green leafy vegetables, cereals, legumes, groundnut and milk (5 times more in cow milk than in human milk).

Often, deficiencies of thiamine and riboflavin may be coexisting. This relationship is now widely recognized.

Etiology

Since both breast milk and cow milk provide sufficient riboflavin for infant's needs, its deficiency usually occurs in children on restricted protein intakes or with dominant protein malabsorption state.

Its deficiency may also occur in infants under phototherapy because of its being subject to photo-degradation.

Clinical Features

Manifestations include angular stomatitis, cheilosis (fissuring of lips), nasolabial seborrhea and, occasionally, magenta (purplish-red, smooth) tongue. There may occur corneal injection (vascularization) at the limbus, leading to excessive lacrimation, photophobia, eye pain and later interstitial keratitis.

Diagnosis

Diagnosis is essentially clinical. Laboratory investigations include:

1. Urinay excretion of riboflavin less than 30 μg/24 hours.
2. Excretion of less than 125 μg of riboflavin/g of creatinine in a random urine sample.
3. Increased erythrocyte glutathione reductase activity after the addition of flaving adenine dinucleotide (FAD).

Treatment

Therapy consists in administering riboflavin, 3 to 10 mg orally or 2 mg intramuscularly daily for a few days. This should be followed by 10 mg orally daily for about three weeks.

With this regimen, response is good. Complete recovery occurs provided that adequate intake of vitamin B_2 is ensured in the weeks and months ahead.

Prevention

In order to prevent riboflavin deficiency, it should be ensured that the daily diet provides at least 0.6 mg riboflavin per 1,000 kcal. It is advisable to administer supplements of riboflavin (the whole B-complex may be still better) to the infants and children belonging to vulnerable categories.

NICOTINIC ACID DEFICIENCY

Nicotinic acid (niacin) is also involved in the carbohydrate metabolism and plays vital role in the functioning of the skin, gastrointestinal tract, central nervous system and hemopoietic system.

This vitamin may be obtained either from the natural food sources or from the tryptophan endogenously. The natural food sources include milk, liver, pork, cheese, yeast, cereals, etc.

Etiology

Nicotinic acid deficiency is usually encountered in children receiving a maize diet as staple, in chronic diarrhea, in malabsorption states, and in anorexic states.

Clinical Features

The disease caused by nicotinic acid deficiency is called *pellagra*. It usually occurs in children of school-going age.

The characteristic lesions are seen over the exposed areas of the skin, such as limbs, neck ("Casal necklace") and cheeks. It is worth noting that the lesions are symmetrical, of desquamating pigmentary dermatitis type and are aggravated by sunlight.

There is a widespread gastrointestinal inflammation, leading to red and sore tongue, dysphagia, nausea, vomiting and diarrhea.

Just like diarrhea, dementia is encountered much less in childhood than in adults. Most children with pellagra are, no doubt, quite apathetic.

Anemia as also other signs of malnutrition are usually present.

Diagnosis

It is purely clinical.

At times, severe protein-energy malnutrition in the form of kwashiorkor may warrant differentiation. Remember that in kwashiorkor the skin lesion tend to be around pressure sites and flexure surfaces in the trunk, groin and knee rather than over the exposed parts as is typical of pellagra.

Treatment

Nicotinamide, 50 to 300 mg daily in divided doses orally, given for two weeks followed by adequate supply of B-complex vitamins in diet brings about complete recovery.

Prevention

The disease may be prevented by providing a balanced diet containing 5 to 10 mg daily supply of nicotinamide.

PYRIDOXINE (VITAMIN B_6) DEFICIENCY

Pyridoxine along with pyridoxal and pyridoxamine (vitamin B_6) play a vital role in the metabolism of proteins and fatty acids. It is claimed to have a role in blood formation, in proper functioning of the nervous system and in conversion of tryptophan into nicotinic acid.

Its natural sources include liver, egg yolk, meat, wheat germ, soyabean, yeast, peas, pulses and cereals. It is found in only small quantity in most vegetables and milk.

Etiology

Pyridoxine deficiency of nutritional origin is rare in childhood—in fact, in humans as such. Deficiency may, however, complicate prolonged isoniazid or cycloserine therapy in tuberculosis or penicillamine therapy in Wilson disease.

Pyridoxine-responsive convulsions and anemia have been described. Pyridoxine-dependecy inborn errors of metabolism, e.g. homocystinuria, cystathioinuria, xanthurenic aciduria, kynureninase deficiency and hyperoxaluria, are also reported.

Clinical Features

The manifestations include convulsions and microcytic-hypochromic anemia refractory to iron therapy. Growth retardation and gastrointestinal symptoms like diarrhea may occur. Seborrheic dermatitis around nose and eyes, and sensory neuropathy occur only uncommonly in children. Cheilosis and glossitis are infrequent in childhood.

Diagnosis

High sense of suspicion of vitamin B_6, deficiency in infants with persistent convulsions, provided that hypoglycemia, hypocalcemia and birth injury have been excluded, would help to diagnose this condition. Such an infant should receive 50 to 100 mg of pyridoxine intravenously. If the response is gratifying, diagnosis is quite probable. The confirmation of diagnosis may be done by the tryptophan loading test.

The same applies to anemia refractory to iron deficiency.

Treatment

Administration of 5 mg of pyridoxine intramuscularly followed by 0.5 mg daily orally for two weeks causes complete recovery.

BIOTIN DEFICIENCY

Biotin is produced by a number of micro-organisms. Hence, its deficiency is rare.

Etiolopathogenesis

Most common cause of biotin deficiency is parenteral nutrition. Secondly, it may occur in children consuming raw egg white. The latter is supposed to contain a substance, *avidin,* that is a biotin antagonist. Thirdly, it may be encountered in babies whose mothers are biotin deficient.

There is an accumulation of organic acids in the body. As a result, the child develops organic aciduria, especially propionic acid and dicarboxylic acid.

Clinical Manifestations

These include skin lesions such as orofacial lesions, brawny dermatosis and alopecia, and neurologic symptoms in the form of somnolence, hallucinations, hypotonia and hyperesthesia.

Treatment

Clinical and biochemical response to administration of biotin (10 mg) establishes the diagnosis suspected on the basis of clinical presentation and presence of organic aciduria.

Prevention

The parenteral hyperalimentation, being the most common cause of biotin deficiency, addition of biotin in the parenteral nutrition prevents its deficiency to a large extent.

VITAMIN B_{12} (COBALAMIN) DEFICIENCY

Vitamin B_{12} is synthesized from cobalamin, mainly in animal sources. After ingestion, it is released in the acidity of the stomach. Here it combines with the intrinsic factor and R proteins. In the duodenum, the pancreatic proteases break down the R proteins. It is absorbed in the distal ileum. Physiologic requirement is 1-5 mcg/day.

Etiology

It results from:

1. Inadequate dietary intake.
2. Deficiency of intrinsic factor in the stomach.
3. Malabsorption.
4. Absence of vitamin B_{12} transport protein.

Table 102.1 list the important causes of vitamin B_{12} deficiency.

Table 102.1: Important causes of vitamin B_{12} deficiency

Inadequate Intake
- Strict vegetarianism
- Infants of mothers who are deficient in vitamin B_{12}

Intrinsic Factor Deficiency
- Congenital pernicious anemia
- Gastric surgery

Malabsorption
- Inflammatory bowel disease
- Celiac disease
- Tropical sprue
- Surgical excision of terminal ileum
- Fish tapeworm (*Diphylbothrium latum*)

Absence of Vitamin B_{12} Transport Protein
- Transcobalamin II (TC-II) deficiency (the main transport vehicle for this vitamin)

Clinical Manifestations

These include anemia, generalized weakness, fatigue, failure to thrive, irritability, glossitis, vomiting, diarrhea and jaundice.

Neurologic manifestations (which may occur even in the absence of anemia) include paresthesia, sensory deficit, tremors, hypotonia, developmental delay/regression, seizures and neuropsychiatric symptoms.

Laboratory Diagnosis

Peripheral blood film shows macrocytic anemia with marked macro-ovalocytosis of the RBCs.

Neutrphils are large and hypersegmented. Neutropenia and thrombocytopenia in advanced deficiency may be confused with aplastic anemia or leukemia.

Srum B_{12} level is <100 pg/mL.

Serum LDH activity very high because of poor erythopoiesis.

Serum bilirubin may be somewhat increased (usually 2-3 mg/dL).

Methylmalonic acid excretion in urine (normal 0-3.5 mg/4 hours) is a reliable and sensitive index of vitamin B_{12} deficiency.

Schiling test is indicated when there is no obvious cause for vitamin B_{12} deficiency.

Box 102.1: Schilling Test

Indication: When no detectable cause for vitamin B_{12} deficiency is forthcoming.

Principle: When a normal individual ingests a small amount of vitamin B_{12} + ^{57}Co (an isotope), the radioactive vitamin combines with the intrinsic facor in the stomach secretions and passes to the terminal ileum where it is absorbed. This small amount of radioactive vitamin B_{12} is hardly excreted in urine. Two hours later, a large "flushing dose" (1 mg) of nonradioactive vitamin B_{12} is administered parenterally. Around 10-30% of the radioactive vitamin normally appears in the 24 hours urine.

Procedure and Interpretation: The procedure as described above is followed in the suspected case. If the amount passed in 24 hours hours is < 10%, it could either be intrinsic factor deficiency or malabsorption. To differentiate between the two, along with the second dose of radioactive vitamin, 30 mg of intrinsic factor is also given. In case of deficiency of intrinsic facor (pernicious anemia), normal amount of radioactive vitamin is absorbed and excreted in urine. In case of vitamin B_{12} malabsorption, absorption remains affected and excretion in urine is subnormal i.e. <10%. This is termed positive Schilling test. Whereas Schilling test result remains abnormal even subsequent to therapy, in malabsorption, it reverses to normal following successful treatment.

Diagnosis

When diagnosis is in doubt, a therapeutic trial may be conducted by administering a minidose which should result in a positive hematologic response.

Treatment

Following administration of parenteral vitamin B_{12} (1 mg), a prompt hematologic response usually with reticulocytosis occurs in 2-4 days.

In case of neurologic involvement, 1 mg should be injected intramuscularly daily for at least 2 weeks. Lifelong maintenance is through monthly intramuscular injections of 1 mg.

Though high doses given orally may be effective, it is not the preferred modality on account of uncertainty of absoption of vitamin B_{12}.

FOLIC ACID DEFICIENCIES

Folic acid-rich foods are green vegetables, fruits and meat, especially liver and kidney. Heating or boiling cuts down folic acid content of the food. It is absorbed throughout the small intestine. Normal daily requirement for infants is just 25-35 mcg.

Human milk provides adequate amount of it. Goat's milk is deficient in it.

Etiology

Folic acid deficiency follows:

1. Inadequate folate intake.
2. Folate malabsorption.

3. Folate metabolism disorders (both congenital and acquired).

Table 102.2 list the important causes of folic acid deficiency.

Table 102.2: Important causes of folic acid deficiency

Inadequate Folate Intake
- Pregnant and lactating mothers with folate deficiency
- Enhanced needs during active growing periods
- PEM: Kwashiorkor, marasmus

Malabsorption of Folate
- Chronic diarrheal states, especially celiac disease, tropical sprue
- Diffuse inflammatory conditions
- Previous intestinal surgery
- Anticonvulsant agents e.g. phenytoin, phenobarbital, primidone

Congenital Folate Metabolism Disorders
- Congenital dihydrofolate reductase deficiency
- Congenital methylene tetrahydrofolate reductase deficiency in homocystinuria

Acquired Folate Metabolism Disorders
- Methotrexate
- Pyrimethamine
- Trimethoprim

Clinical Manifestations

These include megaloblastic anemia (in case of LBW infants, having peak incidence at 4-7 months of age) with usual manifestations of anemia, irritability, failure to thrive and chronic diarrhea. In advanced anemia, bleeding secondary to thrombocytopenia may occur.

Serious dysmorphologic effects, especially neural tube defects, in the growing fetus may occur in case the mother is deficient in folic acid.

Laboratory Diagnosis

The blood picture mimics that of vitamin B_{12} deficiency.

Blood film shows macrocytic anemia (MCV > 100 fL) with variation in RBC size and shape (anisocytois and poikilocytosis) and nucleated RBCs.

Other findings include raised reticulocyte count, neutropenia and thrombocytopenia. Neutrophils are large, some having hypersegmented nuclei.

Folic acid level is < 3 ng/mL (normal 5-20 ng/mL).

RBC folate level is reduced (normal 150-600 ng/mL). It is a better index.

Serum lactate dehydrogenas (LDH) is very high.

Bone marrow is hypercellular from erythoid hyperplasia with megaloblastic changes and giant metamylocytes (which are abnormal neutrophilic forms) with cytoplasmic vacuolation and hypersegmented nuclei of the megakaryocytes are seen.

Treatment

Folic acid, 0.5-1.0 mg daily (O) leads to a positive hematologic response within 72 hours. This therapy should be continued for 3-4 weeks for definitive hematologic response. It is advisable to further continue maintenance therapy wih a multivitamin providing 0.2 mg of folate.

Prevention

Periconception administration of 400 mcg of folic acid daily by the mother considerably decreases the incidence of neural tube and other anatomic defects in the baby. It may also reduce incidence of premature labor.

Daily administration of 1 mg of folic acid with 5-100 mg of pyridoxine may reduce incidence of thrombotic events related to slightly high level of cystine in adults. However, supplements of vitamin B_{12} and betadine in small doses need to be given side by side for normalizing homocystine levels.

KEY LEARNING POINTS

- *Thiamine deficiency* causes beriberi which may be of two forms, namely wet beriberi and dry beriberi; occasionally meningic beriberi may be encountered.
- *Riboflavin deficiency* causes, among other manifestations, angular stomatitis, cheilosis, nasolabial seborrhea and magenta tongue.
- *Nicotinic acid (niacin) deficiency* causes pellagra which is characterized by dermatosis of exposed areas of skin, diarrhea and dementia which in children is in only a subtle form (say, mental apathy).
- *Pyridoxine (vitamin B_6 deficiency* may present as seizures, microcytic-hypochromic anemia refractory to iron therapy, growth retardation and diarrhea.
- *Biotin deficiency* manifests in the form of orofacial lesions, brawny dermatosis, alpecia plus neurologic symptoms.
- *Vitamin B_{12}* deficiency causes megaloblastic anemia and neurologic manifestations.
- *Folic acid deficiency* causes megaloblastic anemia and neural tube defects and facial dysmorphism in infants of deficient mothers.
- *Treatment* is in the form of replacement therapy.

FURTHER READINGS

1. Baxter P, Gardner-Medwin D, Kelly T, *et al.* Pyridoxine-dependent seizures: Demographic clinical MRI and psychometeic features and effect of dose on intelligence. *Dev Med Child Neurol* 1996;38:998-9-203.
2. Bowman BA, Russel RM. *Present Knowledge in Nutrition,* 8th edn. Washington: ILSI 2001.
3. Heird WC. Vitamin deficiencies and excesses. In: Kliegman RM, Behrman RE, Jenson HB, Stanto F (eds): *Nelson Textbook of Pediatrics,* 18th edn. Philadelphia: Saunders 2008: 177-190.

103 Scurvy

Suraj Gupte • Shally Sharma

INTRODUCTION

Deficiency of vitamin C (ascorbic acid), though not uncommon in its sub-clinical form, has virtually disappeared in its overt form (scurvy) from the affluent countries. However, its frank cases still continue to be seen from time to time in some parts of India and other developing regions.

The term, *scurvy,* is derived from the Nordic word *skyrbjugr,* meaning swelling or edema. It has also been suggested that the term is derived from the Old Icelandic words *skyrbugr, scarby and skurvic.*

BACKGROUND: OVERVIEW OF VITAMIN C

Table 103.1 provides salient features of Vitamin C

Table 103.1: Salient features of Vitamin C

Sources

Citrus fruits (lemon, orange, guava, Indian goose-berry (amla) and vegetables (tomatoes, potatoes, berries, cabbage, cauliflower, spinach. Heating/cooking has adverse effect on vitamin content of the foodstuff.

Characteristics

Water-soluble, easily oxidized, accelerated by heat, light, alkali, oxidative enzymes, traces of Fe and Fe.

Biochemical Action

An antioxidant maintains Fe and Cu ions in reduced state hydroxylases involved in collagen synthesis, metabolism of choloesterol and neurotransmitters may be needed to maintain folate in a reduced form; facilitates non-hem Fe absorption and Fe transfer from transferritin to ferritin.

Ascorbic acid (Vitamin C), which structurally resembles a monosaccharide sugar, is known to play important role:

- In oxidation of tyrosine and phenylalanine.
- In formation of hydroxyproline.
- In preventing depolymerization of collagen.
- In maintaining integrity of ground substance, and
- In hemopoiesis; enhances absorption of non-heme iron, transfer of iron from transferrin to ferritin, formation of tetrahydrofolic acid.

Contd.

Contd.

- As an important antioxidant (electron donor) in the aqueous milieu of the body.

Deficiency Signs

See text.

Toxicity

Gastrointestinal upset in the form of gastritis and diarrhea; oxaluria.

ETIOPATHOGENESIS

Scurvy may occur in the following situations:

- Primary protein-energy malnutrition, though during periods of gross retardation of growth, overt scurvy may not be seen as is the case with rickets.
- Secondary protein-energy malnutrition as in malabsorption.
- Exclusively artificially-fed infants.
- Even breastfed infants born to mothers deficient in vitamin C.
- Restrictive dietary habits: food faddism, exclusion diets with stress on avoidance of vitamin C-rich sour fruits.
- Vitamin C dependency occurring in newborns accustomed to saturation levels of vitamin C since the mother had been taking very high doses of it during pregnancy to prevent colds, etc.
- Infections which enhance the requirement of vitamin C.

The deficiency results in two major changes:

1. Impaired collagen synthesis, causing defective formation of osteoid and dentine.
2. Modification of the intercellular ground substance that binds the cells of the capillary walls. All this may lead to changes in the calcified tissues and capillary hemorrhages. In addition, there is an impaired wound healing and susceptibility to infections.

CLINICAL FEATURES

Scurvy occurs usually in infants, between the age of 6 months to 2 years. Nevertheless, no age is a bar, including adolescence.

Infantile scurvy is characterized by gross irritability, excessive crying, low grade fever, anorexia, tachypnea, GIT upset and generalized tenderness to touch, more so in the lower limbs. The infant adopts the so-called "frog-position" in which he lies with the lower limbs that are partially flexed at the knees and hips and externally rotated. The posture of the lower limbs gives an impression as though these are paralysed (pseudoparalysis).

The palpable *subperiosteal hemorrhage* into the lower third of the femur may contribute to pain, thus preventing movements of the leg further and strengthening the impression that the limb may be paralysed.

Hemorrhages may occur into the skin and mucous membranes. Hemorrhages into the gums may result in spongy, swollen, bluish purple gums, especially about the erupted teeth. Hemorrhages in the internal organs may cause hematuria, melena, proptosis and subdural swellings. Subperiosteal hemorrhage, usually involving lower third of the femur, may cause a clinically-detectable swelling along the shaft.

Mild to moderate anemia is usual *Scorbutic rosary* may result from posterior displacement of the sternum. Unlike rachitic rosary, it is tender, sharp and angular and has a "step-shaped" configuration, the sternum, being depressed (Fig. 103.1).

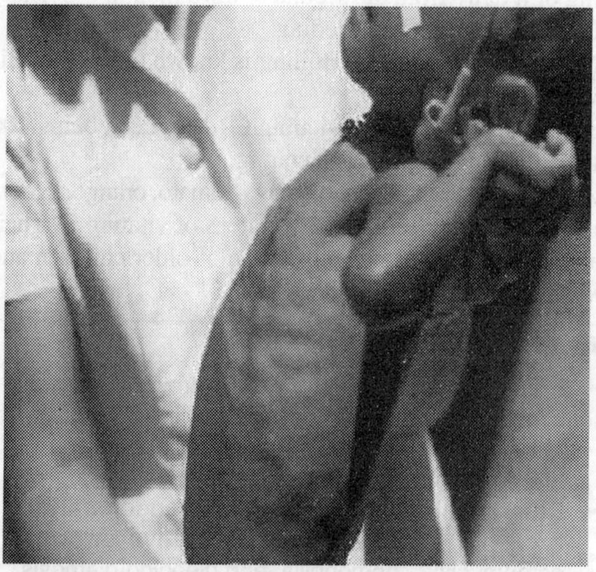

Fig. 103.1: Scorbutic rosary. Note the costochondral beading, which is sharp, angular and tender (See for colour figure Plate 10)

Childhood scurvy presents as follicular hyperkeratosis with development of minute hemorrhages at the root of the hair follicles. Bleeding into the skin, leading to petechiae or even large purpuric swellings, and into gums may occur but subperiosteal hemorrhages are infrequent. "Cork-screw" skin (Fig. 103.2) though less frequent, is characteristic.

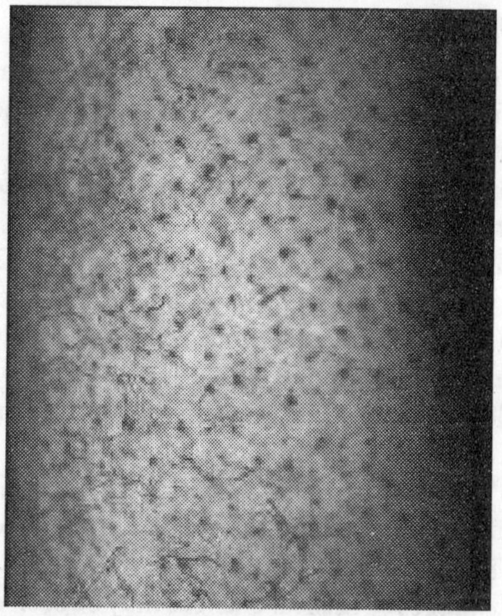

Fig. 103.2: Cork-screw appearance of skin (See for colour figure Plate 10)

Table 103.2: Dermatologic manifestations in scurvy

Initial
- Follicular hyperkeratosis
- Coiling of hair on upper arms, back, buttocks, lower limbs

Later
- Perifollicular erythema and hemorrhages, particularly on legs
- Pupura: Petechia
- Erythematous/bleeding gums
- Stomatitis
- Subperiosteal hematoma (usually in relation to lower third of femur)

Over and above these manifestations, the child may show poor wound and fracture healing, muscle weakness, degeneration of skeletal muscles, cardiac hypertrophy, bone marrow depletion and adrenal atrophy.

DIFFERENTIAL DIAGNOSIS

Pseudoparalysis of scurvy needs to be differentiated from the true paralysis of poliomyelitis. If the child is held at the shoulders and lifted, he will flex his legs and not allow these to touch the ground because of fear of pain in case of scurvy.

In ***poliomyelitis,*** the paralysis is truly flaccid. In this situation, the infant's legs will just fall helpless on the ground rather than be lifted as in scurvy.

Pseudoparalysis may also occur in ***syphilis***, ***suppurative arthritis*** and ***osteomyelitis***. In the former, other signs of the disease are usually present, whereas the latter two conditions are usually unilateral.

Subperiosteal hemorrhage causing swelling over lower end of femur may have to be differentiated from hemarthrosis of hemophilia.

Bleeding into skin and mucous membranes needs to be differentiated from the bleeding diathesis of purpura (Henoch-Schöenlein, idiopathic (immune) thrombocytopenic) and leukemia.

DIAGNOSIS

Following high index of suspicion based on clinical presentation, response to vitamin C is the most acceptable criteria for the diagnosis of scurvy.

The diagnosis may be confirmed by the following investigations:

- Ascorbic acid level in plasma and serum (<0.2 mg/dL), white cells (< 10 mcg/10^{8}) or buffy coat, i.e. platelet layer (usually < 0.1 mg%).
- Excretion of ascorbic acid in urine:
  - Below 1.5 mg after a loading dose of 20 mg/kg by intravenous route 4 hours earlier.
  - No or less than 20% excretion of ascorbic acid in urine after a loading dose of 10 mg/kg by oral route 24 hours earlier.
- *X-ray changes*: Classical changes may be seen especially in the X-ray knee including lower part of femur and upper parts of tibia and fibula (Fig.103.3).

  A dense irregular white line, called *white line of Fraenkel*, appears at the epiphyseal ends of the long bones. Subsequently, adjacent to this line occurs an area of destruction (rarefaction). This area is called *fracture zone*. This is very susceptible to fractures and fissuring. The projection of the white line laterally, away from the limit of the shaft, may lead to formation of a spur or marginal cleft. This is what is known as *Corner sign*. It has great diagnostic value.

The rarefied epiphyseal centers may be sharply outlined. This is termed signet-ring or simply "ringing" of the epiphysis. There may be epiphyseal separation also.

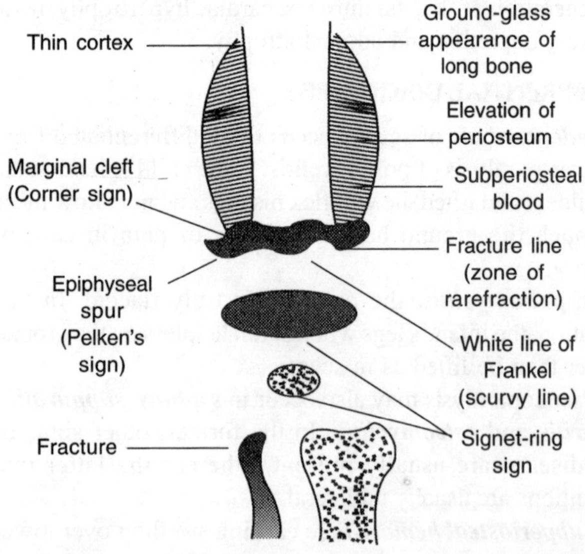

Fig. 103.3: Diagrammatic representation of radiological picture of scurvy

The cortex is thinned because of generalized osteoporosis and the trabeculae have *ground glass appearance*.

Large subperiosteal hemorrhage may lead to lifting of the periosteum. This is seen as a regional increase in the soft tissue density. The affected bone looks like a dumbell or a club. Later, when the hematoma is calcified during healing, it may become clearly visible in the X-ray.

In Menkes (kinky hair) disease, a sex-linked recessive neurodegenerative disorder due to copper deficiency, radiologic changes simulating scurvy may be observed.

TREATMENT

It consists in giving a loading dose of 500 mg of vitamin C followed by a daily dose of 100 to 200 mg daily for several weeks. Oral administration is good enough and should be the preferred choice. Alternatively, orange or tomato juice, around 100 ml daily may be given. The response is somewhat slower than with medicinal vitamin C.

Clinical response occurs rapidly—within 24 to 48 hours. Improvement in the radiological picture takes a week or two. Subperiosteal hemorrhages are likely to take months to disappear.

PREVENTION

Mothers should be encouraged:

- To exclusively breastfeed the babies for the first 6 months.
- To give supplements of vitamin C, providing about 25 mg of it daily from the second or third month, especially in infants on artificial feeding.
- Not to boil fruit juices. Boiling is known to destroy this vitamin.
- To consume additional vitamin C (daily need being 100 to 150 mg) while she is lactating.

Amla (Indian goose berry), guava, tomato, orange, lemon, peas, beans, etc. constitute rich sources of vitamin C. Their intake should be encouraged in case of older children and pregnant and lactating mothers.

KEY LEARNING POINTS

- Frank cases of scurvy, though now uncommon, continue to be seen from time to time.
- Manifestations of infantile and childhood scurvy are on somewhat different lines.
- Differential diagnosis is from pseudoparalysis (poliomyelitis, syphilis, suppurative arthritis, osteomyelitis, hemophilia, and bleeding diathesis.
- Diagnosis is by and large clinical with support from X-ray of knee, including lower part of femur and therapeutic response to vitamin C by mouth.

Specific treatment revolves round oral vitamin C and improvement in overall nutritional status.

FURTHER READINGS

1. Gropper SS, Smith JI, Groff JL. *Advanced Nutrition and Human Metabolism*, 4th edn. Belmont:Thomson Wadsworth 2005.

2. Morelli JG. Nutritional dermatosis. In: Kliegman RM, Behrman RE, Jenson HB, Staton BF (eds): *Nelson Textbook of Pediatrics*, 18th edn. Philadelphia: Saunders 2008: 2767:2769.
3. Naidu KA. Vitamin C in human health and disease is still a mystery? An overview. *Nutr J* 2003;2:7.
4. Olmedo JM, Yiannias JA, Windgassen EB, Gornet MK. Scurvy: A disease almost forgotten. *Int J Dermatol* 2006;45:909-913[Medline].
5. Oumeish OY, Oumeish I. Nutritional skin problems in children. *Clin Dermatol* 2002;19:426-431.
6. Tamura Y, Welch DC, Zic JA, *et al.* Scurvy presenting as painful gait with bruising in a young boy. *Arch Pediatr Adolesc Med* 2000;154:732-735.
7. Zile M, Chenoweth W. Vitamin C (ascorbic acid). In: Kliegman RM, Behrman RE, Jenson HB, Stanton BF (eds): *Nelson Textbook of Pediatrics*, 18th edn. Philadelphia: Saunders 2008: 251-253.

104 Nutritional Rickets

Suraj Gupte • Shally Sharma

INTRODUCTION

Nutritional rickets, predominantly secondary to vitamin D deficiency, continues to be a significant problem globally. It is encountered not only in India and other developing countries but also in the developed word. According to the UNICEF, 25% of infants and children in South-East Asia suffer from rickets.

BACKGROUND: OVERVIEW OF VITAMIN D

Table 104.1 provides the salient features of vitamin D, the most dominant cause of nutritional rickets.

Table 104.1: Salient features of vitamin D

Sources
Cutaneous synthesis employing sunlight (most important source), fish liver oil, fatty fish, egg yolk, milk.

Characteristics
The ultraviolet rays of the sunlight are responsible for converting the 7-dehydrocholesterol that is normally present under the skin, into vitamin D_3 or cholecalciferol. The latter is further converted to 25-hydroxycholecalciferol and 25-hydroxyergocalciferol in the liver. The last two forms are essential for maintenance of adequate calcium and phosphorus concentration in the extra cellular fluid and for the formation of bone matrix. It is now established that 25-HCC is then converted to 1,25-dihydroxy-cholecalciferol. The latter is specifically helpful in promoting synthesis of "calcium transport protein" in the intestinal wall.

Biochemical Action
Essential for formation of the bone matrix.

Deficiency Signs
See text.

Toxicity
Hyperostosis.

ETIOLOGY

Vitamin D deficiency produces rickets by failure of the growing bones to mineralize. Despite such a lot of sunshine, its incidence continues to be high in India and other countries of the Third World. This appears to be due to:

- Poor dietary intake of vitamin D and calcium and phosphorus.
- Poor exposure to sunlight. The latter seems to be related to the widely prevalent practice of covering the infants with loads of clothes and from living in slums and crowded places. Poor exposure to sunlight may also be related to the inactivity of the malnourished children.
- Poor ability of the dark skin to convert 7-dehydro-cholesterol to vitamin D_3 even when enough of sun exposure is available.

Disturbed metabolism, malabsorption state, diarrheal disease and excessive phylate with low calcium and low phosphate content of the diet may well be other causes of rickets in malnourished children.

Our repeated observations of development of rickets in later age-group too, suboptimal intake of calcium and more gratifying response to a combination of vitamin D and calcium than to vitamin D alone in India strongly indicate both vitamin D and calcium (and perhaps phosphate too) deficiency contribute to the continuing high incidence of nutritional rickets in India and other developing countries. Obviously the problem of calcium deficiency (perhaps, in association with phosphate deficiency), in addition to vitamin D deficiency, in etiology of rickets in developing countries needs greater consideration. The preventive as well as therapeutic implications of this observation are vital.

PREVALENCE

Conservatively speaking, vitamin deficiency ricket should be the problem of temperate climate. Paradoxically, howerver, it has more or less disappeared from the temperate zones, except in migrant black population, in bed-ridden institutionalized children and in areas where milk supply is not fortified with vitamin D. This is ascribed to health education, enrichment of milk with vitamin D, wide use of vitamin D concentrates, and better standard of living and better health and medical care.

The problem of rickets in India is much greater than its extent suggested by the descriptions in various texts. In our experience, every other child in the age group 6 months to 5 years attending the children outpatient has evidence of active rickets, which is often missed because of some other dominating presenting problem.

A high proportion of older children too have evidence of old rickets.

Congenital rickets is a rare entity occurring in neonates of mothers suffering from osteomalacia.

CLINICAL FEATURES

Rickets is a disease of rapid growing period. The peak incidence is encountered in the age group 6 months to 2 years. It is uncommon in infants under 3 months of age.

The earliest manifestations are quite vague and nonspecific. These include irritability, restlessness and profuse sweating over the head (more so during sleep).

Major signs encountered in overt rickets are summarized as follows:

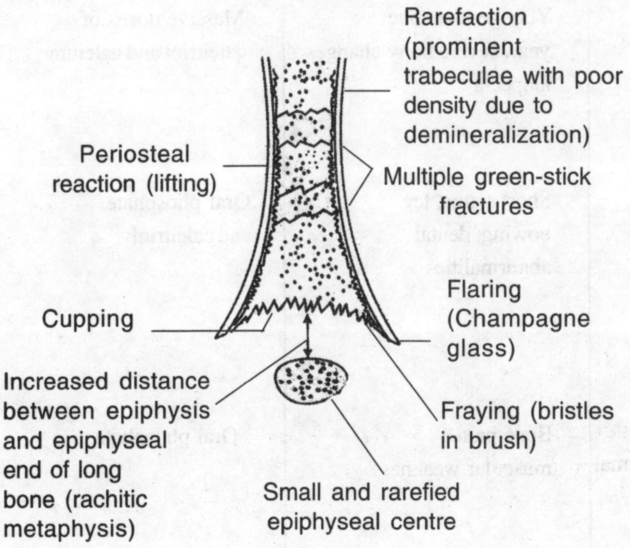

Fig. 104.1: Rickets: Diagrammatic representation of radiologic appearance of radius

Head: Bossing (frontal and parietal, macrocephaly with flattening of vertex (box head), increased size and delayed closure of fontanels, craniotabes (a peculiar softening of occipital and posterior parietal bones which give in like a ping-pong ball under pressure from thumb). At times, craniotabes may be encountered in normal preterm babies. Remember, preterm infants have higher incidence of rickets compared to full-term infants.

Teeth: Delayed dentition.

Thorax: Rachitic rosary (smooth rounded, nontender costochondral beading), pigeon-chest deformity (pectus carinatum), Harrison sulcus or groove (a depression along the insertion of diaphragm into the ribs), flaring of lowers ribs. "Violin-shaped" deformed chest is characteristic. Infrequently, sternum is unusually depressed, the so-called *pectus excavatum*. A concavity at inferior angle of scapula may be detected.

Spine: Scoliosis, Kyphosis.

Limbs: Widening of wrists (Fig. 104.2), ankles (with double malleoli) and other epiphyses due to expansion and cupping of growing ends of bones. Genu valgum (knock knees genu varum (bowlegs) may result.

Miscellaneous: As a result of poor muscle tone and relaxation of ligaments, the child may have delayed milestones, flat feet, pot-belly and some degree of visceroptosis so that liver may become palpable without its having been enlarged.

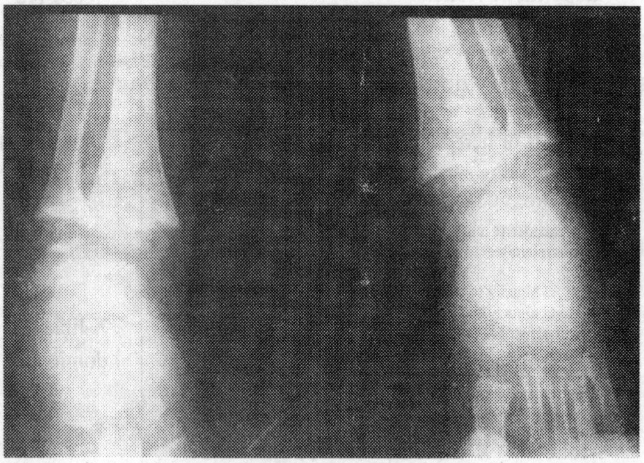

Fig. 104.2: Healing rickets
Note prominent line of preparatory calcification and restoration of joint space

At times, laxity of ligaments may be of such a magnitude that the limbs can be bent in to any position. *Acrobatic rickets* is the name given to this condition. Constipation is often present. Rarely, tetany may accompany rickets due to reduced level of ionized calcium in plasma.

If rickets is not adequately treated in time, bone deformities may be left as scar the so-called "old rickets". Short statute may also follow.

DIFFERENTIAL DIAGNOSIS

Table 104.2 gives salient features of various types of rickets. However, in practice, differential diagnosis revolves around only a few conditions.

Physiologic bowing of the legs seen in some healthy toddlers due to normal deposition of adipose tissue over the lateral aspects is not accompanied by other signs of rickets and disappears in due course of time without any

Table 104.2: Salient features of various types of rickets

Type of rickets	*Causes*	*Inheritance pattern*	*Clinical features*	*Line of treatment*
A. Nutritional rickets of vitamin D-deficiency rickets	Vitamin D deficiency, phosphorus or calcium deficiency (rare), inadequate sunlight exposure, secondary to malabsorption, syndromes [IBD, celiac disease, cystic fibrosis (rarely)]	NA	Skeletal findings, abnormal gait, hypocalcemic tetany/seizures, developmental delay, failure to thrive	Replace the deficient nutrient Vitamin D, calcium and phosphate
B. Vitamin D-dependent rickets Type I or pseudovitamin D-deficiency rickets	Deficiency of renal 25 (OH) D_3-1-alpha-hydroxylase	Autosomal recessive	Younger than two years, hypocalcemic tetany, severe bony changes, seizure	Calcitriol (Rocaltrol)
Type II or hereditary 1-alpha, 25-dihydroxyvitamin D-resistant rickets	Defective interaction between calcitriol and receptor	Autosomal recessive	Younger than one year, severe bony changes alopecia	Massive doses of calcitriol and calcium
C. Vitamin D-resistant rickets Familial hypophosphatemic rickets (X-linked hypophosphatemic rickets)	Impaired proximal renal tubular reabsorption of phosphorus and inappropriately normal calcitriol levels	X-linked dominant	Short statue, leg bowing, dental abnormalities	Oral phosphate and calcitriol
Hereditary hypophosphatemic rickets with hypercalciuria	Impaired proximal renal tubular reabsorption of phosphorus and increased calcitriol	Autosomal recessive, autosomal dominant	Bone pain, muscular weakness	Oral phosphate
D. Miscellaneous Renal rickets	Loss of functional renal parenchyma caused by chronic renal failure leads to mineral derangements and decreased calcitriol production	NA	Bone pain, arthralgias, fractures, muscle weakness, failure to thrive	Vitamin D and phosphate-binding compound
Rickets of prematurity	Multifactorial	NA	Osteopenia, fractures	Replace dietary deficiencies and minimize iatrogenic cuases
Oncogenic rickets	Tumor-induced inhibition of renal 25 (OH)D_3-1-alpha-hydroxylase	NA	Fractures, bone pain, muscle weakness	Treat underlying malignancy

treatment. Similarly, slight valgus position of the feet may cause some degree of *physiologic genu valgum* without any other rickety deformity.

Renal rickets may result from deficiency in the tubular reabsorption of phosphate or cystinosis. In the former condition, called phosphaturic rickets or late rickets, manifestations develop at a later age than is usual in the infantile rickets and it is resistant to usual doses of vitamin D. It is encountered more often in girls but is more advanced when boys are affected. In cystinosis (*Fanconi syndrome*), cystine crystals are found throughout the reticuloendothelial system and there are multiple renal tubular defects (glycosuria, aminoaciduria, tubular acidosis, phosphaturia, potassium loss, and, at times, uricosuria and sodium loss). The rickets associated with this condition needs heavy doses of vitamin D (50 thousand to 3 lakh units/day) for healing.

Pseudodeficiency rickets (*hereditary vitamin D-dependent rickets*), an autosomal recessive disorder involving deficiency of α-25 (OH)2 D_3, is characterized by severe rickets which develop in early infancy but which fail to respond to vitamin D therapy upto 4,000 units/day. It responds to long-term massive doses of it or still better to oral therapy with α-hydroxyvitamin D_3. Hypocalcemia is characteristic of this variety of rickets.

Celiac rickets, in fact rickets associated with any major malabsorption state, is most readily excluded by tests of intestinal absorption and histology.

DIAGNOSIS

Biochemical findings include raised alkaline phosphatase (except in malnourished children), usually normal serum calcium and reduced phosphorus. Today, reduction in the serum 25-hydroxy vitamin D level is considered a sensitive and reliable index of rickets even in malnourished children.

X-ray findings are best seen at the wrist (Fig. 104.3 and 104.4). These include a trio of changes at the the lower ends of radius and ulna.

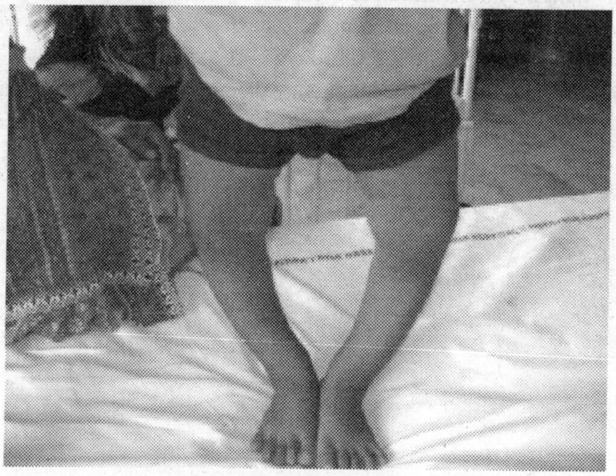

Fig. 104.3: Bow leg deformity

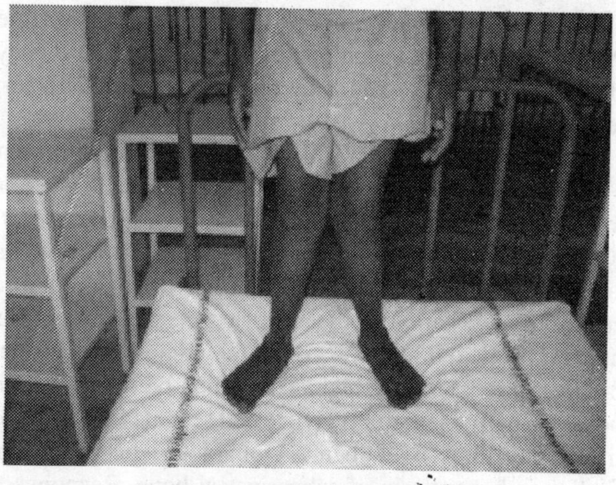

Fig. 104.4: Knock knee deformity

- Cupping (saucer-like depression)
- Flaring/splaying (widening)
- Fraying (rarefaction)

Additional radiologic findings include:

- Long bones giving the "champagne glass" appearance.
- Increase in the distance between the epiphyseal center and shaft of long bones due to radio-translucency of the osteoid.
- Periosteal reaction.
- Prominence of trabeculae.

TREATMENT

Drug Treatment

Specific treatment consists in administering a single massive dose of vitamin D_3 (3,00,000 units upto 1 year of age; 6,00,000 units for later ages) orally or intramuscularly together with supplementary calcium and phosphorus. Though serum alkaline phosphatase and phosphorus followed by calcium tend to return to normal within just 5-7 days, apparent radiological healing is seen in 7 to 14 days. Physical examination findings may normalize within 6 months.

In order to achieve real consolidation of cure, it may be desirable to give additional one or two periodic massive doses of vitamin D as also supplementary calcium and phosphorus in the subsequent months.

Careful monitoring is required for:

- Serum calcium, phosphorus, alkaline phosphatase and calcidiol levels.
- Urine calcium and phosphorus.
- Urine calcium to creatinine ratio to detect hypercalciuria.

Alternatively,

1. 60,000 units of vitamin D_3 daily orally for 10 days.
2. 20,000 units of vitamin D_3 daily orally for 30 days.

A poor response to adequate doses of vitamin D indicates refractory or resistant rickets due to malabsorption state, chronic renal disease (renal rickets), hypophosphatemia, hypocalcemia, Fanconi syndrome or Lowe syndrome. Prolonged anticonvulsant therapy, magnesium deficiency, chronic liver disease, etc. may also lead to unsatisfactory response.

Overdosage (at least 50,000 IU daily for a minimum of 3 weeks) may cause *hypervitaminosis D*. The manifestations resembling the so-called *"infantile cortical hyperostosis"* (Caffey disease) include irritability, anorexia, hypotonia, constipation, polydipsia polyuria, dehydration, anemia, calciuria, metastatic calcification, aortic valvular stenosis, hypertension, retinopathy, cornea cloudiness and growth failure. ESR is usually high. There may be fever. Certain bones (usually mandible, clavicle and scapula) develop soft tissue swellings over them. A characteristic radiologic finding is hyperplasia of subperiosteal bone. Response to withdrawal of vitamin D and calcium and therapy with aluminium hydroxide, cortisone or chelating agent, sodium versenate, is good.

Orthopedic Treatment

Gross orthopedic deformities, especially in adolescents, may occasionally need surgical correction (say, osteotomy).

PREVENTION

- Availability of at least 400 IU of vitamin D through sunshine, diet or supplements must be ensured. Health education to parents against over clothing the infants and young children and proper housing should be given.
- Vitamin D supplements to all exclusively-breastfed infants and vulnerable older children.
- Consumption of high calcium-containing foods by infants and children (Table 104.2).

Table 104.2: Foodstuffs providing calcium

- ***Rich Source***
  - Milk
  - Dairy products (cheese, ice cream, yogurt)
  - Greens (Spinach)
  - Pizza
- ***Poor Source***
  - Chicken
  - Cheeseburger
  - French fries

KEY LEARNING POINTS

- Both vitamin D and calcium (perhaps, phosphate too) appear to be contributing to the continuing high incidence of nutritional rickets in India and other developing countries.
- Diagnosis in a suspected case is confirmed by biochemical findings and X-ray findings.
- Differential diagnosis is from physiologic bowing, renal rickets, celiac rickets and pseudodeficiency rickets.
- Specific treatment is in the form of vitamin D_3 plus supplementary calcium and phosphorus, a poor response poisoning to refractory or resistant rickets.

FURTHER READINGS

1. Bhalala U, Desai M, Parekh P, Mukal R, Chheda B. Subclinical hypovitaminosis D among exclusively breastfed young infants. *Indian Pediatr* 2007;44:897-901.
2. Bisere-Rohrbaugh A, Hadley-Miller N. Vitamin D deficiency in breastfed toddlers. *J Pediatr Orthop* 2001;21:508-511.
3. Cesur Y, Caksen H, Gundem A, Kirimi E, Odabas D. Comparison of low and high dose vitamin D treatment in nutritional vitamin D deficiency rickets. *J Pediatr Endocrinol Metab* 2003;16:1105-1109.
4. Carvalho NF, Kenney RD, Carrington PH, Hall DE. Severe nutritional deficiencies in toddlers resulting from health food milk alternatives. *Pediatrics* 2001;107:E46.
5. DeLucia MC, Mitnick ME, Carpenter TO. Nutritional rickets with normal circulating 25-hyroxyvitamin D: A call for re-examining the role of dietary calcium intake in north American infants. *J Clin Endocrinol Metab* 2003;88:3539-3545.
6. Fitzpatrick S, Sheard NF, Clark NG, Ritter ML. Vitamin D-deficient rickets: A multifactorial disease. *Nutr Rev* 2000;58:218-222.
7. Kutluk G, Cetinkaya F, Bask M. Comparisons of oral calcium, high dose vitamin D and a combination of these in the treatment of nutritional rickets in children. *J Triop Pediatr 2002*;48:351-353.
8. Nield LS, Mahajan P, Joshi A, Kamat D. Rickets: Not a disease of the past. *Am Family Phys* 2006:74:1-12.
9. Peng LF, Serwint JR. A comparison of breatfed children with nutritional rickets who present during and after the first year of life. *Clin Pediatr* 2003;42:711-717.
10. Shah BR, Finberg L. Single-day therapy for nutritional vitamin D-deficiency rickets: A preferred method. *J Pediatr* 1994;125:487-490.

105 Failure to Thrive

Anupama Chawla

INTRODUCTION

Failure to thrive (FTT) is a description of interrupted growth caused by innumerable medical, nutritional, behavioral, or environmental disease states. The immediate cause of failure FTT is malnutrition. Underlying causes are often categorized as organic and non-organic etiologies. However, organic etiologies are frequently compounded by psychosocial factors which diffuse the lines of categorization.

DEFINITION

No single definition exists for failure to thrive, reflecting the complexity and diversity of its presentations. Often weight less than the expected weight for a measured length is loosely used to describe failure to thrive. However, this criteria alone could lead to the inclusion of healthy infants. For a child to be labelled as having 'failed to thrive', the assessment must be based on several growth points plotted on the standard age- and sex-appropriate growth charts. To be characterized as having 'failed to thrive', a child must meet at least two of the following criteria:

1. Weight progressing in a downward deviation across at least two major percentile lines on the standard chart.
2. Weight less than 90% of the expected weight for measured length.
3. Weight below the third percentile of expected weight for age.
4. Actual weight loss.

NORMAL GROWTH PATTERNS AND ERRONEOUS DIAGNOSIS OF FAILURE TO THRIVE

In order to diagnose an abnormal, one needs to have knowledge of the normal. In general, term infants lose 5% to 10% of their birth weight and regain their birth weight by 2 weeks. They double their birth weight by 4-5 months of age and triple it by 1 year. They double their height by 3-4 years of age. The size of an infant at birth is related more to maternal and intrauterine influences than to genetic factors. In the first years of life, there often is a change in growth velocity, both in weight and height, as the result of genetic factors.

The new WHO Child Growth Standards confirm that children born anywhere in the world and given the optimum start with adequate nutrition in life have the potential to develop within the same range of height and weight. Naturally, there are individual differences among children, but across large populations, regionally and globally, the average growth is remarkably similar. For example, children from India, Norway and Brazil all show similar growth patterns when provided healthy growth conditions in early life. The new standards prove that differences in children's growth to age five are more influenced by nutrition, feeding practices, environment, and healthcare than genetics or ethnicity. The new WHO standards are based on the breastfed children as the norm for growth and development. This brings consistency for the first time between the tools used to assess growth, and national and international infant feeding guidelines, which recommend breastfeeding as the optimal source of nutrition during infancy.

Growth patterns often erroneously labelled as failure to thrive include growth characteristics of infants born with intrauterine growth retardation (IUGR), constitutional growth delay, familial short stature, and the breast fed infant.

The different outcomes observed in growth patterns of *IUGR infants* most likely reflect multiple factors and variations associated with the duration of intrauterine insult. Children with *constitutional growth delay* are often described as "slow growers" and "late bloomers". These children usually have a deceleration of growth in the first 2 years of life; subsequently grow along a curve that parallels the normal curve until well beyond the age at which the usual adolescent growth spurt occurs. *Familial short stature* is defined as genetic short stature. Affected patients remain short throughout life. They also readjust their growth percentiles to their genetic potential by 2 to 3 years of age. Their bone age is not delayed as it is in constitutional growth delay. *Breast fed infants* may gain weight at a slower rate than infants who are formula fed. Despite their slow weight gain, these infants double their birth weight by 4-6 months of age and triple their birth weight by 1 year.

ETIOLOGY

Table 105.1 provides the list of causes of FTT.

The differential diagnosis of failure to thrive has traditionally been categorized as organic versus non-organic causes (Table 105.1). However, the delineation is often not so clear. Organic causes are often compounded by psychosocial factors.

Table 105.1: Causes of failure to thrive

Oropharyngeal
Oakatak abomaly
Pierre Robin syndrome
Central nervous system
Cerebral palsy
Fetal alcohol syndrome
Intracranial tumors, cysts, hematoma
Neuromuscular disorders
Cardiac
Congenital heart defects
Pulmonary
Bronchopulmonary dysplasia
Chronic infection (e.g., secondary to cystic fibrosis)
Gastrointestinal
Defect eased intake
Oropharyngeal disorders
Cerebral palsy
Chronic vomiting
Gastroesophageal disorders
Cerebral palsy
Chronic vomiting
Gastroesophageal reflux
Malrotation
Pseudo-obstruction
Increased intracranial pressure
Chronic diarrhea
Celiac disease
Cystic fibrosis
Giardiasis
Microvillus inclusion disease
Abetalipoproteinemia
Inflammatory bowel disease
Short bowel syndrome
Autoimmune enteropathy
Chronic liver disease
Selective enzyme deficiency
Enterokinase
Sucrase-isomaltase
Genitourinary
Renal tubular acidosis
Fanconi syndrome
Endocrine
Hypothyroidism
Hypopituitarism
Diabetes mellitus
Diabetes insipidus
Congenital adrenal hyperplasia
Growth hormone deficiency
Congenital infections
Syphilis
Cytomegalo inclusion virus
Rubella
Toxoplasmosis
HIV infection
Metabolic disorders
Malignancies
Iatrogenic
Prolonged use of steroids
Chromosomal disorders
Turner's sydnrome
Immunodeficiency disease
Severe combined immunodeficiency
Digeorge syndrome
HIV infection
Psychosocial Deprivation
Maternal depression
Maternal deprivation
Economic forces
Social stresses
Unwanted pregnancy
Marital stress
Poverty
Family losses
Chronic illness in the family
Job loss or demands

EVALUATION

Assessment of FTT should be in a systematic manner (Table 105.2)

History

The assessment of a child with failure to thrive requires a careful recording of history with special emphasis on nutritional intake (24-hour diet recalls and 3-5 day food intake diary are helpful), any chronic symptoms, caretakers involved, and social stresses. The common biologic insult in all children with failure to thrive, regardless of cause, is malnutrition. Children with failure to thrive have incurred malnutrition due to one of the following reasons:

1. Not being offered adequate calories.
2. Inability to consume adequate calories.
3. Inability to retain adequate calories; or
4. An energy expenditure rate that exceeds energy intake.

The *medical history* should include a careful review of systems. Keeping the differential diagnosis in mind (Table 105.1) pertinent questions should be asked to help direct the search for an underlying organic etiology. A neurological cause may be suspected if there has been developmental delay, loss of achieved milestones or deviation of head circumference across two percentiles.

Shortness of breath, pallor, and sweating during feeds suggest underlying cardiac disease.

Table 105.2: Assessment of infants with failure to thrive

Document failure to gain weight
Obtain history (birth, medical, dietary and social history)
Physical examination:
- Note any specific abnormality
  - Oropharyngeal defects
  - Cardiac defects
  - Respiratory compromise
  - Cerebral palsy
  - Organomegaly especially hepatomegaly.

If suspicious of non-organic failure to thrive
- Social history
- 3-Day calorie counts
- Consider hospitalization to document weight gain with adequate nutrition

If suspicious of organic failure to thrive

Perform laboratory studies	To screen for
Complete blood count, leukocyte differential platelet count, erythrocyte sedimentation rate, C-reactive protein	Anemia, inflammatory causes
Serum electrolites bicarbonate, arterial blood pH, liver profile	Renal and hepatic disease
Urine pH, specific gravity, glucose, protein, microscopic examination	Tubular acidosis, diabetes mellitus, diabetes insipidus, urinary tract infection
Serum immunoglobulins/HIV testing	Immunodeficiency
Sweat chloride test	Cystic fibrosis
Antigliadin, antiendomysial, tissue transglutaminase antibody	Celiac disesae
Somatomedin C/bone age, thyroid function tests	Endocrine disease
Plasma amino acids/urine organic acids	Metabolic defects

Failure to thrive is common in children with congenital heart disease and influences the metabolic response to injury and outcome after corrective cardiac surgery. Energy imbalance is a major contributing factor.

Gastroesophageal reflux (GER) is common in children during the first year of life. In severe cases aversion to feeds has been attributed to GER. The infant experiences severe discomfort, secondary to acid reflux induced by the intake of formula. This learned association may lead to persistent food aversions and growth failure despite appropriate reflux therapy. GER during infancy is seen in many infants with failure to thrive who also have other health problems such as respiratory disease, neurological problems, and acidosis secondary to renal or metabolic disease. Therefore, caution must be sought when attributing failure to thrive exclusively to GER disease.

Cystic fibrosis is of concern in a child with repeated episodes of bronchitis or pneumonia and failure to thrive. These children may also have malabsorption, reflected by the presence of oily, foul smelling stools. It is no longer a disease of the west. Children from the Indian subcontinent and Pakistan have been diagnosed to have cystic fibrosis with classical clinical features. Diagnosis is often delayed and the disease is advanced at the time of diagnosis mainly because of lack of awareness, and unavailability of testing in the rural areas.

Unexplained fevers, need for repeated courses of antibiotics may indicate underlying immune deficiency e.g. infection with HIV and AIDS or congenital immunodeficiency.

Metabolic disorders affecting amino acid and fatty acid metabolism may present with failure to thrive and chronic vomiting. Hypoglycemia, metabolic acidosis and hyperammonemia in a child with failure to thrive, are suggestive of underlying metabolic disorders.

Obstructive sleep apnea is an under-recognized cause of poor growth, perhaps because it interferes with nocturnal growth hormone production.

A social history should be reviewed carefully. It is important to identify the child's primary caretakers keeping in mind that the family structure has changed significantly over the past couple of decades. More families have needed to have two working parents or, in single parent families, that parent working full time to provide for the children. Multiple caretakers are often involved. Psychosocial stressors and lifestyle changes involving loss of job, family, financial hardships should also be identified.

The *Nutritional history* must be thorough. A twenty-four hours recall can provide some insight but is not accurate or reflective of day-to-day variations in intake. It is recommended that one obtain 72 hours prospective charting of the food intake for evaluating the caloric intake. This should include weekend and week days and days with variable caregivers if multiple caregivers are involved. Formula mixing, length of breast feeds, number of feeds a day, number of ounces consumed in 24 hours are all helpful questions in assessing caloric intake.

Examination

The malnourished child has decreased subcutaneous fat (as evidenced by loss of fat on the shoulders, buttocks and over the rib cage), bony prominences, protuberant abdomen flat buttocks, muscle wasting and poor tone. These children also have brittle, thin, coarse hair.

Anthropometric measurements must be obtained and plotted. Serial measurements to trend the parameters are very important as opposed to a single point measurement (Fig. 105.1). Weight is the first indicator to decline followed by height and lastly head circumference. An isolated decline in weight suggests acute malnutrition and a decline in all three indices is suggestive of chronic malnutrition.

Fig. 105.2 illustrates how to calculate ideal weight.

Congenital malformations must be noted. Even minor congenital anomalies such as low set ears, body asymmetry,

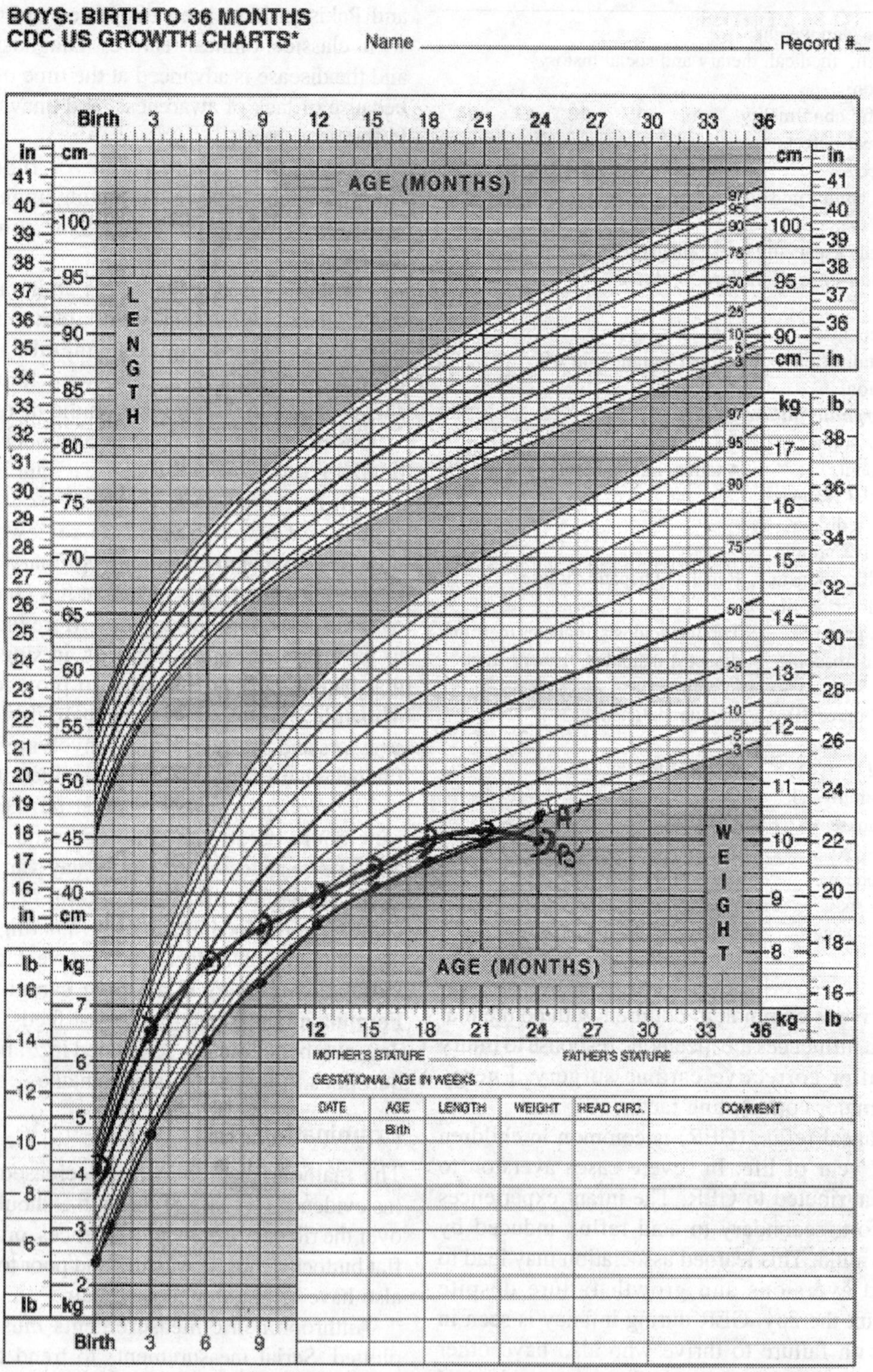

Fig. 105.1: Importance of growth trends: A standard growth chart clearly illustrates the importance of evaluating weight trend rather than a single point measurement. Patient A and B are of the same weight at 2 years of age and in fact up until that point patient B has been weighing more than patient A at each point measurement. However patient B has been falling off the weight percentiles and is failing to thrive. Patient A is gaining weight steadily and is most likely normal

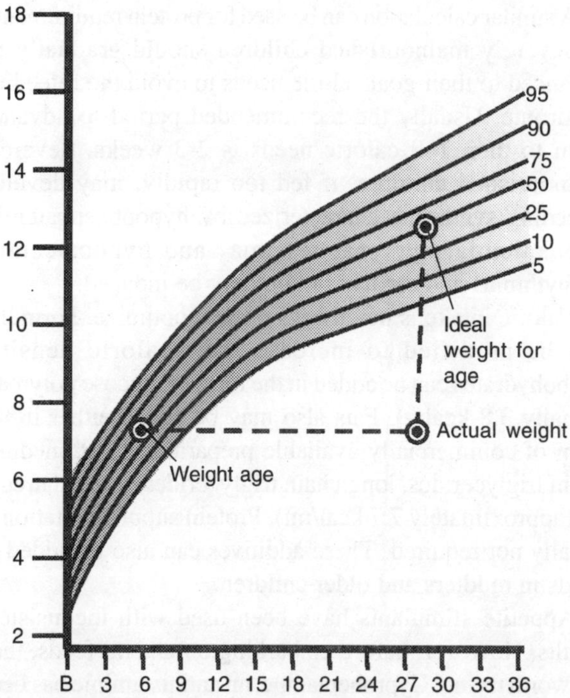

Fig. 105.2: Illustration to calculate the ideal weight for age and weight age based on the actual weight. Ideal weight for age is the 50th percentile weight for that age. Weight age is the age at which the child's current weight would be at the 50th percentile. In the above figure the actual weight is 8 kg at 2 years of age. Therefore weight age is 6.5 months and his ideal weight for his age is 12.5 kg

and extra digits may be associated with developmental delays and consequent poor caloric intake with failure to gain weight.

Every organ system should be carefully examined. Signs of chronic disease such as clubbing should be noted. Cyanosis may be present as a sign of pulmonary or more importantly congenital heart disease. Lymphadenopathy may indicate congenital immune deficiency or disseminated tuberculosis. Abdominal distension is often seen in malabsorptive syndromes for e.g. celiac disease, cystic fibrosis. Hepatomegaly may be seen in congenital heart disease with failure or may be secondary to fatty infiltration seen in malnutrition. Hepatosplenomegaly may imply a storage disorder.

Neurological examination to assess age appropriate development is important. Failure to achieve age appropriate milestones is a sensitive marker of underlying neurological disorder, especially if these delays can be documented prior to the child failing to gain weight. Children with developmental delays may have mental retardation and underlying neurological disorder. However, children with severe malnutrition may not achieve developmental milestones.

The neglected malnourished child often appears apathetic, and lacks interest in his or her environment. A child's general appearance should be examined for signs of neglect such as poor hygiene, unwashed skin and clothes.

Laboratory Evaluation

The history and physical examination should determine which laboratory studies are warranted. In children with specific abnormalities, the evaluation should be organ specific. Table 105.2 outlines certain guidelines to assist in the evaluation of children with failure to thrive.

Useful screening studies include complete blood count, serum electrolytes, hepatic panel and urine analysis. Anemia may be the result of malnutrition, malabsorption and decreased utilization of iron in chronic disease states. In the anemic child lead toxicity should be screened for as this can lead to anemia and failure to thrive. Children with malnutrition and iron deficiency have been shown to have increased lead absorption.

Simultaneous measurement of serum electrolytes and urine analysis for specific gravity, glucose, protein and microscopic examination will screen for diabetes mellitus and insipidus, urinary tract infections and renal tubular defects.

In children with chronic diarrhea, infectious causes should be screened for. Stool for ovum and parasites as well as stool for *giardia* antigen should be obtained. The *giardia* specific stool antigen test is more sensitive and specific than routine ovum and parasite screening when looking for *giardia* infection. The *giardia lamblia* infection can result in significant malabsorption and failure to thrive. If no infectious cause is determined then chronic conditions with malabsorption should be considered.

Cystic fibrosis should be suspected if failure to thrive is associated with chronic diarrhea, recurrent respiratory infections or recurrent pancreatitis. Cystic fibrosis is increasingly being recognized in children in the developing world. A sweat chloride should be performed to screen for cystic fibrosis.

If celiac disease is suspected then celiac antibodies (antigliadin antibody IgA and IgG, endomysium antibody and tissue transglutaminase antibody) are helpful screening tools (Would refer to the chapter on celiac disease here).

Hepatic enzyme screening helps screen for chronic liver disease. Metabolic disorders may present with abnormal liver enzymes, acidosis and an elevated anion gap on electrolyte screening. Plasma amino acids and urinary organic acids are useful screening tests for metabolic defects.

In children with failure to thrive and recurrent infections or opportunistic infections congenital immunodeficiencies and human immunodeficiency virus (HIV) infection should be suspected. Serum immunoglobulins and HIV testing should be performed.

If all above tests are normal and unrevealing, and malabsorption is suspected, then stool studies for 72-hour fecal fat study, stool elastase (a pancreatic enzyme), stool pH and reducing substances should be assessed. These tests help screen for fat and carbohydrate malabsorption. If either fat or carbohydrate malabsorption is determined, then further evaluation of pancreatic function and intestinal disaccharidases function respectively is warranted.

Imaging studies should be based on clinical history. A chest radiograph will help confirm suspected cardiac or pulmonary disease. An echocardiogram may be warranted if congenital heart disease is suspected. An upper gastrointestinal barium study should be obtained if the child has chronic vomiting and failure to thrive. If the barium study is unrevealing and the child is continuing to have forceful vomiting episodes especially unrelated to meals or in association with headaches or seizures then an intracranial space occupying lesion should be suspected. A magnetic resonance imaging study of the brain would be the most sensitive study to look for these lesions.

Endocrine evaluation should be considered if the height is more significantly affected than the weight to screen for thyroid disease and growth hormone deficiency.

If 'non-organic failure' to thrive is suspected, then its confirmation requires ruling out an underlying organic etiology and demonstrating a positive growth response to increased caloric intake.

MANAGEMENT

Therapy is directed at the underlying organic cause if determined but more acutely to malnutrition itself and its complications.

The fluid and electrolyte disturbances if present should be corrected.

The goal of nutritional treatment is to promote compensatory catchup growth to restore weight and height. Catch-up growth is defined as acceleration of growth that occurs when a period of growth retardation ends and measured parameters begin to climb across percentiles towards expected height and weight percentiles for age. During periods of catch-up growth, a child requires 150-200% of the calories required for their weight and age.

Farrel has suggested the following formula to calculate the calories needed for catch-up growth:

$$\text{Energy requirement for catch up growth (kcal/kg/day)} = \frac{\text{Calories required for weight age} \times \text{Ideal weight for age (kg)}}{\text{Calories required for weight age} \times \text{Ideal weight for age (kg)}}$$

Table 105.3: Caloric requirements/kg body weight

Age	*Kcal*
0-6 months	108
6-11 months	98
1-3 years	102
4-6 years	90
7-10 years	70
11-14 years	55

Illustrates the calories per kilogram required at a particular age.

A similar calculation can be used for protein requirements.

Severely malnourished children should gradually be advanced to their goal caloric needs to avoid the refeeding syndrome. Usually the recommended period to advance them to their full caloric needs is 2-3 weeks. Severely malnourished children, if fed too rapidly, may develop refeeding syndrome characterized by hypophosphatemia, hypokalemia, hypomagnesemia and hypocalcemia. Arrhythmias and cardiac failure may be induced.

Caloric intake is not always easy to optimize. Formulas can be modified to increase their caloric density. Carbohydrates can be added in the form of glucose polymers (usually 3.8 kcal/g). Fats also may be added either in the form of commercially available preparations e.g. medium chain triglycerides, long chain triglycerides or regular corn oil (approximately 7.7 kcal/ml). Protein supplementation is usually not required. These additives can also be added to foods in toddlers and older children.

Appetite stimulants have been used with inconsistent results. However, before embarking on enteral feeds, they are worth trying. Cyproheptadine, an antihistaminic has been used especially in children with chronic illness. Recommended dose is 0.5 mg/kg/day in 3 divided doses to a maximum of 4 mg four times a day. Megestrol acetate has been used but because of its higher side effect profile its use is limited to severe chronic illness like cancer and cystic fibrosis.

If an adequate amount of calories cannot be delivered by mouth, enteral feedings through a nasogastric tube or a gastrostomy tube should be considered. This may especially be required in children with congenital heart disease, where the ability to take in adequate calories is compromised by the energy expended in sucking and swallowing. Very often this intervention may be required until corrective surgery is performed.

Parenteral nutrition is rarely required unless there is severe gastrointestinal compromise.

LONG-TERM CONSEQUENCES OF FAILURE TO THRIVE

There are few long-term studies on the effects of nutritional deprivation and failure to thrive on ultimate growth and development. However, almost all studies have shown some long-term deficiencies in growth and development. Reiss *et al.* evaluated 61 children with non-organic failure to thrive diagnosed in infancy. These children were evaluated 5 years after their initial presentation and compared to age, sex and social status matched controls. The group with history of failure to thrive had gained less weight and was shorter. They also had more learning difficulties and significant developmental delays. Children who caught up faster, had better school performance.

The critical period for growth is under 2 years of age

and significant nutritional insults before this age, are likely to have long-term adverse effects on growth. This makes it imperative for the involved physician to recognize the underlying correctable or treatable etiologies. Corrective intervention of the underlying organic etiology is the single most effective tool that has been shown to significantly improve nutritional intake, decrease energy expenditure, resulting in marked acceleration of growth. One example is in the children with congenital heart disease where the age and time of corrective surgery affects the potential for nutritional recovery. Significant improvements in weight and growth occur within months after corrective surgery. Another example is in the children with cystic fibrosis where early diagnosis, enzyme supplementation, pulmonary therapy and nutritional intervention, has significantly improved the growth of these children.

However, in children with non-organic failure to thrive, the outcome is often suboptimal. The question remains whether these infants could have a yet unidentified, therefore untreated, organic explanation for their failure to thrive.

KEY LEARNING POINTS

- Denotes interrupted growth caused by several medical, nutritional, behavioral or environmental factors.
- At least two of the four standard criteria must be satisfied before the diagnosis is made.
- Evaluation should be in a systematic manner, based on history and examination (especially anthropometry), and laboratory tests.
- Treatment is directed at underlying organic cause, if determined, but more specifically to malnutrition.
- Goal of nutritional therapy being promotion of compensatory catchup growth to restore weight and height.

FURTHER READINGS

1. Aldeen WE, Hale D, Robinson AJ, Carroll K: Evaluation of a commercially available ELISA assay for detection of *Giardia lamblia* in fecal specimens. *Diagn Microbiol Infect Dis* 1995; 2:77-79.
2. Baudon JJ, Johanet C, Absalon YB *et al.* Diagnosing celiac disease: A comparison of human tissue transglutaminase antibodies with antigliadin and endomysium antibodies. *Arch Pediatr Adolesc Med* 2004;158: 584-588.
3. Behavioral and nutritional treatment to improve energy intake and growth in toddlers and preschool-aged children with cystic fibrosis. *Pediatrics* 2006;118:432-433.
4. Bithoney WG: Elevated lead levels in children with non-organic failure to thrive. *Pediatrics* 1986, 78:891-895.
5. Bottaro G, Volta U, Spina M *et al.:* Antibody pattern in childhood celiac disease. *J Pediatr Gastroenterol Nutr* 1997, 24: 559-562.
6. Careaga MG, Kerner JA. A gastroenterologist's approach to failure to thrive. *Pediatr Ann* 200; 29:558-67.
7. Casey P: FTT: A reconceptualization. *J Dev Behav Pediatr* 1983,4:63-66.
8. Chase HP, Martin HP: Undernutrition and child development. *N Engl J Med* 1970;282:933-939.
9. Chawla A: Failure to thrive. In: Brandt L (ed): *Clinical Practice of Gastroenterology*. Philadelphia: Current Medicine 1999: 1466-1471.
10. Dawson P. Normal growth and revised growth charts. *Pediatr Rev* 2002;23:255-256.
11. Dickstein S, St Andre M, Sameroff A, Seifer R, Schiller M. Maternal depression, family functioning, and child outcomes: A narrative assessment. *Monogr Soc Res Child Dev* 1999; 64:84-104.
12. Elmer E, Gregg GS, Ellison P: Late results of the 'failure to thrive' syndrome. *Clin Pediatr* 1969;8:584-589.
13. Farrell MK: Failure to Thrive. In: Wyllie R, Hyams JS (eds): *Pediatric Gastrointestinal Diseases*. Philadelphia: Saunders 1993:271-280.
14. Gahagan S, Holmes R. A stepwise approach to evaluation of undernutrition and failure to thrive. *Pediatr Clin North Am* 1998; 45:169-187.
15. Homnick DN, Marks JH, Hare KL, Bonnema SK. *Pediatr Pulmonol* 2005: 40:251-256.
16. Kabra SK, Kabra M, Lodha R *et al.*, Clinical profile and frequency of delta f508 mutation in Indian children with cystic fibrosis: *Indian J Pediatr* 2003;40:612-619.
17. Lodha R, Upadhyay A, Kapoor V, Kabra SK. Clinical profile and natural history of children with HIV infection: *Indian J Pediatr* 1,2006; 73:201-204.
18. Maggioni A, Lifshitz F. Nutritional management of failure to thrive. *Pediatrr Clin North* Am 1995,42:791-810.
19. Marchand V, Baker SS, Baker RD. *Gastrointest Endosc Clin North Am* 1998 ;8:669-703.
20. Mezoff AG, Gremse DA, Farrell MK: Hypophosphatemia in the nutritional recovery syndrome. *Am J Dis Child* 1989; 1992:111-112.
21. Nydegger A, Bines JE. Energy metabolism in infants with congenital heart disease. *Nutrition* 2006; 22:697-704.
22. Powell GF, Low J: Behavior in nonorganic failure to thrive. *J Dev Behav Pediatr* 1983, 4:26-33.
23. Raghuveer TS, Garg U, GRAF WD. Inborn errors of metabolism in infancy and early childhood: An update. *Am Fam Physician* 2006:1:1981-90.
24. Reiss S, Beller B, Villa Y, Spirer Z: Long-term follow up and outcome of infants with non-organic failure to thrive. *Irr J Med Sci* 1995,8:483-489.
25. Rostom A, Dube C, Cranney A *et al.* The diagnostic accuracy of serologic tests for celiac disease: A systematic review. *Gastroenterology* 2005; 128: S38-S46.
26. Sameroff A, Chandler MJ: Reproductive risk and the continuum of caretaking casualty. In: Horowitz PD (ed): *Review of Child Development Research.* Chicago: University of Chicago Press 1978.
27. Schwartz D. Failure to thrive: An old nemesis in the new millennium. *Pediatr Rev* 2000;21:257-264.
28. World Health Organisation. *WHO Release on New Child Growth Standards.* Geneva: WHO 2006.
29. Williams EF, Woo P, Miller R *et al.:* The effects of adenotonsillectomy on growth in young children. *Otolaryngol Head Neck Surg* 1991; 104:509-514.

106 Obesity

Rossy Aulakh • Gurmeet K Chaudhry • Tejinder Singh

INTRODUCTION

Obesity is a condition of abnormal or excessive fat accumulation in adipose tissue, to the extent that health may be impaired. The terms *"obese"* and *"overweight"* often are used interchangeably. Technically, "obesity" is the upper end of "overweight".

OBESITY: GLOBAL EPIDEMIC

Obesity is emerging as a global epidemic. The increase in childhood and adolescent obesity has resulted in increases in obesity or overweight in adults. Overweight 10 to 14 year olds are 20 times more likely to be overweight in their third decade of life than if they were of normal weight as young adolescents. Approximately 80% of overweight adolescents become overweight adults. This tracking of obesity from childhood to adulthood is of primary importance and, if an accurate predictor is used, would allow for the targeting of appropriate subjects for intervention such as those who will continue to be obese rather than focusing on those who will reduce their percentage of body fat spontaneously. The calculated global prevalence of overweight (including obesity) in children aged 5-17 years is estimated by the International Obesity Task Force (IOTF) to be approximately 10%, but this is 'unequally distributed' with prevalence ranging from over 30% in Americas to <2% in sub Saharan Africa. According to WHO (2000) atleast 50% of adults and 20% of children in UK and USA are currently overweight. Over the past 25 years the prevalence of obesity or overweight doubled in American children ages 6 to 11 years and tripled in adolescents' ages 12 to 17 years. A 75% relative increase in obesity in adolescents is noted from 1970 to the present and currently 25% of American adolescents are identified as obese. Prevalence of overweight amongst Australian children has increased from 11% in 1985 to 20% in 1995. Childhood obesity has tripled in Canada in last 20 years. Obesity does not seem to have spared developing countries either. Thailand, Iran, Nigeria and Brazil have all reported unprecedented levels of obesity with trends that are substantially rising every year. An Indian study had shown the prevalence of overweight (including obese) adolescents ranged from 22% in better off schools to 4.5% in lower income group schools. In a Delhi school with tuition fees more than Rs. 2500 per month, the prevalence of overweight was 31%, of which 7.5% were frankly obese. In Pune the figures for overweight children are 24% in a well off school and 6% in a 'corporation' school.

Though more studies are needed to understand the precise prevalence of overweight and obesity in India, school-based data demonstrates an obesity range of 5.6% to 24% for the children and adolescents of India.

OBESITY: DEFINITION

Obesity is not equivalent to overweight; obesity denotes excess body fat, whereas overweight might relate to fat or other tissue in excess with relation to height. What should determine the presence of obesity? In adults, morbidity and mortality are related to adiposity, and cut-offs can be determined related to such complications; in adults, presently a BMI of 25 is considered overweight and a BMI of 30 is considered obese. In children, morbidity and mortality are not usually related proximately to body fat, although the increasing findings of morbidity in childhood may assist in determining such cut-off in future. Thus, standard and convenient statistical cut-offs are used: 85th percentile BMI for "overweight", or the more acceptable term, at risk for obesity, and the 95th percentile for obesity.

The crucial periods for persistence of obesity appear to be:

i. Gestational period.
ii. Adiposity rebound age (5-7 years).
iii. Adolescence.

Obesity compounds a common adolescent problem of low self-esteem and can disrupt psychosocial development, interfering with the normal process of adolescence, a timeless journey that prepares the child for adulthood. Not all obese infants become obese children, and not all obese children become obese adults. However, the prevalence of obesity increases with age among both males and females and there is a greater likelihood that obesity beginning even in early childhood will persist through the life span.

INDIANS AT HIGH RISK; OUR SPECIAL CONCERNS

The prevalence of diabetes, CHD and other life-style disorders is increasing alarmingly in India, and is affecting much younger populations than the West. In transitional economies such as in India obesity and malnutrition often coexist (double burden of disease) causing confusion in health messages. In fact, frank obesity may not be as high in India as in the West, but the body composition and metabolism of Indians make them more prone to adiposity and its consequences. The fat is typically located centrally, and around visceral organs where it is metabolically more dangerous than peripheral fat. Recent Pune studies have demonstrated the 'thin fat Indian phenotype' with evidence of hyperinsulinemia even at birth. Moreover, recent longitudinal studies in India have highlighted the deleterious effect of accelerated weight gain in childhood 'crossing of centiles' especially in LBW babies. It is now evident that our traditional understanding of concepts of 'catch up growth', weight gain in pregnancy and birth weight may need redefining.

CAUSES OF EPIDEMIC IN INDIA

India is in the midst of an escalating epidemic of life-style disorders associated with childhood obesity. The causes include:

a. ***Changes in life-style ('urbanization'):*** With improving standards of living, and availability of food in plenty, the upper class societies of India in recent years have urbanized to western levels. The components of life-style changes are:
   - ***Unhealthy eating patterns, wrong choices of food:*** Traditional micronutrient rich foods are being replaced by energy dense highly processed micronutrient poor foods. All celebrations and festivals seem to be centered on rich foods.
   - ***Sedentary pursuits:*** Television and movie watching, video games, internet gazing and telephone gossip sessions are now important activities of children and these replace the time earlier utilized for physical activities.
   - ***'Obesogenic' schools and tuition classes:*** An important factor for obesity in India is intense competition for admissions to schools and colleges with flourishing tuition classes right from nursery levels! Children are forced to use their playtime for additional studies.
   - ***Inadequate play areas:*** Due to unsafe roads (traffic, crime) children are discouraged from walking or cycling to school. Motorized vehicles are popular and they are perceived to be quicker and safer for transport. As against food as rewards, ironically exercise is meted out as a punishment—'100 sit ups', 'run around the field'.

b. ***Genetic constitutional predisposition:*** The factors responsible could be:
   - The previously malnourished populations have a tendency to accumulate fat more intensely in an attempt to store for future starvation'.
   - Modern environment may have unmasked previously silent obesogenic genes 'thrifty genotypes.
   - Stunting in childhood may increase the risk of central obesity especially in transitional economies.
   - High rate of gestational diabetes in pregnant women causing higher birth weights in babies leading to intergenerational effects of obesity in childhood and its attendant problem.
   - Familial patterns of eating, exercise and behavior.

c. ***Other factors:***
   - ***Lack of prolonged and exclusive breast-feeding:*** Breastfeeding is associated with a significantly lower rate of obesity and hypertension in later life. It is not clear if early introduction of energy dense supplements in infancy has contributed to childhood obesity in India.
   - The high glycemic index of our predominantly carbohydrate diet may be responsible for hyperinsulinism, weight gain and eventual type 2 diabetes.
   - Yet other factors controlling body weight regulation such as low body metabolic rate (BMR) and probably governed by hypothalamus–these factors as of now are all speculative.

CAUSES OF OBESITY

As with adult-onset obesity, childhood obesity has multiple causes centering on an imbalance between energy in (calories centered from food) and energy out (calories expended in the basal metabolic rate and physical activity). Childhood obesity most likely results from an interaction of endogenous and exogenous factors:

I. Endogenous Factors

a. ***Heredity:*** Since not all children who eat non-nutritious foods, watch several hours of television daily, and are relatively inactive develop obesity, the search continues for alternative causes. Heredity has recently been shown to influence fatness, regional fat distribution and response to overfeeding. In addition, infants born to overweight mothers have been found to be less active and to gain more weight by age three months when compared with infants of normal weight mothers, suggesting a possible inborn drive to conserve energy.

b. ***Medical causes:*** These include Cushing's syndrome, prolonged use of corticosteroids, hypothalamic lesions (trauma, tumor, tuberculosis, sarcoidosis), Prader-Willi syndrome, Laurence-Moon-Beidl syndrome and various other endocrine disorders (hypothyroidism, hypopituitarism, hyperinsulinemia, hypercortisolism). Other medications that can induce weight gain include anticonvulsants, neuroleptics, depomedroxyprogesterone acetate and tricyclic antidepressants.

II. Exogenous Factors

a. ***The family:*** The risk of becoming obesity greatest among children who have two obese parents. This may be due to powerful genetic factors or to parental modelling of both eating and exercise behaviors, indirectly affecting the child's energy balance.

b. ***Low energy expenditure:*** The average child spends several hours each day watching television; the time, which in previous years might have been devoted to physical pursuits. Obesity is greater among children and adolescents who frequently watch television, not only because little energy is expended while viewing but also because of concurrent consumption of high calorie snacks. Only about one-third of elementary children have daily physical education, and less than one-fifth have extracurricular physical activity programs at their schools.

c. ***Environmental factors:*** There are many environmental factors that contribute to obesity in our modern culture. They are diverse in origin and applicability to individual patients, but collectively tend to explain many of the reasons we have an increasing problem in obesity. There are *calories of culture* and cuisine as quite simply, food is a way of life. Moreover, the food that comprises that way of life tastes very good yet is often quite unhealthy. There are *calories of cost* that are also significant. Fatty foods and those high in starch are frequently inexpensive

Table 106.1: Endogenous causes of childhood obesity

Hormonal causes	*Diagnostic clues*
Hypothyroidism	Increased TSH, decreased thyroxine (T_4) levels
Hypercortisolism	Abnormal dexamethasone suppression test; increased 24-hour free urinary cortisol level
Primary hyperinsulinism	Increased plasma insulin, increased C-peptide levels
Pseudohypoparathyroidism	Hypocalcemia, hyperphosphatemia, increased PTH level
Acquired hypothalamic	Presence of hypothalamic tumor, infection, syndrome trauma, vascular lesion
Genetic syndromes	Associated characteristics
Prader-Willi	Obesity, unsatiable appetite, mental retardation, hypogonadism, strabismus
Laurence-Moon/Bardet-Biedl	Obesity, mental retardation, pigmentary retinopathy, hypogonadism, spastic paraplegia
Alström	Obesity, retinitis pigmentosa, deafness, diabetes mellitus
Börjeson-Forssman-Lehmann	Obesity, mental retardation, hypogonadism, hypometabolism, epilepsy
Cohen	Truncal obesity, mental retardation, hypotonia, hypogonadism
Turner's	Short stature, undifferentiated gonads, cardiac abnormalities, webbed neck, obesity, 45, X genotype
Familial lipodystrophy	Muscular hypertrophy, acromegalic appearance, liver enlargement, acanthosis nigricans, insulin resistance, hypertriglyceridemia, mental retardation
Beckwith-Wiedemann	Gigantism, exomphalos, macroglossia, visceromegaly
Sotos'	Cerebral gigantism, physical overgrowth, hypotonia, delayed motor and cognitive development
Weaver	Infant overgrowth syndrome, accelerated skeletal maturation, unusual facies
Ruvalcaba	Mental retardation, microcephaly, skeletal abnormalities, hypogonadism

Table 106.2: Genes affecting fat mass

Central expression	*Peripheral expression*
Leptin receptor	Leptin
Melanocortin receptor-4 (MC4R)	Bardet-Biedl
α-melanocyte stimulating (α-MSH)	Dunnigan partial lipodystrophy
Prohormone convertase-1 (PC1)	Perilipin
Melanocortin receptor-3 (MC3R)	Diacylglycerol acyl transferase (DGAT)
Neuropeptide receptor-5 (NPY5R)	Lipin-1
Agouti gene related protein (AgRP)	Hgmic
Melanocyte concentrating hormone (MCH)	Protein tyrosine phosphatase-1B
Tubby (TULP1)	β-3 adrenergic receptor

compared to leaner cuts of meat, fresh fruits and vegetables. There are *calories of community* that are produced when children are not allowed to play; neighborhoods are simply not safe enough or appropriate facilities do not exist for the encouragement of physical activity among youth. *Calories of convenience* are found in the single serving foods, prepackaged, and frequently high in fat; these are meals that make up a significant portion of particularly young children's and school-aged children's diet. *Calories of complacency* occur when a parent simply concedes to child's demand of consuming calorie dense sweet foods like cookies. The *calories of chronic disease* may be seen in children who have physical limitations yet continue to eat in a normal fashion and become overweight. *The calories of computers, televisions and video games* generate in the snacks that frequently accompany these activities as well as the loss of physical exertion such activities will replace. Adolescents and younger children in response to sales pitches generate the calories of commercialism. *Calories of competition* refer to eating habits, and may involve both weight gain and weight loss associated with competitive sports. *The calories of chaos* occur in situations where there is simply not adequate control and supervision over dietary process.

d. ***Breastfeeding:*** Armstrong J *et al.* had suggested that breastfeeding is associated with a reduction in childhood obesity risk. The prevalence of obesity was significantly lower in breastfed children, and the association persisted after adjustment for socioeconomic status, birthweight and sex.

Neurophysiology of Feeding

Numerous biophysical factors impinge on eating behavior. The arcuate and paraventricular nuclei in the ventromedial hypothalamus are parts of a system integrating body composition with energy intake and expenditure. Afferent neural (vagal and catecholaminergic) stimuli and hormonal stimuli (e.g., insulin, cholecystokinin, leptin and glucocorticoids) related to metabolic status are received in the hypothalamus, where they modulate the release of peptides known to affect food intake and efferent signals to the hypothalamic-pituitary axis (resulting in endocrine mediation of fuel disposition) and the autonomic nervous system (resulting in energy expenditure and insulin release). Although there has been considerable interest in dietary composition and weight fluctuations as determinants of body composition, these factors do not have major roles in the pathogenesis of obesity (Fig. 106.1).

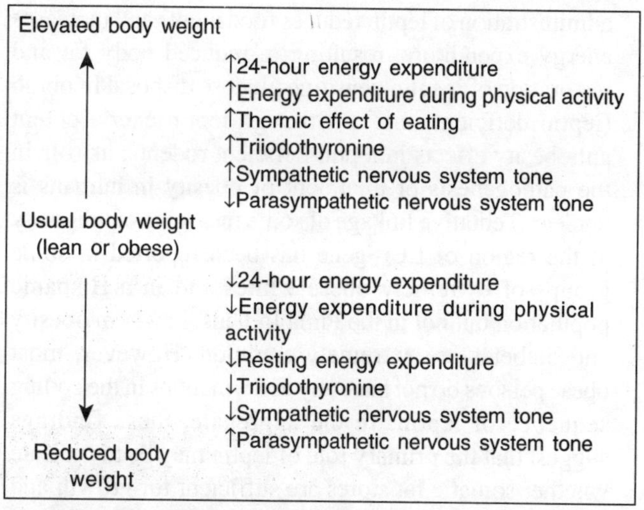

Fig. 106.1: Metabolic changes after change in weight

Metabolic Changes After Weight Gain or Loss

Chemical mediators of energy homeostasis: These include:

a. ***Insulin:*** Plasma insulin concentrations are proportional to the adipocyte volume. Insulin gains access to the central nervous system through a saturable transport system and reduces food intake by inhibiting the expression of neuropeptide Y, enhancing the anorectic effects of cholecystokinin and inhibiting neuronal norepinephrine reuptake.

b. ***Cholecystokinin:*** Cholecystokinin, a peptide secreted from the duodenum in the presence of food, reduces food uptake. There are two types of cholecystokinin receptors: type A predominates in gastrointestinal system and type B predominates in the brain. The anorectic effect of cholecystokinin is blocked by abdominal vagotomy, suggesting that the primary site of action of cholecystokinin is in the periphery. Cholecystokinin does not cross the blood-brain barrier—further evidence that duodenal cholecystokinin does not directly affect central nervous systems of energy homeostasis. However, cholecystokinin is synthesized in the brain, and intracranial administration of cholecystokinin results in a feeling of satiety.

c. ***Other endocrine and peptide signals:*** Numerous other hormones modulate fat storage through their effects on energy intake (e.g., glucocorticoids and glucagon), energy expenditure (e.g., androgens and thyroid and growth hormones), or a partitioning of stored energy between lean tissue and fat. Other gut peptides, including gastrin-releasing peptide, neuromedin B, enterostatin, and amylin, may also contribute to the regulation of energy balance in humans.

d. ***Leptin:*** Leptin, encoded by the Lep gene, is synthesized in and secreted from adipose tissue and is a potential afferent signal of fat stores. In humans this gene is referred to as LEP. Systemic or intracerebroventricular administration of leptin reduces food intake and increases energy expenditure, resulting in reduced body fat and restoration of insulin-sensitive glucose disposal in ob/ob (leptin deficient) mice. Although leptin exerts potent antiobesity effects in leptin-deficient rodents, its role in the pathogenesis or treatment of obesity in humans is unclear. Tentative linkage of some measures of adiposity to the region of LEP gene has been reported in some groups of extremely obese whites and in a Hispanic population but not in the Pima Indians, in whom obesity and diabetes are extremely common. However, most obese persons do not have any abnormalities in the coding sequence of leptin. In the aggregate, these findings suggest that the primary role of leptin may be to indicate whether somatic fat stores are sufficient for growth and reproduction. If the stores are inadequate—as reflected by a decline in plasma leptin concentrations to level below a threshold that may be genetically and developmentally set—the result is hyperphagia, low energy output and infertility. Plasma leptin concentrations above this threshold may have a minimal physiologic effect or none. Hence, obese humans with high plasma leptin concentrations have neither hypophagia nor hypermetabolism.

e. ***Neuropeptide Y:*** Neuropeptide Y links afferents reflecting the nutritional status to the organism from the endocrine, gastrointestinal, and central and peripheral nervous systems to effectors of energy intake and expenditure. The peptide is synthesized by cell bodies in the arcuate nucleus of the hypothalamus and transported axonally to the paraventricular nucleus, where the highest concentrations are found. Neuropeptide Y is also synthesized and released from the adrenal gland and sympathetic nerves, but it does not cross the blood-brain barrier. Neuropeptide Y is a potent central appetite stimulant. The expression of neuropeptide Y mRNA is increased by insulin and glucocorticoids and decreases by leptin and estrogen. Despite evidence of physiologic importance of neuropeptide Y in energy homeostasis, neuropeptide-knockout mice have normal body fat and food intake, with normal hyperphagia when food is withheld. These findings highlight the extraordinary redundancy of systems regulating caloric storage.

METABOLIC EFFECTS OF WEIGHT PERTURBATION

The responses of both lean and obese humans to experimental perturbation of body weight support the hypothesis that body fat is regulated; making it unlikely that behavior can be the sole determinant of obesity. The 24-hour energy expenditure per unit of lean body mass is similar in lean and obese subjects at their usual body weight. Small decreases in body weight result in declines in energy expenditure that persist despite a caloric intake that is sufficiently reduced to maintain the lower weight. Thus, a formerly obese person requires approximately 15 percent fewer calories to maintain a "normal" body weight than a person of the same body composition who has never been obese. Some adults and children who later become obese have lower rates of energy expenditure than non-obese persons. In addition, both formerly obese adults and those who later become obese oxidize fat more slowly than do obese adults or non-obese adults who later do not become obese, making the formerly or subsequently obese more prone to accumulate fat. The observation that a decreased expenditure for energy and increased propensity to store fat may precede the development of obesity suggests that the extra body fat in the obese person in some way corrects for low energy expenditure.

Futile cycles: In animals, some regulation of energy balance is achieved through metabolic cycles that consume ATP without performing useful biochemical work (futile cycles)—for example, simultaneous lipolysis and glyceride synthesis in fat cells and glycolysis and gluconeogenesis in the liver. Although small changes in energy expenditure through these cycles could theoretically affect body weight over time, there is little evidence that the cycles are important in energy homeostasis on humans (Fig. 106.2).

MEASUREMENT OF OBESITY

1. ***Body mass index (BMI):*** Body weight is reasonably correlated with body fat, but is also highly correlated with height. Therefore, weight adjusted for height squared (body mass index, BMI) is a useful index to assess overweight and is a fairly reliable surrogate for adiposity. BMI also correlates with markers of secondary complications of obesity, including current blood pressures, blood lipids and with long-term mortality. A limitation of BMI however, is that it cannot differentiate an obese individual from a muscular one. It also cannot locate the site of fat e.g., people with 'central obesity' may have normal BMIs. Still, it remains the most practical way of measuring and comparing obesity for clinical and epidemiological purposes. As per WHO classification (for adults): BMI > 25 is overweight while BMI > 30 is classified as obesity. However, as these WHO criteria may underestimate obesity in Asians, the International Obesity Task Force (IOTF) has proposed the standards for adult obesity in Asia and India as: BMI > 23 as overweight and BMI > 25 as obesity. Obesity in children and adolescents is defined as total body weight more than 25 percent fat in boys and more than 32 percent in girls.

BMI reference charts in children: Unlike BMI values in adults that are age and sex independent, BMI values in children vary greatly with age and sex. At birth the median BMI as low as 13 kg/m^2, increasing to 17 kg/m^2 at age 1, decreasing to 15.5 kg/m^2 at age 6, then increasing to 21 kg/m^2 at age 20. The two BMI charts that can be

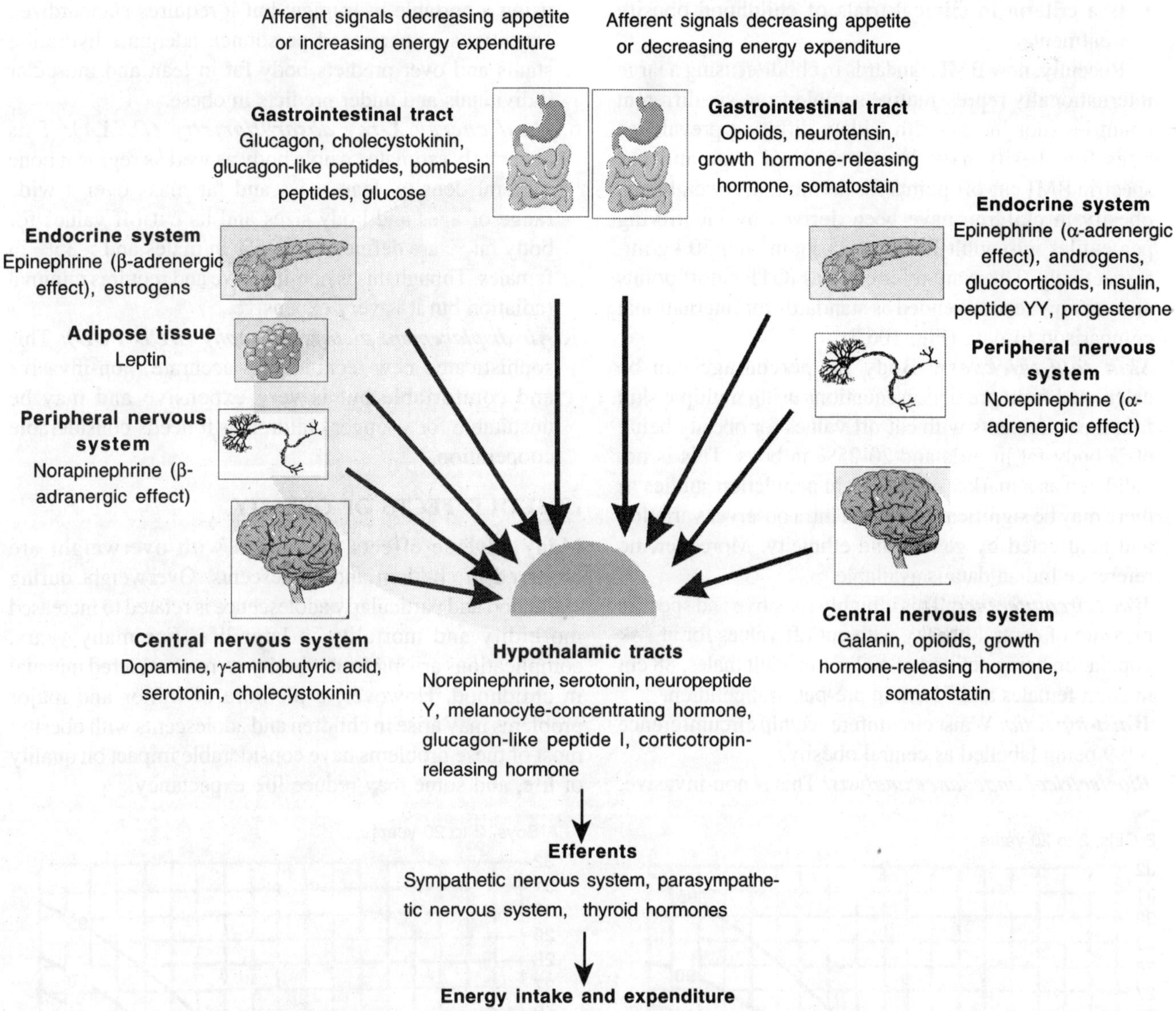

Fig. 106.2: Molecules that affect energy intake and expenditure

used as a reference, for Indian children, as of now, therefore are:

The NCHS/CDC charts from USA:

The American Obesity Association uses the 85th percentile of BMI for age and sex as a reference for overweight and the 95th percentile for obesity in children. Healthcare professionals use the following established percentile cutoff points to identify underweight and overweight in children.

The 95th percentile of BMI is used as criteria for obesity because it:

- Corresponds to a BMI of 30 which is obesity in adults. The 85th percentile corresponds to a BMI of 25, adult overweight.
- Is recommended as marker for when children and adolescents should have an in-depth medical assessment.
- Identifies children that are very likely to have obesity persist into adulthood.
- Is associated with elevated blood pressure and lipids in older adolescents, and increases their risk of diseases.

Table 106.3: Percentile cutoff points for weight-related problems

Underweight	BMI-for-age < 5th percentile
Normal	BMI-for-age 5th percentile to < 85th percentile
At risk of overweight	BMI-for-age 85th percentile to < 95th percentile
Obesity	BMI-for-age ≥ 95th percentile

- Is a criteria for more aggressive treatment.
- Is a criteria in clinical trials of childhood obesity treatments.

Recently, new BMI standards in children using a large internationally representative sample from six different countries (not India), with widely differing prevalence rates for obesity have been published. Age and sex specific BMI cut-off points for defining overweight and obesity in children have been derived by identifying percentiles into adult BMIs of 25 kg/m^2 and 30 kg/m^2, respectively. These are referred to as IOTF cutoff points and are now recommended as standards for international comparison to data (Fig. 106.3).

2. ***Skin fold thickness:*** Body fat percentage can be calculated from prediction equations using multiple skin fold measurements with cut-off values for obesity being 30% body fat in girls and 20-25% in boys. This is not validated as a marker of obesity in population studies as there may be significant inter and intra observer variation and is affected by gender and ethnicity. Moreover, no reference Indian data is available.
3. ***Waist circumference:*** This is highly sensitive and specific measure of central obesity with cut off values for at risk population being defined as 102 cm in adult males, 88 cm in adult females and 71 cm in pre-pubertal children.
4. ***Waist-hip ratio:*** Waist circumference/hip circumference > 0.9 being labelled as central obesity.
5. ***Bioelectrical impedance analysis:*** This is non-invasive, safe, cheap and reliable estimation of body composition using a portable instrument but it requires standardized conditions, experienced personnel, adequate hydration status and over predicts body fat in lean and muscular individuals and under predicts in obese.
6. ***Dual energy X-ray absorptiometry (DEXA):*** This accurately estimates whole body as well as regional bone mineral density, lean mass and fat mass over a wide range of ages and body sizes and its cut off values for body fat % are defined as > 25% in males and > 35% in females. Though this is non-invasive and requires minimal radiation but it is very expensive.
7. ***Air displacement plethysmography (BOD-POD):*** This sophisticated new technique is accurate, non-invasive and comfortable but is very expensive and may be unsuitable for younger children as it needs considerable cooperation.

HEALTH EFFECTS OF OBESITY

Many adverse effects associated with overweight are observed in children and adolescents. Overweight during childhood and particularly adolescence is related to increased morbidity and mortality in later life. For many years, complications arising from obesity were considered unusual in childhood. However, a plethora of minor and major problems may arise in children and adolescents with obesity; most of these problems have considerable impact on quality of life, and some may reduce life expectancy.

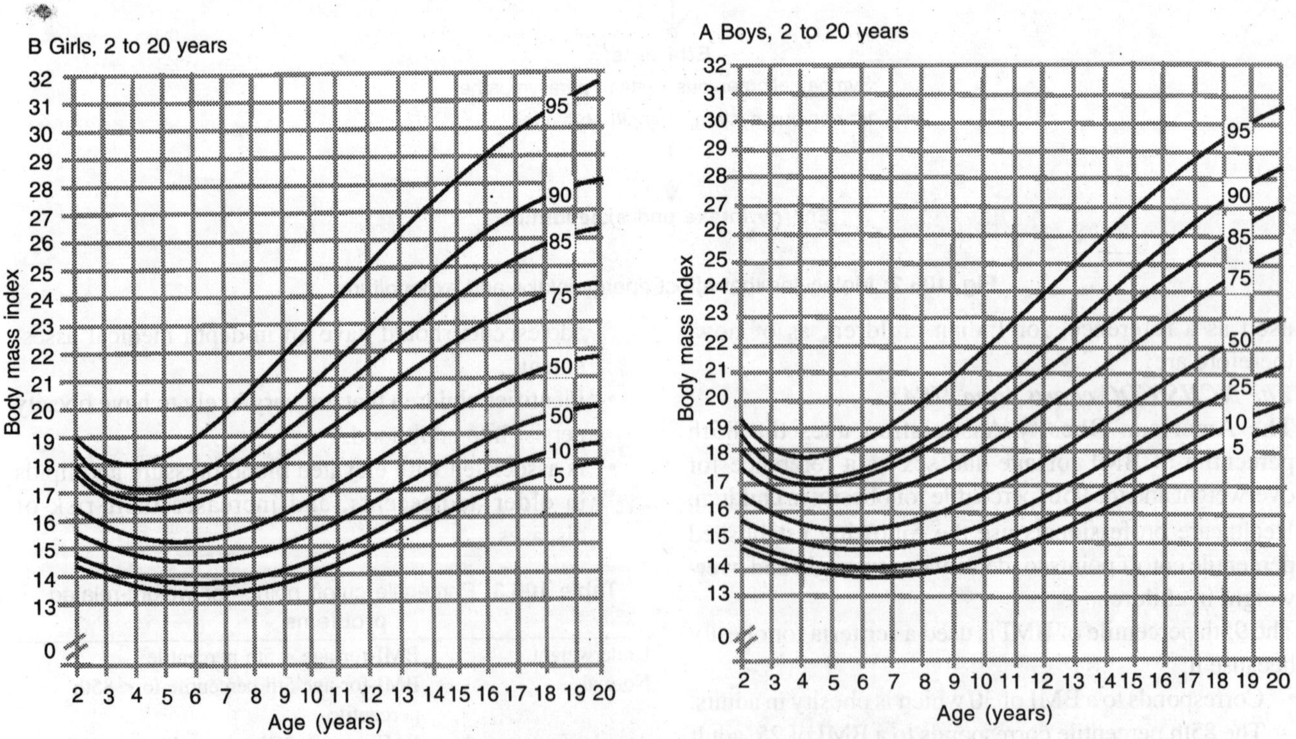

Fig. 106.3: Body mass index and percentiles
The charts were compiled by the centers for Disease Control and Prevention on the basis of combined data from several nationally representative surveys of the U.S. population that were collected between 1963 and 1980

I. Acute Complications

a. ***Sleep apnea and sleep-disordered breathing:*** These are common in children and adolescents with obesity; in some cases, the apnea is accompanied by neurocognitive dysfunction. Tonsillectomy and adenoidectomy and/or bilevel positive airway pressure/continuous positive airway pressure (BIPAP/CPAP) may be beneficial in patients with reduced oxygenation or carbon dioxide retention.

b. ***Pseudotumor cerebri:*** It may occur with increased frequency in children with obesity; the pathogenesis of this condition is unclear.

c. ***Orthopedic disorders:*** These include genu valgum, slipped capital femoral epiphysis, and tibia vara, are observed more commonly in children with obesity. Excess weight in young children can cause bowing of the tibia and femurs; the resulting overgrowth of the proximal tibial metaphysis is called Blount disease.

d. ***Liver dysfunction:*** Elevated plasma concentrations of transaminases, is observed in 20% of children with obesity; the liver dysfunction most commonly reflects hepatic steatosis, but cirrhosis may develop in rare instances. One recent study indicates that vitamin E supplements may be effective in reversing this so-called steatohepatitis, suggesting that the disorder reflects a relative state of vitamin E deficiency. Cholelithiasis is more common in adults with obesity than in adults with normal weight. Although gallstones are unusual in childhood, nearly one half of all cases of cholecystitis in adolescents are associated with obesity. Cholecystitis may be even more common during rapid weight loss, particularly with very controlled-energy diets.

e. ***Emotional and psychosocial sequelae:*** Anecdotal evidence suggests that depression and eating disorders are common in children and adolescents referred to obesity clinics. Prejudice and discrimination against individuals with obesity are ubiquitous within US culture; even young children have been found to regard their peers who have obesity in negative ways. Social isolation, peer problems, and lower self-esteem frequently are observed.

f. ***Cardiovascular effects:*** Obesity during childhood and adolescence is associated with a number of ***cardiovascular risk factors***, including hyperinsulinism and insulin resistance, hypercholesterolemia, hypertriglyceridemia, reduced levels of HDL, and hypertension. A hallmark of insulin resistance is acanthosis nigricans, the presence of which indicates an increased risk of type 2 diabetes. Adolescent girls with obesity also demonstrate a hyperandrogenic profile, consisting of elevated serum concentrations of androstenedione, dehydroepiandrosterone-sulfate (DHEA-S), and testosterone, as well as reduced levels of sex hormone-binding globulin. The clinical picture resembles that of polycystic ovary syndrome (PCOS). The excess androgens are of adrenal and ovarian origin and may be related, at least in part, to increased serum concentrations of insulin and insulin growth factor 1 (IGF-I). Among sexually mature adolescents, changes in serum lipids and androgens seem to correlate more strongly with body fat distribution than with absolute weight. Thus, adolescents with central obesity (i.e., android or abdominal fat pattern) are more likely to manifest these cardiovascular risk factors than individuals with peripheral obesity (i.e., gynoid or gluteal pattern). In prepubertal children, however, the cardiovascular risk factors correlate better with body weight than with body fat distribution. The increasing prevalence of obesity in childhood and adolescence, accompanied by insulin resistance, appears to explain the increasing incidence of type 2 diabetes in adolescents, particularly in minority populations.

II. Long-term Complications

a. ***Adulthood obesity:*** Obesity during childhood and adolescence is associated with an increased risk of ***obesity during adulthood***, with its attendant long-term health risks. This increased risk appears most pronounced for adolescent males with moderate-to-severe obesity. The long-term implications of obesity during infancy and early childhood on subsequent health are less clear. In general, the proportion of children with obesity who have obesity as adults increases with increased age at onset of obesity, such that 26-41% of preschoolers with obesity have obesity as adults, compared to 42-63% of school-aged children. Additionally, the higher the degree of obesity during childhood, the higher is the risk of adult obesity. One study indicates that 18-year-old adolescents with a BMI at or above the 95th percentile have a 66-78% risk of being overweight at age 35 years.

b. *Diabetes mellitus:* The dramatic increase in the prevalence of ***type 2 diabetes*** among adolescents with obesity is likely to be accompanied by a host of diabetic-related complications in adulthood and a reduction in life span. The epidemiological data, although limited, indicate that adolescent obesity is associated with increased morbidity and mortality in later life. An increased risk of death from all causes and from coronary artery disease (CAD) has been observed consistently in males, but not in females, who had obesity during adolescence. In a follow-up of the Harvard Growth Study, the risk of morbidity from CAD and atherosclerosis was increased among men and women who had been overweight (BMI >75th percentile) as teenagers. Gout and colorectal cancer increased among men who had obesity as adolescents, and arthritis increased among women who had obesity as adolescents. Many of these adverse health outcomes appear to be independent of adult weight, suggesting a direct effect of adolescent obesity on adult health and mortality.

c. ***Psychosocial dysfunction:*** Seen in individuals who have obesity in childhood and adolescence is a serious concern. Among teens and young adults who were tracked after 7 years, overweight females were found to have completed less schooling, were less likely to have married, and had higher rates of household poverty compared to their nonoverweight peers. For overweight males, the only adverse outcome was a decreased likelihood of being married.

Thus, if one is obese, you're more likely to develop a number of potentially serious health problems. These may include:

High blood pressure: As one puts on weight he gains mostly fatty tissue. Just like other parts of the body, this tissue relies on oxygen and nutrients in your blood to survive. As demand for oxygen and nutrients increases, the amount of blood circulating through your body also increases. More blood travelling through your arteries means added pressure on your artery walls. Weight gain also typically increases the level of insulin, a blood-sugar-controlling hormone, in your blood. The increase in insulin is associated with retention of sodium and water, which increases blood volume. In addition, excess weight often is associated with an increase in heart rate and a reduction in the capacity of blood vessels to transport blood. All of these factors can increase blood pressure.

Diabetes: Obesity is a leading cause of type 2 diabetes. Excess fat makes one's body resistant to insulin, the hormone that helps the body maintain a proper level of a sugar (glucose) in blood.

Abnormal blood fats: A diet high in saturated fats— red meat and fried foods, for example—can lead to obesity as well as elevated levels of low-density lipoprotein ("bad") cholesterol. Obesity is also associated with low levels of high-density lipoprotein ("good") cholesterol and high levels of triglycerides. Triglycerides are the form in which most fat exists in food as well as in body. Over time, abnormal blood fats can contribute to atherosclerosis—the buildup of fatty deposits in arteries throughout the body. Atherosclerosis puts one at risk of coronary artery disease and stroke.

Coronary artery disease: This is a form of cardiovascular disease. It results from the buildup of fatty deposits in arteries that supply the heart. Over time these deposits can narrow the heart's arteries, so less blood flows to your heart. Diminished blood flow to the heart can cause chest pain (angina). Complete blockage can lead to a heart attack.

Stroke: Obesity is associated with atherosclerosis— the buildup of fatty deposits in arteries throughout the body, including arteries in the brain. If a blood clot forms in a narrowed artery in brain, it can block blood flow to that area of brain. The result is a stroke. Being obese thus, raises the risk of a stroke.

Osteoarthritis: This joint disorder most often affects the knees, hips and lower back. Excess weight puts extra pressure on these joints and wears away the cartilage that protects them, resulting in joint pain and stiffness.

Sleep apnea: This serious condition causes a person to stop breathing for short periods during sleep and to snore heavily. The upper airway is blocked during sleep, which results in frequent awakening at night and subsequent drowsiness during the day. Most people with sleep apnea are overweight, which contributes to a large neck and narrowed airways.

Cancer: Many types of cancer are associated with being overweight. In women, these include cancers of the breast, uterus, cervix, ovaries and gallbladder. Overweight men have a particularly higher risk of cancers of the colon, rectum and the prostate.

Fatty liver disease: When one is obese, fats can build up in his liver. This fatty accumulation can lead to inflammation and scarring of the liver. Such scarring can cause cirrhosis of the liver, even if one is not a heavy alcohol drinker.

Gallbladder disease: Because overweight people may produce more cholesterol, which can be deposited in the gallbladder, the risk of gallstones is higher in obese people. Fast weight loss—more than 3 pounds a week—also can increase the risk of gallstones.

Gout: Obesity is also considered to be a risk factor for gout (Table 106.1).

EVALUATION OF OBESE CHILDREN

Evaluation of obesity in childhood is important for several reasons. First, it offers the best hope for preventing disease progression with its associated morbidities into adulthood. Second, while genetic and hormonal causes of obesity are rare, they do warrant consideration in obese children. In addition, obesity has a negative impact on the self-esteem of children and adolescents, which may have significant implications for long-term happiness and success in life. Finally, directed sessions that emphasize healthy eating and exercise habits for children and their families may have lasting effects on the lifestyle of these patients.

Assessment of Obese

a. ***History:***

- Short stature or a reduced rate of linear growth in a

Table 106.1: Consequences of childhood obesity

Immediate effects and complications (usually in severe obesity):	
Psychosocial stress Respiratory embarrassment Obstructive airway disease Restrictive airway disease (most severe, Pickwickian S) Pseudotumor cerebri Cholelithiasis (and cholecystitis)	Blount's disease Slipped femoral epiphysis Flat feet Hepatic steatosis Endocrine effects Increased skeletal growth Early puberty (reduced final growth)
Co-morbidities: Dyslipedemias Hypertension Insulin resistance syndrome (Syndrome X) Childhood type 2 diabetes mellitus Ovarian hyperandrogenism (hirsuitism, oligomenorrhoea and infertility ± ovarian cysts) Reduced bone density Raised creactive protein/systemic inflammation	
Future risks: Adult obesity Coronary heart disease and cerebrovascular disease Type 2 diabetes mellitus Osteoporosis	

Table 106.2: Characteristics of idiopathic and endogenous obesity

Idiopathic obesity	*Endogenous obesity*
>90 percent of cases	<10 percent of cases
Tall stature (usually >50th percentile)	Short stature (usually <5th percentile)
Family history of obe1sity common	Family history of obesity uncommon
Mental function normal	Often mentally impaired
Normal or advanced bone age	Delayed bone age
Physical examination otherwise normal	Associated stigmata on physical examination

child with obesity suggests the possibility of growth hormone deficiency, hypothyroidism, cortisol excess, pseudohypoparathyroidism, or a genetic syndrome such as Prader-Willi syndrome.

- A history of dry skin, constipation, intolerance to cold, or fatigability suggests hypothyroidism.
- Polyuria and polydipsia may be noted if the adolescent with obesity develops overt diabetes (Table 106.2).
- A history of damage to the CNS (e.g., infection, trauma, hemorrhage, radiation therapy, seizures) suggests hypothalamic obesity with or without pituitary growth hormone deficiency or pituitary hypothyroidism. A history of morning headaches, vomiting, visual disturbances, and excessive urination or drinking also suggests that the obesity may be caused by a tumor or mass in the hypothalamus.

b. ***Physical examination:***

- Two particularly useful clinical measures are the rate of linear growth and the timing of puberty. Most patients who have familial or diet-induced obesity grow at a normal or excessive rate and enter puberty at the appropriate age; many mature more quickly than children with normal weight, and bone age commonly is advanced. In contrast, growth rate and pubertal development are diminished or delayed in growth hormone deficiency, hypothyroidism, cortisol excess, and a variety of genetic syndromes. Conversely, growth rate and pubertal development are accelerated in precocious puberty and in some girls with PCOS.
- Clinical clues that suggest a hormonal etiology for childhood obesity include the following:
  - Weight gain out of character for the family.
  - Obesity in a short child.
  - Progressive weight gain without a comparable increase in linear growth.
  - Dry skin, constipation, intolerance to cold, and fatigability.

- Accumulation of fat in the neck and trunk but not in the arms or legs.
- Purple striae (stretch marks).
- Hypertension.
- Inappropriate sexual development at an early age.
- Excess facial hair, acne, and/or irregular menses in a teenage girl.
- Headaches, vomiting, visual disturbances, or excessive urination and drinking.

Treatment with certain drugs or medications:

- Selective accumulation of fat in the neck, trunk and purple striae suggest an excess of cortisol, particularly if the rate of linear growth has declined.
- The appearance of signs of sexual development at an early age suggests that the weight gain is caused by precocious puberty. On the other hand, excessive facial hair, acne, and irregular periods in a teenage girl suggest that the weight gain may be caused by cortisol excess or PCOS. Obesity itself may be accompanied by facial hair, irregular menses and hypertension.
- ***Measurement of BMI*** represents the first step in assessment and treatment. The term "obesity" is applied when BMI of a child exceeds the 95th percentile for children of the same age and sex, and the term "at risk for overweight" is applied to children or adolescents whose BMI is between the 85th and 95th percentiles. The crossing of major growth percentile lines upward is an early indication of risk. Less than 5 percent of children cross two major percentile lines upward on the growth charts of the Centers for Disease Control and Prevention after four years of age. Thereafter, children who cross major percentile lines upward may be at increased risk for overweight (Table 106.3).

Table 106.3: Assessment of childhood overweight

Calculate body mass index: Divide the weight in kilograms by the square of the height in meters.
Family history: Identify obesity in first-degree relatives.
Evaluate history of cardiovascular disease; type 2 diabetes, or cancer in first-degree relatives.
Diet: Identify caretakers who feed the child.
Identify foods high in calories and low in nutritional value that can be reduced, eliminated or replaced.
Activity: Identify barriers to physical exercise.
Evaluate time spent in play.
Evaluate school recess and physical education (frequency, duration and intensity).
Assess after school and weekend activities.
Assess screen time (television, computer and video games).
History and review of systems.

Although visceral fat increases the likelihood of morbidity in adults and youth, no widely accepted clinical measure of central adiposity yet exist in youth.

The family history of obesity and obesity-related diseases and the dietary and activity patterns should routinely be assessed. The signs and symptoms that are most frequently associated with a congenital or endocrine abnormality underlying overweight are hypogonadism, short statue, dysmorphic features, a somatic abnormality and mental retardation. The history and physical examination should also address potential complications of overweight.

c. ***Laboratory testing:***

- Fasting and 2-hour postprandial glucose and insulin levels and hemoglobin A1c (for evaluation of insulin resistance and glucose tolerance).
- Fasting lipid panel for detection of dyslipidemia.
- Thyroid function tests.
- Serum leptin.
- Adrenal function tests, when indicated, to assess the possibility of Cushing syndrome.
- Karyotype (with fluorescence in situ hybridization [FISH] for Prader-Willi [15q-]), when indicated by clinical history and physical examination.
- Growth hormone (GH) secretion and function tests, when indicated.
- Assessment of reproductive hormones (including prolactin), when indicated.
- Serum calcium, phosphorus, and parathyroid hormone levels to evaluate for suspected pseudohypoparathyroidism.

d. ***Imaging studies:*** MRI scan of the brain with focus on the hypothalamus and pituitary, when clinically indicated.

e. ***Procedures:*** Sleep studies to detect sleep apnea.

Some experts for all overweight children have recommended a fasting profile of lipoprotein, insulin and glucose levels. Elevated levels of liver enzymes, which usually indicate hepatic steatosis, occur in approximately 10 percent of overweight children and adolescents in the general population. As with all screening tests, clinicians should decide whether testing is likely to alter the course of treatment they prescribe. The American Diabetes Association recommends a fasting plasma glucose test for children 10 years of age or older who have a BMI at or above the 85th percentile and two of the following risk factors: a family history of type 2 diabetes in first-degree or second degree relatives, nonwhite race, and conditions associated with insulin resistance (e.g. acanthosis nigricans, hypertension, dyslipidemia or polycystic ovarian syndrome) (Table 106.4).

CONTROLLING THE OBESITY EPIDEMIC—PREVENTION AND ITS TREATMENT

Atleast 1 in 10 urban middle class children in India is

Table 106.4: Clinic based approach to childhood obesity

BMI	*Clinical evaluation*	*Assessments*	*Comments*
>95th centile NCHS	Rule out underlying causes* e.g., Hypothyroidism (1-2/1000 children), Prader Willi (1/25000 population), Cushing's syndrome	Developmental Delay, Short Stature, Dysmorphism, Abnormal genitalia	All are relatively rare conditions and have distinctive clinical features *May require referral to Endocrinologist
>95th centile NCHS	Look out for severe complications* (See Table 36.1)	Blurred optic disks, Breathing difficulties, Painful walking, Abdominal pain	Rare, but some severe complications are potentially fatal *Appropriate reference to experts
>75th centile, NCHS and family history of obesity/related morbidities	Screen for co-morbidities such as hypertension (25% obese children)	Blood pressure	Comorbidities are very common (upto 30%)
	Dyslipidemias (20% obese children)	Lipid profile	Further investigation and referral according to findings
	Polycystic ovaries (20% obese children)	Blood sugar levels	
	Childhood Type II Diabetes Mellitus	Fasting insulin	
	Insulin Resistance Syndrome	USG	
All overweight and obese children	Assess for Psychological disorders e.g., Depression, Binge eating, Bulimea	Counsellors	Could be cause or effect of obesity

overweight. If we allow this epidemic to continue, we will top the world in diabetes and CHD earlier than estimated. The cost of treating obesity and its associated complications will consume a major chunk of our resources, which we can ill afford. Only community-based approaches can address such large numbers of affected children. Obesogenic lifestyles behaviors are less well developed in children and therefore more amenable to change. An overwhelming body of evidence now indicates that prevention must begin in childhood to reduce the burden and cost of obesity in society.

In India, public health efforts so far, have been directed towards improving nutrition. Obesity treatment campaigns will have to be carefully worded to avoid conflicting messages and deleterious results. However, the only way to cut short the escalating epidemic appears to be prevention of obesity and other lifestyle problems in childhood itself.

Strategies and Aims: Public Health Approach

As a public health approach, essentially all children, adolescents and families should benefit from counselling to prevent excess weight gain and obesity.

I. Life Style Approach

a. ***Healthy eating patterns:*** Emphasis should be on nutrition rather than 'dieting'. It is essential to maintain healthy components of traditional diets and guard against heavily marketed energy dense foods. The strategy should be to recognize and eliminate risk features of high calorie intake such as frequent snacking, eating out frequently, and celebrating with food and drinks.

A simple Indianised message based on recommendations of AHA could be: "think of a day's food composition as a 'Thali' wherein 50% is full of vegetables, salads and fruits. A quarter should be made up of cereals such as rice and/or chapatis and the remaining quarter should be protein based. Fried, snacks and sweet dishes are only for a very few special occasions (Fig. 106.4).

b. ***Increase physical activity levels:*** Children should be encouraged to be active not only for weight control but also for general well-being. The WHO recommends atleast 30 minutes of cumulative moderate exercise (equivalent to walking briskly) for all ages; plus for children, an additional 20 minutes of

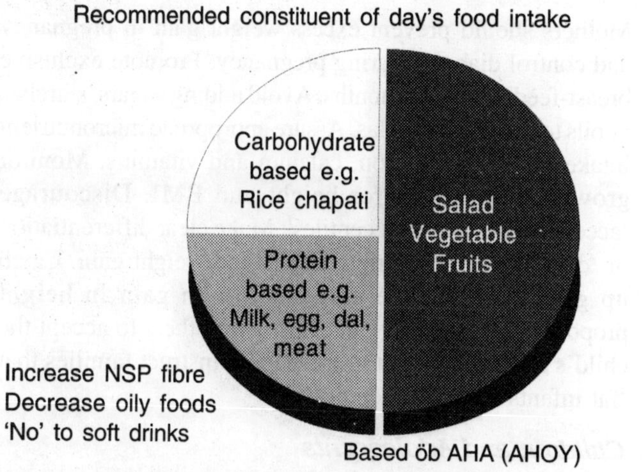

Fig. 106.4: Showing recommended constituents of day's food intake in a 'Thali' based visual

vigorous exercise (equivalent to running), three times a week. These recommendations are basically for prevention of CHD; prevention of obesity may require more physical exertion. In general, moderate to vigorous activities for a period of atleast one hour a day may be more practical recommendation for all school going children.

c. ***Decrease sedentary behavior:*** This is perhaps even more important. Avoid overfeeding stunted populations—assess stature and prevent feeding excess calories with low weight for age but normal weight for height, i.e., 'stunted children'. Most PEM prevention programs (school mid-day meals) use food supplements that provide ample energy and protein but may be deficient in micronutrients. Such programs may induce weight gain in underweight children while length deficit may not be reversed, thereby creating a risk of obesity.

'Target' populations most in need of interventions; in India this would probably mean urban children from higher and mid socio-economic status. Targeting avoids confusing messaging directed towards opposite segments of society.

'Tailor the interventions' to suit the specific needs of the community.

Address 'behavior change'—consideration of socio-cultural and ethnic issues is important in suggesting diets and activity.

Focus on involvement of entire family indeed the entire community for better results.

Build supportive infrastructure e.g., safe playgrounds, transport and town planning.

Confront vested interests e.g., advertising of colas.

II. Special Strategies to Target Specific Age Groups

Infants and Young Children

Mothers should prevent excess weight gain in pregnancy and control diabetes during pregnancy. Promote exclusive breast-feeding for six months. Avoid adding sugars, starches or oils to feeding formulas. Assure appropriate micronutrient intake especially of iron, calcium and vitamins. Monitor growth with weight for height and BMI. Discourage 'accelerated crossing of centiles'. Make clear differentiation of 'catch up growth' from accelerated weight gain. Catch up growth should be associated with gain in height proportional to weight gain. Instruct mothers to accept the child's appetite and not to force feed. Instruct families that 'fat infants make fat adults'.

Children and Adolescents

The fat rebound age (5-8 years) and adolescence are particularly high risk periods for accumulating fat. Strategies for prevention include. Promote active lifestyles including at least one hour of vigorous play per day. Limit television viewing and other sedentary activities to <2hr/day. Promote sensible eating—increase fruit and vegetables and restrict energy dense sweets and soft drinks. Modify environment to promote physical activity e.g., safe roads for cycling, jogging. Celebration should be in the form of outdoor play/picnics rather than fast food joint parties. Educate about the evils of alcohol/tobacco to adolescents.

Channels of Interventions/Health Education Include:

a. ***School based programs:***

Schools are probably the ideal medium of intervention as they are central to children's lives and information can be relatively quickly dissipated through this channel. Aspects to be considered are: Training of teachers in lifestyles, nutrition and activity. Introduction of ideal school meals or provision of canteens offering only healthy options based on Indian foods. Introduction of 'nutrition and physical education' in school curriculum. These activities should become compulsory and/or a 'scoring subject' with marks to be added to total grades.

After-school games should be encouraged. Obese children should not be teased, targeted or bullied or isolated. Involve parent associations. School health check ups should monitor BMI along with height and weight annually.

b. ***Media involvement:***

Another powerful channel especially for upper and middle class societies is media coverage. Regular columns and supplements have already started making a mark.

c. ***Health centers/doctors/other professionals:***

- It is important for doctors and other health professionals to think 'prevention of obesity' at all visits and incorporate relevant health education.
- Incorporate BMI charts/IOTF cut offs and waist circumference in routine health records. Monitor BMI every year, particularly for children from high-risk families.
- Identify children with BMI>75th centiles (and with accelerated crossing of centiles) for frequent monitoring and 'life style' interventions.
- Discourage parent's obsession with food intake and pleas for tonics.
- The pediatrician plays an important role in the prevention of obesity. From birth on, feeding a child always involves a dual task—namely, offering food in appropriate amounts and gearing it to the child's expression of his needs. Only in this way can he develop discriminating awareness and become active in establishing self-regulation. ... If a child is fed when he is hungry, played with when he needs attention, and encouraged to be active when he is restless, he is not likely to grow up inhibited and passive or overstuffed

and helpless, unable to control his eating because every discomfort is misinterpreted as a need to eat.

d. ***Governmental authorities:*** Both health and infrastructure authorities should be responsible for devising national strategies. Encouraging food outlets/restaurants to serve healthy choices. Providing safe exercise opportunities. Regulate advertisements aimed at children and insist on food labelling. Consider taxation on 'fatty food' or alternatively reduce taxation/promote production of fresh food and vegetables.

e. ***Paternal involvement: Tips for Parents***
- Respect your child's appetite: Children do not need to finish every bottle or meal.
- Avoid pre-prepared and sugared foods when possible.
- Limit the amount of high-calorie foods kept in the home.
- Provide a healthy diet, with 30 percent or fewer calories derived from fat.
- Provide ample fiber in the child's diet.
- Skim milk may safely replace whole milk at 2 years of age.
- Do not provide food for comfort or as a reward.
- Do not offer sweets in exchange for a finished meal.
- Limit amount of television viewing.
- Encourage active play.
- Establish regular family activities such as walks, ball games and other outdoor activities.

MANAGEMENT OF ESTABLISHED OBESITY

Whereas the public health campaign is to be targeted to the society as a whole, individual or clinic based approach is necessary for the treatment of the obviously obese child.

I. Individual Approach

Treatment is more likely to be successful in children than adults.

Goals of Therapy

Medical goal: It should be resolution of complications and co-morbidities such as hypertension and hyperlipidemias.

Behavioral goal: Achievement of healthy eating and activity patterns is primary to achievement of ideal body weight.

Weight goal: Weight maintenance rather than weight loss (unless moribund obesity) in young children—'let the child grow into his weight'. Prolonged weight maintenance will allow a gradual decline in the BMI as the child grows in height.

General Approach to Therapy

Institute small, gradual and permanent changes, not short-term diets in exercise programs aimed at rapid weight loss. Involve the family and all caregivers in the treatment programs. Intervention should begin early (later than 3 years but earlier than adolescence). Clinicians should encourage and emphasize and not criticize.

II. Group Weight-Loss Programs

Even when you decide the best way to lose weight comes from eating low-calorie foods in moderate amounts, you don't have to go it alone. Commercial group programs can support your efforts, giving you eating plans and reinforcement from others on the same path.

Principles of Therapy

Theoretically, obesity management is energy balance (eat less and exercise more). These include:

1. ***Dietary Therapy***

Limiting energy intake of growing children can result in decreased linear growth velocity in obese children and is therefore risky. Dieting could also increase prevalence of inadequate nutrients, such as iron, calcium, zinc and vitamins A, C and E. High degrees of parental dietary control may in fact have adverse psychosocial effects on young children with treatment failures. Hence the aim should be provision of well balanced healthy meals with a healthy approach to eating. Several different dietary studies have shown successful reduction of caloric intake and improved eating behaviors. The advice usually centers on reducing calories from fat, saturated fats, cholesterol and sugars (high density foods) while increasing fruits, vegetables and whole grain cereals (lower density foods). Counting of calories can be tedious and inaccurate and it is more advantageous to supply indigenous versions of Food Guide Pyramids or Epstein's traffic light diets. Trials of hypocaloric diets, protein modified fasts, fibre supplementation and anorectic drugs have been shown to be by and large, ineffective in children in the long range. Consultation with a dietitian/nutritionist that specializes in children's needs is often a valuable part of obesity treatment. Nutrition consultants can outline specific and appropriate nutritional needs for healthy growth.

As with adults, a nutrition consultant may or may not recommend reducing the number of calories the child eats and implementing strategies like learning to read nutrition labels and the food guide pyramid, selecting proper portion sizes, and prepared foods. Some eating behaviors that nutrition consultants typically encourage include taking smaller bites, chewing food longer, and to avoid eating too quickly by putting the utensil down between bites.

To lose weight and keep it off, eat moderate amounts of nutrient-rich, low-fat, low-calorie foods. Follow these fundamentals of healthy eating:

Think 'energy density': Energy density is the number of calories in a given volume of food. One shouldn't eat a food that's energy dense, such as fat which one can't eat much without consuming a lot of calories. On the other hand, eat a food with low energy density, including most vegetables and some fruits, and one can consume a huge amount for few calories. For example: A tablespoon of butter has the same number of calories as 20 cups of leaf lettuce. Which would leave one feeling fuller? Choose low-energy-dense foods, which include a lot of fresh fruits and vegetables.

Choose healthy foods: Healthy foods include vegetables, fruits, grains and lean sources of protein, including beans, fish, low-fat dairy products and lean meats. These foods optimize nutrition and taste and promote a healthy weight. Eat a variety of healthy foods in lieu of junk foods.

Choose the right carbohydrates: Nutrition experts generally agree that 45 percent to 65 percent of your total daily calories should come from carbohydrates. Butone has to be choosy about those to eat. Steer away from simple carbohydrates, such as table sugar and other sweeteners, and limit fruit juice, which is a type of carbohydrate concentrated in calories. Instead, try to eat plenty of complex, high-fiber carbohydrates, such as whole-grain bread and pasta, brown rice, and other grains, such as oatmeal.

Cut back on sweets. Limit candies, cakes, cookies, muffins, pies, doughnuts and frozen desserts. They're a large source of calories. Better dessert choices include angel food cake, vanilla wafers, fig-bar cookies, low-fat frozen yogurt, sorbet or sherbet.

Reduce fat: Because fat has more than twice the calories of carbohydrate and protein ounce for ounce, reducing the fat content of one's diet is an important way to cut calories. Foods high in fat include most fast foods, pastries, red meats, full-fat dairy products, oils, margarine, butter, salad dressings and mayonnaise. Current dietary guidelines recommend that healthy Americans get between 20 percent and 35 percent of total calories from fat, with less than 10 percent of the total calories coming from saturated fat sources.

Watch portion sizes: Serving sizes may be smaller than one may think. A single 2-1/2-ounce serving of fish or poultry, for example, is about the size of a deck of cards. A 2-ounce serving of cheese or 1 teaspoon of butter is about the size of four dice. A small apple or a medium orange are comparable in size to a tennis ball. A hockey puck is about the size of one-half a bagel or a slice of whole-grain bread. It's especially important to watch serving sizes when eating out because many restaurants serve oversized portions.

Count calories: Read food labels. Foods that are low in fat can sometimes be very high in calories. Processed foods—most products other than fresh foods—often have hidden fat and sugar. Cut back on sugary soft drinks. They're high in calories.

Healthy Weight Pyramid: To help simplify what you should eat, Mayo Clinic has developed the Mayo Clinic Healthy Weight Pyramid—a tool to help you manage your weight and improve your health. The strengths of the Mayo Clinic Healthy Weight Pyramid are:

- It emphasizes weight management.
- Fruits and vegetables are located at the bottom of the Mayo Clinic pyramid as opposed to the bread, cereal and starch group because these foods are very low in calories and high in health-enhancing properties. The Mayo Clinic pyramid doesn't limit the intake of whole, fresh or frozen fruits and vegetables.
- The Mayo Clinic Healthy Weight Pyramid emphasizes healthier choices within each of the five food groups. That's because not all foods within a group provide the same health benefits even though they may contain the same number of calories.
- Daily physical activity is located in the middle of the Mayo Clinic pyramid to emphasize its central role in both managing weight and improving health.

2. ***Physical activity:*** Moderate physical activity is recommended for children every day for at least 60 minutes. If a child is unable to meet that goal, than an individualized program should be designed according to fitness level, using the general guideline as an ultimate goal.
3. ***Behavior therapy:*** Behavior therapy involves changes in diet and physical activity habits to one that promote a healthy weight. Some behavioral therapy strategies for children and adolescents should include parent and family involvement.

   Some behavioral therapy strategies for children are to:

   - ***Record diet and exercise patterns*** in a diary to keep track of types and amount of foods eaten and exercise performed as well as the location and time that foods are eaten and exercise takes place. The diary is useful to determine any problem areas in eating and exercise behavior.
   - ***Identify high-risk situations*** (such as having too many high-calorie foods in the house), and consciously avoid them. Watching TV during meal times is another high-risk situation that encourages eating every time the TV is on.
   - Reward specific positive actions. Examples of such actions include meeting an exercise duration goal or eating less of a certain type of food.
   - Rewards for achieving goals can be decided by children and parents together, and should revolve around something that encourages positive behavior. For example, giving sporting equipment as a reward may encourage more physically active behavior.
   - Avoid using food as a reward, especially high-calories foods. Making them a reward may only make them more desirable. Parents and health professionals should regularly use verbal praise.

- Change unrealistic goals and false beliefs about weight loss and body image to realistic and positive ones.
- The family can work as a team to set weekly activity goals. Making a contract and having every family member sign it encourages commitment to a goal. Parents can also help a child adopt or maintain a positive attitude about new behaviors in addition to helping the child cope with any negative remarks from peers.
- Develop a ***social support network*** (family, friends or neighbors) that can encourage weight loss in a positive and motivating manner.
- ***Motivate oneself:*** No one can make someone lose weight. In fact, increased external pressure—often from people close to oneself—may only make matters worse. Likewise, trying to lose weight to satisfy someone else rarely works either. Make diet and exercise changes to please oneself.
- ***Make lifestyle changes a priority:*** As one is planning to launch new weight-related lifestyle changes, other pressing problems in your life should be resolved so that one can be sure of being focused on the matter at hand.
- ***Have a plan:*** Work out a strategy that will gradually change the habits and attitudes that may have undermined one's past efforts to lose weight. Choose a definite start date. Consider how often and how long one will exercise. Determine a realistic eating plan that includes plenty of water, fruits and vegetables. Write everything down: When and where will one do the steps in his plan? How will one's plan fit into his schedule? What are the potential roadblocks, and how will one deal with them?
- ***Set small goals:*** Remember that one is in this for the long haul. One's making lifestyle changes, and the goals he has written down are the first steps in that direction. Anything one undertakes too intensely or too vigorously will often become uncomfortable, and one is more likely to give it up.
- ***Surround oneself with good examples:*** As one sets his goals, it helps to surround oneself with good examples. Magazines on "Health", and "Healthy Diets" include plenty of real-life stories, healthy and easy recipes, exercise tips and interesting facts about fitness.
- ***Avoid food triggers:*** Distract oneself from desire to eat with something positive, such as calling a friend. Practice saying no to unhealthy foods and big portions. Eat when one is actually hungry—not when the clock says it's time to eat. When one eats, he should focus on eating. Serve one's meals on smaller plates to make less food seem like more. In general, store food out of sight and don't keep junk foods around.
- ***Keep a record:*** It is also recommended that one keeps a food and activity diary periodically, so he can reinforce good habits and discover any behaviors that may need improvement. Remember that success isn't defined only by actual weight lost. In fact, one must be sure to track other important health parameters such as blood pressure, cholesterol levels and overall fitness.
- ***Focus on the positive:*** Rather than focusing on what one can't eat, focus on what one can eat. Look at what new tastes and activities one can discover that will enhance your health.
- ***Don't give up:*** One will have setbacks. Don't expect perfection. But don't give up. Use relapses to get back on track. Motivate oneself with healthy, nonfood rewards when one reaches his goals.

  Dealing with obesity may mean taking a hard look at how one lives and making some tough changes. It may be helpful to talk to a weight-loss specialist or others trying to lose weight. They may be able to help one to think of food and exercise in a new light. Limiting energy intake of growing children can result in decreased linear growth velocity in obese children and is therefore risky. Dieting could also increase prevalence of inadequate nutrients, such as iron, calcium, zinc and vitamins A, C and E. The aim should be provision of balanced healthy meals with a healthy approach to eating. The advice usually centers on reducing calorie intake from fat, saturated fats, cholesterol and sugars while increasing fruits, vegetables and whole grain cereals. Counting of calories can be tedious and inaccurate and it is more advantageous to supply indigenous versions of Food Guide Pyramids or Epstein's traffic light diets. Trials of hypocaloric diets, protein modified fasts, fiber supplementation and anorectic drugs have been shown to be by and large, ineffective in children in the long range.
- Addition of physical activity and reduction in sedentary behavior, both improve long-term outcome. The important components of behavioral therapy include treatment of families as a whole, identification of problem behaviors and their modifications, and 'tailor' made advice and support component. Parenting skills recommended in treatment plans are praising the child's behavior, never using food as reward, establishing firm daily family meal and snack times, providing only healthy options, removing temptations and being a good role model.

4. ***Drug Treatment:*** These drugs are yet not approved for use to treat obesity in children. However, clinical trials are underway. The use of anorectic drugs for the treatment of obesity has a checkered history. In general,

anorectic agents have little or no effect on weight gain in the absence of a controlled diet and exercise program. The drugs have modest effects on total body weight, with long-term weight losses amounting to 2-10 kg in patients with obesity, and the responses of individuals to drug therapy vary considerably. Most of the weight loss resulting from drug therapy is achieved within the first 6 months of treatment, with subsequent maintenance of the reduced weight or slight regain of weight. Unfortunately, discontinuation of the drug therapy is accompanied by rebound weight gain and loss of the selective advantage over placebo.

Of more concern, the drugs may have potentially serious adverse effects, particularly in patients with psychiatric disorders. For example, adrenergic agents, such as phentermine, phenylpropanolamine (withdrawn from US market), mazindol (withdrawn from US market), ephedra, and sibutramine, may cause dry mouth, insomnia, nervousness, diaphoresis, hypertension, nausea, and constipation. Tolerance to most adverse effects is achieved within 2 weeks of continuous treatment. Contraindications to the use of noradrenergic agents include angina and other forms of atherosclerotic disease, cardiac arrhythmias, hyperthyroidism, and/or the concomitant use of MAOIs.

The serotoninergic preparations, fenfluramine and dexfenfluramine, recently were withdrawn from the commercial market because of their association with valvular heart disease and primary pulmonary hypertension. These drugs also were associated with drowsiness, insomnia, tremor, and short-term memory loss. High doses of fenfluramine and dexfenfluramine are neurotoxic in rats and monkeys, raising concerns about the long-term use of other serotoninergic preparations, such as fluoxetine, in children.

Essentially, no information exists regarding the use of anorectic agents in children. In general, do not use anorectic drugs routinely for the prevention or treatment of obesity in childhood or adolescence. Indeed, do not administer anorectic drugs to prepubertal children until carefully controlled clinical studies are performed to assess their safety and efficacy. Administer anorectic drugs only after the patient has failed to respond to vigorous attempts to modify behavior, diet, and family interactions. Unless prohibited by a specific investigational protocol, all adolescents who are administered anorectic agents should receive concurrent nutritional and family counselling and should implement a plan of regular exercise and physical activity.

Medications for Weight-loss

Prescription weight-loss drugs aren't for people who just want to lose a few pounds for cosmetic reasons. They're for people with a BMI of 30 or higher or for those with a BMI of 27 or greater who have health problems that would likely improve with weight-loss. The two main prescription weight-loss medications are:

- Sibutramine (Meridia).
- Orlistat (Xenical).

Over-the-Counter Products

Over-the-counter (OTC) diet products promise to help you shed pounds by raising your metabolism or suppressing your appetite. Their side effects, however, can be dangerous.

- Ephedra (ma-huang).
- Metabolite.
- Chitosan.
- Chromium.
- Garcinia (hydroxycitric acid).
- St. John's wort.
- 5-hydroxytryptophan (5-HTP).
- Herbal laxatives and diuretics.
- Caffeine.
- Pyruvate.

Thus if you're troubled by your weight, talk to your doctor. OTC diet drugs can't help you with anything beyond short-term, temporary weight-loss—if that. These diet products are more harmful than helpful.

5. ***Surgery:*** Surgical procedures such as gastric bypass have been performed successfully on adolescents. However surgery for adolescents is usually considered only when severe medical conditions are present that can improve with the surgery.

Surgery for Weight-Loss

If you've tried diet and exercise to lose weight but remain seriously obese (a BMI of 35 or higher) and have weight-related health problems as a result, weight-loss surgery (bariatric surgery) may be the next best step.

The most common operations fall into one of two categories:

Stomach surgery: The first uses a band or staples to create a small pouch at the top of your stomach, where food enters from your esophagus—the tube from your mouth to your stomach. The stomach pouch can hold only about an ounce or two of food, though this can later expand to several ounces. After the operation, you can eat only small portions of food at a time without feeling nausea or discomfort.

Stomach surgery plus intestinal bypass: The second type of surgery also creates a small pouch, but adds a bypass around part of your small intestine, where most of the calories from foods that you eat are absorbed. This surgery does double duty. It reduces what you can eat, and it reduces the calories your body absorbs.

Here are some of the specific operations, representing these two categories:

Vertical banded gastroplasty (VBG): This is an example of the first category of weight-loss surgery, which is designed to partition the stomach into two parts. Using a surgical stapler, the surgeon divides your stomach into upper and lower sections. The upper pouch is small and empties into the lower pouch, which is the rest of your stomach. At the dime-sized opening where the upper pouch empties into the rest of your stomach, the surgeon wraps the tissue with a piece of nonexpandable plastic. This banding of the opening between the upper stomach pouch and the rest of the stomach helps prevent the opening from stretching.

Gastric bypass: This weight-loss surgery is an example of the second category of surgery—creating a small pouch and adding a bypass around part of your small intestine. The surgeon staples your stomach all the way across the top, leaving a tiny pouch. Then the surgeon cuts the small intestine and sews a part of it directly onto the upper pouch. This redirects the food, bypassing most of your stomach and the first section of your small intestine. Food flows directly into the middle section of your small intestine, limiting your body's ability to absorb calories. Even though food never enters the lower part of your stomach, the stomach stays healthy and continues making digestive juices that flow into your small intestine. Some surgeons can perform gastric bypass by inserting laparoscopes—tiny, tubular instruments with a small camera attached—through small incisions made in the abdomen.This is called laparoscopic gastric bypass. Performing the operation laparoscopically can help decrease your hospital stay and lead to a quicker recovery. There also appear to be fewer wound-related problems with laparoscopic gastric bypass than with the traditional "open" gastric bypass. Not everyone is a candidate for laparoscopic gastric bypass, so consult your doctor.

When appropriate, weight-loss surgery can result in dramatic improvements in weight and health. In the first year or two, most people lose upto 50 percent of their excess weight. Generally, those who follow dietary and exercise recommendations keep most of that weight off long-term.

However, weight-loss surgery does have side effects. Complications such as pneumonia, blood clots and infection can occur with any type of surgery. Rapid weight loss can result in gallstones in about one-third of people who have obesity surgery. A hernia or weakness, which may require surgery to correct, may develop at the site of your incision.

At first after surgery, if you eat too much or too fast, you'll experience nausea and other symptoms, called dumping syndrome. Over time, you'll be able to increase your food intake.

Surgery for weight reduction isn't a miracle procedure, and there are side effects and potential complications. Though you can expect to lose weight and keep it off, you still need to eat healthy foods and remain active.

Liposuction: Not a weight-loss plan. Liposuction is cosmetic surgery, not a weight-loss plan. The surgeon inserts a narrow tube under your skin through tiny incisions, and then suctions out fat cells. It's most commonly used to trim the outer thighs and abdomen. Though liposuction has improved to allow surgeons to remove some fat during the procedure, this body-shaping procedure isn't a treatment.

Intensive Therapy

Yanovski reviewed the limited data on intensive therapies that have been proposed and tried in children. These include (a) severe energy restriction below 1000 kcal/day (b) drugs-fenfluramine, metformin, sibutramine, leptin, octreotide and (c) bariatric surgery such as gastric bypass and gastric stapling. Although initial weight loss can be dramatic, most of these approaches are fraught with significant adverse consequences and need constant long-term monitoring.

Table 106.5: Possible targets of future treatments for obesity

Target of treatment	*Goal*
• Adipocyte transcription factors (peroxisome proliferator-activated g2)	Decrease differentiation of adipocytes from fibroblasts.
• Tumor necrosis factor	Interfere with insulin action and ameliorate insulin resistance.
• Specific endogenous anorectic substances	Develop pro-satiety agents.
• Primary signals regarding body composition or central control of energy balance	Alter central mechanisms for regulating body weight rather than appetite or energy expenditure
• Specific genes (leptin receptor, leptin and antisense neuropeptide Y	Manipulate promoters to increase expression of satiety factors (e.g. leptin) or decrease expression of appetite stimulants (e.g. neuropeptide Y)

None of these treatment modalities can be successful without positive behavioral changes (Table 106.5).

Follow-Up

Regular follow-up is indicated for the following reasons:

- Reinforcement of nutritional goals and exercise objectives.
- Identification of social and emotional barriers to therapy.
- Family support and counselling (if indicated).
- Assessment of growth, pubertal development, and reproductive function.
- Assessment of glucose tolerance and fasting lipid levels.
- Identification and management of obesity-related acute and chronic complications.

Obesity is increasing at a high rate in developed and developing countries. Steps to alter this trend in growing body weight have failed. The reason for this failure has been inadequate teaching of healthful dietary practices to children in early grades, overemphasis of the importance of greater weight and stature during infancy and adolescence, lack of a national unified anti-obesity program, and failure to commit to long-term health practitioner support for those individuals needing help to lose weight. Food promotion by industry and the physician's fear of childhood wasting and failure to thrive has created an environment in which almost everyone in developed countries suffers from excess calories, saturated fat, and protein. Failure to change our priorities and current dietary practices will result in continued increases in overweight, chronic diseases and associated costs.

The increased prevalence of obesity highlights the need of programs for its prevention. In the obesity prevention programs calorie and nutrient intake, emotional and social cues related to food intake must be considered. Thus, in order to prevent development of obesity modifying the nutritional factors it would be necessary: increasing breast-feeding in terms of percentage and duration; modifying wrong weaning patterns decreasing protein intake and increasing fat intake until 2 years of age; modifying toddler and school age children eating habit decreasing fat intake and increasing carbohydrates and fiber intakes, helping parents and/or guardians to understand the real needs of their children without using food as form of gratification, reward, and/or consolation for every negative feelings and situations; asking governments, consumer unions, food industries, and mass media to reduce and regulate non-nutritional food advertisings during children television time.

Childhood obesity is thus a serious nationwide health problem requiring urgent attention and a population-based prevention approach so that all children may grow-up physically and emotionally healthy.

KEY LEARNING POINTS

- Obesity, defined as overweight with abnormal deposition of fat in the tissues to the extent that health may be impaired in one or the other way, is now emerging as a global epidemic.
- India is now in the thick of "double burden" with obesity and malnutrition often coexisting.
- Acute complications of obesity include sleep apnea, sleep-disordered breathing, pseudomotor cerebri, emotional and psychologic problems and cardiovascular effects.
- Long-term complications include adulthood obesity, diabetes mellitus, hypertension, stroke, gallbladder disease, cancer, etc.
- A complete assessment, based on history and physical examination, laboratory testing, imaging studies, sleep studies, etc is warranted depending on individual merits of the case.
- Controlling obesity epidemic needs public health approach and special strategies to target specific age groups.
- Principles of treatment include dietary therapy, increase in physical activity, drug therapy and surgery.

FURTHER READINGS

1. Armstrong J, Reilly JJ, *et al.* Breastfeeding and lowering the risk of childhood obesity. *Lancet* 2002; 359 (9322): 2003-2004.
2. Armstrong J, Reilly JJ. Child Health Information Team. Breast-feeding and lowering the risk of childhood obesity. *Lancet* 2002; 359: 2003-2004.
3. Barker DJP. Mothers, babies and health in later life. London: Churchill Livingstone 1998.
4. Bavdekar A,Yajnik CS, Caroline HD, Bapat S, *et al.* Insulin resistance syndrome in 8-year old Indian children—Small at birth, Big at 8 years, or both? *Diabetes* 1999; 48: 2422-2429.
5. Bhargava SK, Sachdev HPS, Fall CHD, Osmond C, *et al.* Relation of serial changes in childhood body-mass index to impaired glucose tolerance in young adulthood. *New Eng J Med* 2004; 350: 865-875.
6. Bhatia V. IAP Task Force for C Childhood Prevention of Adult Diseases: Insulin resistance and type 2 diabetes mellitus in childhood. *Indian Pediatr* 2004; 41: 443-457.
7. Bhave S, Bavdekar A, Otiv M. IAP National Task Force for Childhood Prevention of Adult Diseases: Childhood obesity. *Indian Pediatr* 2004; 41: 559-575.
8. Cole TJ, Bellizzi MC, Flegal KM, Dietz WH. Establishing a standard definition for child overweight and obesity worldwide international survey. *BMJ 2000*; 320: 1240-1243.
9. Dabelea D, Hanson RL, Lindsay RS, Pettitt DJ, *et al.* Intrauterine exposure to diabetes conveys risks for type 2 diabetes and obesity: A study of discordant sibships. *Diabetes* 2000; 49: 2208-2211.
10. Dietz WH, Robinson TN. Overweight children and adolescents 2005; 352(20): 2100-2108.

11. Dietz WH. Overweight in childhood and adolescence. N Engl J Med 2004; 350: 855-857.
12. Edmunds L, Waters E, Ellist EJ. Evidence based management of childhood obesity. BMJ 2001; 323: 916-919.
13. Freedman DS, Kahn LK, Dietz WH, Srinivasan SR, *et al.* Relationship of childhood obesity to coronary heart disease risk factors in adulthood: The Bogalusa Heart Study. Pediatrics 2001; 108: 712-718.
14. Higgins PB, Gower BA, Hunter GR, Goran MI. Defining health-related obesity in prepubertal children. *Obes Res* 2001; 9: 233-240.
15. Himes JH. Agreement over anthropometric indicators identifying the fattest adolescents. *Int J Obes Relat Metab Disord* 1999; 23(suppl):18-21.
16. Ikeda JP, Mitchell RA. Dietary approaches to the treatment of the overweight pediatric patient. *PCNA* 2001; 48: 955-968.
17. Kapil U, Singh P, Pathak P, Dwivedi SN, Bhasin S. Prevalence of obesity amongst affluent adolescent school children in Delhi. *Indian Pediatr* 2002; 39: 449-452.
18. Kurpad AV, Swaminathan S, Bhat S. IAP National Task Force for Prevention of Adult Diseases. The effect of childhood activity on prevention of adult diseases. Indian Pediatr 2004; 41: 37-62.
19. Lobstein T, Baur L, Uauy R. Obesity in children and young people: A crisis in public health. Report to the WHO. Published by IASO International Obesity Task Force, London 2004.
20. Mei Z, Grummer-Strawn LM, Thompson D, Dietz WH. Shifts in percentiles of growth during early childhood: Analysis of longitudinal data from the California Child Health and Development Study. *Pediatrics* 2004; 113: e617-e627.
21. Nelson EAS, Baur LA. Childhood obesity. In: Gupte S (ed): *Recent Advances in Pediatrics*, New Delhi. Jaypee 2002; 86-99.
22. Obesity: Preventing and managing the global epidemic. Report of a WHO Consultation. Geneva, World Health Organization 2000 (WHO Technical Report Series, No. 894).
23. Popkin BM, Richards MK, Montiero CA. Stunting is associated with overweight in children of four nations that are undergoing the nutrition transition. *J Nutr* 1996; 126: 3009-3016.
24. Robinson TN, Dietz WH. Weight gain: Overeating to obesity. In: Rudolph CD, Rudolph AM, editors. Rudolph's Pediatrics, 21st ed., NY McGraw-Hill, 2003: 476-481.
25. Rosenbaum M, Leibel RL, Hirsch J. Obesity. *N Eng J Med* 1997; 8: 396-407.
26. Stice E, Cameron RP, Killen JD, Hayward C, Taylor CB. Naturalistic weight-reduction efforts prospectively predict growth in relative weight and onset of obesity among female adolescents. *J Consult Clin Psychol* 1999; 67: 967-974.
27. Styne DM. Childhood and Adolescent Obesity. *PCNA* 2001; 48: 823-847.
28. Uauy R, Kain J. The epidemiological transition: The need to incorporate obesity prevention into nutrition programmes. *Public Health Nutr* 2002; 5: 916-919.
29. WHO/IASO/IOTF. The Asia Pacific Perspective: Redefining Obesity and its treatment. Health Communications Australia Pvt Ltd. 2000.
30. Willams CL, Hayman LL, Daniels SR, Robinson TN, *et al.* Cardiovascular Health in Childhood–A statement for health professionals from the Committee on Atherosclerosis, Hypertension and Obesity in the Young (AHOY) of the Council on Cardiovascular Disease in the Young. American Heart Association (AHA) Circulation 2002; 106: 143-160.
31. World Health Organization. Annual global move for health initiative. A concept paper. WHO: Geneva 2003.
32. Yajnik CS, Lubree HG, Rege SS, Naik SS, *et al.* Adiposity and hyperinsulinemia in Indians are present at birth. *J Clin Endocrinol Metab* 2002; 87: 5575-5580.
33. Yanowski JA. Intensive therapies for pediatric obesity. *PCNA* 2001; 48: 1041-1054.

107 Exclusion Diets

CE Abraham

INTRODUCTION

The term, *exclusion (elimination) diets*, refers to the diets in which different foods or groups of foods are excluded either on account of allergy or intolerance. Sometimes, the excluded items may be reintroduced, to see whether they are causing the symptoms as in case of gluten-induced enteropathy (celiac disease). Patients often start by cutting out some of the foods, which most often cause intolerance, such as wheat or dairy. They may overdo and on their own progress to cutting out other foods such as citrus fruit, gluten-containing foods such as barley and rye, and caffeine-containing drinks such as coffee, at times inviting troubles.

The term, *trigger foods*, denotes the foods that trigger the symptoms. These triggers will be different in every sufferer. Nevertheless, there are some foods, which seem to cause problems in many sufferers. These include:

- Alcohol.
- Artificial sweeteners - sorbitol seems to be a particular offender.
- Carbonated drinks.
- Coffee.
- Dairy.
- Fried foods.
- Oils.
- Poultry skin and dark meat.
- Red meat.

ADVERSE EFFECTS ASSOCIATED WITH EXCLUSION DIET

The most important adverse effects is fair chances of nutritional deficiencies because patients are actively avoiding whole food groups. It is, therefore, important that they make sure they are still receiving the nutrition they need.

It can be very helpful to work with a qualified nutritionist who can advice about the best way to use exclusion diets safely.

The nutritionist is also able to advise on substitute foods for any trigger foods such as using gluten-free flour for baking or the use of rice or potatoes as food staples rather than bread.

DAIRY-FREE DIET

The *dairy-free diet* means cutting out all obvious dairy products such as milk, cheese and butter. In case of subjects very sensitive to dairy products, it may also become important to cut out ingredients made from dairy products such as whey and casein.

Lactose intolerant children are allergic to lactose in the milk, as they don't have sufficient amounts of the enzyme *lactase* to properly digest lactose. They may be able to eat products such as hard cheese with no ill effects, because they only contain low levels of lactose. Nevertheless, they certainly need to either avoid products such as milk or use soymilk or other substitutes.

For a completely dairy-free diet, the following foods should be avoided:

- Milk, cheese, butter.
- Cream cheese, cottage cheese.
- Sour cream, ice cream.
- Chocolate and other candy that contains milk.
- Malted milk.
- Some cereals which contain milk powder.
- Whey, casein, or foods that contain any of these ingredients.

This list being incomplete, it is mandatory to check food labels regularly and learn which ingredients contain dairy products and which are safe.

Any long-term problems with this diet? Because dairy-products are a good source of calcium, people who avoid most dairy products may need to take a calcium supplement.

GLUTEN-FREE DIET

Gluten is a protein found in wheat, barley and rye. Gluten-free means avoiding all of these foods, which are commonly found in everyday foods such as bread and pasta, as well as sauces and many processed foods. A gluten-free diet is not the same as a *wheat-free diet*, where wheat alone must be excluded, but the gluten-containing barley and rye can still be eaten freely

In celiac disease the lining of their intestine is actually damaged by gluten. The symptoms should disappear on a gluten-free diet.

Oats are somewhat controversial on a gluten-free diet, because some people who have celiac disease seem to be able to eat them without symptoms, and others do not. Oats do contain a protein, which is similar to gluten. However, oats are often processed in a factory alongside wheat and other gluten-containing foods, and so become contaminated with small amounts of gluten.

What foods are avoided? Well, patients should avoid all wheat, barley and rye (and sometimes oats as well), but they must also take care to avoid gluten in a wide range of other foods. Some food items which may contain gluten include:

- Soups.
- Sausages.
- Processed meats such as slices of ham.
- Ready meals.
- Crisps and potato chips.

Some people find that they can eat small amounts of gluten without any problems, and so would not need to worry about things such as potato chips which would probably only use gluten in the flavorings.

Any long-term problems with this diet? Totally eliminating gluten from the diet is not easy, and it does require vigilance to make sure that gluten does not sneak into the diet. However, many patients do benefit from a gluten-free diet and so it can be worth the effort.

A wide variety of specially made gluten-free foods including breads, cakes and pasta are often more expensive than their gluten-filled equivalents and may not taste quite the same.

Gluten-free flour too is available.

EXCLUSION DIETS IN INFLAMMATORY BOWEL DISEASE

Though it is common for the physician or the parents to impose one or the other exclusion diet on the child suffering from IBD, the practice is not well founded. According to current belief:

- Dietary restrictions should generally be avoided, the exceptions being intestinal obstruction or specific abnormalities of digestion or absorption.
- *Lactose-free* or low-lactose diet in the presence of established lactose malabsorption. Lactose-free (primarily milk-free) diet is indicated in only severe lactose intolerance in IBD children. Yoghurt is an excellent alternative. Soya-based formula, especially when supplemented with methionine, too is a good option.
- In patients with strictures it may be prudent to avoid such fiber containing food as broccoli, raw carrot, grapes, nuts, seeds, mushrooms, popcorn, celery and all fruits with skins as they are potentially able to cause obstruction. It is important to warn patient to chew their foods well if strictures are present. Some patients may need top 2 rely on liquids as the sole source of nutrition if strictures or narrowing do not allow passage of normal foods.
- Children, having undergone new *ileostomies, need* to avoid the high fiber foods for a period of 2-4 weeks to allow post-operative swelling to subside. Fiber-containing foods typically are added back slowly beginning with water-soluble fibers (e.g. oatmeal, banana, rice and apple sauce) followed by insoluble fibers (wheat, bran, corn or nuts) as tolerated.
- *Low oxalate diet* is required in patients with terminal ileum resection or with significant fat malabsorption, because these patients have the propensity for oxalate kidney stones.

EXCLUSION DIET IN LACTOSE INTOLERANCE

Transient lactose intolerance often is an indication for a diet that excludes high lactose i.e. milk. In case of lactose intolerance, clinically the infant passes very frequent loose, watery stools (with acidic pH) and develops perianal erythema. Stool pH is <5.5. The suggested line of treatment is to reduce the lactose load either by:

- Lactose-free milk i.e. formula or soya milk.
- Substitute milk by yoghurt.
- Add mashed banana to the milk feed.

Evidence is now available that babies fed on soy protein-based formula grow satisfactorily.

EXCLUSION DIET IN ALLERGY

Though around 15% of the population reports having had adverse food reactions, true prevalence of food allergy is rather low, ranging from 1% to 4% in random population and about 6% in pediatric population. About 25% of children with eczema may have food allergy.

Since there is as yet no laboratory studies that help identify foods responsible for cell-mediated allergy, exclusion diets followed by food challenges are the only means to establish the diagnosis.

Exclusion diet, or elimination diet, is a diet in which likely allergens or other foods to which a patient may be sensitive are avoided. Elimination diets are commonly used both for:

- Confirming other diagnostic tests, like RAST tests and prick tests; and
- Pinpoint impossible food intolerances. Exclusion diets should only be tried under a doctor's care. These diets are generally safe, but allergists are able to recommend when elimination diets are appropriate, advise how they

can be effectively carried out, and interpret their results properly.

A. For Diagnosis

While other diagnostic tests rarely return false negatives (that is, if they indicate that a patient is not allergic to a given food, the patient has at least a 95 percent likelihood of indeed not being allergic), they are fairly likely to return false positives. Unless the patient experienced anaphylaxis before taking diagnostic tests, allergists will often recommend an elimination diet (to see if symptoms improve) followed by a *double-blind food challenge test* (one in which neither the doctor nor the patient is aware of whether the patient is eating the likely allergen) to confirm test results.

Exclusion diet may be recommended as a diagnostic tool in its own right. In some cases, for example, when a child who is being exclusively breastfed shows symptoms of a food allergy, it can be difficult to discern which foods might be causing allergic symptoms. An elimination diet in which likely allergens are removed and then added back one by one may be useful as a diagnostic tool.

B. For Therapeutics

Experience has shown that an exclusion diet is the only known effective therapeutic strategy in food allergy e.g. food-induced enteropathy, cow milk protein allergy, lactose intolerance etc.

Management of food allergy in infants and children requires education about dietary avoidance and consideration for nutritional deficiencies that may result. The pediatrician plays a central role in identifying children with food allergy and for continued monitoring of food-allergic patients for growth and development. Indeed, a review of the child's growth chart with emphasis on growth velocity is the most efficient way to monitor children with food allergies. For comprehensive nutritional management, the pediatrician may benefit from the additional assistance of a dietitian and an allergist in many cases:

- For a definitive diagnosis (elimination diets, oral challenge).
- When there are multiple maternal dietary restrictions during breastfeeding.
- When food groups or multiple foods are avoided (especially without a complete formula).
- To determine appropriate substitutions of allergenic foods with safe foods.
- To determine the nutritional adequacy of the diet in the face of poor growth.
- To educate the family regarding the words/terms/ indicators that are used on food labels to indicate the presence of an allergen.

HOW EXCLUSION DIETS WORK

The mechanics will work in one of two ways, depending on whether the likely allergen is known. In cases where a particular food is suspected to cause an allergic reaction or intolerance, the said food is strictly avoided for a period of time. If avoiding the food causes the symptoms to subside, and ingesting some in a double-blind food challenge causes them to return, impression about allergy is corroborated.

TYPES OF EXCLUSION DIETS IN FOOD ALLERGY

In case the cause of allergic symptoms is unclear, allergists use several different types of elimination diets to narrow down the range of foods that might be causing symptoms. Since 90 percent of food allergies are caused by the eight *most common food allergens*, one option is to eliminate *any of these foods* that may be problematic. This type of diet does not have a specific name. If this doesn't yield results, the allergist/pediatrician may recommend a "few foods" diet or a "rare foods" diet.

The "Few Foods" Diets

The so-called "oligoallergenic diet" consists of a small number of foods (rice, pears, lamb, turkey) which are deemed unlikely to cause an allergic reaction. This diet is eaten for a period of time. In case this diet is employed as a diagnostic tool, foods are gradually added back one at a time to see if symptoms reappear.

The "Rare Foods" Diet

This diet excludes all foods that are currently part of the child's diet in favor of foods he has either never eaten at all, or has never eaten regularly. The logic behind this is that foods that are not a regular part of the diet are unlikely to cause ongoing allergic symptoms. Else, rare foods diets are very similar to few foods diets.

EXCLUSION DIETS AND ECZEMA

In addition to their use as a diagnostic tool, exclusion diets are commonly used for patients with eczema. Many patients with eczema have food allergies or sensitivities, and patients will commonly eliminate these foods to alleviate eczema.

LIFESTYLE CHALLENGES WITH EXCLUSION DIETS

An important challenge of an elimination diet, especially a rare foods or few foods diet, is finding ways to prepare foods without using ingredients that the child may have used frequently. Flour, milk and margarine are some of the common foods the child may not be allowed to use. The pediatrician must provide the family a list of resources and recipes along with his instructions for carrying out the diet.

HEALTH ISSUES WITH EXCLUSION DIETS

Undoubtedly, prolonged employment of exclusion diets can be risky in infants and young toddlers on account of its adverse effect on their growth and development. Not just that! The breastfeeding mothers may also suffer from nutritional deficiency states. Studies have demonstrated that long-term elimination diets are associated with failure to thrive in infants and nutritional inadequacy in mothers.

Researchers have expressed concern that long-term diets that eliminate foods that cause minor immediate reactions, when used as a treatment for disorders like eczema, may oversensitize the body to allergens and raise the risk of anaphylaxis.

NUTRITIONAL CONSEQUENCES OF EXCLUSION DIETS

When a food or a food group is eliminated, one must consider:

- The types of nutrients that are potentially lost;
- Whether other components of the diet are adequate to fulfill nutritional needs; and
- Whether additional dietary alterations are needed to fulfill the lost nutrients.

In case the allergy is to a food group that is a major contributor to the diet, such as in cow milk allergy, all dairy products should be avoided. Therefore, calcium, phosphorus, riboflavin, pantothenic acid, vitamin B_{12}, vitamin A, and vitamin D will need to be supplied from other sources. Supplementation with appropriate amounts of calcium and vitamin D are important to individuals with milk allergy at any age. It is difficult to obtain adequate calcium from nondairy foods. There are, however, alternative drinks (soy and rice) and juices that are enriched with calcium. Milk-free calcium supplements can also be considered for use with milk-allergic children.

Use of calcium-fortified juices that come in "juice box" form could result in unexpected problems because contamination with milk protein has been noted in several different products in juice box form, presumably from cross-contact during processing. Juices that are from bottles, cans, and/or frozen concentrates are not as commonly contaminated.

Intake of residual foods must be considered to determine whether an adequate amount of, for example, vitamin A, is provided and whether it is necessary to increase the intake of foods high in vitamin A.

Yet another issue of concern for children with multiple food allergies is the distribution of carbohydrates, protein, and fats in the diet. Modifications in food choices should be made to ensure sufficient macronutrient and energy intake. A grain-allergic child should be evaluated to ensure adequate intake of carbohydrates from alternative foods. This is because enough intake of carbohydrates is a must to prevent ketosis.

KEY TO SUCCESS OF EXCLUSION DIETS

Success of exclusion diets depends on two main factors, namely:

- Adherence; and
- Nutritional adequacy.

Either of these factors may be adversely affected unless intelligent and creative choices are made to allow diversity of taste and texture in addition to nutrition. The exclusion of even a single food protein may require that a large number of products with diverse nutritional and social advantage be excluded from the diet.

Let's take an instance of allergy to wheat. All commercial breads, cereals, baked goods, and pastas need to be eliminated. Wheat is not only a main ingredient for a large number of products, it is also one of the common starches used in many processed foods. In this situation, the use of alternative grains (e.g., rice, oat, potato, barley) as flour in baked goods may provide a solution. Use of commercial products with alternative grains such as crackers, cakes, and pastas made of rice, corn, potato, or quinoa can also provide normalcy and convenience to the diet of the allergic child on a wheat-restricted diet.

All this may seem fine theoretically. Nevertheless, the practical difficulties in execution of the exclusion diets are endless.

KEY LEARNING POINTS

- *Exclusion diets* are the diets from which different foods or food items are excluded either on account of allergy or intolerance e.g. gluten-free diet, dairy-free diet, lactose-free diet, etc.
- *Trigger foods* are the foods that trigger the symptoms in vulnerable subjects e.g. carbonated drinks, artificial sweeteners, red meat, etc.
- Strict adherence to a certain exclusion diet is difficult, thereby causing difficulties in achieving the desired outcome.
- Prolonged exclusion diets can be risky, including risk of nutritional deficiencies and growth failure.

FURTHER READINGS

1. Gupte S. Elimination diet: A case for caution against overindulgence. *Eur Med* 2002;7:123-125.
2. Warinr P, Championn H. *Urticaria*, Philadelphia: Saunders 1974.
3. Barbi E. Fatal Allergy as a Possible Consequence of Long-Term Elimination Diet. *Allergy* 59.6 (2004): 668-69. Accessed on May 21, 2007.
4. Lockey, Richard F, Samuel C. Bukantz, and Jean Bousquet. *Allergens and Allergen Immunotherapy*. 3rd edn. New York: Marcel Dekker, 2004: 331-334.
5. Mofidi S. Nutritional Management of Pediatric Food Hypersensitivity. *Pediatrics* 111.6 (2003): 1645-53. Accessed on May 20, 2007.
6. Sinagra JL. Unnecessary Milk Elimination Diets in Children with Atopic dermatitis. *Pediatr Dermatol* 24.1 (2007): 1-6. Accessed on May 21, 2007.
7. Niggemann E, Heine RG. Who should manage infants and young children with food induced symptoms? *Arch. Dis. Child* 2006; 9: 379-382.
8. Hill DJ, Roy N, Heine RG, Hosking CS. Effect of a Low-Allergen Maternal Diet on Colic Among Breastfed Infants: A Randomized, Controlled Trial. *Pediatrics* 2005; 116: e709 - e715.

108 Enteral Nutrition

Swati Kolpuru • Karoly Horvath

INTRODUCTION

Enteral nutritional support should be considered if the recommended daily requirement is not likely to be met on account of problems such as swallowing dysfunction, food refusal, or gastrointestinal diseases for:

- One to three days in infants.
- Three to five days in children; and
- More than seven days in older children and adults.

Feeding through tubes placed in the stomach or small intestine is useful not only to provide adequate nutritional support, but also to provide additional calories for catch-up growth. In certain clinical situations, tubes are used primarily for the administration of fluids or medications.

In the case of short-term problems, orogastric and nasogastric tubes are used. Nevertheless, if long-term feeding is necessary, tubes placed endoscopically, radiologically or surgically are recommended.

The basic rule is that if the intestine works, then it should be used. It should be the preferred modality over parenteral nutrition that is not only cumbersome and expensive but also carries risk of serious complications.

This review attempts to encompass the indications, contraindications, different techniques, sites, and complications of enteral tube feeding. In addition, it also provides a general guideline for formula selection for tube feeding in children.

ADVANTAGES

- Safer than parenteral nutrition.
- Easier to administer.
- More physiologic.
- Supplies gut-preferred fuels like glutamine, glutamate, and short-chain fatty acids; also provides other beneficial compounds, such as fibers, fructo-oligosaccharides and probiotics that are absent from parenteral formulations.
- Maintains the mucosal integrity of the small and large intestines and prevents atrophy not only of the intestinal mucosa but also the pancreas. It also preserves the normal function of the gut-associated immune system.
- Prevents cholelithiasis by stimulating gallbladder motility.
- Less expensive than parenteral nutrition.

CLINICAL INDICATIONS/CONTRAINDICATIONS

Enteral nutrition through tube feeding is used in various clinical settings. Tube feeding is needed in the neonatal period to meet the nutritional needs of premature babies. Children with gastrointestinal diseases, such as short-bowel syndrome, inflammatory bowel disease, malabsorption, severe intestinal dysmotility, chronic liver disease, eosinophilic gastroenteritis, hepatic failure also require enteral feeding. It is used in children with nongastrointestinal diseases, including congenital heart disease, pulmonary diseases (e.g. cystic fibrosis, bronchopulmonary dysplasia, respiratory failure), in cases with renal insufficiency, neurological disability, malnutrition/failure-to-thrive, feeding disorders, cancer, post-bone marrow transplantation, trauma and burns.

The only absolute contraindications of enteral feeding are intestinal obstruction and a non-functioning gastrointestinal tract. Relative contraindications include severe vomiting, enteric fistula, severe diarrhea, and significant intestinal dysmotility. In other clinical situations, certain enteral feeding methods are not indicated, e.g. nasogastric tube placement is contraindicated in children with critical illness, facial fractures, and severe coagulopathy or esophageal strictures.

Table 108.1 summarizes the indications and contraindications of tube feedings. Table 108.2 lists the clinical conditions and diseases in which enteral tube feeding is a reasonable approach.

SELECTION OF THE TUBE FEEDING METHOD

The selection of access and site for enteral feeding depends upon the following factors:

- Expected length of tube feeding (short-term or long-term).
- Site of tube insertion and the target organ of tube feeding (nasal or oral entry, stoma entry, gastric, duodenal or jejunal feeding).

Table 108.1: Indications and contraindications of the various tube feedings

Tube feeding	*Indication*	*Contraindication*
Nasogastric tube	Short-term feeding in patient with no reflux and normal gastric motility	Facial injury; nasal tumor, polyp, trauma, severe coagulopathy; sinusitis, pharyngeal or esophageal obstruction
Orogastric tube		Pharyngeal or esophageal obstruction
Nasojejunal tube	Short-term feeding in patient with significant reflux, risk of aspiration or and abnormal gastric motility; critical care patients	Facial injury; nasal tumor, polyp, trauma, severe coagulopathy; sinusitis, pharyngeal or esophageal obstruction
Orojejunal tube		Pharyngeal or esophageal obstruction
Gastric tube	Long-term feeding in patient with no reflux and normal gastric motility	Gastroparesis, gastric outlet obstruction, gastric surgery that precludes gastric feeding
Jejunal tube	Long-term feeding in patients with significant reflux and risk of aspiration; critical care patients with long-term feeding needs; altered mental status, removal of stomach	Small bowel ischemia, diarrhea
Gastrojejunal tube		

Table 108.2: Clinical conditions and the typical tube feeding used

Disease	*Tube feeding*
Prematurity	Orogastric or orojejunal
Swallowing dysfunction	
Food Refusal	
Oro-motor dysfunction (Inability to process the food in the pharynx)—sucking and swallowing abnormalities	Nasogastric, gastrostomy; if severe reflux: nasojejunal, gastrojejunal or gastrostomy
Pharyngo-esophageal dysfunction (the food stays in the pharynx and results in aspiration)	Nasogastric, gastrostomy; if severe reflux: nasojejunal, gastrojejunal or gastrostomy
Aspiration only with clear liquids	Nasogastric, gastrostomy
Food refusal (usually after long-term withdrawal of oral feeding in infants)	Gastrostomy
Proximal GI tract obstruction (e.g. head and neck injury, malignancy)	Gastrostomy
Inadequate caloric intake	Nasogastric, gastrostomy
Gastrointestinal ***Dysfunction/Disease***	
Severe gastric dysmotility	Nasojejunal, gastrojejunal or jejunostomy
Pancreatitis	Nasojejunal
Inflammatory bowel disease	Nasogastric, gastrostomy
Chronic liver disease (e.g. biliary atresia)	Gastrostomy

Contd.

Contd.

Superior mesentery artery syndrome	Nasojejunal
Short bowel syndrome	Gastrostomy
Severe food allergy and eosinophilic gastroenteritis	Nasogastric
Acute Events	
Acute respiratory distress in critically-ill patients	Nasojejunal
Trauma	Nasogastric, gastrostomy
Burns	Nasogastric, gastrostomy
Postoperative stage	Nasogastric, nasojejunal
Chronic, non-gastrointestinal ***Diseases***	
Metabolic diseases	Gastrostomy
Cancer patients	Gastrostomy
Acquired immune deficiency disease	Gastrostomy
Neurological impairments	Gastrostomy
Bone marrow transplant	Nasogastric
Severe congenital heart disease	Nasogastric, gastrostomy
Chronic renal disease	Nasogastric, gastrostomy
Bronchopulmonary dysplasia	Nasogastric, gastrostomy
Cystic fibrosis	Nasogastric, gastrostomy

- Method of formula administration (bolus feeding, gravity or continuous feeding).

The above factors depend on the following:

- Patient's diagnosis (e.g. severe reflux, failure to thrive, chronic illness, neurological impairment).
- Physical examination (e.g. severe scoliosis, surgical scar in epigastrium, etc.).
- Past medical history.
- History of allergy (e.g. in case of latex allergy, silicon tubes should be used; allergy to milk or soy protein requires use of special hypoallergenic formulas).
- Feeding history: Previous nutritional interventions, volume of oral intake and tolerance to the feeding regimen (e.g. if a patient was able to tolerate nasogastric feeding, gastrostomy tube placement for long-term feeding is a reasonable approach).
- Surgical history (e.g. previous abdominal surgery; ventriculoperitoneal shunt, pacemakers, splenectomy etc.).
- Prior imaging studies (upper gastrointestinal studies to rule out esophageal stricture, malrotation or other anatomical problems).
- Result of past pH probe study.
- Previous endoscopy histology results.
- Risk of aspiration (e.g. jejunal feeding or transpyloric feeding preferred over gastric feeding in this situation).
- Patency, motility and function of the gut (e.g. jejunal feeding preferred over gastric feeding if there is history of gastroparesis).
- Age of the patient (e.g. orogastric feeding is preferred in neonatal age group as they are obligate nasal breathers).

A variety of tubes are available for each form of enteral feeding. Feeding tubes are usually made of polyethylene, polyurethane or silicone. Because latex allergy had become more prevalent in the last decade, patients with suspected or proven allergy should not receive tubes containing latex.

Short-term Tube Feeding

In patients requiring short-term feeding (usually less than 30 days), nasally placed tubes (nasogastric or nasojejunal tubes depending on the indication) are recommended because of their low cost, ease of placement, and lower complication rate.

Long-term Tube Feeding

If the tube feeding is needed for more than 30 days, gastrostomy tubes represent the most common method for enteral nutrition support. A G-J tube or a jejunostomy tube may be indicated for specific clinical scenarios, which will be discussed later.

Nasogastric Tube Feeding

Nasoenteric tubes (NETs) technically refer to any feeding tube that is placed nasally beyond the esophagus. Nasogastric tube (NGT) is the easiest method of enteral feeding. If tube is needed for only a few days, polyethylene tubes can be inserted. However, small and soft silicon nasogastric tubes are generally preferred as they provide more patient comfort, and possibly results in less local complications, gastroesophageal reflux and aspiration pneumonia. The NGT can be easily placed at the bedside.

Larger caliber tubes are used when decompression of

the stomach, monitoring gastric pH or administration of thicker medications are needed in addition to the feeding.

Nasally-placed tubes can cause local irritation, epistaxis, otitis media and sinusitis. Rare complications are gastrointestinal bleeding, and esophageal perforation

In infants and young children, the NG tubes may be changed once a month; in older school-age children, they may be placed every night and taken out in the morning.

For NGT feeding, increased gastric residuum should alert attention to recheck the residuum in an hour but should not lead to automatic cessation of feeding.

Nasojejunal Tube (NJT) Feeding

Nasojejunal feeding or transpyloric feeding is indicated whenever there is a risk of aspiration, history of significant reflux, evidence of gastric dysmotility, acute pancreatitis, or superior mesenteric artery syndrome. Transpyloric feedings are an invaluable and well-tolerated method of feeding in critically-ill children. Tubes placed into the third portion of the duodenum or passing the ligament of Treitz are associated with a decreased risk of aspiration.

All transpyloric feeding requires the use of a feeding pump, which increases the cost of enteral feeding. The NJ tubes are more difficult to maintain and use than NG tubes.

In the absence of any contraindication, gastric feeding is preferred to jejunal feeding because it is more physiological. Gastric feeding permits the action of lingual lipase, and initiates protein digestion in the stomach. In addition, gastric acid also has bactericidal activity.

Gastrostomy Tube (GT) Feeding

When a patient requires prolonged tube feeding (more than 30 days) gastrostomy should be considered. However, before the placement of a permanent feeding tube, it is necessary to prove that the patient tolerates the feeding regimen with a temporary nasogastric tube. GT can be placed in endoscopically, radiologically or surgically.

Indications

- Young children who require long-term administration of unpalatable medications or dietary components.
- Children who did well with nasogastric feeding and needs long-term feeding.
- Neurological diseases.
- During facial reconstructive surgery for congenital malformations.
- Maxillofacial trauma or facial tumors.
- Swallowing study demonstrating aspiration with clear liquids due to dysfunctional swallow.

Jejunostomy Tube (JT) Feeding

The main indications for the use of jejunostomy tube feeding includes aspiration, gastroparesis, insufficient stomach size due to previous resection, postoperative feeding after major procedures and superior mesentery artery syndrome.

If a long-term postpyloric feeding is required, jejunostomy tube placement is considered. In patients who already have a gastrostomy tube, another option is to convert it to a gastrojejunostomy (GJ) tube. Alternatives are endoscopic, radiological or surgically-placed jejunostomy tube. JT feeding is administered continuously with a normal osmolality formula in order to avoid hyperosmolar diarrhea. Bolus feeds must not be given via JT as it results in vomiting, distention and diarrhea.

Formula Administration Methods

Enteral feedings can be delivered as a bolus, gravity feeding or as continuous feeding by using a feeding pump. Bolus and gravity feeding is used in gastric feeding only, while continuous feeding is an option with every type of feeding.

Bolus feeding or intermittent feeding is the administration of formula, usually by syringe within a 5-15 minutes period every few hours.

Advantages of intermittent feedings:

- Do not require infusion pumps.
- More convenient for the caregiver.
- Permits patient mobility.
- More physiologic.

Disadvantages of intermittent feedings are higher incidence of diarrhea, vomiting, aspiration pneumonitis and reflux.

Gravity feedings can be delivered *via* intermittent or continuous drip. The rate of delivery is less accurate than with bolus feeding and usually requires the use of a bag. Bolus and gravity feeding share similar risk of reflux and aspiration.

Continuous feedings require a feeding pump with a source of power. It allows for accurate control and delivery of the formula either via an intermittent or continuous schedule. Compared with intermittent feedings, continuous intragastric feeding is safer with fewer episodes of diarrhea and less risk of aspiration.

Infants who cannot tolerate bolus feeds are switched to continuous gastric or duodenal/jejunal feeds. Continuous feeds are also appropriate when patients cannot tolerate a high infusion rate or bolus feeds.

If the clinical situation permits, continuous feeding can be converted into intermittent feeding. No defined protocol exists for this change. The feeding should be gradually compressed depending on the patient's age and condition.

Continuous feeding is associated with less thermal energy loss. Additionally, caloric goals can be achieved quickly with continuous feeding. Of note, a continuous duodenal perfusion of liquid formulas has been shown to cause sequestration of bile acids as a result of incomplete emptying of the gallbladder.

TECHNIQUES OF TUBE PLACEMENT

Orogastric or Nasogastric Tube Placement

The first step in nasogastric intubation is estimating the length of the tube to be inserted. A simple method to calculate this length is to extend the distal end of the tube from the tip of the patient's nose to the earlobe and then from there to the xiphoid process with the addition of 10-15 cm (4-6 in). A more accurate measurement for the distance between the nares and gastroesophageal junction is the formula used for pH probe placement:

$$0.25 \times \text{height (cm)} + 5 \text{ cm}$$

The nares should be checked for obstruction and the tube passed down the more patent side. For patient comfort, topical vasoconstrictors, such as phenylephrine (Neo-Synephrine 0.5%), or oxymetazoline (Afrin 0.05%) may be sprayed into the nasal passages, at least 3 to 5 minutes before the procedure. In order to avoid gagging, the nares, nasopharynx and oropharynx should all be anesthetized at least 5 minutes before the procedure. However, in infants the local anesthetic may trigger cough and laryngeal spasm.

The tube is then lubricated with viscous lidocaine or lidocaine jelly and is inserted along the floor of the nose. Mild resistance may occur in the posterior nasopharynx, but only gentle pressure should be required to overcome this resistance. Bleeding or dissection into retropharyngeal tissue may occur if force is used.

Flexing the neck also tends to direct the tube into the esophagus. Excessive choking or gagging or any coughing, change in voice, or the appearance of condensation in the lumen of the tube are signs of misplacement into the trachea and a prompt withdrawal into the oropharynx is necessary. In patients who cannot co-operate or cannot cough (e.g. infants with chronic aspiration) extra-precautions should be taken.

The pharynx should be inspected to exclude a coiling of the tube. A tube position lateral to the midline suggests correct position in the esophagus. Once the tube is in the esophagus, it should be advanced rapidly to the previously determined depth.

Confirmation of Tube Placement

Before securing the NG tube, its position should be confirmed.

- X-ray is the most definitive way to confirm the position of an NG tube.
- Injecting approximately 20 cc of air through the tube and auscultating in the epigastric region for a gurgling sound is a simple way of confirming tube placement in the stomach at the bedside. If the patient burps immediately after air instillation, the tube is probably in the esophagus and needs to be advanced further.
- If the patient is able to talk, the tube most likely is not coiled in the pharynx or in the trachea.
- Aspirating gastric contents is also an acceptable way of checking the tube placement.

Nasojejunal Tube Placement

Successful placement of a nasojejunal tube depends on an individual's skill and experience. The tube placement can be attempted at the bedside, under fluoroscopic view, or endoscopically. Simple bedside placement is the preferred method. The initial phase of tube placement is the same as the nasogastric tube placement. Endoscopically or fluoroscopically-guided tube placement should be reserved for those patients for whom bedside techniques have not been successful.

Nasojejunal tubes are available from 8F to 16F in diameters and in 90 to 240 cm in lengths. Some tubes have a removable stylet or a weighted tip. Most of these tubes have radio-opaque markers. Tubes with multiple side holes are less likely to become clogged. There are special tubes with double lumen and double port to allow access to both the stomach and small intestine.

Transpyloric placement (duodenum, jejunum) of feeding tubes can be difficult and time consuming. There is no significant difference in the passage rate between tubes with or without weighted tips. In one study, patients were placed in right lateral decubitus position and track of the tube into the small intestine was followed by auscultation. This technique resulted in a successful transpyloric placement in 83% of the 103 patients, but only 44 of 103 of the tubes (43%) were in the preferred position, which is the third portion of the duodenum or beyond.

Prokinetic medications that increase the antral motility such as erythromycin and metoclopramide are used for blind and fluoroscopic insertions. Erythromycin stimulates gastric migrating motor complexes via the release of motilin, which then increases gastric motility. Metoclopramide is a cholinergic agonist and dopamine antagonist. It increases the amplitude of gastric contractions and promotes synchronization of peristalsis. In a study comparing weighted vs. unweighted 8F tubes, metoclopramide was given as an intravenous bolus 10 minutes before tube placement. The combination of preinsertion metoclopramide treatment and unweighted tubes was significantly better, and after 4 hours, 84% of unweighted tubes passed into the duodenum compared to 36% of the weighted tubes.

Although intravenous prokinetic administration may help, experience of the health care worker correlates better with successful tube placement than the administration of medications. In an antroduodenal motility report metoclopramide failed in 3 patients. Subsequently they got erythromycin (3 mg/kg as infusion an hour before tube placement). Five other patients received erythromycin first. All 8 tubes passed into the duodenum.

Ozdemir *et al.* reported 88% success with the use an external magnet to direct a tube with a magnetic end through the pylorus.

If the blind insertion is not successful, fluoroscopic guidance may be used to advance the feeding tube into the jejunum, with a success rate of 86 to 90%. If the fluoroscopic attempts fail, nasojejunal tube can be placed with endoscopic guidance, which has a success rate as high as 98%.

Maintenance of chronic transpyloric jejunal feeding catheters is more difficult then the NG tubes. Upto one-third of patients require reinsertion because of jejunostomy tube malfunction or misplacement.

Gastrostomy Feeding Tube Placement

Gastrostomy is the most frequently used method for long-term enteral feeding. It can be placed endoscopically, radiologically and surgically. Endoscopic placement is the recommended method over surgery, as it is faster, cheaper and permits feeding within few hours after the procedure. The contraindications of non-surgical placements are:

- Large ascites.
- Inability to bring the anterior gastric wall in apposition to the abdominal wall.
- Inability to localize the insertion site with finger palpation and transillumination.
- Coagulopathy.
- Neutropenia.
- Portal hypertension.
- Gastric varices.
- Hepatomegaly.
- Morbid obesity.
- Pharyngeal or esophageal obstruction.
- GI tract obstruction.
- Gastrointestinal fistulas.
- Microgastria or partial gastrectomy.

Percutaneous Endoscopic Gastric (PEG) Tube Placement

Antibiotic prophylaxis (e.g. ceftriaxone, cefazolin) is recommended 30 minutes prior to the procedure. A standard upper gastrointestinal endoscope is introduced into the stomach. After air insufflation, the stomach is slightly distended. With the combination of insufflation, transillumination and finger indentation on the abdominal wall, a site for PEG placement is identified. In most cases, the insertion site is along an imaginary line drawn from the umbilicus to the left axillary line in the subcostal region, and it is at the junction of the upper and the middle third of this line. After an aseptic field is created, local anesthetic (1% lidocaine) is injected into the selected area. The anesthetic syringe is advanced into the stomach lumen and can be seen by the endoscope. Next, withdraw the needle aspirating for air as the needle is removed. The appearance of air bubbles while the needle tip is in the wall may indicate the presence of an intervening hollow organ between the stomach and abdominal wall. If the illumination and the indentation are good and there is no suspicion of intervening bowel loop, a skin incision is made to accommodate the PEG tube. The length of incision depends on the size of feeding tube.

The next step is the insertion of a trochar through the incision into the stomach. It should be done with a brief, forceful thrust so that the trochar does not push the anterior gastric wall away from the anterior abdominal wall. A guide wire is then advanced through the trochar into the stomach where it is grasped with a snare or forceps and withdrawn along with the endoscope through the mouth. The PEG tube (12-20 Fr) is hooked to the guidewire, lubricated with sterile jelly and is pulled through the mouth and esophagus into the stomach, and through the abdominal wall. The endoscope is passed again to inspect for mucosal trauma and to evaluate the PEG tube's position against the anterior abdominal wall of the stomach.

The discomfort and pain after PEG placement can be managed usually with acetaminophen (through G-tube or rectal suppository) or with intravenous non-steroid anti-inflammatory drugs. Intravenous narcotics should be avoided for pain as they may induce a pharmacologic ileus.

One modification of the placement described above is the push technique, in which a wire is inserted percutaneously over which the feeding catheter is threaded into the stomach and through the abdominal wall.

An external plastic positioner (crossbar) secures the PEG outside and prevents the inward migration of the tube into the stomach. It also keeps the tube in a close approximation to the skin and inner part proximal to the stomach wall. Once the PEG is fixed in place, the tube, which is approximately 3 feet long, is cut and an adapter is attached to its end.

A "one-step button" tube is available (Surgitek one-step button) as another option for initial placement. If it is used the thickness of the abdominal wall should be assessed before the insertion. The button tube is compressed and, which opens after "peeling off" the plastic line. Whichever tube is used, the attached adapter usually has ports for feeding pumps and syringes used for the administration of formula and medications.

There is no uniformly accepted recommendation for the time when the tube feeding can be started after PEG placement. In our practice, we start infusing small volume of formula 8 hours after the procedure if the intestinal motility is normal, and there is no significant gastric residuum. The volume is increased every 2-3 hours and given as continuous feeding. Usually the patients reach the full volume of feeding within 24 hours after the procedure. Our protocol includes the ventilation of the tube for 6 hours and a repeat dose of antibiotic 6 hours post procedure. If the patient does not tolerate the feeding, it should be stopped and restarted at the initial volume 3 hours later. Once the abdominal wall edema resolves, the plastic crossbar is repositioned to provide a good fit against the abdomen. The gastrostomy site can be cleaned with soap and water or alcohol pad. Full strength hydrogen peroxide should be avoided as it contributes to the formation of granulation tissue.

Complications of Gastrostomy Placement

The possible complications of PEG tube placement include *hemorrhage, infection, intestinal perforation, and peritonitis*. Hemorrhage is a rare and results from the puncture of a vessel in the gastric wall. It can be stopped with increased traction on the internal bumper to tamponade the tract bleeding temporarily. Radiographic study should be performed in those patients who develop abdominal pain, vomiting, fever, and abdominal distention to evaluate for the above complications.

Since PEG placement requires the passage of the tube through the mouth, it is not a sterile procedure. The risk for tube-site infection therefore is greater compared to open gastrostomy. Administration of prophylactic antibiotic therapy reduces the incidence of infection and is cost-effective. Peristomal wound infection is the most common complication of PEG placement. Treatment usually includes local care and rarely systemic antibiotic therapy. Special circumstances such as necrotizing fasciitis often requires surgical debridement in addition to IV antibiotic therapy.

Peritonitis soon after PEG placement occurs in less than 1% of patients. It is usually due to the premature removal of the tube before the gastrocutaneous tract has healed. Leakage around a properly fixed tube is unlikely. The perforation of another viscus, especially the colon during the procedure, also may cause perforation. Because of the high mortality associated with bowel perforation, prompt diagnosis and treatment are important. Post-PEG procedure pneumoperitoneum is common, and it occurs in more than one-third of the cases. Therefore the presence of free air on abdominal X-ray cannot be used to diagnose perforation. If the PEG tube is still present, radiographic study with instillation of a water-soluble contrast medium through the tube will localize the tip of the tube and rule out a leak.

Colo-cutaneous fistulas are rare complications of PEG placements. They are usually not detected until months after the initial placement, often when the first tube is replaced. In these cases, feeding causes severe diarrhea that resembles the formula. Contrast administration under fluoroscopy is the best method to recognize this complication and it is usually treated surgically.

"Buried bumper syndrome" is another complication of PEG placement. This complication can occur with PEG tubes that have rigid internal bumpers. If too much pressure is maintained between the inner and outer bumpers, pressure necrosis and ulceration occurs leading to tube migration slowly from the stomach into the gastrocutaneous tract.

Removal of Gastrostomy Tube

Several methods are used to remove PEG tubes, depending on the configuration of the inner bumper. Some tubes are designed such that they can be directly pulled through the stoma, whereas stiff or rigid bumpers are best managed by endoscopic removal. Among the many available tubes, we prefer using the Cor-Pak tube system. It has a collapsible intragastric disk (bumper), which is easy to remove by traction without the need for endoscopy. Additional advantage of the Cor-Pak system is that it can be converted to gastrojejunal feeding, at the time of PEG placement or later if needed. Simply cutting the tube externally at skin level and allowing the tube to pass in the stool is not recommended, as it may cause obstruction and require surgical intervention. When the skin level tube is in site, we pass a small (5Fr) feeding tube through it and aspirate gastric fluid to confirm the proper positioning. If there is any doubt we recommend checking the tube by injecting contrast material through the tube under fluoroscopy.

Replacement of Gastrostomy Tube

The initial PEG tube is changed after 2-3 months when a good tract has been formed. Skin level gastrostomy tubes (e.g. button-type) are commonly used as PEG replacement devices placed in the mature tract. The balloon replacement gastrostomy tubes are available in sizes from 12 Fr to 24 Fr, usually the same diameter as the PEG tube. If there is some leaking around the PEG, upgrading to a 2 Fr thicker button tube is recommended. The length of the tube can be assessed with a measuring device before the insertion of the skin level tube.

Subsequent replacement of the balloon gastrostomy tubes is simple and may be performed by trained nurses or caregivers through the established gastrostomy tract. Once the tube is advanced into the stomach, the balloon is inflated with 5 to 10 ml of water.

Percutaneous Radiological Gastric (PRG) Tube Placement

Gastrostomy tubes can be placed under fluoroscopy. PRG is less expensive than surgical or endoscopic placement. Using a technique similar to PEG placement, the gastrostomy tube is pulled or pushed over a fluoroscopically-placed guide wire. In one study the success rate for PRG placement was 98% in a group of patients in whom PEG was unsuccessful or who were not candidates for the PEG procedure.

Open Surgical Gastric Tube Placement

In one study, the cost of a PEG was $ 700 less than operative gastrostomy. This advantage, however, narrowed to approximately $100 if the tube required repeat endoscopy for a tube change and skin level device insertion.

Fewer side effects are associated with PEG tube placement than with surgical GT placement. Patients can be fed sooner with a PEG, and general recovery is quicker.

In most pediatric cases, the surgical gastrostomy placement is combined with fundoplication in patients with intractable reflux or aspiration.

Surgical placement of a gastrostomy tube may be required when PEG or PRG is contraindicated or not available. It can be accomplished with either open or laparoscopic technique. Surgical gastrostomy also should be used when PEG cannot be performed safely (e.g. in patients with extensive intra-abdominal adhesions or if an intestinal loop is positioned in between the stomach and abdominal wall).

Jejunostomy Feeding Tube Placement

Endoscopic Jejunal Feeding Tube Placement

It is more difficult and time consuming to place a jejunal tube. Contraindications are the same as PEG placement, and are listed above.

Jejunal feeding is preferred in patients who require postpyloric feeding because of risk for aspiration, or have significant duodenogastric dysmotility, pancreatitis or superior mesentery artery syndrome. Jejunostomy is most commonly used to reduce the risk of aspiration. It is frequently used in critically-ill patients to avoid total parenteral nutrition (TPN). Aspiration cannot be fully prevented with jejunal feeding, however, its incidence is substantially reduced when combined with gastric decompression.

Percutaneous endoscopic jejunostomy and gastrojejunostomy were originally reported in 1984. Both indirect and direct methods are available.

The indirect endoscopic method is used when the patient has an existing PEG tube. The jejunal tube is inserted through the gastrostomy (PEG/J). The jejunal tube is then advanced into the jejunum either over a guide wire or pushed into the jejunum with the endoscope. A simple technique is to attach a suture at the end of the tube. The tube is then inserted into the stomach and grasped by forceps. The endoscope is advanced into the small bowel with the tube along its side. Once in position, the suture is released and the endoscope is slowly removed to avoid withdrawal of the jejunal tube.

The advantage of the combined tube is that the gastric port can be used for gastric decompression, and the jejunal port is used for feeding. Use of 10 to 12 F jejunal tubes substantially decreases the possibility of tube clogging.

Direct endoscopic jejunostomy can be performed if stomach is removed or altered. Usually an enteroscope or pediatric colonoscope is used for this procedure. The endoscope should be advanced into the jejunum near the ligament of Treitz. The abdominal wall is illuminated and a percutaneous endoscopic jejunostomy tube is inserted with a technique similar to that for PEG placement. Success rates with this approach have been in the range of 72 to 100%, with minimal complications.

Percutaneous Radiologic Jejunostomy (PRJ) Tube

The percutaneous jejunostomy (PRJ) feeding tube is placed under fluoroscopic guidance. The tube can be inserted through an existing gastrostomy tube and advanced into the jejunum over a guide wire (indirect method). It can be inserted into the jejunum by direct percutaneous puncture near the ligament of Treitz.

Surgical Jejunostomy

Open surgical and laparoscopic techniques have been used with success to obtain jejunostomy access.

Some disadvantages of jejunal tubes are that, jejunal feeding tubes can easily be dislodged requiring frequent X-ray to confirm its position. Also bolus feedings cannot be given through jejunal tube, a higher rate of the formula administration can cause diarrhea, and there is a higher incidence of formula intolerance manifesting as diarrhea, nausea and cramps.

COMPLICATIONS OF TUBE FEEDING

Tube feeding patients should be monitored especially in the initial stages for gastric residuals, reflux, vomiting, pulmonary symptoms, abdominal distention, urinary output, and stool frequency and consistency.

Common Complications

Clogged Tube

Acid precipitation of feeding formulas is an important factor in the occlusion of gastrostomy and NG feeding tubes.

Tubes are easily clogged if:

- Caliber of the tube is small.
- Length of the tube is long.
- Tube is in the stomach.
- Feeding is continuous as opposed to bolus feedings.
- Gastric residual volume is measured frequently.
- Medication is administered through the tube.
- Bulking agents such as psyllium fiber or resins, such as cholestyramine are given through the tube.

Recommendations to prevent clogging are:

- Administer medications orally whenever possible.
- Flush the tube every 6 to 8 hours if on continuous feedings and also after every feed and medication administration.

Management

- Instill warm water and clamp the tube for a few minutes, then instill air.
- In a prospective study the best declogging agent was a pancreatic enzyme concentrate mixed with bicarbonate to optimize the pH.
- If applying the declogging solution with a syringe fails, a catheter can be passed through the tube to directly apply the solution at the clog.
- Most clogged-tubes should be replaced. Tubes that have been unclogged by using force should be radiographed after water-soluble contrast injection to check for internal leaks.

Complications at the Insertion Site

Local Irritation

Transnasally-placed tubes can cause nasopharyngeal erosions, soreness of the nose, sinusitis and otitis media. Changing the side of tube may resolve these problems.

Leakage at the Tube Site

Leaking of gastric juice around the tube site indicates that the internal part is not covering the tract completely. It leads to maceration and irritation of the skin predisposing to local infection, abscess formation and also promotes the development of granulation tissue.

Management

- Inflate the balloon so that it sits firmly on the surface covering the tract. If needed, change to a bigger size tube.
- Apply an antacid on the surface to prevent maceration.
- Treat granulation tissue with silver nitrate at the time of dressing changes.

Dislodged G-tube

Gastrocutaneous tracts may close in as little as 24 hours; thus, dislodged tubes should be replaced promptly. A Foley catheter can be used temporarily to maintain the patency of the fistulous tract.

Bleeding

Bleeding is a rare complication in the tube tract. If it occurs the external bumper should be tightened against the abdominal wall to compress the PEG tube tract. The compression should be released within 48 hours to avoid PEG tube tract wound breakdown. Surgical intervention is rarely necessary.

Ulceration

Ulcers may develop below the internal PEG tube bolster or on the gastric wall. Loosening of the external bolster releases the bolster from the gastric mucosa and aids healing. Ulcers occur more frequently with rigid bolsters.

Deterioration of Material of the Tube

Deterioration can be recognized if there is pitting, ballooning, and a characteristic smell. It does not present significant risk to the patient; however, the tube can break, develop leaks or come out while the patient is sleeping. If the later occurs, the tube site shrinks within an hour and often tract dilatation is necessary to insert the same size tube. In our practice, we replace the low profile tubes every 3-4 months. Microscopic examinations have demonstrated that fungal colonization is an important cause of PEG failure.

Complication at the End of the Tube

Nasogastric, nasojejunal and gastrojejunal feeding tubes may get displaced during a procedure, during patient care, coughing, etc. When dislodgement of the feeding tube is suspected, feeding should be stopped immediately and a radiograph obtained to verify the position of the tube prior to restarting the feeding.

Gastric Feedings

- Plastic and larger diameter tubes may cause esophageal and gastric erosions especially if they are used to check gastric residuum.
- Dislodgement: Non-endoscopic replacement of a dislodged tube/button is contraindicated in the absence of a mature tract. Nasogastric tube can be replaced at the bedside.
- A gastrostomy tube may migrate in the stomach and obstruct the gastric outlet if the external crossbar is not properly positioned. This can present with vomiting, high residual volume or as formula regurgitation.

Jejunal Feedings

- Jejunal tubes are more prone to dislodgement due to difficulty anchoring them.
- Small intestinal ischemia and necrosis may develop. It is more likely to occur in patients who are hemodynamically-unstable.
- Large feeding volume or formulas with high osmolality can cause abdominal distention, pain, tenderness, and diarrhea.

Nutritional complications

Refeeding Syndrome

Refeeding syndrome may manifest in patients who previously had limited oral intake or in whom feeding is introduced rapidly. It occurs in approximately 25% of these patients. The signs of refeeding syndrome are glucose intolerance, fluid retention, and electrolyte imbalance with hypophosphatemia, hypomagnesemia, and hypokalemia. These signs are usually observed during the first few days after initiation of feeding. In these patients, the daily monitoring of electrolyte concentrations should be continued until nutritional goals are achieved and the electrolytes and glucose to stabilize. If the condition is left untreated, paralysis, respiratory failure, and even death can occur.

Aspiration

Aspiration is a risk in children with severe gastroesophageal reflux disease who are on nasogastric or gastrostomy feeding. Confirming the position of the tube radiographically both before initiating the feeding or when displacement is suspected, can reduce the incidence of aspiration. Reflux precautions, including the elevation of the head of the bed by 20-30 degrees during feeding, and using continuous feeding, decreases the risk of aspiration.

In high-risk patients, nasojejunal, gastrojejunal or jejunostomy feeding can be used temporarily. In refluxing patients, funduplication with gastrostomy tube provide a long-term resolution to avoid aspiration.

Table 108.3 provides a short troubleshooting guideline for tube feeding.

TUBE FEEDING FORMULA SELECTION

Feeding should not be started until the proper placement of the feeding tube is verified. The most important goal of the tube feeding is to meet the nutritional needs of the patient.

The formula selection depends on the age, clinical diagnosis and gastrointestinal function of the child. In general, "intact" formulas containing unaltered components (proteins, carbohydrates, fat) are suitable for most patients and "elemental" or "predigested" formulas

Table 108.3: Tube feeding troubleshooting

Problem	*Possible causes*	*Possible solution*
Diarrhea	Too rapid feeding	Slow feeding
	Intolerance to formula	Change formula
	Too concentrated formula	Add pedialyte or water and gradually increase the concentration in 3-5 days
	Medications	Check for stool C. difficile
Cramping	Cold formula	Room temperature formula
	Tube in wrong place	Reposition
	Too fast feeding	Slow
Constipation	Inadequate fluid	Use more water to flush along with medicines
	Low fiber diet	Increase fluids, add prune juice or change to a fiber containing formula
	Lack of activity	Improve activity
Vomiting	Too rapid feedings	Slow feeding
	Tube too large	Use smaller sized tube
	Improper tube placement	Reposition
	Large residual matter in stomach	Change to continuous drip infusion Use isotonic formula Change to jejunal feeding Consider adding a prokinetic agent
	Formula too concentrated	Dilute the formula
	Medications given with feeding	
Nausea	During feeding may indicate delayed gastric emptying	Stop feeding; resume when improved
	Stomach distention	
	Too cold formula	
Reflux	Large residual matter in the stomach	Elevate head of the bed Thicken feeds (add cereal to the formula)

Contd.

Contd.

	Physiological reflux	Ranitidine and metoclopramide can be used
Clogged tubes	Inadequate irrigation	Order tube irrigation, especially after feeds and medications
	Insoluble precipitates	Try a catheter-tipped syringe filled with water, held high to facilitate movement of fluid. If needed inject 1 ml of papain solution
Aspiration	Tube displacement	Verify placement
	Regurgitation	Change to jejunal or duodenal feeding

are suitable for patients with specific clinical needs, such as malabsorption, critical illness, or other gastrointestinal impairment.

There are new components added to formulas in the last few years. These include nucleotides, soluble fiber, glutamine, arginine, and fructo-oligosaccharides.

When *selecting the appropriate formula*, the factors to consider include the following:

- Age and medical condition.
- Protein, calorie and volume requirements.
- History of food intolerance or allergy.
- Gastrointestinal function.
- Formula characteristics (e.g. osmolality, viscosity, nutrient content, convenience and cost).

As a general rule adult formulas for enteral nutrition can be used in children >10 years of age. Below 10 years of age, formulas specially made for children are recommended. Age-specific formulas exist for premature infants, term infants, toddlers, and children upto 10 years of age. Infants under 12 months should be given breast milk, a standard infant formula or a special infant formula. For most children 1-10 years of age, pediatric enteral formulas (e.g. Pediasure, Resource, Kindercal) are designed specifically to meet their nutrient requirements. Figure 108.3 provides a general guideline for formula selection in infants.

In premature infants, who are unable to co-ordinate sucking, swallowing, and breathing, orogastric (or nasogastric) tube feeding is preferred initially. Breast milk or special formula is given by continuous infusion or bolus delivery every two to three hours. Healthy premature infants tolerate bolus feeding, while infants with pulmonary problems or gastrointestinal abnormalities may tolerate continuous feeding better.

Protein and calorie requirements are age-dependent. In certain clinical situations higher protein intake is necessary (e.g. intestinal loss) or higher caloric intake is required for a catch-up growth.

Infants with intolerance to milk and/or soy protein should get hydrolyzed, hypoallergenic formula or if this is not tolerated amino acid based formula.

The presence of gastrointestinal disease may require special formulas, e.g. medium chain triglyceride (MCT) containing formulas used in patients with pancreatic, biliary, or intestinal diseases when the digestion and absorption of long-chain fatty acids is impaired or when there is problem in the lymphatic flow.

The availability and price of special formulas can be a limiting factor in the selection. Generally, it is better to use original formulas without modifications in order to avoid errors. After estimating energy needs, if additional nutrients are needed, the tube feeding formulas can easily be supplemented with fats, carbohydrates or lipids.

Sometimes caregivers modify formulas without physician approval. This may result in altered caloric or protein intake (e.g. mixing formula with juice reduces protein content, etc.). It is important to reassure caregivers that the appropriately selected formulas will meet their child's nutritional needs.

TYPES OF FORMULAS

Complete or Standard Formulas

Standard formulas are nutritionally complete and made of complex proteins, fats, carbohydrates, and contain adequate vitamins and mineral supply. They are for patients who have normal digestion and absorption with inability to ingest adequate calories and nutrients. The advantages of complete formulas are that they have low osmolality, do not contain lactose, and are palatable, easy to use, and sterile. Some of the complete formulas have fiber, which helps regulating bowel movements and prevents constipation, which is frequent in neurologically-damaged or postoperative patients.

Elemental Formulas

One form of elemental formulas or hypoallergenic formulas are made from hydrolyzed (predigested) protein. Other elemental formulas have only amino acids. In addition, they usually have different ratios of medium-chain triglycerides essential fatty acids, vitamins and minerals.

Elemental formulas require less digestion, results in lower stool volume and less stimulation of bile and pancreatic secretions. The disadvantage of elemental formulas is that they are hyperosmolar so that a higher infusion rate may cause cramping and osmotic diarrhea. Since they are much more expensive than standard formulas, they should not be given to children with normal digestive function and no food allergies.

The most frequent clinical indications for the use of elemental formulas include short gut syndrome, malabsorption syndromes, severe food allergies, inflammatory bowel disease and gastrointestinal fistulas.

Home-Prepared Formulas

Home-prepared, blenderized formulas can be administered through short gastrostomy tubes and cost less than standard commercial formulas. However, they require more time to prepare and they are not sterile with risk of being nutritionally incomplete. They can only be used with a close supervision of a nutritionist. This is used more in developing countries. Home-made preparations are more viscous and may contain chunks, which could easily block the tube.

Modular Formulas

Modular formulas contain only specific nutrients. They are added to commercial or home-prepared formulas to meet special nutrient needs. Examples of modular formulas are the following:

- Medium-chain triglycerides (e.g. MCT oil) provide fat calories in an easily digestible and absorbable form.
- Readily digested carbohydrates (e.g. Moducal or polycose) used for additional calories.
- Protein and specific amino acid preparations (e.g. Casec or ProMod).

Special Formulas

There are various specialized formulas that are available for children with special needs, such as premature infants, children with renal failure or inborn errors of metabolism. These formulas should be selected by the treating physician and dietitian who are familiar with the products and their particular uses.

MONITORING PATIENTS ON LONG-TERM TUBE FEEDING

- Weigh every other day until stable, then weekly for acute care and monthly for long-term care. Daily weights may be required in intensive care settings. Monitor weight for height. Evaluate the need for reducing caloric intake in case of low energy needs due to low activity and adjust the calories accordingly.
- Basic electrolytes plus calcium, magnesium, and phosphorus, complete blood count initially, then every 10 days. It should be ordered more frequently in intensive care situations. Test monthly or at least quarterly in long-term home care.
- Albumin initially, then every month.
- Monitor serum glucose readings until feeding is at goal rate and blood sugars are stable.
- Evaluate if formula is meeting the requirements for fluids, calories, protein, vitamins, minerals and electrolytes.
- Replace the tubes as needed.

KEY LEARNING POINTS

- Enteral tube feeding is widely used both in inpatient and outpatient setting in patients who otherwise cannot meet adequate nutritional requirements for various reasons.
- There are several methods of enteral feeding.
- Once the decision is made to tube feed, determine the most appropriate feeding route.
- Determine requirements for fluid, calories, protein, vitamins, minerals and electrolytes.
- Determine most appropriate type of formula and method of delivery.
- Carefully monitor the patients on tube feeding and make changes in the type, amount, method of delivery and additional supplements as needed.
- Most important part is to teach caregivers appropriate techniques for tube feeding, stoma and skin care and to watch for signs of complications.
- Complications can usually be avoided if care is taken.
- Patients should constantly be monitored for intolerance, complications, and assessed for a possible return to oral feeding.

FURTHER READINGS

1. Cunningham J. Body composition and nutrition supporting pediatrics:What to defend and how soon to begin. *Nutr Clin Pract* 1995;10:177-182.
2. Heiselman D, Hofer T, Vidovich R. Enteral feeding tube placement success with intravenous metoclopramide administration in ICU patients. *Chest* 1995;107:1686-1688.
3. Ho S. Radiological percutaneous gastrostomy. *Clin Radiol* 2001;56:902-910.
4. Iber F, Livak A, Patel M. Importance of fungus colonization in failure of silicone rubber percutaneous gastrostomy tubes (PEGs) *Dig Dis Sci* 1996;41:226-231.
5. Kirby DF, MH Delegge, Fleming CR. American Gastroenterological Association Technical Review on Tube Feeding for Enteral Nutrition. *Gastroenterology* 1995;108:1282-1301.
6. Komenaka I. Erythromycin and position facilitated placement of postpyloric feeding tubes in burned patients. *Dig Surg* 2000;17:578-580.
7. Lockett M. Percutaneous endoscopic gastrostomy complications in a tertiary-care center. *Am Surg* 2002;68:117-120.
8. Ozdemir B. Placement of nasoenteral feeding tubes using magnetic guidance:Retesting a new technique. *J Am Coll Nutr* 2000;19:446-451.

109 Parenteral Nutrition in PICU

Anil Gautam • Praveen C Sobti

INTRODUCTION

Despite the well-recognized importance of nutrition in periods of illness, it is often a neglected or underaddressed area in the management of critically ill patients. Special considerations in infants and young children make nutrient metabolism in response to systemic stress different from adults. These are variable caloric requirements, high growth velocity, immaturity of organs and decreased energy stores. Studies in adults have shown that malnutrition is associated with increased morbidity, infections and mortality. Although few studies have been conducted specifically in critically ill children, there is evidence that patients in the pediatric intensive care unit (PICU), especially younger than 2 years, are at risk of developing protein-energy malnutrition (PEM). Also, malnourished children have longer hospitalizations, increased morbidity and mortality.

FALLOUT OF STARVATION IN THE CRITICALLY ILL

Tables 109.1 and 109.2 depict the impact of starvation and factors contributing to nutritional imbalance in critically ill patients respectively.

Table 109.1: Impact of starvation

- Negative nitrogen balance, further weight loss
- Morphological changes in the gut
  - Mucosal thickness ↓
  - Cell proliferation ↓
  - Villous height ↓
- Functional changes
  - Increased permeability
  - Decreased absorption of amino acids
- Enzymatic/hormonal changes
  - Decreased sucrose and lactose
- Impact on immunity
  - Cellular - Altered T cell function
    - Mitogenic proliferation
  - Humoral - Decreased complement, opsonins, secretory IgA
  - Increased bacterial translocation

The goal of nutritional support in PICU is to minimize the deleterious effect of catabolism following acute injury and to promote anabolism. Knowledge of basal energy requirement and escalation due to the catabolic stress are keys for successful nutritional support, both enteral and parenteral.

Table 109.2: Nutritional imbalance in critically ill

Catabolic factor	*Anabolic factors*
• Epinephrine	• Growth hormone
• Cortisol	• Insulin
• Glucagon	• Nutritional support
• Starvation	– Enteral
• Cytokines	– Parenteral
• Gut injury/stress ulceration	

Metabolic Stores

Children, like adults, rely upon metabolism of proteins, lipids and carbohydrates to meet the demands of catabolic stress. The metabolic reserves of neonates, children and adults are mentioned in Table 109.3 as a per cent of total body weight.

Table 109.3: Body composition of neonates, children and adults as percentage of total body weight

Age	*Percent protein*	*Percent fat*	*Percent carbohydrate*
Neonates	11	14	0.4
Children (age 10 years)	15	17	0.4
Adults	18	19	0.4

Carbohydrates do not serve as stores for the time of stress and remain relatively constant. Fat stores increase somewhat gradually with age with premature babies having even further reduced stores. The most significant macronutrient is protein which is present as twice or even thrice in amount as a metabolic source in adults as compared to children. Besides having decreased stores, the baseline requirements in children and neonates are higher than adults as shown in (Table 109.4).

Table 109.4: Recommended energy and protein requirements in healthy humans

Age	*Protein (g/kg/d)*	*Energy (kcal/kg/d)*
Neonates	2.2	120
Children (age 10 years)	1.0	70
Adults	0.8	35

This inverse relationship between requirement and stores is due to higher body surface area and increased need for growth itself. Thus, the child and neonate in particular is potentially more susceptible to the deleterious effects of catabolic stress of illness.

METABOLIC RESPONSE TO ACUTE INJURY

The physiologic response to acute injury has been characterized by 3 phases:

1. **Initial hypermetabolic response:** This is the first response triggered by acute insult. It usually lasts only minutes to hours and is related to the activation of sympathetic nervous system.
2. **Ebb phases:** This second response is characterized by transient or persistent decrease in metabolic rate. Its duration is chiefly determined by the severity and duration of the etiologic stress and lasts until adequate tissue perfusion is restored.
3. **Flow phase:** The third phase of acute injury is characterized by a hypermetabolism lasting for days to weeks after resuscitation. This is the state most often seen in critically ill children after admission to PICU. It is further subclassified into catabolic period where body tissue is degraded to provide substrate for the hypermetabolism and a late anabolic period where there is restoration of tissue energy protein reserves. Clinically, there is increased cardiac output and minute ventilation, decreased gut motility, loss of brush border enzymes and mucosal integrity resulting in stress ulceration and a myriad of cellular and humoral responses.

Ultimately, in children who recover, anabolism ensures with positive nitrogen balance resulting in tissue repair and resumption of growth.

Protein Metabolism

Proteins are composed of amino acids and continuously degraded and synthesized in a process called 'protein turnover'. Ninetyeight percent of the amino acids reside in proteins and the rest as free endogenous pool. Protein degradation releases amino acids which are again reutilized for anabolism thus contributing to the protein turnover. The protein turnover is high in critically ill patients, more so in neonates and young children. In fact, seriously ill patients with extensive burns and those with respiratory insufficiency requiring mechanical support, may have double the protein turnover as compared to normal subjects.

As the protein degradation predominates over synthesis during critical illness, patients go into net negative nitrogen balance which may be clinically evident by weight loss and skeletal muscle wasting. One of the stimulants for muscle breakdown is the production of glucose from amino acids (gluconeogenesis), glucose being the most important substrate fuel for energy metabolism in brain, blood cells, kidneys and elsewhere. However, dietary glucose supplementation does not prevent this catabolic cascade, thereby suggesting need for protein/amino acid supplementation in sick patients. Since children have limited muscle mass and protein reserves, prolonged illness can have serious consequences. If the catabolic stressor continues unchecked, progressive loss of diaphragmatic and intercostals muscles may cause respiratory failure while cardiac muscles loss may result in life threatening arrhythmias once 1/3rd of the lean body mass is dissipated. Evidence suggests that amino acid supplementation improves protein balance by resulting in increased synthesis, since degradation remains constant.

The type and specific composition of amino acids formulas which best increase protein balance is however yet to be established. Moreover, different diseases may accentuate certain specific amino acid requirements e.g. proline in burns and histidine, cystine, taurine and proline in infants less than 6 months. Roughly, the quantity of protein administered should be 3-4 g/kg/d for LBW infants, 2-3 g/kd/d for term babies and 1.5 g/kg/d for older children. Adequate protein intake increases protein synthesis, promotes wound healing and preserves skeletal muscle mass. In fact, it is the single most important nutritional intervention in intensive care. Conversely overzealous and excessive administration (> 6 g/kg/d) may result in toxicity, particularly in neonates, manifested as azotemia, fever, visual disturbances and lower IQ.

Energy Metabolism

Increase in energy requirement during acute illness closely parallels elevated protein requirement. Resting energy needs may be determined directly by measuring heat released by the patient at rest wherein the patient is placed in a thermally isolated chamber and heat released is measured over a prolonged period. This is not easily applicable and is more of theoretical interest. The indirect methods use calculations based on quantity of O_2 consumed, CO_2 produced by the body over a specific time period, and a correction factor based on urinary nitrogen excretion rate. These are accurate aculeate but involve lot of sophisticated equipment and are not practical in developing countries. In practice therefore, the recommended dietary caloric intake for healthy children can serve as useful reference starting point in critically ill patients. Moreover nutritional assessment of the child base on anthropometric measures, biochemical markers like retinal binding protein and prealbumin (half lives 0.5 and 2 days, respectively – to assess/monitor acute hyper-metabolism) and albumin (half life 20 days to monitor/assess chronic malnutrition) can also be used. Sequential clinical examinations, daily weight and dietary evaluation are other helpful aids while calculation energy needs of the patient.

Table 109.5: Distribution of calories needs in healthy growing infants and children

Age (years) kcal/kg/d	*BMR Total kcal/kg/d*	*Activity kcal/kg/d*	*Growth*	
VLBW	47	15	97	130
< 1	55	1	40	110
1	55	35	20	110
2	55	45	5	100
5	47	38	2	87
10	37	38	2	77

Table 109.6: Increased in resting energy expenditure with physiologic stress

Condition	*Increase in EE (%)*
Fever	12% per °C above 37°C
Cardiac failure	15 – 25
Major surgery	20 – 30
Burns	Upto 100
Severe sepsis	40 – 50

Over feeding, calories, however, does not have any benefit. It cannot reverse the obligate hyper metabolism and is associated with increased mortality. Also, it can result in synthesis of excess fat and development of fatty liver.

Carbohydrates

Adequate glucose supply is vital for functioning of RBCs, brain and various other body tissues as it serves as the principal substrate. Glucose turnover may increase upto 3 times in injury and illness. However, provision of dietary glucose does not prevent gluconeogensis and so catabolism of muscle proteins continues. A combination of glucose and amino acids, on the other hand is effective in improving protein balance. Excess glucose provision is more detrimental as it leads to carbon dioxide production, causing increased ventilatory burden on the child. In adult patients, dextrose delivery of 4 mg/kg/min has been reported as optimal. Infants and children utilize glucose ranging from 8-13 mg/kg/min. Critically sick children tolerate maximally upto 8-10 mg/kg/min while malnourished children may tolerate higher rates.

Lipid Metabolism

Lipids are also metabolized at a faster rate during illness. Approximately 30-40% of the released fatty acids are oxidized for energy suggesting that free fatty acids are prime source of energy in sick patients. The glycerol released along with free fatty acids from triglycerides can be converted to pyruvate, which in turn, may be used as a precursor in gluconeogenesis. To obviate the essential fatty acid deficiency in sick infants, provision of linoleic acid and linolenic acid at 4.5% and 0.5% of total calories, respectively, is recommended.

Administration of fats in excess of patent's ability to metabolise may result in hyper triglyceridemia. Due to possible adverse effects of lipid administration, lipid supplementation in ill neonates and children is usually started at 0.5 g/kg/d and increased over 4-5 days upto 2-4 g/kg/d.

TOTAL PARENTERAL NUTRITION (TPN) IN PICU

Optimal use of TPN has resulted in higher survival of critically ill children. Also, improvements in techniques for artificial nutrition have led to an improved quality of life for long-term TPN-patients. Indications for parenteral nutrition are described in (Box 109.1).

The WHO recommends that wherever possible the energy requirements of patient should be based on its expenditure. The requirements for preterm infants are higher than for older children because of elevated metabolic rates, high percentage of metabolically active tissue, low carbohydrates and lipids stores, high evaporated losses and immature GI system. The goal is to provide adequate calories for proper growth, which is determined by maintenance of child's respective growth percentile for age and gender.

Box 109.1: Indications for parenteral nutrition

- Prematurity
- Abdominal surgery e.g. for malrotation
- Congenital defects, e.g. gastroschisis (defect within the abdominal wall) or tracheoesophageal fistula
- Chronic intestinal pseudo-obstruction
- Autoimmune enteropathy, severe diarrhoea or microvillus atrophy
- Short bowel syndrome
- Pancreatitis
- Respiratory distress syndrome
- Post chemotherapy complications, such as inflammation of membrane surfaces

Fluid Requirements

These are based on sum of maintenance, repair of dehydration and replacement of ongoing losses. Maintenance fluid requirements are calculated as follows:

1-10 kg	100 ml/kg/d
10-20 kg	1000 ml + 50 ml for each kg > 10 kg
> 20 kg	1500 ml + 20 ml for each kg > 20 kg

It is important to consider medications, flushes, drips, pressure lines and other IV fluids while calculating total fluids planned.

Protein Requirements

Amino acids are essential for growth and formation of tissue. 10% amino plasma is readily available amino acid/protein source for parenteral supplementation. Its caloric density is 4 kcal/g but as it is not optimal to use protein as a caloric source, the protein caloric content of hyper alimentation fluids is generally not calculated.

Carbohydrates

These are normally provided in PN formulations as glucose which is readily used by all body tissues. Between 40-45% of calories in PN should be from carbohydrate source. Carbohydrate intolerance is not uncommon in infants because of low glycogen reserve in liver and a diminished capacity for gluconeogenesis. Carbohydrate, as a sole source of energy, will lead to steatosis, increased carbon dioxide production and fatty acid deficiency. Parenteral nutrition can be administered over < 24 hours in older children but must be tapered over 1-2 hours to prevent rebound hypoglycemia. Blood glucose measurements should be checked 15-60 min after discontinuation of a parenteral feed. Maximum concentration of dextrose that can be safely administered through a peripheral line is 12.5%. Higher concentration should be given through a central venous catheter to prevent thrombophlebitis.

Lipid

Lipids provide between 35-40% of the non-nitrogen calories in parenteral nutrition. Lipids may be decreased in sepsis or if bilirubin level exceeds 200 mmol/l because lipoprotein lipase activity is reduced. Between 0.5-1.0 g/kg/d of lipid is required to prevent essential fatty acid deficiency in infants and children. The lipid emulsions currently available are isotonic and are suitable for PN administration because of their low osmolarity. Lipids are an important component of PN as a source of energy dense calories, providing 2 kcal/ml. Intra lipid 20% is the most commonly used lipid source. It is a soybean oil, containing long chain triglycerides emulsified with egg yolk phospholipids. 10% emulsions are not recommended because of high phospholipids to triglyceride ratio which can lead to elevated plasma triglycerides and hyper phospholipidemia. Newer lipid substrates that combine soyabean oil, olive oil and omega 3 fish oils are in development. Omega 3 enriched emulsions contain arachidonic acid and docosahexanoic acid, which are important for the development of brain and retina.

Electrolytes

Electrolytes are added to PN according to patient's individual requirements, based on blood chemistry. Differences in body water composition and immature renal functions are two factors that make a neonate more susceptible than older children or adults to dehydration and electrolyte imbalances. In comparison with adults, water accounts for a much larger percentage of body weight in neonates, with approximately 80% being extra cellular fluid. Sodium is restricted during first few days after birth to allow contraction of extra cellular fluid. Renal immaturity in premature infants results in inability to concentrate urine, and the concomitant use of diuretics leads to increased sodium requirements. Sodium is usually given at a dose of 3-4 mmol/kg/d in premature infants and 2-3 mmol/kg/d in older children. Potassium is also given at a dose of 2-3 mmol/kg/d. There is evidence of sodium depletion in patients failing to thrive, especially if urine sodium falls below 10 mmol/l. Parenteral nutrition is also supplemented with calcium and organic phosphate. Besides this vitamin and trace elements are added based on recommended daily requirements.

Complications of TPN are either metabolic or mechanical. Cholestasis is a common complication of long-term artificial feeding and is often associated with sepsis, over feeding and lack of enteral feeding. Cyclical PN and trophic feeding may reduce this complication. Minimal enteral or trophic

Table 109.7: PN suggested guidelines for initiation and maintenance

Substrate	*Initiation*	*Advancement*	*Goals*	*Comments*
Dextrose	10%	2-5%/d	Max. 25%	Increased as tolerated consider insulin if hyperglycemia
Amino acids	1 g/kg/d	0.5-1.0g/kg/d	2-3g/kg/d	Maintain calorie: nitrogen ratio at ~200:1
20% lipids	1 g/kg/d	0.5-1.0 g/kg/d	2-3 g/kg/d	Only use 20%

Box 109.2: Parameters to be monitored while the patient is on TPN

Initial monitoring

Complete blood count, serum sodium, potassium, calcium, urea, magnesium, phosphate, bilirubin, albumin, alanine trasaminase, alkaline phosphates and blood glucose.

Daily (for first week)

Weight, blood glucose (in each shift), electrolytes.

Weekly

Urea, electrolytes, calcium, magnesium, phosphate, bilirubin and alanine transaminase, triglycerides, CBC.

feeding of 1-10 ml/hr dependent on age of child is recommended to maintain intestinal mucosa integrity, reduced bacterial translocation and prevention of biliary cholestasis. Cyclical PN involves the PN being infused over a shorter period of time (12-16 hours over night). Catheter related sepsis is the more frequently seen complication and *Staphylococcus epidermidis, Staph. aureus, Enterococcus* and *Candida albicans* are the common causative organisms. Treatment is with antibiotics.

Enteral vs Parenteral Nutrition—Which is Best?

The optimum method of providing nutrition to the critically ill has been controversial for many years. Most believe that enteral nutrition is the preferred method of feeding whenever possible because it is more physiologic and has reduced rate of complications compare with TPN. Patients have a lower prevalence of GI bleeding and infection, a shorter duration of mechanical ventilation, and an improved mortality rate. There is data both in pediatric as well as adult literature which support the institution of protocols to improve time to reach target caloric needs. Also recent evidence suggests that protocol based early, aggressive enteral nutrition in the pediatric intensive care unit improves time to goal feeding and results in fewer complications associated with enteral feeding such as vomiting and constipation.

Although gut use is preferable, PN can be used for indications as described earlier and also concomitantly with enteral feeds if GI intolerance limits intake. PN should be started in a timely manner if caloric needs cannot be reached despite concerns related to complications as meeting the nutritional requirements of sick patients takes precedence over such issues. Moreover, by attending to strict aseptic precautions during handling of central venous catheters and preparation of TPN, sepsis related complications can be decreased. In cases of clinical equipoise, cost should be taken into account as PN is much more expensive. This is particularly important in developing countries like India.

NEWER CONCEPTS

The concept of 'immunonutrition' or immunomodulation by use of fish liver oils, branched chain amino acids, arginine and glutamine is an area of active research and investigation branched chain amino acids are considered to have a role in hepatic encephalopathy as these postulated to minimize protein catabolism during stress, are not metabolised by liver and serve as an energy source for muscles. This has been based on observations that severity of hepatic encephalopathy correlates with degree of decrease in branched chain amino acids. However, there has not been convincing evidence where their use has affected outcome favorably, clearly indicating that more research is required. Glutamine is an other area of recent interest. It is the most abundant amino acid in plasma and muscle and the major energy source of the gut. Its use in TPN has been shown to improve intestinal atrophy associated with standard TPN in animal models. Better survival, shorter hospital stay and increased nitrogen balance has been demonstrated in transplant recipients. Also its use in TPN in neonates has shown promising results and may become an important potential nutrient in the future.

CONCLUSION

Nutritional support of critically sick children poses many challenges. Our ability to accurately measure and predict the child's metabolic state during acute stress is still sufficient, significant advances are nonetheless being made in the nutritional support of these children through use of enteral and parenteral route resulting in improved clinical outcome. However, more research is clearly indicated in the pediatric population.

Key Learning Points

- Start nutrition early.
- Enteral route is preferred when available.
- Set goals for the individual patient.
- Dose nutrients compatible with existing metabolism.
- Appropriate monitoring is essential.
- Avoid overfeeding.
- Attention to aseptic precautions helps.

FURTHER READINGS

1. Albarano TP, Pettignano R, Asfaw M, Easley K. Use of a feeding protocol to improve nutritional support through early, aggressive, enteral nutrition in the pediatric intensive care unit. *Pediatr Crit Care Med* 2006; 7: 1-5.
2. Atkinson S, Siefful E, Bihari D. A prospective randomized, double blind, controlled clinical trial of enteral immunonutrition in the critically ill. Guy's hospital intensive care group. *Crit Care Med* 1998; 26: 1164-1172.
3. Bower RH, Cerra FB, Bershadsky B *et al.:* Early enteral administration of a formula (Impact) supplemented with arginine, nucleotide and fish oil in intensive care unit patients: Results of multicenter, prospective, randomized, clinical trial. *Critical Care Med* 1995; 23: 436-449.
4. Briassoulis GC, Zavras NJ, Hatzis TD. Effectiveness and safety of a protocol for promotion of early intragastric feeding in critically ill children. *Pediatr Crit Care Med* 2001; 2: 113-21.
5. Cerra FB. The hypermetabolism organ failure complex. *World J Surg* 1987; 11: 173-181.
6. Chapman G, Curtas S, Meguid M. Standardized enterol ordus attain caloric goals sooner: A prospective study. *JPEN* 1992; 16: 149-151.
7. Chawals WJ, Fernandez ME, Charles BJ *et al.:* Serum visceral protein levels reflect protein – caloric repletion in neonates recovering from major surgery. *J Pediatr Surg* 1992; 27: 317-320.
8. Chellis MJ, Sanders SV, Webster H *et al.:* Early enteral feeding in the pediatric intensive care unit. *JPEN* 1996; 20: 71-73.
9. Committee on Nutrition, European Society of Pediatric Gastroenterology and Nutrition: Comment on the content and

composition of lipids in infant formulas. *Acta Paediatr Scand* 1991; 80: 887-896.

10. Cuthbertson D, Tilstone WJ. Metabolism during post injury period. *Adv Clin Chem* 1969; 12: 1-55.
11. Fomon SJ, Haschke F, Zeigler EE, Nelson SE. Body composition of reference children from birth to age 10 years. *Am J Clin Nutr* 1982; 35: 1169-1175.
12. Forbes GB, Bruining GJ. Urinary creatinine extraction and lean body mass. *Am J Clin Nutr* 1976; 29: 1359-1366.
13. Galanos AN, Pieper CF, Kussin PS *et al.*: Relationship of body mass index to subsequent mortality in seriously ill hospitalized patients. Support Investigators. The study to understand prognosis and preferences for outcome and risks of treatment. *Crit Care Med* 1997; 25: 1962-1968.
14. Goldman HI, Freudenthal R, Holland B *et al.*: Clinically effects of two different levels of protein intake on low birth weight infants. *J Pediatr* 1969; 74: 881-889.
15. Goldman HJ, Liebman OB, Freudenthal R *et al.*: Effects of early dietary protein intake on low birth weight infants: Evaluation at 3 years. *J Pediatr* 1971; 78: 126-129.
16. Heird WC, Kashyap S, Gomez MR. Protein intake and energy requirements of the infant. *Somin Perinatal* 1991; 15: 438-448.
17. Holliday MA. Metabolic rate and organ size during growth from infancy to maturity and during late gestation and early infancy. *Pediatrics* 1971; 47(1) Supp 2: 1691.
18. Keshen TH, Miller RG, Jahoor F, Jaksic T. Stable isoatopic quantitation of protein metabolism and energy expenditure in neonates on and post extracorporeal life support. *J Pediatr Surgery* 1997; 13: 958-963.
19. Long CL, Kinney JM, Geiger JW. Non-suppressability of gluconeogenesis by glucose in septic patients. *Metabolism* 1976; 25: 193-201.
20. Marik PE, Zaloga GP. Early enteral nutrition in acutely ill patients. A systemic review. *Crit Care Med* 2001; 29: 2264-2270.
21. Meis SJ, Dove EL, Bell EF *et al.*: A gradient layer calorimeter for measurement of energy expenditure in infants. *Am J Physiol* 1994; 266: R1052-1062.
22. Moore FA, Feliciano DV, Andrassy RJ *et al.*: Early enteral feeding compared with parenteral, reduces postoperative septic complications. The results of a metaanalysis. *Ann Surg* 1992; 216: 172-183.
23. Nanii G, Siegel JM, Coleman B *et al.*: Increased lipid fuel dependence in critically ill septic patient. *J Trauma* 1984; 24: 14-30.
24. Peltignano R, Heard M, Davis R *et al.*: Total enteral nutrition versus total parenteral nutrition during pediatric extracorporeal membrane oxygenation. *Crit Care Med* 1998; 26: 358-363.
25. Pollack A, Cowett RM, Schwartz R, Oh W. Glucose disposal in low birth weight infants during steady state hyperglycaemia: Effects of exogenous insulin. *Pediatrics* 1978; 61: 546-549.
26. Pollack MM, Smith D. Protein energy malnutrition in hospitalized children. *Hosp Formul* 1981; 16(1): 1189-90, 1192-1193.
27. Pollack MM, Wiley JS, Kanter R, Holbrooke PR. Malnutrition in critically ill infants and children. *JPEN* 1982; 6: 20-24.
28. Rivera A Jr, Bell EF, Dier DM. Effect of intravenous amino acids on protein metabolism of preterm infants during first 3 days of life. *Pediatr Res* 1993; 33: 106-111.
29. Seale JL, Rumpler WV. Synchronous direct gradient layer and indirect room calorimetery. *J Appl Physio* 1997; 83: 1775-1781.
30. van Lingen RA, van Goudoever JB, Luijendijit IHT *et al.*: Effects of early amino acid demonstration during total parenteral nutrition on protein metabolism in preterm infants. *Clin Sci* 1992; 82: 199-203.
31. Villet S, Chiolwe RL, Bollmann MD *et al.*: Negative impact of hypocaloric feeding and energy balance on clinical outcome in ICU patients. *Clin Nutr* 2005; 24: 502-509.

110 Total Parenteral Nutrition (TPN)-Associated Cholestasis

Shanthy Sridhar • Anupama Chawla

INTRODUCTION

Total parenteral nutrition (TPN) has been one of the most innovative techniques introduced into pediatrics in the last 50 years. TPN remains the main source of protein and calories for infants and children who cannot meet their nutrition goals by oral or enteral route.

INDICATION OF TPN

TPN is an intravenous nutrition used when oral feeding or using the gut is not feasible, or when the digestive system cannot absorb nutrients due to chronic illness. Indications of TPN therapy are summarized in Table 110.1.

Table 110.1: Indications for TPN

- Prematurity and low birth weight
- Respiratory distress syndrome in preterm infants
- Congenital malformations (Abdominal wall defects—Gastroschisis and omphalocele, extensive atresia)
- Abdominal surgery (Malrotation, short gut syndrome)
- Chronic intestinal pseudo obstruction
- Autoimmune enteropathy, severe malabsorption or microvillous atrophy
- Pancreatitis
- Inflammatory bowel disease
- Post-chemotherapy complications: Severe graft versus host disease

TPN: AN UNSAFE BLESSING

There is no doubt that the extensive use of TPN has extended the life of children born with severely malformed or malfunctioning guts, however its use is not free from complications. Experimental studies have shown that total parenteral nutrition has severe metabolic and endocrine consequences on the developing intestine and hepatic function as well.

TPN associated cholestasis has historically been a significant cause of morbidity and mortality in infants and children. The first documented case of TPN associated cholestasis was noted in a preterm infant and reported in 1979. Reported incidence vary widely from 7.3% to 84%. More recent studies, indicate that about 40-60% of TPN dependent children will develop some degree of liver dysfunction during the therapy.

Metabolic complications of TPN have been long described, but the underlying pathophysiology is not fully understood. These biochemical abnormalities are usually mild to moderate and tend to resolve with discontinuation of the TPN therapy. In some cases these biochemical changes are severe and the hepatic pathological changes are not totally reversible. In the most severe cases, TPN use in infants and children has been shown to be associated with cholestasis and hepatic fibrosis, progressing to the development of portal hypertension in children with biliary cirrhosis, leading to progressive liver failure.

Total intravenous nutrition necessitates considerable clinical and pharmaceutical expertise and laboratory support to minimize biochemical, bacteriological, and surgical complications. TPN is best formulated, prepared and administered by personnel experienced in nutrition support. Infusates must be prepared aseptically. Experienced nursing care must be available to prevent and resolve catheter related problems.

ETIOLOGY OF TPN RELATED CHOLESTASIS

Several risk factors (Table 110.2) have been identified as causative factors in the development of TPN related cholestasis. Pathogenesis remains multifactorial related to TPN composition, duration of TPN therapy, concurrent enteral feeds, and underlying liver disease. The pathogenesis is much broader in infants and neonates, as compared to older children and adults. Preterm infants are more vulnerable to toxic liver injury due to the immaturity of their enzyme system. The degree and the severity of liver dysfunction often correlates with associated comorbid conditions like, recurrent catheter related sepsis, ascending cholangitis and bacterial translocation.

Patients exclusively fed on parenteral nutrition have been shown to have their gut hormone secretion suppressed. Experimental studies have shown that lack of enteral

Table 110.2: Risk factors contributing to TPN cholestasis

- Prematurity and low birth weight
- Prolonged duration of PN
- Short gut syndrome
- Lack of enteral feeding
- Reduced entero hepatic circulation
- Recurrent sepsis
- Manganese and copper toxicity
- Lipid emulsions
- Amino acid formulations

nutrition has severe metabolic and endocrine consequences on the developing intestine and the hepatic function. Gastrointestinal hormones like gastrin, motilin, secretin, glucose dependent insulinotrophic polypeptides, glucagons and intestinal vasoactive peptides levels often remain low in parenterally fed children. These hormones play a vital role in improving intestinal maladaptation, by enhancing gut motility, improving gut permeability and promoting growth and maturation of the gut epithelium.

Lack of enteral hormones may also lead to poor gall-bladder contractility and impaired intestinal peristalsis leading to intestinal stasis. Intestinal stasis is often associated with bacterial overgrowth and sepsis. Endotoxin release from gram negative bacteria often leads to bacterial translocation and production of the toxic metabolites like lithocholic acid. Preterm infants have decreased bile formation secondary to diminished enterohepatic circulation which often results in decreased hepatic uptake of bile acid and bile salts synthesis. Impaired gut motility further decreases bile synthesis and bile flow resulting in biliary sludge leading to cholestasis.

Hepatic glutathione levels are often depleted in premature infants as compared to term infants and adults. Glutathione enhances the tissue antioxidant capacity by decreasing the oxidative stress induced liver dysfunction. Glutamine becomes essential during metabolic stress to replenish the tissue. Glutathione levels which have become depleted. Supplementation of glutamine has shown to decrease the

Table: 110.3: Guidelines for monitoring on TPN therapy

Laboratory Test	*Frequency of determination*
Serum Electrolytes	
(Na+, K+, Cl-, CO_2/HCO_3)	Daily until stable then weekly
Minerals (Ca,PO_4,Mg)	Daily until stable then weekly
Blood urea nitrogen	Daily until stable then weekly
Creatinine	Daily until stable then weekly
Total protein	Weekly
Serum albumin	Weekly
Glucose	Daily until stable then weekly
Liver function tests	Weekly
Triglycerides	As needed
Carnitine levels	As needed

incidence of sepsis and oxidative stress induced hepatic dysfunction seen in some of the patients receiving total parenteral nutrition. Therefore glutamine deficiency resulting in depleted glutathione levels may be a contributing factor in the induction of hepatic dysfunction and cholestasis.

The relationship between lipid emulsions and cholestasis has been reported in adults and children. The mechanism remains purely speculative. Intravenous lipids are well-known to cause hepatic accumulation of phospholipids, phytosterols and/or production of inflammatory cytokines in the liver. Phytosterol in newborn piglet model is known to decrease bile flow across the bile canalicular membrane. The phytosterol derived from the soya-oil and/the soya-lecithin oil used to make the intravenous lipid emulsions, tends to be elevated in children with TPN related cholestasis. An increase in cholesterol content of the cell membrane has also been documented. This reduces the fluidity of the cell membrane and impairs the function of the integral membrane proteins. This alteration often leads to impaired bile transport across the canalicular membrane resulting in cholestasis.

Other components of TPN have been incriminated in the pathogenesis of TPN-associated cholestasis. Infusion of amino acid solution has been shown to decrease bile flow in the experimental model. Incidence was related directly either to the cumulative volume of amino acid solution administered, or the composition of amino acid infusate. There seems to have been a higher incidence of TPN-associated cholestasis reported in the pre trophamine (a neonatal specific amino acid solution introduced in the late 80's to early 90's) era. The goal for developing infant solutions was to normalize plasma amino acid patterns similar to those of 30-day-old human milk fed term infants. Pediatric specific formulations like trophamine and aminosyn PF are also known to improve nitrogen retention, growth and attenuate TPN-associated cholestasis. Hepatotoxicity has been related to the deficiency of some of the essential amino acids in TPN infusates (Taurine and/or Cysteine). Cysteine remains a conditionally essential amino acid in the preterm population due to low hepatic cystothianase levels. Cystothianase enzyme is essential for the conversion of methionine to cysteine and taurine. Administration of cysteine requires special consideration as solubility factors prevent the addition of cysteine in the standard ready to use amino acid preparations. Taurine in experimental models has been shown to increase bile flow and inhibit formation of lithocholate. Taurine and cysteine are synthesized from methionine in pediatric and adult population, but this conversion is limited in the preterm infants. Intravenous methionine is not an option as it has been known to be hepatotoxic in experimental model.

Lately, there seems to be a trend towards early and aggressive increments in the use of amino acid solution in the preterm population during the first week of life. These increments are often made to promote positive nitrogen balance and the protein intake is often advanced rapidly even before sufficient carbohydrate and fat calories are administered. Often due to fluid restriction in preterm infants, and immature glucose homeostasis, one is unable to provide sufficient carbohydrate and fat calories. It is still not clear if the concept of "protein sparing" effect is compromised when protein calories are advanced, while providing suboptimal non-protein calories. This leads to utilization of protein for energy expenditure, and it has been speculated as a contributing factor resulting in TPN-associated cholestasis. Parenteral nutrition with high glucose loads may lead to insulin resistance and further development of hepatic steatosis.

Trace elements like copper and manganese used in TPN therapy are known to be hepatotoxic. Copper and manganese are mainly excreted in the biliary system and their clearance is shown to be impaired in patients with hepatocellular dysfunction.

CLINICAL FEATURES

Early clinical sign of cholestasis is a rapid rise in direct bilirubin levels seen as early as 2 weeks following initiation of parenteral nutrition therapy. Clinical icterus becomes apparent when the direct bilirubin levels exceed 2dl. Rise in direct bilirubin is usually followed by a rise in alkaline phosphatase and hepatic transaminases. This is usually not seen until 4-6 weeks following the start of TPN therapy. Gamma glutamyl transpeptidase (GGT) levels and sulphated bile acids in particular might be helpful early markers of TPN related cholestasis. Enlarged liver and spleen may or may not be present. In severe and prolonged cholestasis clinical signs of portal hypertension may be evident with the evidence of collateral circulation visible across the abdominal wall. Cirrhosis may set in with impending liver failure and often present with bleeding from their stoma and catheter sites.

Hypoalbuminemia has been reported in the adult population with long-standing TPN use. The studies done on infants and children do not elicit this. Cirrhosis has been reported as early as four months after initiation of TPN therapy. Biochemical markers of liver dysfunction often do not correlate with the histopathological findings. Patients with cirrhosis often have evidence of ascites and coagulopathy. Death may result from multisystem organ failure.

TYPES OF TPN ASSOCIATED CHOLESTASIS

Two types of parenteral nutrition associated cholestasis have been described: uncomplicated and complicated forms.

The uncomplicated form is usually milder; it occurs most commonly in premature infants and is characterized by an early rise in serum bilirubin and a rise in GGT within 1-4 weeks of initiation of TPN therapy. Liver biopsy in the uncomplicated cases shows evidence of hepatocellular and canalicular cholestasis, bile duct proliferation with peri portal fibrosis and extramedullary haematopoiesis. With the introduction of enteral feeds and cessation of TPN therapy the biochemical indicators of hepatocellular dysfunction and cholestasis often resolve within a 4-6 week period. These patients rarely need a liver biopsy for management.

The complicated form of TPN associated cholestasis is more severe, and commonly seen in children with major intestinal disorders and intestinal failure who require TPN support for over 3 months duration. The clinical course is characterized by a rise in serum bilirubin levels and liver enzymes as early as 1-2 weeks of initiation of TPN therapy and tends to be prolonged. In some severe cases, TPN use and related cholestasis may last for more than 12-18 months. The clinical condition often prevails and the biochemical markers remain elevated for upto 6 months even after the cessation of parenteral nutrition. The condition in some cases may be irreversible progressing to cirrhosis and hepatic failure. Lack of enteral feeding and bouts of gram negative sepsis often compounds the situation in these patients. These patients are more prone to gut stasis, gallbladder stasis and bacterial translocation leading to hepatic steatosis, cholestasis and fibrosis.

These patients with complicated cholestasis have an enlarged liver and spleen and in severe cases have clinical evidence of portal hypertension with evidence of collateral circulation across the abdominal wall. Ascites may or not be clinically evident.

Liver biopsy in complicated cases often shows evidence of intracellular and canalicular cholestasis, macrophage hyperplasia with portal fibrosis (stage-1) and inflammation. Fibrosis often extends from the portal area into the hepatic lobule (stage-2), and then extends later to the adjacent hepatic lobule as septae with bridging fibrosis (stage-3), progressing to cirrhosis (stage-4).

Stage 1 and 2 fibrosis usually is a self-limited condition and resolves when the parenteral nutrition is discontinued. The clinical symptoms and biochemical markers tend to resolve completely however fibrosis may remain indefinite. It is unclear if there is any clinical significance of the persisting fibrosis to long-term outcome. Stage 3 and 4 fibrosis is irreversible in most cases and these patients often end up with bowel and/or liver transplant.

STRATEGIES TO REDUCE PARENTERAL NUTRITION ASSOCIATED CHOLESTASIS

Macronutrient Monitoring

Judicious and appropriate use of macronutrients is the key in preventing parenteral nutrition associated cholestasis. Patients on parenteral nutrition should be closely monitored for various metabolic derangements like hyperglycemia, hypertriglyceridemia and metabolic acidosis. Liver functions should be monitored on a weekly or biweekly basis.

Parenteral nutrition with high glucose loads may lead to insulin resistance and further development of hepatic steatosis. Maintaining GIR (glucose infusion rates) within the recommended range for age will help in preventing hyperglycemia. Blood glucose should be monitored closely for hyperglycemia at least on a daily basis especially in preterm infants. In the presence of cholestasis lipid intake is often limited to no more than 1-2 grams/kg/day to prevent essential fatty acid deficiency while minimizing the accumulation of phytosterols. Carnitine is essential for efficient oxidation of long chain fatty acids. Carnitine levels are found to be low in patients receiving long-term parenteral therapy. Carnitine deficiency may result in hypertriglyceridemia. If hypertriglyceridemia persists despite limiting the fat intake then carnitine deficiency should be investigated and supplementation should be considered.

Micronutrient Monitoring

When TPN use is needed for less than 4 weeks duration, the only micronutrient that should be considered is zinc. If TPN use is more prolonged, over 4 weeks duration then other trace elements needs to be supplemented. Total removal of trace elements from parenteral formulation often results in zinc deficiency. Clearance of trace elements especially manganese and copper is significantly compromised in cholestasis. Deposition of copper has been observed in the liver of children with cholestatic disease, and manganese deposits have been found in the brains of adults receiving total parenteral nutrition. Monitoring serum levels of manganese and copper may be useful in determining the need for their supplementation.

Bacterial Overgrowth

Bacterial overgrowth with anaerobic bacteria is commonly seen in children with short gut and bowel resection. These patients often have impaired intestinal peristalsis which promotes bacterial overgrowth and translocation. Lack of enteral feeding also enhances bacterial overgrowth and bacterial translocation. Enteral feeds should be initiated as soon as feasible. Metronidazole has been used to inhibit colonic bacterial overgrowth. However studies have shown no benefit of antibiotic therapy in decreasing the incidence of cholestasis and its treatment.

Probiotic use has resulted in preferential colonization of the gastrointestinal tract with a variety of favorable gram-positive micro organisms like Lactobacilli and Bifido bacteria. In addition to regenerating healthy flora they may also reduce pathological alterations in cellular permeability, potentially reinforce the mucosal barrier defenses against deleterious agents, and inhibit the translocation of other bacteria. These lactic acid producing bacteria usually do not undergo translocation. Early initiation of enteral feeds has been shown to help prevent gut atrophy, decrease gut permeability, inhibit bacterial translocation and help shorten the duration of TPN therapy. Enteral feeds stimulate gallbladder contractility and enhance bile flow minimizing biliary stasis and the formation of biliary calculi.

Prevention of Central Line Sepsis

Prevention of central line catheter sepsis and thrombosis is essential for children receiving TPN. Aseptic techniques must be followed for every dressing change. The importance of these sterile techniques must be emphasized to the parents. The parents must be adequately trained and demonstrate competency before these children are discharged from the hospital. TPN infusate tubing must be interrupted with adequate filters to prevent bacterial contamination.

Interventions like low dose antibiotics and thrombolytic therapy have shown to be effective in reducing the incidence of line sepsis in certain case reports however a prospective large muticenter trial is warranted before it is recommended for its widespread use.

Cyclic TPN

Cyclic TPN is often recommended for metabolically stable children. Cyclic TPN is used by infusing TPN over 12-18 hours instead of 24 hours continuously. Continuous infusion of hypertonic dextrose solution results in high circulating insulin levels, enhanced lipogenesis, and excessive glycogen deposition in the hepatocyte, resulting in fatty infiltration with increased risk for hepatocellular dysfunction. Cyclic TPN with the interruption of high glucose flow for a period of time decreases circulating insulin levels and also helps in mobilization of fat and glycogen stores. Children should be monitored for nausea, vomiting and hypoglycemia while on cyclic TPN.

Pharmacotherapy

Cholecystokinin (CCK) is known to induce gallbladder contractility with increase in intra hepatic bile flow. This has been used in children to treat the parenteral nutrition induced hyperbilirubinemia. The dose is 0.02-0.04 microgram per day in two to three divided doses. The more recent study using CCK-OP (octreo peptide) failed to show any beneficial effect in reducing neither the incidence nor the severity of TPN associated cholestasis. CCK use is not recommended routinely.

Glutamine supplementation in TPN solutions has shown to increase production of immunoglobulin A levels and enhance gut immunity and promote gut development. Its use in preventing cholestasis in patients on long-term TPN therapy is not clearly established and needs further evaluation.

Use of ursodeoxycholic acid at 30 mg/kg/day in three divided dose has been shown to increase bile flow and reduce formation of biliary sludge. Its mechanism of action includes the exchange of hydrophobic bile acids for hydrophilic bile acids, leading to an improvement in bile flow. Large control studies are needed to determine its clinical effectiveness. However with its relative safe profile and with little else to offer as pharmacotherapy to these cholestatic children it is unlikely that a large study with a control group will be forthcoming. Phenobarbital given at 3-5 mg/kg/day in two divided doses has shown to enhance bilirubin conjugation and increase bilirubin elimination.

Vitamin Supplementation

Rickets and osteoporosis has been documented in children with longstanding parenteral nutrition and cholestasis. Balancing of calcium and phosphorus salt intake in TPN infusates is essential in alleviating some of the long-term bone diseases seen in patients with long-term TPN therapy and cholestasis. Fat soluble vitamins (ADEK) are now available in the prescription form. Daily supplementation of fat soluble vitamins (A,D,E,K) in recommended doses is found to be beneficial.

INVESTIGATIONS

The rapid rise in direct bilirubin in children on parenteral nutrition therapy often warrants a thorough investigation to exclude other cause of cholestasis. Anatomic, metabolic, infectious causes might mimic TPN induced cholestasis. Cholestasis from parenteral nutrition is a diagnosis of exclusion and should only be attributed to TPN after other causes have been ruled out. The investigations should be approached in a staged manner (Table 110.4). This approach is helpful in excluding other possible etiologies of cholestasis. In complicated cases, liver biopsy should be considered earlier in the course of evaluation so that some of the irreversible complications can be prevented.

CONCLUSION

Fortunately TPN related cholestasis is more often a reversible condition. Bilirubin levels and liver functions tend to improve with initiation of enteral feeds and resolve by 1-2 weeks following discontinuation of the parenteral nutrition. With the introduction of enteral feeds, discontinuation of parenteral feeds, adequate oral/enteral caloric intake, bile acid therapy and supplementation of fat soluble vitamins, cholestatic children can be managed effectively. In children with severe form of cholestasis despite the clinical and biochemical reduction of signs and symptoms, the hepatic fibrosis may not regress completely. The long-term significance of persistent fibrosis remains unclear. Children with intestinal failure, dependent on total parenteral nutrition should be considered for early bowel transplant surgery before the development of irreversible hepatic dysfunction.

Table 110.4: Stepwise evaluations of TPN-associated cholestasis

Evaluation of Neonatal Cholestasis:
- Clinical Evaluation (History, Physical Exam)
- Fractionated bilirubin
- Liver function tests (Total and Direct bilirubin levels, alkaline phosphatase, Transaminases and 5 alpha nucleotidase)
- Index of hepatic synthetic function (serum albumin and prothrombin time)
- Screen for Hepatitis A, Hepatitis B and Hepatitis C
- Torch Panel: Screen for Toxoplasmosis, Rubella infections, Cytomegalovirus, Herpes virus)
- Thyroid studies (TSH and T4)
- Urine organic acids profile
- Plasma amino acid profile
- Qualitative serum and urine bile acid assay
- Alpha-1 Antitrypsin levels (and phenotype)
- Sweat Chloride Test

Imaging Studies:
- Abdominal ultrasound (gallbladder and common bile duct abnormality)
- HIDA scan
- Endoscopic retrograde cholangiogram
- Percutaneous trans hepatic cholangiography
- Intraoperative cholangiogram

Histological evaluation:
- Liver biopsy.

KEY LEARNING POINTS

- TPN, a blessing for children born with severely malformed or malfunctioning gut, may cause severe complications including cholestasis.
- Among the risk factors for development of TPN-associated cholestasis figure premaurity and LBW, recurrent sepsis and prolonged duration of TPN.
- Earliest manifestation is a rapid rise in conjugated bilirubin levels some 2 weeks after starting TPN.
- Two forms are: complicated and uncomplicated.
- Judicious and appropriate use of macronutrients, micronutrient (especially zinc) monitoring, prevention of central line sepsis, and cyclic TPN are the key to its prevention.
- A reversible condition that usually responds to stoppage TPN and introduction of enteral feeds, bile acid therapy and supplementation with fat soluble vitamins.

FURTHER READINGS

1. Adamkin DD, Radmacher P, Rosen P. Comparison of a neonatal versus general-purpose amino acid formulation in preterm neonates. *J Perinatol* 1995;15:108-113.
2. Bhave S, Bavdekar A. Paediatric parenteral nutrition in India. *Indian J Pediatr* 1999;66: S 141-S145.
3. Bindl L, Lutjohann D, Buderus S Lentze MJV Bergman K. High plasma levels of phytosterols in patients with parenteral nutrition: A marker for liver dysfunction. *J Pediatr Gastroenterol Nutr* 2000;31:313-316.

4. Daniel H. Teitelbaum, Thomas F. Tracy, Jr, Moustafa M. Aouthmany, Adolfo Llanos, Morton B. Brown, Sunkyung Yu, Marilyn R. Brown, Robert J. Shulman, Ronald B. Hirschl, Patricia A. Derusso, Jeanne Cox, Jacqueline Dahlgren, Jonathan I. Groner, and Peter J. Strouse: Use of cholecystokinin-octopepetide for the prevention of parenteral nutrition associated cholestasis. *Pediatrics* 2005; 115: 1332-1340.
5. Deirdre A Kelly. Intestinal failure-associated liver disease: What do we know today? *Gastroenterology* 2006;130: S70-S77.
6. Javid PJ, Collier S, Richardson D, Iglesias J, Gura K, Lo C, Kim HB, Duggan CP, Jaksic T. The role of enteral nutrition in the reversal of parenteral nutrition-associated liver dysfunction in infants. *J Pediatr Surg* 2005;40:1015-1018.
7. Kaufmann SS. Prevention of Parenteral nutrition associated liver disease in children. *Pediat Transpl* 2002;6:37-42.
8. Sobdheimer JM; Asturias E; Cadnapaphornichai M: Infection and cholestasis in neonates with intestinal resection and long-term parenteral nutrition. *J Pediatr Gastroenterol Nutr* 1998; 27:131-37.
9. Steven Okeefe. Bacterial overgrowth and liver complications in short bowel intestinal failure patients. Editorial. *Gastroenterology* 2006; 128:S67-69.
10. Stuart S. Kaufmann, Gabriel E. Gondolesi and Thomas M. Fishbein. Parenteral nutrition associated liver disease: *Seminars in Neonatol* 2003;375-381.
11. Teitelbaum DH, Tracy T. Parenteral nutrition-associated cholestasis. *Semin Pediatr Surg* 2001;10:72-80.
12. V Colomb, A. Jobert-Giraud, F. Lacaille, O. Goulet, J.C. Fournet and C Ricour. Role of lipid emulsions in cholestasis associated with long-term parenteral nutrition in children. *J Parenter Enteral Nutr* 2000;24: 345-350.
13. Whitfield PD, Clayton PT, Muller DPR. Effect of intravenous lipid emulsions on hepatic cholesterol metabolism. *J Pediatr Gastroenterol Nutr* 2000: 6: 538-546.
14. Kaufman SS, Loseke CA, Lupo JV, Young RJ, Murray ND, Pinch LW, Vanderhoof JA. Influence of bacterial overgrowth and intestinal inflammation on duration on parenteral nutrition in children with short bowel syndrome, *J Pediatr* 1997; 131: 356:361.
15. Kubota A, Okada K Imura H. The effects of Metronidazole on TPN associated liver dysfunction in neonates. *J Pediatr surgery* 1990; 25; 618-621.
16. Eijsink VG, Axelsson L, Diep DB, Havarstein LS, Holo H, Nes IF. Production of class II bacteriocins by lactic acid bacteria: An example of biological warfare and communication. *Antonie Van Leewenhoek* 2002; 81: 639-654.

111 Immunonutrition: A Step Ahead

Jyoti Suvarna • Sandeep B Bavdekar

INTRODUCTION

Nutrition has been used to complement the healing process since time immemorial. Even without the scientific backup of double-blinded randomized studies, grandmother's remedies, herbal teas and a host of other remedies have been used to augment and complement the healing processes in various medical conditions. An avalanche of nutritional products available in the market (claiming to promote health and to cure various diseases) bears testimony to man's faith in the nutrition as a mode of therapy. A number of individuals unhappy with the effects of modern medicines are also looking upon this modality as a natural way to combat various disorders.

The medical fraternity has also used nutritional therapy to complement the treatment of various disorders. Nutrient enemas to provide nutritional support had been used as far back as 3500 years ago. This field has grown by leaps and bounds since then. Nutrition was originally visualized as a modality to provide energy, proteins, and essential micronutrients, to offset muscle wasting and starvation-induced immune depletion in patients. Dudrick and co-workers flagged off the modern era of clinical nutrition with the development of intravenous hyperalimentation, followed by the development of chemically defined diet by Greenstein and coworkers. Total parenteral nutrition (TPN) was considered as an all purpose panacea. But soon the scientific fraternity realized that there are certain nutrients (that can have pharmacological effects on the immune system) which can be used to the patient's advantage. Thus, apart from providing calories and essential nutrients, one could also use nutrients to modulate the immune and the inflammatory response.

The role of several specific nutrients including macronutrients, vitamins and trace elements in augmenting or modulating the immune system has been the focus of studies for the last 20 years. The mode of action could be through their effects on the mucosal barrier, cellular defense mechanism, local/systemic inflammatory response, etc. The need of the hour is to study and identify nutrients as primary treatment agents.

This communication offers an overview of the work done in the field of immunonutrition, the factors that determine its efficacy and provide a peek at the current status of knowledge in this evolving field. It should, however be conceded that the vast majority of work has been carried out in adults and that there is a need to check if it could be applied to infants and children.

CONCEPT OF IMMUNONUTRITION

Immunonutrition is the process of studying the potential of specific nutrients to modulate the activity of the immune system and the use of diets for enhancing immune function. Certain molecular compounds, while being dietary components, also have a favorable influence on some aspect of immune response. They are added to standard nutritional support solutions for deriving immunological benefits and are termed "immunonutrients". These immunonutrients may be given in supranormal doses enterally or parenterally, to achieve a pharmacological effect for modulating the response to surgery, trauma or infection. Although many nutrients are potential immunonutrients, the most commonly used and researched upon immunonutrients are arginine, glutamine, omega-3 polyunsaturated fatty acids and nucleotides.

HOST RESPONSE TO INJURY AND INFECTION

In response to challenges like injury or infection, the body recruits the immunological system to induce an array of metabolic and chemical changes. The chief among them is the activation of the T- and B-lymphocytes, and the systemic inflammatory response engineered by the proinflammatory cytokines- interleukin-1, interleukin-6 and tumor necrosis factor- alpha. Cytokines increase the catabolism of the body proteins and fat to provide nutrients for the immune system. Other mediators like the chemokines, anti-inflammatory cytokines, growth factors, nitric oxide, eicosanoids and free radicals are also released. The timing of the mediator release and the amount of these mediators available in circulation or at the site, determine the inflammatory response and ensuing effects.

Central to the inflammatory changes is the activation of the nuclear transcription factors such as nuclear factor kappa B (NFkB) and activator protein-1 (AP-1). NFkB plays a key role in inflammation (promoted by oxidant molecules) and AP-1 in cellular immune function. Increased NFkB activation in patients with sepsis is associated with increased mortality rates. Prevention of NFkB activation can thus be exploited for treatment. Antioxidants prevent the activation of the NFkB activation by decreasing the oxidative stress and omega-3 fatty acids decrease the activation by stabilization of the transcription factor complex.

ENTERAL FEEDING, IMMUNITY AND IMMUNONUTRITION

The gastrointestinal tract, besides being an organ for digestion, absorption and utilization of nutrients, is an important immunological organ. Patients with gastro-intestinal diseases are at an increased risk for immunological problems not only due to the disease process *per se* but also because of therapeutic interventions undertaken. Several gastrointestinal diseases are associated with a breach in the mucosal lining and often manifest with anorexia and altered nutritional requirements which further compromise the tract's immune function. Many patients, especially if they are very sick, are treated with limitation or even proscription of enteral feeding resulting in mucosal atrophy. Mucosal lesions whether suffered as a consequence of disease process or due to therapeutic or diagnostic interventions (including withholding enteral feeds), lead to a breach in the mucosal lining, which in turn, results in an increased permeability to bacteria and bacterial exotoxins. The resultant endotoxemia and bacteremia can trigger off a local and/or systemic inflammatory response syndrome (SIRS) that carries the risk of multiple organ failure and high mortality.

The clinicians should be aware of this vital relationship between gastrointestinal mucosal integrity and future course of illness. They should maximize their efforts at maintaining the gastrointestinal mucosal integrity in critically ill or other patients to allow the host immunity to be maintained or enhanced. One of the principal ways of doing this is through continuation of enteral feeds. The goal of enteral therapy is not only to provide adequate caloric and protein requirements, but also to continue to stimulate the mucosal lining so as to prevent gut mucosal atrophy and, thereby, prevent all the consequent complications related to breach in the gut integrity. In addition to the obvious benefits stated above, enteral feeding is available at a much lower cost, is more physiological and is associated with lower incidence of complications as compared to parenteral nutrition. TPN should be resorted to only when a true contraindication to enteral feeding exists e.g. perforation, total obstruction, proven mesenteric ischemia and toxic megacolon. It could also be employed in conjunction with enteral nutrition when nutritional requirements cannot be met fully by enteral administration, alone.

Immunonutrients such as arginine, glutamine, omega-3 fatty acids, RNA nucleotides and fiber exert their effect by helping maintain gut integrity, by stimulating the immune system and by preventing bacterial translocation from the gut into the circulation.

The immune system is profoundly affected by poor nutritional status, illnesses and states with hypercatabolism e.g. sepsis, surgery and trauma. The latter group of diseases is associated with malnutrition and this complication further adds to the adverse effects on the immune system. Protein-energy malnutrition (PEM) can suppress essentially all arms of the immune system, including B-cell, T-cell, macrophage, neutrophil functions and complement activation. It also adversely affects regeneration processes and compromises host's position in his fight against infection. The associated deficiency of specific trace elements and vitamins also contributes to derangement of the immune status. It should be remembered that even overnutrition and obesity are associated with altered immune status.

APPLICATION OF IMMUNONUTRITION IN VARIOUS DISORDERS

Sepsis

Sepsis is a complex syndrome characterized by hypercatabolism and an initial hyperinflammatory response that is followed by immune suppression. Hyperinflammatory response leads to a simultaneous activation of pro-inflammatory and pro-coagulant processes in response to microbial insult. The syndrome is associated with release of proinflammatory cytokines and pro-coagulant substances and formation of reactive oxygen and nitrogen species and adhesion molecules from the immune cells or damaged endothelium. These processes and events can cause severe tissue damage and immunosuppression and are responsible for the increased morbidity and delayed recovery associated with sepsis. It is being postulated that immunonutrition provides a means of modulating the inflammatory response to injury and infection, and thereby help in improving the clinical outcome. Early institution of therapy with immuno-nutrition is aimed at decreasing the proinflammatory responses, abolishing or decreasing hyperinflammation and preventing the occurrence of compensatory immuno-supression subsequently. Studies have shown that although immunonutrition may not decrease mortality, it does decrease infection rates, duration of hospital stay and requirement of ventilatory support. Omega-3 poly-unsaturated fatty acids have a direct immunoenhancing effect, glutamine acts by influencing the anti-oxidant status and suppressing the inflammation, and nucleotides exert direct effects on lymphocyte proliferation.

The effects of immunonutrition in critically ill patients may be different from those in patients undergoing elective surgery.

Trauma

Trauma and sepsis share a similar pathophysiology. Severe trauma threatens the life of victims directly and indirectly *via* immunological deregulation that follows severe trauma and results in sepsis and multi-organ failure. Early immunomodulation, in the form of institution of immunonutrition in patients with severe trauma, has been undertaken in anticipation of beneficial effects such as amelioration of the early hyper-inflammatory phase, reduced incidence of SIRS and multiple organ failure and reduction in the use of antibiotics and in duration of hospital stay.

Surgery

Major surgery is followed by a period of immune-suppression that increases the risk of morbidity and mortality due to infection. Gastrointestinal tract surgery is followed by formation of microvascular thrombi, gut hypoperfusion and mucosal lesions that disrupt the mucosal barrier. Improving the immune function with immunonutrition before and during this period may reduce the incidence of infectious complications, especially if the patient is malnourished, as well.

Many studies have shown that early preoperative and/or postoperative enteral immunonutrition is associated with beneficial immunological effects.

Inflammatory Bowel Disease

Chronic gastrointestinal inflammatory diseases like ulcerative colitis or Crohn's disease are associated with decreased oral intake, malabsorption, accelerated nutrient losses, increased nutritional requirements and drug-nutrient interactions. These result in nutritional and functional deficiencies. It has been postulated that correction of nutritional deficiencies and steps aimed at modulation of inflammatory response could exert a positive influence on the disease activity. Although the first aim of nutritional rehabilitation could be achieved through institution of feeding either by enteral and parenteral route, the former carries the advantages of lower complication rate and lower costs in patients who can tolerate enteral feeds. Immunonutrition is an important therapeutic alternative, modulating inflammatory processes and changing the eicosanoid synthesis profile. It induces remission in adult subjects and promotes growth in children with inflammatory bowel disease. Early reports suggest that enteric-coated sustained release fish oil capsules may help sustain remission in patients with Crohn's disease.

IMMUNONUTRITION AND PREVENTION OF CANCERS

As early as 1863, Rudolf Virchow observed the presence of leucocytes in tumor tissues and suggested a role for chronic inflammation in the origin of cancers. This postulation has been confirmed by our understanding of the pathogenesis of cancers in the recent years. Inflammatory processes result in release of pro-inflammatory cytokines and formation of reactive oxygen and nitrogen species. Although anti-inflammatory effects usually follow such actions rapidly, excessive production of pro-inflammatory cytokines, or their production in the wrong biological context may lead to perpetuation of inflammation over time. In certain situations, chronic inflammation increases the risk of developing cancer, for e.g. increase in risk for developing colorectal cancer in inflammatory bowel disease, esophageal cancers in Barrett's esophagus, and pancreatic cancer in chronic pancreatitis.

Chronic inflammation occurs either when the perpetuating factor remains or when the process of resolution fails. The reactive oxygen and nitrogen species produced can damage DNA and contribute to tumorogenesis. The inflammatory response activates the transcriptor factor NFkB, which regulates many pro-inflammatory cytokines, adhesion molecules, chemokines, growth factors, and other inflammatory mediators like cyclooxygenase-2 (COX-2). NFkB also promotes cellular proliferation of the tumor cells and protects them from apoptosis. Activation of NFkB has been reported in cancers of breast, colon, pancreas, thyroid, bladder and skin. COX-2 leads to release of prostaglandins, which favor cancer development and progression. Thus inflammatory responses may play a decisive role in the initiation, progression (cell division, neo-vascularization and angiogenesis), and perpetuation of the tumor. A multitude of avenues like pharmacotherapy and immunotherapy have been tried, to temper down the inflammation and in turn, restrict or destroy the tumor. Immunonutrition may provide a less invasive alternative to immunotherapy and pharmacotherapy, for prevention of cancers associated with chronic inflammation.

A number of nutrient zinc, epigallacatechin gallate (EGCG), omega-3 polyunsaturated fatty acids, probiotics and prebiotics, all act differently to modulate the immune response, but all seem to have the potential to protect the host from the development of cancer and its progression. A better understanding of the innate or adaptive immunity and its regulation, may pave the path to better dietary management of cancer for cancer patients and the general public.

IMMUNONUTRITION AND FACTORS AFFECTING ITS EFFICACY

Type of Immmunonutrient

The requirement of adequate nutrition and specific immunomodulating nutrients, to maintain the gut integrity and function, is common to all sick patients. But the extent of gut failure, bacterial translocation, failure of cellular defense mechanisms, balance between inflammation and anti-inflammatory actions, regional and systemic generation of reactive oxygen species (ROS), varies from patient to patient and from time to time in the same patient. The use of a cocktail of multiple nutrients in a heterogeneous group of patients may lead to the loss of any benefit (or harm) achieved from the therapy. Tailoring the immunonutrient use as per the underlying pathophysiological processes in a given individual may help yield better results. For example, a patient undergoing elective surgery demonstrates minimum cytokine activation and some postsurgery immunosuppression leading to infections and morbidity. In such a scenario, arginine that stimulates the cellular defense mechanism, may fit the bill. However, in a critically ill patient, the process is much more complex with an exaggerated inflammatory response (with excess of reactive oxygen species, lipid mediators and nitric oxide), and cellular immune dysfunction. Here we require immunonutrients that will augment the cellular defense, ameliorate the reactive oxygen species and the oxidative stress, without increasing the inflammatory response. In such a situation glutamine and antioxidant strategies could prove more useful. Use of immunonutrients like arginine that will augment the inflammatory process could prove deleterious in such cases. Studies focusing on single nutrients tested in homogenous populations would chart a more definite path for the use of specific immunonutrients.

Dose of Immunonutrient

There is a dearth of literature on the dosage requirements. At least, some of the treatment failures in immunonutrition could be related to inadequate doses. Meta-analysis has shown that a higher dose of glutamine showed a greater response. Clinical benefits with arginine were seen in patients receiving an arginine concentration of at least 12 g/L. Immunonutrients are at present being added to voluminous amounts of standard enteral nutrition solutions. Sick patients, many a times, have problems with tolerating the enteral feeds. These factors may result in suboptimal intake of nutrient supplement with consequent suboptimal therapeutic benefit or even failure. Providing immunonutrient separately would simplify its administration and would ensure its intake even food tolerance is a problem.

Route of Administration

The debate of enteral *versus* parenteral immunonutrition continues. Although parenteral therapy can be resorted to when enteral administration is not possible, enteral immunonutrition can be given to all intensive care patients with a fully functioning gastrointestinal tract.

Timing of Immunonutrition

Studies have shown that pre- and perioperative immunonutrition is more advantageous than only post-operative immunonutrition.

Nutritional Status

Preoperative enteral nutrition benefits malnourished patients more than well nourished patients and the benefit is increased by using immunoenhancing diets which reduce the duration of the hospital stay and complication rates.

Genetic Variability

Different genotypes differ in their response to immunonutrition. Many genes have single base variations in their promoter regions (single nucleotide polymorphism-SNP) which decide the amount of gene produced when the activation occurs. These SNP for the cytokines and other inflammatory chemicals would decide the outcome of the disease of the patient and hence the response to the immunonutrition. More studies are warranted to decide the genotype suitability for immunonutrition and specific immunonutrients.

Gender Variability

Gender seems to affect the response to immunonutrition. For example, critically ill female patients in ICU have a better prognosis than their male counterparts. However in ICU patients receiving immunonutrition, the frequency of infectious complications and duration of ICU stay are decreased in such a manner that male patients seem to fare better than female patients admitted in the ICU. The reason for this phenomenon remains to be elucidated. It is thought that arginine load leads to relatively much higher levels of growth hormone in females, which in turn is responsible for hyperglycemia. It is believed that hyperglycemia has a negative effect on the clinical outcome. In addition increased levels of interleukin-1 and arginine may lead to excessive amounts of nitric oxide production, and exacerbation of the inflammatory process and systemic inflammatory response syndrome.

IMMUNONUTRIENTS

Glutamine

Glutamine is a precursor for nucleotide synthesis, a substrate for liver gluconeogenesis and an important fuel source for cells with rapid turnover (such as gastrointestinal epithelia, lymphocytes, fibroblasts and reticulocytes). It is a precursor for nucleotide synthesis and for glutathione synthesis which is a major link in the anti-oxidative defense mechanism. It is a non-essential amino acid under normal circumstances.

Under catabolic stress, humans show an increased efflux of glutamine from the skeletal muscle, where it is normally stored. Visceral organs, enterocytes, T-lymphocytes and macrophages utilize glutamine mobilized from muscle and plasma as a source of fuel. Catabolic states are also characterized by increased metabolic demand for glutamine. To make the matters worse, most parenteral solutions do not contain glutamine, as the amino acid is highly unstable in standard protein solutions. Thus, severely ill patients whose nutrition is supported solely by parenteral route are at risk of developing glutamine deficiency state due to inadequate supply of glutamine, mobilization of the amino acid from the stores and increased needs. Hence, in catabolic states, glutamine is regarded as "a conditionally essential nutrient". Considering the fact that glutamine is vital for the rapidly dividing cells like lymphocytes and gastro-intestinal mucosal cells, it is not surprising that its depletion contributes to the development of immunosuppression in critically ill patients. Studies have documented that:

- Use of glutamine results in amelioration of mucosal atrophy, enhanced healing of gastrointestinal mucosa damaged due to radiotherapy or chemotherapy and reduction in the number of episodes of bacterial translocation from the gut to the systemic circulation. Glutamine decreases negative nitrogen balance and maintains muscle mass and gut integrity in very low weight babies and in patients after major surgery. Glutamine-enriched TPN improves net nitrogen balance, reduces third space fluid accumulation and shortens the length of hospital stay in bone marrow transplant recipients. Enterally administered glutamine decreases the incidence of sepsis in premature neonates and reduces the incidence of pneumonia, bacteremia and severe sepsis in critically ill patients. Parenteral glutamine administration reduces the incidence of infections in bone marrow transplant recipients and induces a change in the pattern of mortality in patients in intensive care units. These clinical benefits seem to be related to improvements in intestinal integrity and cellular immune function. Use of glutamine is associated with better survival rates, lowered incidence of intra-abdominal abscesses, lesser infection rates, reduced hospital costs and decrease in the duration of antibiotic usage. Novak *et al.* conducted a systematic review and meta-analysis of studies to determine the role of glutamine in surgical and critically ill patients. Eight trials in surgical patients showed a decrease in the infection rates and length of hospital stay, without an effect on the mortality. Six trials in critically ill patients (three with parenteral and three with enteral glutamine) showed better survival and fewer infectious complications. When the enteral and parenteral trials were considered separately, parenteral therapy seemed to result in better survival and shorter ICU stay; however the data was inadequate to evaluate the effect on infections.
- Although many *in vitro* and *in vivo* studies suggest an important role for glutamine in the maintenance and repair of gastrointestinal mucosa; larger well-designed randomized trials are needed to confirm this finding. The use of glutamine supplementation in conditions like prematurity, short bowel syndrome, immuno-compromised status secondary to HIV infection or chemotherapy/radiotherapy, and the efficacy of parenteral versus enteral glutamine need to be investigated with larger number of well-controlled studies.

Arginine

Arginine is a non-essential amino acid that has a wide range of biological actions that are beneficial to the body. Like glutamine, arginine becomes a "conditionally essential amino acid" during catabolic states like sepsis and trauma. For many mammals, arginine is essential for normal growth and development of the young ones and is regarded as non-essential only in the fully-grown adults.

Arginine owes it immunomodulatory functions to two major metabolic pathways: the arginase pathway and the nitric oxide synthesis pathway. In the arginase pathway, arginine is converted to urea and ornithine. This pathway generates polyamines, which are known to augment lymphocyte mitogenesis, enhance cell division and DNA replication and regulate cell cycle. In addition, the arginine-dependent macrophage-mediated tumor cell cytotoxicity is mediated through induction of arginase.

Arginine is the sole substrate for nitric oxide synthesis. This pathway is mediated by nitric oxide synthetase and results in the formation of nitric oxide and citrulline. Nitric oxide is one of the most versatile molecules. It plays an important role in smooth muscle relaxation and in regulation of blood flow, coagulation pathway, immune function and intestinal secretions. It plays a vital role in disease states such as gastroesophageal reflux, pyloric stenosis, sepsis, hypertension and cirrhosis. In addition, nitric oxide produced by human intestinal epithelial cells inhibits the growth, encystation, and excystation of *Giardia lamblia*. Nitric oxide can have both anti- and pro-inflammatory effects. Anti-inflammatory and homeostatic effects are observed with small amounts of nitric oxide, whereas pro-inflammatory effects are seen with large amounts of nitric oxide. The use of inhaled nitric oxide especially in the management of post-operative pulmonary hypertension, respiratory distress syndrome and other cardiopulmonary problems in pediatric ICUs is gaining momentum. Reduced serum levels of arginine and glutamine have been documented in premature infants with necrotizing enterocolitis. Arginine supplementation is also associated with a dramatic decrease in the incidence of necrotizing enterocolitis in low birth babies.

Supplementation with arginine in postoperative patients results in beneficial effects on T-cells: It increases the mitotic response of peripheral lymphocytes to standard stimuli and accelerates wound healing with increase in wound tensile strength and collagen deposition. Arginine supplementation also inhibits the growth of tumors by up-regulating natural killer and lymphokine-activated killer function. Supplementary dietary arginine enhances lymphocyte cytotoxic mechanisms and acts synergistically with interleukin-2 (IL-2) immunotherapy in the treatment of certain tumors. Tumor response to arginine appears to depend on the immunogenecity of the particular tumor and on the requirements of arginine by that tumor as a growth substrate. Clinical benefits with arginine immunonutrition is seen only when the arginine concentration is at least 12 g/l. Addition of arginine as the lone supplement in the enteral solution did not provide any beneficial effects to ICU patients.

Two groups have provided a meta-analysis of studies of supplementation with commercial formulas containing arginine and other additives. One analysis of 12 trials with 1557 patients showed shorter hospital stay, lower infection rates, and shorter duration of ventilator care in those fed with the formula; however there was no effect on the mortality. The second analysis of 22 trials involving 2419 patients showed lesser infectious complications and decrease in the length of hospital stay. Patients undergoing surgery did better than the critically ill patients. A higher mortality was seen in patients who were very sick, although they were shown to have fewer infectious complications. Data that is available today suggests that arginine has a great potential as an immunomodulator, especially in catabolic conditions like post-operative stress, sepsis, trauma, and certain tumors. More number of well controlled trials is required to define the use of arginine in different clinical conditions.

Nucleotides

Dietary nucleotides play a vital role in T-cell function and cell mediated immunity. RNA appears to have immuno-stimulatory properties and RNA-enriched enteral diets increase the maturation and phenotypic expression of T-cells. Studies in rodents have shown that addition of nucleotides to the diet augments immune responses to fungal infection. Nucleotide-deficient diets are associated with reduced cell mediated immunity and hampered T-cell activation, the defects that are reversed with addition of nucleotides to the diets.

Studies in cancer patients undergoing surgery showed an enhancement of natural killer (NK) cell cytotoxicity and increased disease-free duration in patients supplemented with polyadenylic and polyuridylic acid. Nucleotides are in abundance in the breast milk and are perhaps play an immunomodulatory role in infants. Data showing the effects of nucleotide supplementation in children is limited. Carver *et al.*demonstrated that breastfed infants and infants receiving diet supplemented with nucleotides have higher levels of NK cell cytotoxicity and IL-2 production by macrophages as compared to unsupplemented controls. It may, however, be conceded that the clinical extrapolations in terms of higher growth or reduced frequency of infections could not be demonstrated. Sanchez-Pozo and co-workers showed that lecithin cholesterol acyl transferase and apoprotein A-4 concentrations rise following nucleotide supplementation in pre-term infants. This suggests that nucleotides play a role in the postnatal maturational changes in the hepatic handling of cholesterol and lipids. The role of nucleotides as semi-essential nutrients in infants (especially the premature infants) needs to be evaluated. Early studies indicate that they may have an important role to play in intermediate metabolism, in modulation of immune response and in gut maturation.

Omega-3 Fatty Acids

Two essential fatty acids, linoleic acid (omega-6 fatty acid-found in cooking oils-safflower, soy, corn, sunflower oil, lean meat and fish, and lipid emulsions of parenteral solutions) and linolenic acid (omega-3 fatty acid-found in fatty fish oils–salmon, tuna, herring fish oil) have a significant impact on the immune system. Linoleic acid (omega-6 fatty acid) is a precursor of arachidonic acid, which forms 4-series leukotrienes, 2-series eicosanoids, thromboxane A2 and prostaglandin E2. Leukotriene B4 is a potent neutrophil chemotactic agent and helps in neutrophil adhesion. Thromboxane A2 is a potent bronchoconstrictor and promotes platelet aggregation. Prostaglandin E2 contributes to superoxide generation and increases suppressor T-cell activity, reducing cell mediated immunity. Thus omega-6 fatty acids are pro-inflammatory, but limit the immune system's ability to clear the insult. Linolenic acid (omega-3 fatty acid) is a precursor for docosahexaenoic acid and eicosapentaenoic acid, which form the 3-series prostaglandins and thromboxanes, and 5-series leukotrienes. These products have much lesser biological activity than the omega-6 products. They are less effective in promoting inflammation and immunosuppression as compared to omega-6 fatty acids. Omega-3 fatty acids may also have an indirect action through the inhibition of the activation of the tumor necrosis factor- alpha and nuclear factor-k B, which mediate inflammation.

It has been suggested that the provision of omega-3 fatty

acids to immunonutrition solutions may be important for dampening the pro-inflammatory effects of arginine added to these solution. Fish oils may be useful in the treatment of atopic dermatitis and they slow down the process of IgA nephropathy and prolong the survival in patients with untreatable cancers. Several studies have shown that addition of medium chain triglycerides to TPN achieves more reduction in the production of TNF by stimulating monocytes as compared to what addition of long chain triglycerides to TPN is able to achieve.

Taurine

Taurine plays an important part in membrane stabilization, osmoregulation, antioxidation, calcium homeostasis, apoptosis, bile salt formation, stimulation of glycolysis and glycogenesis, growth modulation and vision. Along with glutamine and arginine it has intestinal protective effects during periods of stress. It is present in high concentrations in most tissues especially in the pro-inflammatory cells like the neutrophils and the lymphocytes and is regarded as a semi-essential amino acid. Normally humans have an inherent capacity to maintain endogenous taurine levels from dietary methionine and cysteine. However during various stressful conditions like cancer, sepsis and post-operative states, decreased levels have been observed.

Taurine constitutes 76% of the free amino acid pool in the neutrophils. The neutrophil modulating action of taurine is mediated through its interaction with the respiratory burst enzyme, myeloperoxidase. The hydrogen peroxide – myeloperoxidase – chloride system generates HOCL.Taurine combines with this HOCL, to form taurine chloramine, which has the following functions:

a. It has bactericidal activity.
b. It modulates the HOCL induced tissue damage.
c. It is an immunomodulator.
d. It regulates the pro-inflammatory mediator release by the macrophage.
e. It behaves as a neutrophil derived signalling molecule which puts the brakes on the production of inflammatory mediators by the macrophages and the neutrophils, and stalls the perpetuation of the inflammatory process.
f. It has cyto-protective function by virtue of its bactericidal action and preservation of cellular function in the face of physiologic stress.
g. It maintains the phagocytic and microbicidal activity in aged neutrophils due to its membrane stabilizing effects and its anti-oxidant effects.
h. It inhibits neutrophil apoptosis via the maintenance of calcium homeostasis.

More than 50% of the free amino acid pool of the lymphocytes is composed of taurine. It has a protective role in the lymphocytes due to its membrane stabilizing effect and prevention of calcium influx. T-lymphocytes are more susceptible to age related decline in the proliferation compared to B-lymphocytes. Taurine tones down the age related decline in the T-cell proliferation and modulates the macrophage mediated T-cell activation via its action on class 2 Major Histocompatibility Antigen.

Role of taurine in sepsis and surgical trauma: The initial host response to sepsis or surgical trauma is mediated through the activated neutrophil. Therefore the advantages of taurine are through its myriad actions on the neutrophils, and taurochloramine formation, as already stated above. In the immediate post-operative period, a spurt in the release of free radicals in the neutrophils, translates into an increase in the levels of taurine in the neutrophils. The taurochloramine among its other actions confers microbicidal action and limits the host cytotoxicity. Gray *et al.* has shown a decrease in taurine levels in cancer patients and post-operative patients. Further studies with pre-operative taurine supplementation and corresponding effect on the septic outcome needs to be investigated.

In a post-ischemia setup, activated neutrophils and pro-inflammatory cytokines mainly constitute the post-ischemic reperfusate, which give rise to localized, and distal endothelial injury and distant organ injury like Adult Respiratory Distress Syndrome (ARDS), and Multiple Organ Dysfunction Syndrome (MODS). Taurine modifies this through the actions already stated. It decreases the lipid peroxidation and cell damage during the reperfusion period.

Taurine is capable of influencing programmed cell death depending on the apoptic stimulus. It has been shown to decrease the bleomycin induced pulmonary fibrosis and reduce cytotoxicity induced by various poisons. Thus apart from a plethora of medical conditions in which taurine is used, like congestive cardiac failure, psoriasis, pulmonary fibrosis, cholestasis associated with total parenteral nutrition and post operatively, taurine can be used as an immuno-nutrient by virtue of its action on various limbs of the immune system. Taurine is regarded as a conditionally semi-essential amino acid in preterms and neonates and is currently used to supplement most infant foods.

Vitamins and Minerals

Antioxidants play an important role in cytokine production, phagocyte function, cell-mediated responses and immunoglobulin production. These minerals and vitamins interact and complement each other facilitating immune-competence at all levels.

Zinc

Zinc is required as a catalytic, structural and regulatory ion for enzymes, proteins and transcription factors. It is an important component of the cell membrane structure and function, and being an antioxidant, it protects from lipid peroxidation. It is a component of several metalloenzymes like alkaline phosphatase, carboxypeptidases, thymidine kinase, and DNA- and RNA- polymerases. It plays a role in DNA synthesis and repair, maintenance of red cell integrity and in bone and liver metabolism. Its role in DNA synthesis and in regulating gene expression makes it especially important for cells having a rapid turnover like hemopoietic cells, thymic tissue, gastrointestinal mucosal cells and cells of the immune system. Matrix metalloproteinases (MMPs) are a family of zinc dependent proteinases that perform the degradation of the extra cellular matrix which play a key role in the invasiveness and metastasis of beast cancer. These MMPs play a role in tumor invasion, migration, host immune escape, extravasations, angiogenesis and the tumor growth. Zinc deficiency has detrimental effects on B- and T-cell function, efficiency of phagocytosis, cytokine production, chemotactic function of neutrophils, monocytes, macrophages and delayed cutaneous hypersensitivity reactions. It is therefore, not surprising that acrodermatitis enteropathica, a congenital disorder of zinc metabolism related to its defective absorption and transport, manifests with recurrent infections especially with candida albicans, as one of its features.

Zinc is important for the conversion of prethymulin to thymulin, in the thymus. A low level of functionally active thymulin in Down's syndrome causing thymic dysfunction was postulated to be due to deficiency of zinc. Prolonged zinc deficiency results in a substantial decrease in the thymus size, depletion of the T- cells from spleen and lymph nodes and reduced pre-B and immature B-cells in the bone marrow. Licastro *et al.* showed that, after four months of zinc supplementation, there was normalization of zinc and thymulin levels, normalization of lymphocyte proliferation and neutrophil function, and improved DNA repair in patients with Down's syndrome. However other studies have failed to substantiate these findings. Many clinical trials showed improved outcomes in children with gastrointestinal diseases, when supplemented with zinc. The benefits are especially noteworthy in children with low levels of zinc or in those with high dietary phytate intake. Zinc supplementation has been shown to decrease the number of watery stools and duration of acute diarrhea, improve intestinal permeability, reduce duration of illness in children with persistent diarrhea, and lower the probability of continuing diarrhea, treatment failure and death. There are ongoing studies that are examining the role of zinc supplementation in preventing childhood mortality in developing countries. The aspect of combining zinc with standard oral rehydration solutions in the treatment of acute diarrhea is also under scrutiny. Further studies are needed to find the mechanism behind this and to identify patient population whose dietary requirements are higher than expected. It is important to realize that excessive zinc can lead to copper deficiency, anemia, growth retardation and depressed immunity.

Selenium

Selenium is a trace element that plays an important role in maintaining the integrity of muscles and nervous system. It also has antioxidant activity by virtue of being a part of the glutathione-peroxidase complex, though its role in immunocompetence is less well defined. It has synergistic actions with vitamin C and vitamin E. Selenium deficiency was noticed in children receiving long-term intravenous nutrition, when it was not a routine practice to add trace minerals to intravenous nutrition fluids.

Vitamin A

Vitamin A plays an important role in cellular differentiation and immune modulation and has anti-tumorogenic capabilities. The extensive involvement of body epithelial surfaces in diseases like measles and protein calorie malnutrition leads to a fast depletion of this vitamin. Administration of vitamin A increases IgG production and lymphocyte counts, without any changes in the complement activity or interleukin-2 production. Children with even mild deficiency of vitamin A are at an increased risk for diarrhea, respiratory infections and death. A large number of clinical trials carried out in various parts of the world have demonstrated the therapeutic efficacy of vitamin A supplementation. Vitamin A supplementation reduces mortality amongst children with diarrhea or respiratory diseases. A meta-analysis of trials showed that vitamin A supplementation helped achieve a 30% decrease in the mortality in infants and young children. A study conducted in Bangladesh showed that vitamin A supplemented group showed a significantly enhanced improvement in clinical recovery from acute shigella infection. A study in Brazil showed improvements in the number of episodes of diarrhea (especially severe episodes) in the vitamin A-supplemented group. A study carried out in India showed that the supplemented children aged less than 23 months suffered from lesser number of episodes of measles and older children when supplemented with vitamin A had lesser episodes of diarrhea and fever. Children with pneumonia receiving vitamin A had fewer episodes of diarrhea in the one-year follow-up in a study conducted in Tanzania. A decrease in all-cause mortality and diarrhea-specific mortality was seen in HIV-infected children after vitamin A supplementation. Vitamin A deficient status was shown to be associated with impaired gastrointestinal barrier function, which could be reversed with administration of a large dose of vitamin A in a study carried out in Indian infants. There is sufficient data to indicate that vitamin A supplementation is of paramount importance for decreasing the morbidity and mortality associated with certain clinical conditions in developing countries.

Vitamin E

Vitamin E is the main membrane-bound antioxidant and free radical scavenger, which prevents lipid peroxidation damage. Excessive tissue damage related to local inflammatory reactions and excessive production of free oxygen radicals is known to occur in various disorders such as necrotizing enterocolitis (NEC), ulcerative colitis and Crohn's disease. There have been some reports that indicate that antioxidants and recombinant dismutase are able to modulate these inflammatory reactions. Larger controlled studies are needed to confirm these preliminary findings.

Iron

Iron prevents anemia and helps in normal somatic growth and normal neurophysiologic development. It also plays an important role in immune function, as demonstrated by the increased susceptibility to infections in children with iron deficiency anemia. Animal studies indicate that iron deficiency affects the immune system at various levels (impaired bactericidal activity and cell mediated immunity, decreased NK cell function, decreased B-cell responses). Young children with iron deficiency showed T-cell dysfunction, decreased IL-2 levels and impaired cell-mediated immunity. However, paradoxically excessive iron induces tissue damage through its oxidant potential. Increased levels of free iron are associated with a risk of overwhelming sepsis, as iron a factor essential for bacterial growth, becomes easily available to them.

Polyphenols: EGCG

Polyphenols are a group of chemicals that are not essential for human health. However, they may play a beneficial role in human nutrition by virtue of their antioxidant, anti-mutagenic and anti-inflammatory properties. Certain polyphenols may decrease the expression of the pro-inflammatory cytokines and adhesion molecules from the endothelial cells and reduce monocyte adhesion. One of the polyphenols popularly used is the epigallocatechin-3-gallate (EGCG), which is found in green teas. They are known to possess significant anti-inflammatory and chemo-preventive properties. EGCG inhibits the tumor necrosis factor-alpha and blocks the activation of the nuclear factor-kB.

Probiotics

Probiotics are live micro-organisms in fermented foods that promote good health, through establishing an improved balance in intestinal micro-flora. They have been used for their health promoting benefits for times immemorial. The use of probiotics in the modern era was sparked off by the Nobel prize-winning scientist Elie Metchnikoff's observation that the long life span of Bulgarian peasants was a result of consumption of fermented milk products. Since probiotics do not permanently colonize the intestine they should be in sufficient quantities to maintain adequate levels in the colon. They should also be of human origin and be able to adhere to the intestinal enterocytes. The commonly used micro-organisms include various species of lactobacilli (L. acidophilus, L. bulgaricus, L. casei), bifidobacterium, streptococcus thermophilus and saccharomyces boulardii.

Several general mechanisms have been cited to explain the beneficial effects of these organisms. They probably enhance the mucosal immune defenses and also protect the host from colonization by pathogenic microorganisms. They also probably reduce the chances of microbial translocation by competing with them for receptor sites on the intestinal surface. Their ability to reduce colonization could be related to competition for intraluminal nutritive substances, crowding out effect, production of antibiotic substances and enhancement of host immune defenses (by means of adjuvant effect, increased polymeric immunoglobulin A production and cytokine stimulus). They can also exert beneficial effects on non-immunological host defenses by strengthening intestinal tight junctions, increasing mucous secretions, enhancing motility and producing metabolic products (amino acids such as arginine and glutamine and short chain fatty acids) that secondarily function as protective nutrients, generating hydrogen peroxide and by decreasing luminal pH and redox potential making it difficult for the pathogenic bacteria to colonize and grow.

Several well-controlled studies have shown encouraging results, but there are methodological difficulties in demonstrating actual colonization by the added live bacteria directly. Reports suggest that the human derived GG strain of lactobacillus casei is able to shorten the duration of diarrhea and help eradicate recurrent Clostridim difficile colitis unresponsive to multiple courses of conventional antibiotics in children. Saavedra *et al.* showed that supplementation with bifidobacterium bifidum and streptococcus thermophilus shortened the duration of shedding of rotavirus in chronically hospitalized children. Majamaa and co-workers demonstrated that use of lactobacillus GG was associated with an enhanced rotavirus-specific immune response. In a pediatric intensive care unit with a high incidence of NEC, premature infants given probiotics had a lower incidence of disease as compared to the controls. A clinical trial with non-pathogenic E. coli in patients with ulcerative colitis showed that the clinical outcome with its use was comparable with that associated with the use of anti-inflammatory agent mesalamine. Probiotics also improve lactose tolerance when added to ferment dairy products like yoghurt, thereby decreasing gas and cramping and decrease in the exhaled hydrogen levels. This enables patients to consume calcium and protein-rich food, which they would otherwise avoid.

Recent clinical studies suggest that probiotics may provide beneficial effects for patients with inflammatory bowel disease. A study in Finland showed that probiotics used along with protein hydrolysate (hypoallergenic formula) can decrease intestinal inflammation, mucosal barrier permeability and clinical symptoms in infants with allergic dermatitis. These findings need to be confirmed with larger studies.

Although probiotics are generally recognized as safe, the possibility of overloading the ability of the intestinal barrier to contain the added yeast should be kept in mind. The case of a one-year-old immunocompetent infant, who developed fungemia and septicemia with saccharomyces boulardii, while receiving this probiotic for the treatment of severe gastroenteritis and dehydration, is an eye opener. Eight patients in Mayo Clinic have showed positive blood cultures for lactobacilli following liver transplantation and imunosuppression. Factors like bowel decontamination routines, bile stasis, drastic changes in the colonic flora, intravenous vancomycin, and biliary anastomosis can result in translocation and dissemination of these organisms that are usually considered as non-pathogenic.

Prebiotics

Prebiotics are non-digestible food ingredients that provide beneficial effects to the host by selectively stimulating the growth and activity of one species or a limited number of species of bacteria in the colon. Unlike the probiotics, which introduce exogenous bacteria into the human colon, prebiotics stimulate the preferential growth of a limited number of health-promoting commensal floras already residing in the colon. For example, oligosaccharides in the human milk facilitate the growth of bifidobacteria and lactobacilli in the colon.

The use of fructose oligosaccharides and inulin-type fructans provides bifidogenic action on the human endogenous flora. Both inulin (group of fructose polymers-fructans) and fructose oligosaccharides are found in many plant foods like wheat, onion and banana. Prebiotics act through the following mechanisms: They are preferred as substrates by the bifidobacteria. They also bring about changes in the luminal pH and other factors that preferentially favor the growth of bifidogenic activity. Their use in infants with NEC or short bowel syndrome and in older patients with colitis or Crohn's disease needs to be probed. Pierre *et al.* found in their study that addition of fructo-oligosaccharides to food reduced the incidence of colonic tumors associated with multiple intestinal neoplasia. Prebiotics have been added to yoghurt in an effort to combine the prebiotic and probiotic effects (termed as a synbiotic effect). Prebiotics by virtue of their chemical structure are not absorbed in the small intestines, but are fermented into gases, combustible gases and short chain fatty acids in the colon. This makes them a preferred sugar replacement in diabetics.

Breast Milk

Any discussion on immunonutrition would be grossly inadequate if one fails to mention the immunonutritive role of breast milk. The breast milk has numerous nutrients and other substances that assume an immunonutritive role. These include secretory IgA, IgG, IgM, IgE, IgD, lactoferrin, macrophages, bifidus factor, T- and B-lymphocytes, anti-adherence substances, lysozymes, interferon, epidermal growth factor, nerve growth factor, insulin-like growth factor, amino sugars, fatty acids, taurine, glutamine, cortisol and thyroxine.

No wonder then that breastfeeding is associated with decreased incidence of gastrointestinal and respiratory infections in the first two years of life. Oligosaccharides in the breast milk inhibit the adhesion of pneumococci and hemophilus influenzae to the pharyngeal and buccal epithelial cells. This protects breastfed infants from infections caused by these pathogens.

Iron is an essential element required for the growth of gram-negative bacteria. These organisms require the element for their multiplication, metabolic pathways and virulence. Lactoferrin in the breast milk binds with iron making it unavailable to these potentially pathogenic bacteria. This favors the growth of lactobacilli and bifidobacteria, which foster an acidic environment in the gut, further inhibiting the growth of enteropathogens.

In addition, breast milk shows lymphocyte transforming activity resulting in the production of alpha-interferon. The decrease in the levels of the myeloperoxidase and beta-glucuronidase activity induced by breast milk tends to help modulate the inflammatory reactions mediated by neutrophils. The milk contains a multimeric alpha-lactalbumin complex that binds with potential pathogens offering protection to the babies.

Box 111.1 gives details of available immunonutrition preparations.

FUTURE

On the basis of the available data, immunonutrition seems to have immense potential for decreasing the morbidity and mortality amongst critically ill individuals, those with gastro-intestinal diseases, immune deficiency disorders, polytrauma, sepsis or severe infections. It could be of great importance in cancer prevention as well. Carbohydrates especially the complex or slowly absorbed ones, seem to have a role in immunomodulation. They have been shown to alter the flora of the small bowel and colon through stimulation of the short chain fatty acids production. More studies are required to

Box 111.1: Available Immunonutrient Preparations

Reconvan (Fresenius–Kabi)

Constituents:

Calories: 420 KJ / 100 Kcal / 100 ml

Protein: 5.5 g (22 %)

Glutamine: 1 g; Arginine L: 0.6 g

Carbohydrates: 12 g (48 %)

Sugars: 0.7 g; Lactose: <0.01 g

Fats: 3.3g (30 %)

Saturated fatty acids: 2 g; Mono-saturated fatty acids: 0.2 g; Cholesterol: < 6 mg;

Polyunsaturated fatty acids: 1.2 g Medium chain triglycerides: 1.9 g

EPA: 0.15 g

DHA: 0.1 g

Fiber: 0 g

Vitamins: A, D, E, K, B1, B2, B6, B_{12}, C, Niacin, Pantothenic acid, Biotin, Folic acid, Beta-carotene and Choline

Minerals: Zinc, Selenium, Iron, Sodium, Potassium, Chloride, Calcium, Magnesium, Phosphorus, Copper, Manganese, Iodide, Fluoride and Chromium

Essential amino acids: Lysine, Threonine, Methionine, Phenylalanine, Tryptophan, Valine, Leucine and Isoleucine

Conditionally essential amino acids: Glutamine, Arginine, Tyrosine, Cysteine and Histidine

Non-essential amino acids: Glycine, Alanine, Proline, Serine, Glutamic acid, Aspartic acid and Aspargine

Adult Doses:

Complete nutrition: 1.5 lit/day

Critically ill patients: 10 ml/hour and increase every hour by 10 ml /hour

Omegaven (Fresenius-Kabi)

Constituents:

Calories: 470 KJ /112 Kcal/100 ml

Highly refined fish-oil comprising of

Eicosapentaenoic acid: 1.25- 2.82 g;	Docosahexaenoic acid: 1.44- 3.09 g
Myristic acid: 0.1- 0.6 g;	Palmitic acid: 0.25- 1 g
Palmitoleic acid: 0.3-0.9 g;	Stearic acid: 0.05- 0.2 g
Oleic acid: 0.6- 1.3 g;	Linoleic acid: 0.1- 0.7 g
Linolenic acid: 0.2 g;	Octadecatetraenoic acid: 0.15-0.45 g
Eicosaenoic acid: 0.05- 0.3 g;	Arachidonic acid: 0.1-0.4 g
Docosaenoic acid: 0.15 g;	Docosapentaenoic acid: 0.15- 0.45 g
Alpha-tocopherol: 0.015-0.0296 g;	Glycerol: 2.5 g

Adult Dose:

10-20 % of total lipid intake, 1-2ml /kg with an infusion rate of not more than 0.5 ml/kg/hour

Dipeptiven 20 % (Fresenius–Kabi)

Constituents: N2- L- Alanayl-L-Glutamine: 20 g / 100ml

Dose: 0.3 g / kg for all age groups

Glutammune (Fresenius–Kabi)

Constituents:

L-Glutamine: 10 g/sachet

Dose: 2- 40 g/day in 3- 6 divided doses (adult)

Contd.

Contd.

Impact (Novartis)

Constituents:

Calories: 420 KJ / 100 Kcal / 100 ml

Protein: 5.6 g (22 %)

Carbohydrates: 13.16 g (53 %)

Low lactose: <0.01 g

Fats: 2.82 g (25 %)

Saturated fatty acids: 60 % of the fats

Polyunsaturated fatty acids: 23 % of the fats

Monosaurated fatty acids: 17 % of the fats

Fiber: 1.1 g

Vitamins: A, D, E, K, B_1, B_2, B_6, B_{12}, C, Niacin, Pantothenic acid, Biotin, Folic acid, Beta-carotene and Choline

Minerals: Zinc, Selenium, Iron, Sodium, Potassium, Chloride, Calcium, Magnesium, Phosphorus, Copper, Manganese, Iodide, Fluoride and Chromium

Essential amino acids: Lysine, Threonine, Methionine, Phenylalanine, Tryptophan, Valine, Leucine and Isoleucine

Conditionally essential amino acids: Glutamine, Arginine, Tyrosine, Cysteine and Histidine

Non-essential amino acids: Glycine, Alanine, Proline, Serine, Glutamic acid, Aspartic acid and Aspargine

Contains:	L- Arginine	1.35 gm/100 ml
	L-glutamine	0.36 gm/ 100 ml
	Omega 3 fatty acids	0.34 gm/100 ml i.e. 12.4 % of the fat
	Omega 6 fatty acid	0.25 gm/100 ml i.e. 9.92 % of the fat

RNA nucleotides

Gluten Free

Adult Doses:

1 Sachet (61 g) is to be dissolved in 206 ml of boiled and cooled water.

3 sachets per day for 3 days pre-op and 3 sachets per day post-op. For ICU cases 3 sachets per day.

Critically ill patients: 10 ml /hour and increase every hour by 10 ml/hour.

EPA: Eicosapentaenoic acid; DHA: Docosahexaenoic acid.

elucidate the clinical relevance of these findings. During periods of stress, like post-operative states, severe trauma, gastrointestinal disorders etc. there is a possibility of restriction and at times proscription of diet. It has been postulated that this deprives the normal bacteria in the gut of a secure environment and a regular supply of food. As a result of this, these bacteria may show virulent characteristics for self preservation, which may harm the host. This further underlines the need for enteral nutrition.

It should, however, be conceded that although the idea of immunonutrition is not new, a lot of work needs to be done for establishing its efficacy and safety. The scientific data available regarding the use of immunonutrition for individual disorders, and the use / efficacy of individual immunonutrients, is scanty at its best and more prospective controlled studies may have to be undertaken to get the correct picture. It is also important to note that most of the data pertains to use of immunonutrition in adults and there is hardly any data about its use in children and infants. Young infants and children have diseases that are peculiar to their age group. They also have metabolic, physiological and immunological processes that are unique. Hence, it may be inappropriate to extrapolate data obtained from studies carried out in adults to infants and children. This makes it imperative for researchers to take special interest in studying the use of immunonutrition in infants and children. Here a mention of needs and priorities of children in developing countries would not be out of place. Infectious diseases in the background of widespread malnutrition continue to besiege children in the developing countries. As immunonutrition has been shown to be effective in these very processes, it is of great significance to children here. More work is needed to identify the nutrients that would help in specific conditions.

Preliminary data also suggests that all genotypes might not be equally sensitive to the effects of immunonutrition. This phenomenon offers a fascinating prospect for research: identifying the genotype and phenotype (response to injury, degree of inflammation, etc.) that would derive the maximum benefit from these interventions. This would bring in strategies tailor-made based on gene polymorphism. In the interim period it is necessary to disseminate information available to healthcare providers so that they can start using simple and affordable interventions straightaway.

KEY LEARNING POINTS

- Immunonutrition is the process of studying the potentials of specific nutrients to modulate the activity of the immune system and the use of iets for enhancing immune function.
- Immunonutrients (arginine, glutamine, omega-3 fatty acids, RNA nucleotides, fiber, etc.) help maintaining gut integrity, stimulating the immune system and preventing bacterial translocation from the gut into the circulation.
- It finds application in many situations, especially sepsis, trauma, surgery-related problems, IBD and cancers.
- Breast milk assumes an important immunonutritive role because of presence of IgA, IgG, IgM, IgE, IgD, lactoferrin, macrophages, bifidus factor, T- and B-lymphocytes, antiadher-ence substances, lysozymes, interferon, epidermal growth factor, nerve growth factor, insulin-like growth factor, aminosugars, fatty acids, taurine, glutamine, cortisol and thyroxine.
- Further work is warranted to establish the efficacy and safety of immunonutrition.

Acknowledgements

The authors thank Dr Yeolekar ME, Director (ME and H) (G and K), Seth GS Medical College and KEM Hospital, Mumbai for permitting the authors to submit the manuscript.

FURTHER READINGS

1. Andrews J, Griffiths RD. Glutamine: Essential for immune nutrition in the critically ill. *Brit J Nutr* 2002; 87(suppl): S3-S8.
2. Braga M, Gianotti L, Vignali A, Di Carlo V. Pre-operative oral arginine and omega-3 fatty acids supplementation improves the immunometabolic host response and outcome after colorectal resection for cancer. *Surgery* 2002; 132: 805-814.
3. Calder PC. Immunonutrition. *BMJ* 2003; 327: 117-118.
4. Duggan C, Gannon J, Walker AW. Protective nutrients and functional foods for the gastrointestinal tract. *Am J Clin Nutr.* 2002; 75: 789-808.
5. Evoy D, Lieberman MD, Fahey TJ, Daly JM. Immunonutrition: The role of arginine. *Nutrition* 1998; 14: 611-617.
6. Grimble RF. Immunonutrition. *Curr Opin Gastroenterol* 2005; 21: 216-222.
7. Heyland DK, Dhaliwal R. Immunonutrition in the critically ill: From old approaches to new paradigms. *Intensive Care Med* 2005; 31: 501-503.
8. Heyland DK, Novak F, Drover JW, Jain M, Su X, Suchner U. Should immunonutrition become routine in critically ill patients? A systematic review of the evidence. *JAMA* 2001; 286: 944-953.
9. Kieft Hans, Roos AN, van Drunen JDE, Bindels AJGH, Bindels JG, Hofman Z. Clinical outcome of immunonutrition in a heterogenous intensive care population. *Intensive Care Med* 2005; 31: 524-532.
10. Koretz RL. Immunonutrition: Can you be what you eat? *Curr Opin Gastroenterol* 2003; 19: 134-139.
11. Levy J. Immunonutrition. The pediatric experience. *Nutrition* 1998; 14: 627-633.
12. McCowen KC, Bistrian BR. Immunonutrition: Problematic or problem solving. *Am J Clin Nutr* 2003; 77:764-770.
13. Novak F, Heyland DK, Avenell A, Drover JW, Su X. Glutamine supplementation in serious illness: A systematic review of the evidence. *Crit Care Med* 2002; 30: 2022-2029.
14. Philpott M, Ferguson LR. Immunonutrition and cancer. *Mutat Res* 2004; 551:29-42.
15. Redmond HP, Stableton PP, Neary P, Bouchier HD. Immunonutrition: The role of taurine. *Nutrition* 1998; 14: 599-604.
16. Sazawal S, Black RE, Bhan MK, Bhandari N, Sinha A, Jalla S. Zinc supplementation in young children with acute diarrhoea in India. *N Eng J Med* 1995; 333: 839-844.
17. Singh R, Gopalan S, Sibal A. Immunonutrition. *Indian J Pediatr* 2002; 69: 417-419.
18. Schears GJ, Deutschman CS. Common nutritional issues in pediatric and adult critical care medicine. *Crit Care Clin* 1997; 13: 669-690.
19. Stechmiller JK, Childress B, Porter T. Arginine immunonutrition in critically ill patients: A clinical dilemma. *Am J Crit Care* 2004; 13: 17-23.
20. Vanderhoof JA. Probiotics: Future directions. *Am J Clin Nutr* 2001; 73 (suppl): S1552-S1555.

112 Nutritional Support in Liver Disease

Lalit Bharedia • Priyanka Rohtagi (Rastogi)

INTRODUCTION

Malnutrition is a remarkable feature of advanced liver disease. A large proportion of patients with cirrhosis show signs of protein-energy malnutrition (PEM) which is associated with a higher prevalence of complications and poor prognosis.

Malnutrition contributes to poor prognosis and complications. It was selected as a component of the score predicting severity of liver disease and death risk after portacaval anastomosis. Hence, the relevance of a correct diagnosis, a thorough analysis of pathogenic causes and a prompt treatment.

ANTHROPOMETRIC ASSESSMENT OF NUTRITIONAL STATUS IN CHILDREN WITH LIVER DISEASE

In children with chronic liver disease, both acute and chronic malnutrition are nearly universal. There can be various potential causes of malnutrition in liver diseases as shown in Fig. 112.1.

There are, however, few studies that have characterized, in a prospective and chronological fashion, anthropometric information defining the nutritional status in children with differing types of liver disease. Several excellent studies do provide general information about nutritional risks in various types of pediatric liver disease and improve the accuracy of interpreting anthropometric assessment result.

Both acute (wasting) and chronic (stunting) malnutrition are nearly universal consequences of early childhood liver disease.

A comparison of z scores for weight and height erroneously suggested that although children with chronic liver disease are stunted in linear growth, they are well-nourished. This misinterpretation probably results from the increased body weight due to the organomegaly and/or ascites which may exist even when not detected clinically. Reconfirmation of the imprecision of using a weight/height index *versus* a triceps skin-fold (TSF) measurement for nutritional assessments comes from a study done within a month of transplantation of adult patients with end-stage liver disease.

Acute malnutrition, therefore, is best estimated by a triceps skin-fold determination. Although weight-for-height is generally used to ascertain acute malnutrition, in children with chronic liver disease the increase in body weight resulting from the enlargement of the liver and the spleen may mask the extent of weight loss. Chronic malnutrition (stunting), which occurs over a considerable span of time, is best determined by a height/age index.

Nearly all nutritional studies have been cross-sectional or prevalence rather than longitudinal. Future studies are needed to confirm the possible immediate benefit of nutritional intervention in children with chronic liver disease.

There are various factors affecting the interpretation of nutrition assessment tests in patients with end-stage liver disease which have been illustrated in the Table 112.1.

The tool used for the assessment comprises the parameters illustrated in the Table 112.2.

There are many nutritional risk factors associated with chronic liver diseases as illustrated in the Table 112.3.

To understand the nutritional role of liver, effects of the hepatobiliary damage and its management, it is essential to understand the normal nutrient metabolism, the alternations in the nutrient metabolism due to the liver damage and the possible remedial measures to be taken as shown in Table.112.4.

NUTRITIONAL AND LIVER DISEASE

An adequate balanced nutrition is essential to maintain body mass, support organ function and allow growth and development of the infant of child. Any deviation from normal nutrition is likely to affect hepatobiliary function.

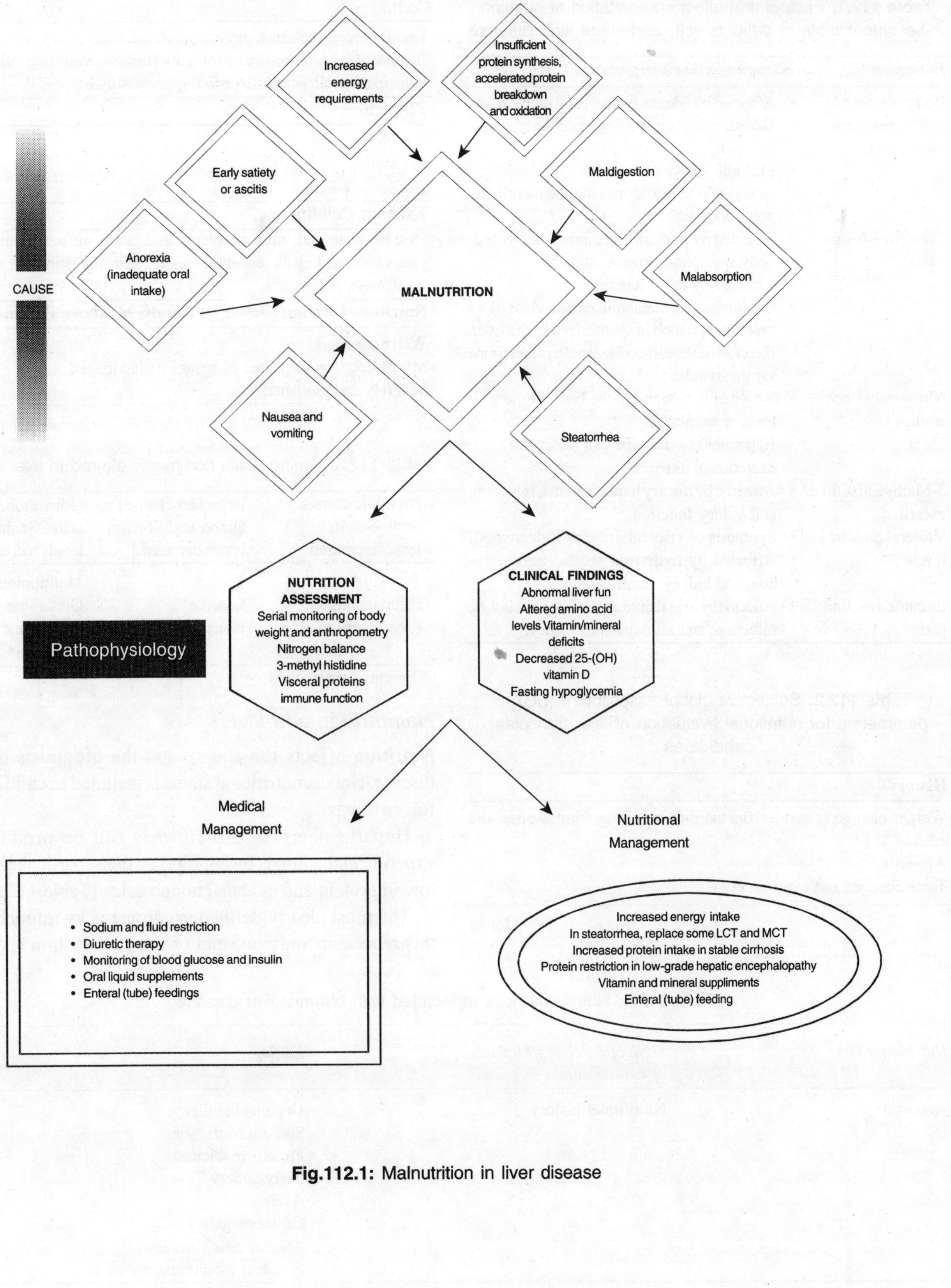

Fig.112.1: Malnutrition in liver disease

Table 112.1: Factors that affect interpretation of nutrition assessment tests in patients with end-stage liver disease

Parameter	*Factors affecting interpretation*
Body weight	• Affected by edema, ascites, and diuretic use.
Anthropometric measurement	• Questionable sensitivity, specificity, and reliability. • Multiple sources of error. • Question if skinfold measurements reflect total body fat.
Creatinine-height index	• Affected by malnutrition, aging, decreased body mass, and protein intake. • Affected by renal function. • Creatinine is a metabolic end product of creatinine, which is synthesized in the liver, therefore severe liver disease alters creatinine synthesis rates.
Nitrogen balance studies	• Nitrogen is retained in the body in the form of ammonia. • Hepatorenal syndrome can affect the excretion of nitrogen.
3-Methyl histidine excretion	• Affected by dietary intake, trauma, infection, and kidney function.
Visceral protein levels	• Synthesis of visceral proteins is decreased. • Affected by hydration status, malabsorption, and kidney insufficiency.
Immune function tests	• Affected by liver failure, electrolyte imbalances, infection, and kidney insufficiency.

Table 112.2: Subjective global assessment (SGA) parameters for nutritional evaluation of liver transplant candidates

History
Weight change (consider fluctuations resulting from ascites and edema) Appetite Taste changes and early satiety
Contd.
Dietary recall (calories, protein, sodium) Persistent gastrointestinal problems (nausea, vomiting, diarrhoea, constipation, difficulty in chewing or swallowing)
Physical
Muscle wasting Fat stores Ascites or edema
Existing Conditions
Disease state and other problems that could influence nutritional status such as hepatic encephalopathy, gastrointestinal bleed, renal insufficiency, infection
Nutritional Rating (Based on Results of Above Parameters)
Well nourished Moderately (or suspected of being) malnourished Severely malnourished

Table 112.3: Amino acids commonly altered in liver disease

Aromatic amino acids–Serum levels increased	Branched-chained amino acids–Serum levels decreased	Other amino acids–Serum levels increased
Tyrosine	Valine*	Methionine*
Phenylalanine*	Leucine*	Glutamine
Free tryptophan*	Isoleucine*	Asparagine
		Histidine*

* Essential amino acid.

Malnutrition and Liver:

Nutrition affects the course and the prognosis of liver disease. Hence, nutritional status is included in child's score for cirrhosis.

Hepatic necrosis and fibrosis can be produced in experimental animals by appropriate diets, particularly those low in protein and essential amino acids (Table 112.5).

The most clearly defined syndrome is kwashiorkor, but this represents only one end of the malnutrition spectrum.

Table 112.4: Nutritional risks associated with chronic liver disease

Nutritional risks	*Signs of deficiency/Methods of assessment*	*Etiology*
Anorexia	Nutritional history	Unpalatable diet Sodium restriction Protein restriction Early satiety Ascites Organomegaly Altered taste sensation Frequent infections/antibiotics
Growth failure	Growth velocity curve Anthropometric measurement	Fat malabsorption 72-hour fecal fat

Contd.

Contd.

	Triceps skin-fold thickness Midarm circumference Midarm muscle mass are (MAMA) History of drugs that bind bile acids or interfere with Mucosal function	
Hypoproteinemia	Assess nutritional intake and distributions of calories, carbohydrates, protein, and fat Clinical examination for edema ascites, muscle wasting Anthropometry	Therapeutic maneuvers to control ascites (e.g. fluid withdrawal) GI protein loss Fecal a1pha-1-antitrypsin excretion and/or clearance Increased catabolism Decreased synthesis due to infection Hepatic dysfunction
Fat-soluble vitamins	Dermatitis, night blindness, rickets/osteomalacia, Serum vitamin A and retinol ester determination (HPLC)	Fat malabsorption, neomycine, cholestyramine, alcoholism, glucocorticoids
Vitamin A	Retinol-binding protein, transthyretin (prealbumin) concentrations Functional assessment, dark field adaptation studies (difficult to perform in children)	
Vitamin E	Edema, peripheral neuropathy, serum vitamin E level (HPLC) Vitamin E/total lipid ratio Vitamin E absorption test Biochemical evidence for vitamin E deficiency Clinical evidence for vitamin E deficiency Neurological dysfunction DTRs diminished Wide-based gait Occular palsy Spinocerebellar degeneration Anemia/hemolysis	Fat malabsorption, cholestyramine
Vitamin D	Assessment of dietary intake of vitamin D and calcium Determine serum 25-OH vitamin D level, absorption study Radiographic studies of bone/bone densitometry Serum alkaline phosphatase Determination/bone fraction Determine 25-OH vitamin D level	Fat malabsorption Increased requirements due to interaction with pharmacologic agents (e.g. phenobarbital, neomycin, cholestyramine)
Vitamin K	Bleeding, prothrombin time/vitamin K challenge clotting factor levels sequestering	Fat malabsorption, cholestyramine Use of antibiotics (neomycin, bile acids)
Mineral deficiency (iron, magnesium and zinc)	Neuromuscular irritability, hypokalemia, hypocalcemia, stomatitis, anemia, malaise, impaired taste acuity, poor wound healing Document adequate supplementation Determination of serum Magnesium level/urinary excretion Serum iron, total iron-binding capacity, ferritin levels Plasma zinc determination	Chronic bleeding Use of bile acid sequestering agents

Contd.

Contd.

	Serum alkaline phosphatase level Urinary excretion	
Proteins	Blood urea may be low in chronic liver disease Blood ammonia may be elevated	Synthesis of plasma proteins, carrier proteins (transferrin) and coagulation factors reduced. Requirements increased in severe viral hepatitis and fulminant hepatic failure.

Table 112.5: Causes of hepatic steatosis

Macrovesicular (large fat droplets in hepatocytes)	*Microvesicular (small fat droplets in hepatocytes)*
Nutritional	
Malnutrition (Kwashiorkor)	Reye's syndrome
Obesity*	
Prolonged parenteral nutrition*	Acute fatty liver of pregnancy
Metabolic diseases	Drugs, e.g. valproic acid, tetracycline, nucleoside analogues
Drug-related	Environmental hepatotoxins
Inflammatory bowel disease	(e.g. phosphorus, petrochemicals)

The liver is often grossly enlarged in children with kwashiorkor, containing 30-50% fat by weight, predominantly in the form of neutral fat or triglyceride. If the malnutrition is severe and of long-standing, hepatic fibrosis may be observed. The hepatic changes in the alcoholic may be, at least in part, nutritional.

In starvation and hunger edema, the liver shrinks, increased lipochrome pigment is seen in the liver cells, but there is no fatty change. Liver biopsies from malnourished children show a reduction in liver protein. Previous malnutrition may 'condition' the liver to toxic and infective agents, but this has not been proved. Increased mortality from viral hepatitis, particularly in pregnancy, may occur in protein-deficient communities.

Fatty Liver

This is defined as fat, largely triglyceride, exceeding 5% of the liver weight. It is caused by failure of normal hepatic fat metabolism either due to a defect within the hepatocyte or to delivery of excess fat, fatty acid or carbohydrate beyond the secretory capacity for lipid of the liver cell. Liver biopsy and imaging procedures, such as ultrasound and CT, are resulting in increasing numbers of patients being identified with excess fat in the liver.

Theoretically fatty liver could accumulate through at least four mechanisms:

1. Increased delivery of dietary fat or fatty acids to the liver. Dietary fat is transported in the circulation mainly as chylomicrons Fig. 112.2. Lipolysis in adipose tissue liberates the fatty acids. These are incorporated into triglyceride within the adipocyte but some fatty acids may be released into the circulation and taken up by the liver. The chylomicron remnants also enter the liver.
2. Increased mitochondrial synthesis of fatty acids or reduced oxidation. Both augment triglyceride production.
3. Impaired export of triglyceride out of the liver cell. Export of triglycerides from the hepatocyte depends upon packaging with apoprotein, phospholipid and cholesterol to form very low density lipoprotein (VLDL). This process may be inhibited. Excess carbohydrate delivered to the liver may be converted to fatty acids.
4. Nonalcoholic fatty liver disease (NAFLD), hepatic steatosis (Fatty liver), and nonalcoholic steatohepatitis (NASH).

Fatty liver can be separated into two categories based on whether the fat droplets in the hepatocytes are macrovesicular or microvesicular (Table 112.5). In addition, fatty infiltration may be accompanied by necroinflammatory activity, a condition designated nonalcoholic steatohepatitis, a form of NAFLD. Although prospective data on natural history are limited, there is increasing evidence that patients may progress through several histologically distinct stages beginning with fatty liver and culminating in cirrhosis with intervening states of steatohepatitis and steatohepatitis with fibrosis.

Parenteral Nutrition and Liver

The use of the vascular system to supply nutrient requirements can be an important and even life-saving therapy. The complications associated with the use of parenteral nutrition can be divided into mechanical, vascular, infectious, metabolic and gastrointestinal.

Hepatobiliary Complications of TPN

Hepatic abnormalities are the most common gastrointestinal complications associated with TPN. However, it is difficult to establish a true causal relationship between the use of TPN and many of the reported liver abnormalities because of the paucity of prospective randomized trials. Many of

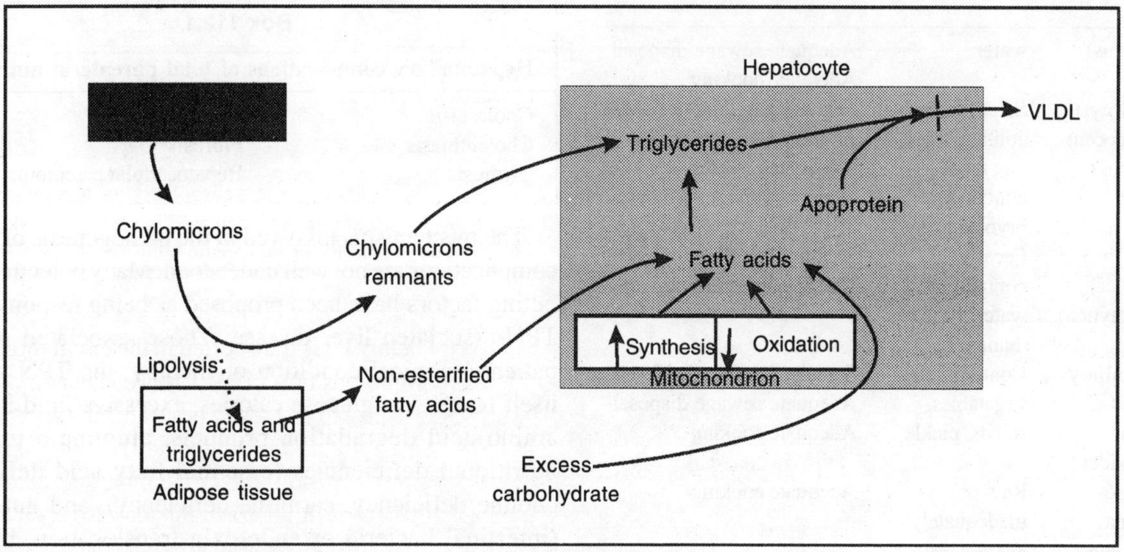

Fig. 112. 2: Factors in fatty liver

the hepatic abnormalities in patients receiving TPN might have been caused by clinical factors unrelated to the use of TPN itself. Patients who require TPN often have serious illnesses that are associated with liver disease or have received hepatotoxic therapy, which can cause liver disease.

Hepatic abnormalities are more frequent and more severe in infants receiving TPN than in adults. The first report of TPN-associated liver disease, published in 1971, was of a premature infant who developed cholestatic jaundice, bile duct proliferation, and cirrhosis after 71 days of TPN therapy. Subsequent studies have shown that cholestasis is the most frequent hepatic complication in TPN-fed infants and correlates directly with decreased gestational age, decreased birth weight, and increased duration of TPN therapy.

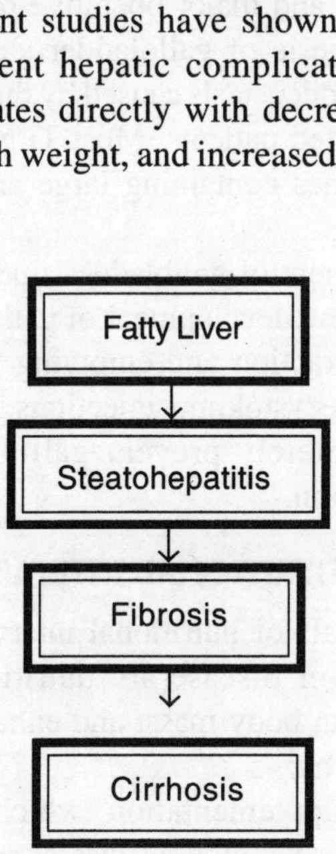

Fig. 112.3: Progression of fatty liver

Obesity and Its Impact on Liver Disease and Transplantation

Obesity is twice as common in patients with cryptogenic cirrhosis compared to those with other chronic liver disease. Obesity is also a negative prognostic predictor in patients with chronic liver disease irrespective of the etiology. In a study of overweight patients with abnormal liver function tests, 30% had septal fibrosis and 11% had cirrhosis, and in this study, BMI>28 was an independent predictor of more advanced liver disease. Obese patients with CC have also been shown to have a relatively lower survival when compared to their age and sex matched controls with hepatitis C virus (HCV) cirrhosis suggesting that the natural history of CC, despite the indolent nature of NAFLD, may be worse than those with HCV cirrhosis. Obesity is also an independent risk factor for the development of hepatocellular carcinoma (HCC) in patients with CC and alcoholic cirrhosis. Post-transplant survival is also affected by obesity. As shown by our group where patients with BMI>35 had a significantly lower 5-year survival compared to less obese transplant recipients.

Hypervitaminosis A and Liver

Vitamin A is a dose-dependent hepatotoxin, and severe liver disease may result from hypervitaminosis A.

Table 112.6: Food-borne liver illness

Disease and organism	*Source*	*Preventive methods*
1. Hepatitis (Hepatitis A	Raw vegetable Contaminated	Sanitary handling of foods Use of pure drinking water

Contd.

Contd.

and E virus)	water	Adequate sewage disposal Adequate cooking
2. Hydatid cyst (Echinococcus granulosus)	Salad, vegetable contaminated dog feces containing embryonated egg	Sanitary handling of foods Adequate sewage disposal Adequate cooking
3. Amebic liver abscess (E. histolytica)	Fecally contaminated water, food or hands	Sanitary handling of foods Use of pure drinking water
4. Hepatobiliary ascariasis (Ascaris lumbricoides)	Contaminated vegetables, salads, pickle	Sanitary handling of foods Adequate sewage disposal Adequate cooking
5. Cholangiocarcinoma (Clonorchis sinensis)	Raw or inadequately cooked fresh water fish	Adequate cooking

Table 112.7: Toxins causing liver illness

Agent	*Type of exposure*	*Nature of liver injury*
1. Pyrrolizidine alkaloids	Herbal and bush teas; contaminated crop	Veno-occlusive disease, cirrhosis
2. Vitamin A	Health tonic; skin disorder (no longer appropriate massive ingestion of liver)	Noncirrhotic portal hypertension, hepatic fibrosis, liver failure with or without cirrhosis, peliosis hepatitis
3. Amanita phalloides, other toxic mushrooms	Accidental ingestion, as little as one mushroom	Fulminant hepatic failure
4. Aflatoxin	Contaminated crops, foodstuffs, groundnuts	Hepatocellular carcinoma (p53 deletions)
5. Arsenic	Nonproprietary medications; contaminated water supply; industrial exposure (pesticides, herbicides)	Hepatic fibrosis, cirrhosis, noncirrhotic portal hypertension, angiosarcoma

The clinicopathologic spectrum of hyper-vitaminosis A-related liver disease includes minor changes with abnormal liver tests and stellate cell hyperplasia, noncirrhotic portal hypertension with perisinusoidal fibrosis, cirrhosis, or fatal chronic liver disease with hepatocellular failure in the absence of cirrhosis.

Gradual improvement occurs after discontinuation of vitamin A ingestion, but deterioration may continue in cases of severe intoxication, particularly when cirrhosis is present. Features of liver failure and established cirrhosis is present. Features of liver failure and established cirrhosis at diagnosis indicate a poor prognosis; most patients die or require hepatic transplantation. There is a need for better public education to prevent hypervitaminosis A.

Box 112.1

Hepatobiliary complications of total parenteral nutrition

Cholestasis	Biliary sludge
Cholelithiasis	Fibrosis
Cirrhosis	Hepatocellular carcinoma

The mechanisms involved in the pathogenesis of hepatic complications are not well understood. Many potential contributing factors have been proposed as being responsible for TPN-associated liver disease: Those associated with the patients' clinical condition or therapy, the TPN solution itself (excessive glucose calories, excessive lipid infusion, amino acid degradation products, aluminum toxicity), nutritional deficiencies (essential fatty acid deficiency, choline deficiency, carnitine deficiency), and gut factors (intestinal bacteria or endotoxin translocation, bacterial overgrowth, bacterial metabolism of bile acids).

Three types of biliary complications have been associated with the use of TPN: acalculous cholecystitis, gallbladder sludge and cholelithiasis. Biliary complications usually occur in patients receiving more prolonged (more than 4 weeks) courses of TPN. Acalculous cholecystitis has been reported to occur in about 5%, cholelithiasis in about 30%, increased risk of cholelithiasis with prolonged total parenteral nutrition and gallbladder sludge in upto 100% of patients receiving prolonged TPN.

The pathogenesis of acalculous cholecystitis is unclear, but it occurs in the setting of bile stasis and increased bile lithogenicity and is associated with major trauma, severe systemic illness, and major operative procedures.

The pathogenesis of gallbladder sludge and stones is related to gallbladder stasis caused by the absence of enteral feeding in TPN fed patients. Most TPN-related gallstones are pigment stones containing large amounts of calcium bilirubinate.

The development of gallbladder sludge appears to be a prerequisite for the development of gallstones. Stimulating gallbladder contraction and emptying with either enteral feedings or cholecystokinin injections has been shown to reduce or completely prevent gallbladder sludge and gallstone formation.

GOALS FOR NUTRITIONAL INTERVENTION

The ultimate goals of nutritional intervention in children with chronic liver disease are nutritional homeostasis, deposition of lean body mass, and enhanced growth. This is accomplished by:

a. Nutritional supplementation, which corrects existing deficits and meets ongoing losses; and
b. Establishing nitrogen deposition while decreasing hepatic encephalopathy.

Special attention must be directed toward infants and

young children, the largest group of young patients requiring liver transplantation.

Nutritional formulas adequate to promote catch-up growth must contain approximately 150% of the recommended dietary allowances (RDA) for height and age. Infant formulas, which contain a balanced lipid composition to maximize absorption in the face of cholestasis and deficient lipolysis (e.g. 40% of lipid calories as medium chain triglycerides) and yet have sufficient linoleic acid to prevent essential fatty acid deficiency, have been recommended. Protein intake adequate to promote growth and to maintain positive nitrogen balance is essential.

Studies that have examined nitrogen balance while reducing hepatic encephalopathy through the use of branch-chain amino acids have conflicting results. The use of branch-chain amino acids in children with liver failure has been recommended, the potential benefits being an increased utilization rate of branch chain amino acids by skeletal muscle, which would promote net energy uptake and possibly reduce the potential for hepatic encephalopathy. To date, the high cost of these formulations and limited information demonstrating efficacy preclude their routine use in children with cholestasis and/or liver disease. Chronic malabsorption and deficiency of fat-soluble vitamins are nearly universal in children with chronic liver disease. Careful assessment of current status and monitoring of vitamin intake to avoid toxicity are essential.

METHOD OF FEEDING IN LIVER DISEASE

Many patients with chronic liver disease are anorexic or suffer from nausea or abdominal distension. Maintenance of an adequate oral intake may prove difficult under these circumstances. Patients should be encouraged to eat, and also to modify, their eating pattern in order to take four to seven small meals throughout the day, including a late night snack, as this reg is better tolerated and improves nitrogen balance and substrate utilization.

It is often difficult, however, to sustain oral intake in patients with persistent anorexia and nausea, or to increase oral intake beyond a certain limit in malnourished patients.

If oral intake remains inadequate despite supplementation, enteral feeding *via* a fine-bore nasogastric tube should be instituted at the earliest opportunity. Depending on the degree of malnutrition, night-time infusions alone may be sufficient to maintain growth. If abdominal distension and vomiting continue then the nasogastric tube can be endoscopically repositioned in the jejunum. Standard, proprietary feeds, providing 1 kcal/ml, are suitable for use in the majority of patients but the volume of feed required to supply daily requirements may be excessive in those who are fluid overloaded. Under these circumstances, more concentrated feeds providing 1.5 or 2.0 kcal/ml can be used, the choice being determined by the amount of protein required. The rate of feed administration and osmolarity can be manipulated to optimize tolerance.

Every attempt should be made to feed these patients either orally or enterally. The use of parenteral feeding should be avoided for a number of reasons. These patients may be fluid intolerant so that the volume infused may need to be restricted to one liter or less. It may also be necessary to modify the amino acid solutions used. In addition many of the formulations used in patients with liver disease are nutritionally incomplete or else contain quantities of amino acids, such as glycine, proline, lysine, threonine, and arginine, which may not be adequately cleared when the liver's ureagenic capacity is limited.

Lipid solutions can be used safely in these patients. Long-chain and medium-chain triglycerides are equally well tolerated. Thus, if patients with liver disease require parenteral nutrition there is no contraindication to providing energy as glucose and fat, the latter constituting 35-50% of the non-protein calories, and nitrogen as conventional amino acids.

Table 112.8: Essential dietary principles in liver diseases

Calories/day	:	1.2-1.4 times resting energy expenditure (REE)
Proteins/day	:	1.2-1.5 g/kg of ideal body weight (IBW)
Fats/day	:	20-40% of non-protein calories
Carbohydrates/day	:	Rest of the calories.

NUTRITIONAL MANAGEMENT OF INDIVIDUAL LIVER DISEASE

Fatty Liver

Fatty liver is known as the disease of the decade, it may or may not be associated with obesity.

Nutritional therapy: Weight management with low-fat diet rich in polyunsaturated and monounsaturated fatty acids is recommended.

Non-alcoholic Steatohepatitis (NASH)/Non-alcoholic Fatty Liver Disease (NAFLD)

Non-alcoholic steatohepatitis (NASH) is thought to be an intermediate stage of the disease which is characterized by the presence of hepatic inflammation, injury and cell death in conjunction with steatosis in the absence of any other attributable causes including alcohol, drugs, or any other identifiable causes. The spectrum of non-alcoholic fatty liver disease (NAFLD) extends from steatosis (fatty liver) without inflammation or fibrosis at the most benign end to cirrhosis at the opposite end.

It represents a spectrum of conditions and is generally associated with obesity, diabetes and hypertension.

Nutritional therapy: Dietary treatment is based on the associated illness. Management involves regular physical exercise, weight maintenance with low fat diabetic diet and salt restriction for hypertension. Saturated fats are to be replaced with polyunsaturated or monounsaturated fats in limited quantity.

Acute Hepatitis

Acute hepatitis is usually a self-limiting inflammatory condition. It is most commonly caused by viruses, and can also be caused by various other agents such as alcohol, drugs, or toxins. Alcoholic hepatitis is frequently accompanied by protein-calorie malnutrition, which increase the risk for clinical severity and poor prognosis.

Nutritional therapy: The principles of diet therapy relate to the liver's function in metabolizing each of the nutrients:

1. *Adequate protein:* Protein is essential for liver cell regeneration. It also provides lipotropic agents such as methionine and choline for the conversion of fats to lipoproteins and removal from the liver, thus preventing fatty infiltration. The diet should supply from 1.2 to 1.5 gms/kg.b.wt./day of high-quality protein.
2. *High carbohydrate:* Sufficient available glucose must be provided to restore protective glycogen reserves and meet the energy demands of the disease process. Also, adequate glucose for energy ensure the use of protein for vital tissue regeneration. The diet should supply from 50 to 55% calories from carbohydrate.
3. *Moderate fat:* A moderate amount of fat makes the food more palatable and therefore encourages the anorexic patient to eat. Some easily used fat, such as whole milk, cream, butter, margarine, mayonnaise, and vegetable oil, is beneficial. The diet should supply about 20 to 25% of the total calories/day.
4. *High energy:* From 1.5 times of the total caloric requirement per day are needed to furnish energy demands of the tissue regeneration process, to compensate for losses from fever and debilitation, and to renew strength and recuperative powers.
5. *Meals and feedings:* The problem of supplying a diet adequate to meet the increased nutritive demands for a patient whose illness makes food almost repellent calls for creativity and supportive encouragement. The food may need to be in liquid form at first, using concentrated commercial or blended formulas for frequent feedings. As the patient improves, appetizing and attractive food is needed. Since nutritional therapy is the key to recovery, a major nutrition and nursing responsibility requires devising ways to encourage the increased amounts of food intake needed. The clinical nutritionist and the nurse will work together closely to achieve this goal.

In the recovery stage after the subacute stage when the enzymes begin to fall, a normal diet is recommended the diet should have normal proteins and normal fat content as tolerated.

Cirrhosis

Studies have shown that there is a direct relationship between calorie intake and mortality in patients with cirrhosis.

Mendenhall's analysis

Calorie intake	*Mortality at 6 months*
< 1000 kcal/day	90%
1000 - 2000 kcal/day	50%
> 2000 kcal/day	20%

It shows that mortality decreases with high calorie diet. Malnutrition is common in cirrhosis and severity of liver diseases is correlated with severity of malnutrition, therefore, it is very essential to feed these patients.

Sample diet plan for a child with Hepatitis

Weight = 10 kg
Sex = Male
Food Habit = Non vegetarian

Table 112.9: Sample diet plan

Food groups	*Amount*	*Household measure*
Cereals	200 g	8 chapatis
Pulses	50 g	2 katon cooked dal
Milk	750 ml	3 glass
Meat	1 piece	
Vegetables	200 g	½ k cooked
Fruits	250 g	2 fruits
Fats	40 g	8 tsp
Sugar	30 g	6 tsp
Nutritive value	Normal	Modified
Total calories	1240 kcals	Increased upto 1½ times 1800 kcals
Proteins	22 g	Increased upto 1½ times 33 gms
Fat	25 g	38 gms

Table 112.10: Sample menu

Early morning	1 cup milk 2 biscuits
Breakfast	1 katori porridge with milk with sugar 1 fruit (Pear)
Mid morning	Sprout chat Sprouted dal + cucumber and potatoes
Lunch	1½ katori vegetable khichdi with veg. raita
Mid afternoon	2 rasgulla
Evening	Fruit juice
Dinner	1 katori rice pulao + dal + 1 katori 1 paneer chapati + 1 katori vegetable
Bedtime	Rice kheer

Chronic liver disease may advance to the chronic stage of cirrhosis.

Nutritional therapy: Therapy is usually aimed at correcting fluid and electrolyte problems and providing nutritional support for hepatic repair as much as possible. Nutritional therapy for cirrhosis should include the following principles:

Optimal general nutrition: The remaining overall diet principles outlined for hepatitis are continued for cirrhosis for the same reasons. Kilocalories, carbohydrates, and vitamins are supplied according to individual need and deficiency. Moderate fat is used. Alcohol is strictly forbidden.

1. *Protein according to tolerance:* In the absence of impending hepatic coma, about 1.2 to 1.5 gms/ kg.b.wt./day of protein is needed to correct severe undernutrition, regenerate functional liver tissue, and replenish plasma protein. However, if signs of hepatic coma appear, protein must be adjusted to individual tolerance.
2. Fats should be about 30 to 35% of the total calories preferably derived from fats rich in unsaturated fatty acids with adequate essential fatty acids.
3. 55-60% of energy as complex carbohydrates with low glycemic index (GI), foods rich in soluble fibers, as according to WHO criteria 60-80% of patients with cirrhosis have impaired glucose tolerance.
4. *Low sodium:* Sodium 2-2.5 g/day is permitted, which would be supplied from 5 gms i.e. 1tsp of the common table salt. Sodium is restricted to help reduce fluid retention. If low sodium affects the palatability of food then low sodium salt preparation can also be used.
5. *Texture:* If esophageal varices develop, it may be necessary to give soft foods that are smooth in texture to prevent danger of rupture and hemorrhage, but the presence of esophageal varices is not a contraindication to the use of nasogastric tubes although they should be used with caution in the presence of post-injection sclerotherapy esophageal ulceration.
6. Liberal amounts of vitamins and minerals with an exception in copper, sodium, iron in cases of Wilson's disease, ascites and hemochromatosis respectively.
7. Fluid as per the ascites status has to be restricted.

NUTRITIONAL MANAGEMENT OF COMPLICATION OF LIVER DISEASE

I. Fluid Retention

Nature of disease: Fluid loss and weight change are directly related to sodium balance in patients with portal hypertension related ascites.

Nutrition: In the presence of avid renal retention of sodium, dietary sodium restriction is essential. The patient and the food preparer should be educated about a sodium-restricted diet by a dietitian. Severe sodium-restricted diets (e.g. 500 mg or 22 mmol/day of sodium) are feasible (but not palatable) in an inpatient setting but are unrealistic for outpatients. The dietary sodium restriction that the author recommends for inpatients and outpatients is 2 g/day (88 mmol/day).

Table 112.11: Suggested nutritional management of persistent cholestasis

Clinical impairment	*Management*
Malnutrition resulting from malabsorption of dietary long-chain triglyceride	Replace with dietary formula or supplements containing medium chain triglycerides
Fat soluble vitamin malabsorption	
Vitamin A deficiency Night blindness, thick skin)	Replace with 10,000-15,000 IU/day as Aquasol A (water soluble)
Vitamin E deficiency (Neuromuscular degeneration)	Replace with 50-400 IU/day as oral α-tocopherol
Vitamin D deficiency (Metabolic bone disease)	Replace with 5,000-8,000 IU/day of D2, or 3-5 ug/kg/day of 25-hydro-cholecalciferol
Vitamin K deficiency (Hypoprothrombinemia)	Replace with 2.5 to 5.0 mg every other day as water-soluble derivative or menadione
Micronutrient deficiency	Calcium, phosphate, or zinc supplementation
Deficiency of water-soluble vitamins	Supplement with twice and recommended daily allowance
Retention of biliary constituents such as bile acids and cholesterol (itch or xanthomata)	Administer choleretics
Progressive liver disease	Interim management (control
Portal hypertension (variceal bleeding, ascites, hypersplenism)	bleeding; salt restriction; spironolactone)
End-stage liver disease (liver failure)	Transplantation

Fluid restriction: An indiscriminate fluid restriction in treating the patient with cirrhotic ascites is inappropriate; hypernatremia may result. It is the sodium restriction, not the fluid restriction, that results in weight loss; fluid follows sodium passively. The chronic hyponatremia usually seen in patients with cirrhotic ascites is seldom morbid. Attempts to rapidly correct hyponatremia in this setting can lead to more complications than occur with hypontremia itself. Indiscriminate fluid restriction serves only to alienate patients, nurses and dietitians.

Bed rest: Although it is traditional to order bed rest, there are no controlled trials to support this practice.

II. Hepatic Encephalopathy

Nature of the disease: As cirrhotic changes continue in the liver, the portal blood circulation diminishes and liver functions begin to fail. The normal liver has a major function of removing ammonia from the blood by converting it to urea for excretion. The failing liver can no longer inactivate or detoxify substances or metabolize others. A key factor involved in the progressive disease process is an elevated blood level of ammonia. The resulting hepatic encephalopathy, sometimes called hepatic coma, brings changes in consciousness, behavior, and neurologic status.

Clinical symptoms: Typical response involves disorders of consciousness and alterations in motor function. There is apathy, confusion, inappropriate behavior, and drowsiness, progressing to coma. The speech may be slurred or monotonous. A coarse, flapping tremor is observed in the outstretched hands. The breath may have a fecal odor.

Basic treatment objectives: The fundamental objective of treatment is two-fold:

1. Removal of the sources of excess ammonia; and
2. Provision of nutritional support.

Medical and nutritional therapy are involved. Parenteral fluid and electrolytes are used to restore normal balance. Two drugs may be used to control ammonia-lactulose and neomysin. Lactulose is a nonabsorbable synthetic disaccharide that reduces the absorption of intestinal ammonia. Neomysin is an antibiotic that reduces the population of urea-splitting organism within the bowel that produce ammonia. To stop bleeding into the intestine as another source of intestinal ammonia, a Sengstaken Blakemore tube may be used.

Nutritional therapy: Special parenteral and enteral nutritional support may include use of branched-chain amino acids. These three essential amino acids leucine, isoleucine, and valine are not catabolized by the liver but are taken up by other tissues. Thus they can be metabolized without depending on healthy liver tissue, as is the case with other amino acids. Solutions of these branched-chain amino acids, for example, hepatamine, have therefore been used successfully to maintain adequate nitrogen balance and reduce the encephalopathy.

General nutritional support for hepatic encephalopathy is based on the following principles of dietary management:

1. *Low protein:* Protein intake is reduced as individually necessary to restrict the dietary sources of nitrogen in amino acids. The amount of restriction will vary with the circumstances. The unconscious patient will receive no protein, but the usual amounts given range from 15 to 50 g/day, depending on whether symptoms of ammonia intoxication are severe or mild. A simple method for controlling dietary protein uses a base meal pattern containing approximately 15 g protein, adding small items of protein foods according to the level of protein desired.
2. *Kilocalories and vitamins:* Adequate energy intake is crucial to the patient's recovery, especially through the impact of caloric intake on liver glycogen reserves and their protective role in the healing process. The amounts of kilocalories and vitamins are prescribed according to need. About 2000 kcal/day is needed to prevent tissue catabolism, which would be as source of more amino acids and available nitrogen and urea. Sufficient carbohydrate is essential as the primary energy source, with some fat as tolerated. Vitamin K is usually given parenterally, along with other vitamins and minerals that may be deficient.
3. *Fluid intake:* Fluid intake-output balance is carefully controlled.

Gallbladder Disease

The basic function of the gallbladder is to concentrate bile 5 to 10 fold and store.

Nutritional preventive measure: There is no specific dietary treatment to prevent cholelithiasis in susceptible individuals. Nutritionally related factors include obesity and severe fasting and these should be corrected where possible. In cholecystitis, dietary treatment includes a low fat diet to prevent gallbladder contractions. Two additional modifications usually found in traditional diets for gallbladder disease concern restriction of foods containing cholesterol and foods labelled "gas formers". Neither modification has a valid rationale. The body synthesizes daily several times more cholesterol than is present in an average diet. Thus restriction of dietary cholesterol has little effect in reducing gallstone formation. Total dietary fat reduction is more to the point. As for the use of so-called "gas formers", such as legumes or cabbage or fiber, blanket restriction seems unwarranted, since food tolerances in any circumstances are highly individual.

Acute Cholecystitis

In an acute attack, oral feedings are discontinued. Parenteral nutrition may be indicated if the patient is malnourished and it is anticipated to be NPO for a prolonged period of time. When feedings are resumed, a low fat diet is recommended to decrease gallbladder stimulation. A hydrolyzed low fat formula or an oral diet consisting of 30 to 45 g fat per day can be given. Studies have failed to show a relationship between dietary cholesterol and gallstone formation.

Chronic Cholecystitis

Patients with chronic conditions may require a long-term low fat diet that contains 25% to 30% of total kilocalories as fat. Stricter limitation is undersirable because fat in the intestine is important for some stimulation and drainage of the biliary tract.

The degree of food intolerance varies widely among individuals with gallbladder disorders, but bloating. It is best to determine with the patient any foods that should be eliminated for this reason.

Administration of water-soluble forms of fat soluble vitamins may be of benefit in individuals with chronic gallbladder conditions or in those in whom fat malabsorption is suspected.

Perioperative nutrition: There is a paucity of data evaluating the usefulness of perioperative nutritional support in patients with liver disease. The results of one PRCT suggested that early postoperative enteral feeding may be beneficial in patients undergoing liver transplantaion. Nasojejunal tube feeding started 12 hours after transplant surgery was well tolerated and allowed increased protein and energy intake during the first 4 postoperative days. Early tube feeding was associated with a significant reduction in postoperative viral infections and a trend toward a decrease in bacterial infections. However, these results may be biased, because one third of the patients who entered the study failed to complete their assigned protocol and were not included in the final analysis. Another PRCT found that pretransplant enteral supplementation improved grip strength and other nutritional parameters but did not affect clinical outcome.

One PRCT evaluated the clinical efficacy of perioperative CPN, given as a BCAA-enriched solution for 7 days before and 7 days after hepatectomy for hepatocellular carcinoma. Patients randomized to receive CPN have better postoperative hepatic function and significantly fewer postoperative complications (mostly pulmonary infection and ascites).

NUTRITIONAL ASPECT OF LIVER TRANSPLANTATION

Liver Transplantation

Better outcome is seen in patients with a good pretransplant nutritional status especially so in the survival rate. So all transplant patients should be well-fed in terms of calories and proteins.

Free Radicals and Antioxidants in Liver Diseases

Although the liver is well endowed with endogenous enzymatic antioxidants, it is also the organ with active microsomal and mitochondrial systems that generate oxygen free radicals during normal metabolic processes. When this balance is upset, tissue damage may occur. Free radical injury has been implicated in a variety of hepatic disorders.

Taking these data into account, a new antioxident solution has been developed (the Carolina rinse solution) for liver allograft preservation that contains antioxidants (e.g., Allopurinol, deferosamine and glutathione), compounds to prevent activation of Kupffer cells, and precursors of ATP generation (adenosine, glucose, and fructose). Improved outcome of allografts after liver transplantation with use of this solution has been reported.

Table 112.12: Nutrition care guidelines for liver transplantation

	Pretransplantation	*Immediate post-transplantation First 2 post-transplantation mo*	*Long-term post-transplantation*
Calories	High calorie (basal + 20% or more)	Moderate calorie (basal + 15-30%)	Weight maintenance (basal + 10-20%)
Protein	Moderate protein (1-1.5 g/kg/day-minimize needed for restriction)	High protein (1.2-1.75 g/kg/day)	Moderate protein (1g/kg/day)
Fat	As needed	20-30% of non-protein calories	Low fat (< 30% of calories)
Carbohydrate	High carbohydrate (complex and simple)	70% of non-protein calorie	Reduced simple carbohydrate
Sodium	2-4 g/day (as indicated)	2-4 g/day (as indicated)	2-4 g/day (as indicated)
Fluid	Restrict to 1000-1500 mL/day (as indicated)		As needed 1200-1500 mg/day
Calcium	800-1200 mg/day	800-1200 mg/day	Daily multivitamin/mineral
Vitamins	Daily multivitamin/mineral supplement to RDA levels; additional water and fat soluble vitamins as indicated	Daily multivitamin/ mineral supplement to RDA levels; additional water and fat-soluble vitamins as indicated	Supplement to RDA levels for first post-transplant year

Table 112.13: Medications commonly used after liver transplantation

Immunosuppressant drug	*Possible nutrition side-effects*	*Proposed nutrition therapy*
Azathioprine	Macrocytic anemia	Folate supplements
	Mouth sores	Soft foods if needed
	Nausea, vomiting, diarrhoea, anorexia, sore throat, stomach pain, decreased taste acuity	Adjust food/meals as needed, monitor intake
Antithymocyte globulin	Nausea, vomiting	Adjust food/meals as needed,monitor intake
Cyclosporine	Sodium retention	Decrease sodium intake
	Hyperkalemia	Decrease potassium intake
	Hyperlipidemia	Limit fat and simple carbohydrate intake
	Hyperglycemia	Decrease simple carbohydrate intake
	Decreased serum magnesium level	Increase magnesium intake; give magnesium supplement
	Nausea, vomiting	Adjust food/meals as needed; monitor intake
Glucocorticoids	Sodium retention	Decrease sodium intake
	Hyperglycemia	Decrease simple carbohydrate intake
	Hyperlipidemia	Limit fat and simple carbohydrate intake
	False hunger	Avoid overheating
	Protein wasting with high doses	Increase protein intake
	Decreased absorption of calcium and phosphorus	Increase calcium and phosphorus intake; give supplement as needed
Muromonab-CD3	Nausea, vomiting, anorexia	Adjust food/meals as needed; monitor intake
Mycophenolate mofetil	GL symptoms, nausea, vomiting diarrhoea	Adjust food/meals as needed; monitor intake
Sirolimus	Possible hyperglycemia	Decrease simple carbohydrate intake
	Possible GL symptoms	Adjust food/meals as needed; monitor intake
	Hyperlipidemia	Limit fat and simple carbohydrate intake
Tacrolimus	Hypertension	Adjust food/meals as needed; monitor intake
	Hyperglycemia	Decrease simple carbohydrate intake
	Hyperkalemia	Decrease potassium intake
	Nausea, vomiting	Adjust food/meals as needed; monitor intake
	GL symptoms (diarrhoea)	Adjust food/meals as needed; monitor intake
15-Deoxysperagualin	GL symptoms	Adjust food/meals as needed; monitor intake

Oxidative stress has been demonstrated in alcohol-induced liver injury because of altered $NADH/NAD^+$ ratios in hepatocytes that favor generation of free radicals from mitochondria and microsomal P_{450} systems and alter ferritin chelation of iron.

The possible use of antioxidant therapy in alcoholic liver disease now is being studied; however, Lieber's group has provided data in nonhuman primates, cautioning against the use of beta carotene in this condition.

Copper and iron storage diseases are strongly linked to oxidant damage of hepatocytes and mitochondria. In Wilson's disease livers removed at liver transplantation, in vivo evidence of oxidant injury and reduced concentrations of vitamin E and glutathione have been demonstrated. The possible use of antioxidants as adjunct therapy, in addition to reducing the iron or copper burden in these disorders, needs investigation. In addition, the possible targeting of antioxidants to the mitochondria should be explored. Recently, an antioxidant "cocktail" (including vitamin E, selenium, deferoxamine, prostaglandin E, and N-acetyl cysteine) apparently has reversed the previously fatal liver failure of neonatal iron storage disease in at least eight infants. Whether such an approach could prove useful in acute iron ingestions in young children awaits trials. Also use of n-acetyl cysteine as an antioxidant in non-paracetamol induced acute liver failure is being studied.

Finally, in cholestatic liver disorders, possible prooxidant compounds are retained in the hepatocyte, such as copper and hydrophobic bile acids. These bile acids seem to be mitochondrial toxins, causing morphologic swelling of mitochondria, inhibition of normal respiration and electron flow through the respiratory chain, and increased H_2O_2 generation by mitochondria. The final consequences of bile acid toxicity consist of ATP depletion, increased intracellular cytosolic calcium levels, protease activation, and cell necrosis. Sokol and co-workers showed that *in vitro* anti oxidants (e.g. SOD catalase, deferoxamine, and alpha tocopherol) protect the isolated hepatocyte from hydrophobic bile acid toxicity. In addition vitamin E treatment to the intact rat prevents hepatic injury and oxidant damage to hepatic mitochondria after the intravenous infusion of taurochenodeoxycholic acid).

The possible role of antioxidant therapy in cholestasis is under investigation. It should be pointed out that the fat malabsorption cosequent to cholestasis leads to malabsorption and deficiency of vitamin E, betacarotene and selenium. This perhaps sensitizes the hepatocyte to oxidative injury.

Galactosemia

This genetic disease, is caused by a missing cell enzyme, *galactose-1 phosphate uridyl transferase* or *galactokinase* which affects carbohydrate metabolism. The missing enzyme controls the conversion of galactose, which is derived from lactose, to glucose. Milk, the infant's first food, contains a large amount of the precursor lactose (milk sugar). After galactose is initially combined with phosphate to begin the metabolic conversion to glucose, it cannot proceed further in the galactosemic infant. Galactose rapidly accumulates in the blood and in various body tissues.

Nutritional therapy is in the form of galactose-free diet. The main indirect source of dietary galactose is the lactose in milk. Therefore all forms of milk and lactose must be removed from the diet. In this instance a galactose free diet is used. Any needed amount of galactose for certain body structures can be synthesized by the body. A soy-base formula, is used. Breast-feeding, of course, cannot be used. Later, as solid foods are added to the infant's diet at about 6 months of age, careful attention must be given to avoiding lactose from other food sources. Parents quickly learn to check labels carefully on all commercial products to detect any lactose or lactose-containing substances.

Liver function improves following exclusion of galactose from the diet unless liver failure or cirrhosis has developed. Galactose elimination is lifelong. The long-term outcome is disappointing. Learning difficulties and growth disturbance are described, and 75% of girls develop ovarian failure. Detection of galactosemia in a neonatal screening program will lead to early detection except for infants who present with fulminant hepatitis. Antenatal diagnosis is possible by chorionic villus sampling.

Hereditary Tyrosinaemia

This autosomal recessive disorder is due to lack of the enzyme fumaryl acetoacetate hydrolase, an enzyme that catalyses the last step of tyrosine degradation. Abnormal metabolites of tyrosine accumulate, which are toxic to both liver and kidney. The main clinical features are progressive live disease and renal tubular abnormalities.

The acute type, usually seen in early infancy, results in death from hepatic failure within the first year of life. The chronic form leads to growth retardation, cirrhosis, severe hypophosphatemic rickets, renal tubular defects and a derangement of tyrosine metabolism with hyperaminoacidaemia. Hepatocellular carcinoma is a complication occurring in over 40% of patients.

The chronic type responds to dietary avoidance of aromatic amino acids and methionine but this does not prevent the liver disease or the appearance of hepatocellular carcinoma. Without liver transplantation death occurs within the first decade of life.

Diagnosis is confirmed by the presence of elevated plasma and urinary tyrosine, phenylalanine and methionine levels and increased levels of succinyl acetone in the urine.

Liver transplantation for both acute and chronic disease can be successful and virtually corrects the metabolic disease. A mild metabolic abnormality persists probably due to continued abnormal renal metabolism but this is not a clinical problem. Because of the high risk of hepatocellular carcinoma with increasing age, liver transplantation should be seriously considered for children aged more than 2 years.

Dietary treatment recommended for tyrosinemia is low phenylalanine and tyrosine diet.

Table 112.14: Phenylalanine and tyrosine content in food items

Eat in moderation		*Avoid*		*Foods allowed freely*	
Beans	Orange	Meat	Chicken	Sugar	Spices
Beetroot	Pineapple	Lamb	Fish	Jam	Fruit juice
Cabbage	Apple	Eggs	Cheese	Squash	Soda
Cauliflower	Melon	Wheat	Wheat products	Cornflour	Custard
Carrot	Grapes	Spinach	Soya	Sago	Oils
Mushroom	Peach	Pulses	Dry fruits	Vinegar	
Cucumber	Pear	Jelly	Ice cream		
Onion	Plum				
Radish	Banana				
Tomato	Turnip				
Milk	Potato				
Corn/wheat	Oats				
Rice	Peas				
Chocolate (milk)					

Hereditary Fructose Intolerance

This autosomal recessive condition is caused by mutations in the gene for aldolase B on chromosome 9[1]. Deficiency of this enzyme impairs the cleavage of fructose 1-phosphate in liver, renal cortex and intestinal epithelium. Exposure to fructose induces cytoplasmic accumulation of fructose 1-phosphate and hence fructose intoxication.

The acute syndrome is marked by abdominal pain, vomiting and hypoglycemia. The chronic syndrome is one of severe metabolic derangement with failure to thrive, vomiting, hepatomegaly and liver and renal tubular dysfunction. Fructosemia, fructosuria and hypophosphatemia are features. Diagnosis is confirmed by the intravenous fructose tolerance test or by direct assay of fructaldolase activities in tissue biopsy samples. Hepatic histology shows similar findings to galactosemia with the ultimate development of cirrhosis.

Treatment is by a diet without sucrose and fructose. Sometimes the symptoms persist in older children and are marked by growth retardation when even more strict fructose restriction may be necessary.

Older children learn to avoid fructose and sucrose and isolated hepatomegaly may be the only abnormality.

Familial Hypercholesterolaemia

This is an autosomal dominant disease due to absence of a gene which codes for the LDL receptor on cell membranes. The liver contains 60% of such receptors. Sufferers have increased plasma total cholesterol and LDL from birth, cutaneous xanthomas develop and most homozygotes die from coronary artery disease before the age of 30.

Hypercholesterolaemia is controlled by reduction in dietary saturated fats and administration of bile acid sequestrants such as cholestyramine. One child has been successfully treated by simultaneous heart transplant for the coronary disease and liver transplant to provide low-density lipoprotein receptors. Follow-up showed decrease in LDL and plasma cholesterol.

Hepatic Porphyrias

Porphyrias are caused by defects in the biosynthesis of ham. Broadly they are classified as hepatic or erythropoietic depending on the major site in which there is excess production of porphyrin or its precursors. Lack of ham results in increased ALA and PBG production because of greater ALA-synthetase activity. The major symptoms and signs are from involvement of the skin and/or neurological system.

The acute hepatic porphyrias include acute intermittent porphyria, hereditary coporphyria and variegate porphyria, which have autosomal dominant inheritance. All are marked by neuropsychiatric attacks with vomiting, abdominal colic, constipation and peripheral neuropathy. All are exacerbated by countless enzyme-inducing drugs including barbiturates, sulphonamides, oestrogens, oral contraceptives, griseofulvin, chloroquine and possibly alcohol.

Hormones are impotrant inducers and women develop attacks in pregnancy and pre-mensturually.

During the attacks, large amounts of the colorless porphyrin precursors, porphobilinogen and delta aminolaevulinic acid (ALA), are excreted in the urine. In all three, an acute attack is treated by glucose loading. Infusions of haematin which repress or inhibit hepatic ALA synthetase may also be valuable.

Ham arginate which suppresses overproduction of ham precursors and improves hepatic oxidative metabolism may be useful.

The fourth type of hepatic porphyria, *porphyric cutanea tarda*, is probably hereditary and may be associated with hepatocellular disease. It is not exacerbated by barbiturates and acute neurological attacks are not seen.

Hepatocellular carcinoma occurs in 8% during long-term follow-up.

Glycogen Storage Disease

Salient Features

- Stored sugar or glycogen cannot be accessed.
- Infants cannot go for longer than 3-4 hours without feeding.
- After 3-4 hours, hypoglycemia occurs.
- Glycogen cannot be broken down but just accumulates in the liver, causing liver enlargement.

Some GSD types cannot be treated, while others are relatively easy to control through symptom management. In more severe cases, receiving an organ transplant is the only option. In the most severe cases, there are no available treatments and the victim dies within the first few years of life.

Of the treatable types of GSD, many are treated by manipulating the diet. The key to managing GSD I is to maintain consistent levels of blood glucose through a combination of nocturnal intragastric feeding (usually for infants and children), frequent high-carbohydrate meals during the day, and regular oral doses of cornstarch (people over age 2). Juvenile and adult forms of GSD II can be managed somewhat by a high protein diet, which also helps in cases of GSD III, GSD VI and GSD IX. GSD V and GSD VII can also be managed with a high protein diet and by avoiding strenuous exercise. Overnight continuous gastric high-carbohydrate feedings; frequent daytime feedings with energy distributed as 65% carbohydrate, 10% to 15% protein, and 25% fat; and supplements of uncooked cornstarch. In GSD III, though glycogenolysis is impeded, gluconeogenesis is enhanced to help maintain endogenous glucose production. In contrast to treatment for GSD I, advocated treatment for GSD III comprises frequent high-protein feedings during the day and a high-protein snack at night; energy is distributed as 45% carbohydrate, 25% protein, and 30% fat. Patients with GSD IV, VI and IX have benefited from high-protein diets similar to that recommended for patients with GSD III.

Table 112.15: The recommended distribution of calories in GSD

	GSD-I	*GSD-II*
Protein	10-15	25%
Carbohydrate	65	45%
Fat	25	30%

Uncooked cornstarch is a complex carbohydrate that provides a slow and continuous glucose source and may delay gastric emptying. Uncooked cornstarch controlled the glucose shifts, resolved most of the symptoms, allowed bolus feedings, and enhanced weight gain in these children.

For GSD cases in which dietary therapy is ineffective, organ transplantation may be the only viable alternative. Liver transplants have been effective in reversing the symptoms of GSD IV.

Prognosis

People with well-managed, treatable types of GSD can lead long, relatively normal lives. This goal is accomplished with the milder types of GSD, such as types VI, IX and X. As the GSD type becomes more severe, a greater level of vigilance against infections and other complications is required.

Wilson's Disease

Normal daily dietary intake of copper is 4 mg of which 2 mg is absorbed and excreted in bile, so that body maintains balance. In Wilson disease only 0.2 to 0.4 mg can be excreted in bile with 1 mg in the urine so that a positive copper balance develops. Diet in Wilson's disease should be of low copper.

Indian Childhood Cirrhosis (ICC)

ICC, though rare these days, is strongly associated with habit of storage and or boiling of milk in copper or brass utensils. Stoppage of use of copper and brass utensils and low copper diet are recommended apart from standard therapy.

Table 112.17: Copper content of diet

> 0.1 mg/portion	*0.1 portion*
High to moderate copper-rich food	Commonly use low copper food
Avoid	Eat
All organ meal	Beef, cheese, paneers, eggs, all dairy products
Soya milks, cocoa soyabeans, lentils and pulses, wheat germ, bran, mushroom	Bread, pastas, wheat flour, all other vegetables except mushrooms all other dried fruits
Dried fruits–raisins, dates, prunes	Lemonade
Mango, pineapple, papaya	Jams, gellies, candies, made from allowed fruits
Mineral water, alcohol chocolates	

Medium-Chain Triglycerides (MCTs)

Medium-chain triglycerides (MCTs) contain only fatty acids with 6-12 carbon atoms. They are rare in nature. They have been fractionated from coconut oil. They are composed of:

75% caprylic acid (8 C)
22-23% caprylic acid (10 C)
1% caprylic acid (6 C)
1% caprylic acid (12 C)

Table 112.16: Summary of various types of GSD with manifestations

Name	*Affected organs system*	*Manifestations*
Type O	Liver, muscle	Enlarged liver with accumulation of fat inside the liver cells (fatty liver); episodes of low blood sugar levels (hypoglycemia) when fasting
von Gierke's disease (Type IA)	Liver, kidney	Enlarged liver and kidney; slowed growth; very low blood sugar levels abnormally high levels of acid, fats, and uric acid in blood
Type IB	Liver, white blood cells	Same as in von Gierke's disease but may be less severe; low white blood cell count; recurring mouth and intestinal infections or Crohn's disease
Pompe's disease (Type II)	All organs	Enlarged liver and heart, muscle weakness
Forbes' disease (Type III)	Liver, muscle, heart, white blood cells	Enlarged liver or cirrhosis; low blood sugar levels, muscle damage and heart damage in some people
Andersen's disease (Type IV)	Liver, muscle, most tissues	Cirrhosis in juvenile type; muscle damage and heart failure in adult (late-onset) type
McArdle disease (Type V)	Muscle	Muscle cramps or weakness during physical activity
Hers' disease (Type VI)	Liver	Enlarged liver; episodes of low blood sugar when fasting; often no symptoms
Tarui' disease (Type VII)	Skeletal muscle, red blood cells	Muscle cramps during physical activity; red blood cell destruction (hemolysis)

Traces of other fatty acids such as linoleic, stearic, and palmitic acids are also present.

Importance of MCTs

Since MCTs are liquid at room temperature, they are more soluble in water than natural triglycerides. MCTs are easily digested by pancreatic lipase and do not require bile salts for absorption. Once absorbed, they enter the portal vein and into the liver as fatty acids and do not go through the lacteal system.

Synthetic MCTs are also popular in the treatment of intestinal diseases, especially malabsorption such as steatorrhea, sprue and pancreatic insufficiency. They are a ready source of energy and prevent starvation from lack of absorbed calories.

Uses of MCTs include:

1. When pancreatic enzymes and/or bile salts are either absent or present in very small amounts.
2. When the lymphatic system has an obstruction especially in the branches leaving the intestinal walls.
3. When the intestinal mucosa is infective.

Problems of MCT Therapy

Because MCTs are easily absorbed, any excessive consumption forces their increased degradation. As a result, formation of acetone, acetoacetic acid and hydroxbutyric acid may increase and acidosis may occur. Patients susceptible to hepatic encephalopathy may react adversely to MCTs that reach the liver directly from the gut.

All vitamins especially the B-complex vitamins should be given in plenty. Sodium may be restricted if swelling is seen. There are restrictions on spices, chillies and oily preparations.

Nutrients and Nutriceuticals

The importance of the liver in the metabolism of ingested nutrients and drugs suggests that hepatic function can be influenced by dietary manipulations. Less obvious is the potential role of specific nutrients in ameliorating the natural history of various chronic liver diseases or toxic exposures. Preliminary evidence supports the use of several nutriceutical agents in the treatment of liver diseases for which conventional therapies are limited.

Silymarin

Silymarin is derived from the seeds of Sily-bum marianum (milk thistle). The extract contains a group of chemical compounds in the flavonoid family. There is a long history of its use in traditional medical systems for treatment of liver disease and manifestations of portal hypertension.

The hepatoprotective effects of silymarin have been demonstrated in animal studies and in cell culture, the principal mechanism of which appears to be the prevention of lipid peroxidation. A randomized trial in patients with alcoholic cirrhosis reported no benefit with regard to either clinical course of the disease of survival of patients over 3 years. The authors of this trial noted the possibility of benefit in patients with hepatitis C, as well as the possibility that the trial was underpowered to detect a clinically meaningful survival benefit.

Cell culture study suggests that silymarin acts independently of the cytochrome P-450 enzyme system, with free radical scavenging the dominant action accounting for hepatoprotection. The possibility of toxic effects on the hepatocyte membrane and cytoskeleton is suggested and requires further investigation.

Antifibrotic effects of silymarin have been shown in a rat model suggesting a role in cirrhosis.

Evidence supporting a role for silymarin in viral hepatitis, drug-induced and toxin-induced hepatitis, and alcoholic liver disease has been summarized. To date, there is no evidence of toxicity in humans. Well-controlled studies of silymarin are small and the populations studied heterogeneous. The historical experience and promising results from studies to date indicate a need for additional well-controlled trials.

Branched-Chain Amino Acids

Impairment in amino acid metabolism in cirrhosis results in accumulation of aromatic ring amino acids and depletion of branched chain amino acids. An imbalance in the amino acid distribution has been implicated in the development of hepatic encephalopathy.

Impairment in amino acid metabolism in cirrhosis results in accumulation of aromatic ring amino acids and depletion of branched-chain amino acids. An imbalance in the amino acid distribution has been implicated in the development of hepatic encephalopathy. There is preliminary evidence that supplementation with branched-chain amino acids benefits patients with chronic hepatic encephalopathy.

Branched-Chain Ketoacids

The ketoacid analogues of branched-chain amino acids offer the putative advantage of providing a substrate for protein synthesis devoid of the amine group. Metabolic advantages of such preparations have been well described, but the evidence of clinical benefit in advanced liver disease is limited. Use of branched-chain ketoacids in patients intolerant of standard protein is reasonable in light of available evidence, although additional study of this intervention is needed.

Vegetable Protein

Benefits from a diet deriving protein from plant sources have been reported to reduce the incidence of hepatic encephalopathy in patients with cirrhosis. Such diets often are poorly tolerated because of their high fiber and high total food volume. To the extent that protein derived from plant sources is tolerated by individual patients, its use is reasonable.

Glutamine

Glutamine is a non-essential amino acid. Because of abnormal intestinal permeability, endotoxemia in cirrhosis accelerates turnover of skeletal muscle. Glutamine is the predominant amino acid in muscle, and its consumption in cirrhosis may result in the need for dietary replacement. Although plausible, the benefits of glutamine supplementation are unproved.

Amino Acids

Cysteine and tyrosine are no essential amino acids the synthesis of which hepatocytes is impaired in chronic liver disease. Inclusion of these amino acids in the diet may become essential when liver disease is advanced.

Vitamins and Trace Elements

Reduction in the serum levels of zinc and selenium attributable to chronic liver disease has been reported in patients with chronic hepatitis C, with or without cirrhosis. Zinc supplementation has been shown to improve hepatic encephalopathy in alcoholic patients. Zinc is also recommended in few subsets of Wilson's disease. Thiamine supplementation is indicated in all alcoholic patients.

Use of a multivitamin supplement is advocated for all patients with chronic liver disease.

KEY LEARNING POINTS

- Malnutrition is a nearly universal component of chronic liver disease in children.
- Etiology is multi-factorial so that careful nutritional assessment, identification of important risk factors, and specific deficiency states and/or excessive losses are essential to good management and for achievement of nutritional rehabilitation.
- Attention to the limited ability of the child with chronic liver disease to withstand a prolonged fast, plus alleviation and treatment of ascites or infection, which may increase energy expenditure or precipitate nutritional deficiencies, are essential.
- The increased success of programs for pediatric liver transplantation has demonstrated the importance of good nutritional rehabilitation prior to transplantation: the pretransplant nutritional status appears to impact on postoperative morbidity, expense, time in hospital and most importantly, survival.

FURTHER READINGS

1. Fan ST, Lo CM, Lai ECS, *et al.* J. Perioperative nutritional support in patients undergoing hepatectomy for hepatocellular carcinoma. *N Eng J Med* 1994; 331:1547-1548.
2. Gupte S, Anderson RA. Pediatric hepatology. In: Gupte S (ed) *The Short Textbook of Pediatrics*, 11th edn. New Delhi: Jaypee 2008:365-402.
3. Hasse JM, Blue LS, Liepa GU, *et al.* Early enteral nutrition support in patients undergoing liver transplantation. *J Parenteral Nutr* 1995; 19: 437-438.
4. Le Cornu KA, McKiernan FJ, Kapadia SA, Neuberger JM. A prospective randomized study of preoperative nutritional supplementation in patients awaiting elective orthotopic liver transplantation. *Transplantation* 2000; 69:1364-1371.
5. Nair S, Mason A, Eason J, Loss G, Perrillo RP. Is obesity an independent risk factor for hepatocellular carcinoma in cirrhosis. *Hepatology* 2002;36:150-155.
6. Nair S, Verma S, Thuluvath PJ. Obesity and its effect on survival in patients undergoing orthotopic liver transplantation in the United States. *Hepatology* 2002;35:105-109.
7. Poonawala A, Nair SP, Thuluvath PJ. Prevalence of obesity and diabetes in patients with cryptogenic cirrhosis: A case-control study. *Hepatology* 2000;32:689-692.
8. Ratziu V, Giral P, Charlotte F, *et al.* Liver fibrosis in overweight patients. *Gastroenterology* 2000;118:1117-23.
9. Ratziu V, Bonyhay L, Di Martino V, *et al.* Survival, liver failure, and hepatocellular carcinoma in obesity related cryptogenic cirrhosis. *Hepatology* 2002;36:150-155.
10. Sharma R. *Diet Management*, 3rd edn. New Delhi: Elsevier 1995: 21-23.
11. Weber FL, Bagby BS, Licate L, Kelsen SG. Effects of branched-chain amino acids on nitrogen metabolism in patients with cirrhosis. *Hepatology* 1990:11:1942-950.

113 Nutritional Support in Diarrhea

Satish K Tiwari • Akash Banga

INTRODUCTION

Diarrhea is defined as the passage of loose, liquid or watery stools, usually more than three times a day. However, more than any absolute number, it is a recent change in the established frequency and consistency of stools which is more important. The recent increase in stool volume may also be significant.

Acute diarrhea is defined by WHO/UNICEF as a diarrheal episode of sudden onset which usually lasts for 3 to 7 days but may last upto 10 to 14 days. An acute diarrhea is almost always infectious in origin in children. In India, rotavirus and enterotoxigenic E. coli account for as many as about half of these episodes.

A diarrhea which starts as an acute episode, is presumably infectious in origin, and lasts at least 14 days is said to be a *persistent diarrhea*. Thus, this definition excludes specific conditions like biochemical, congenital or metabolic disorders and mainly includes persistent infections and acquired malabsorptions. About 3-12% of the acute episodes are known to last beyond 14 days.

THE DIARRHEA MENACE

Diarrhea is one of the most common causes of mortality and morbidity in childhood. About 40% of the global *mortality* due to diarrhea is contributed only by the South-East Asia. In the tropical belt, as many as, 15 to 40% of all deaths among the children below 5 years of age are diarrhea-related. The total *morbidity* of a child due to diarrhea is as high as one-third of the first two years of life. Overall, children are ill with diarrhea for 10-20% of their first 3 years of life.

Even from public health perspective, diarrheal diseases are a major problem especially in the under 5 years of age. In health institutions, upto a third of total pediatric admissions are due to diarrheal diseases and upto 17% of all deaths in indoor pediatric patients are diarrhea related.

WHY IS NUTRITIONAL SUPPORT IMPORTANT?

Inadequate nutrition is leading cause of diarrhea related malnutrition and subsequent mortality and morbidity. The *modus operandi,* in which diarrhea causes malnutrition is multifactorial. The main mechanisms are as follows:

1. Decreased appetite leading to an overall decrease in the food intake.
2. Loss of considerable quantity of macro- and micro-nutrients in the diarrheal stools due to the impairment in the intestinal absorption.
3. Increased catabolism owing to the infection.
4. Decreased or faulty feeding by the parents during the illness due to various misconceptions.
5. Increased severity of diarrhea due to the intraluminal osmotic movement of water owing to the transient malabsorption of carbohydrate (mainly disaccharides) and the consequent increased intraluminal osmotic load. This disaccharide malabsorption is transient, and under no circumstances, warrants discontinuation of feeding. In fact, continued feeding is known to hasten recovery from diarrhea as discussed in the next section.

Diarrhea and malnutrition thus make a dreaded combination. Malnutrition is a risk factor for development of diarrhea and each diarrheal episode further contributes to the existing malnutrition, thus perpetuating the notorious "diarrhea-malnutrition-diarrhea" vicious cycle. Association of malnutrition further increases the risk of mortality and morbidity due to diarrhea. The key factor in breaking this vicious cycle is prevention of diarrhea in a malnourished child—mainly through improved personal hygiene to prevent the fecal-oral transmission; and even more importantly, prevention of malnutrition in a child with diarrhea. This stresses the importance of nutritional support in the child suffering from diarrhea. Various WHO communications have time and again emphasized the importance of nutritional support in diarrhea through the three "F" rules of case management of diarrhea at home, viz:

a. **Fluid intake:** To be maintained and increased.
b. **Feeding:** To be continued.
c. **Follow up:** Explaining the danger signs when to return back immediately and telling the parents when to bring the child back for a routine follow up.

Thus, feeding and nutritional support in diarrhea gain prime importance, especially in a developing nation like India where the already prevalent burden of both malnutrition and diarrheal diseases is large and can further increase due to their coexistence as well as other socio-economic factors like poverty, illiteracy, superstitions, unemployment, poor sanitation, poor personal hygiene, etc. This article focuses on the feeding and nutritional management in acute and persistent diarrhea. Dehydration and fluid therapy including oral rehydration therapy are beyond the scope of this article.

NUTRITIONAL MANAGEMENT IN ACUTE DIARRHEA

The mainstay of nutritional management in an acute diarrhea is continuing feeding which is both quantitatively as well as qualitatively adequate, while the innate immunity and defense mechanisms combat the self-limiting acute diarrheal episode. The feeding recommendations for acute diarrhea are summarized in Table 113.1.

I. Breastfed Infants

Breastfeeding must be continued without any interruptions even during rehydration therapy with ORS. The child should be breastfed *as often as he/she wants, day and night.* The concern about the transient lactose intolerance being significant enough to discontinue feeding is completely misplaced. Continuation of breastfeeding helps in various ways as follows:

- Presence of nutrients in the gut is known to promote absorption of sodium and water and hastens epithelial recovery due to a rapid cell turnover and renewal of intestinal lining. This, in itself, will take care of the transient disaccharide intolerance.
- Continued breastfeeding helps in maintenance of lactation through the prolactin reflex due to the continued stimulation of sensory receptors in and around nipple while suckling and thus prevents future risks of malnutrition due to "not enough milk".
- The anti-infective properties of breast milk may, in fact, shorten the actual duration of symptoms in a diarrheal episode.
- It ensures a continued supply of essential nutrients and thus replaces, at least partly, the nutrients lost in diarrheal stools.
- It acts as a cheap, effective and quality source of substrates for production of calories to combat the catabolic state.
- Infants who are breastfed during acute diarrhea have been shown to have a better weight gain and rarely progress to have persistent diarrhea.
- Breastfeeding also helps in maintaining the hydration. Withdrawal of breastfeeding is known to be associated with a 5 times higher risk of dehydration compared to continuing it.

II. Non-breastfed infants

This distinct group includes young infants who receive their chief nutrition intake from cow's milk or other animal milk or milk prepared from an infant milk formula and who are not yet receiving solid or semisolid complementary foods. Though in past, there was a school of thought that the lactose containing milk should be partially diluted or eliminated from the diet for the first 24 hours of treatment, this is no more recommended. The present recommendations advocate that all those infants whose only nutrition is through animal or formula milk should be given full strength milk without dilution as soon as dehydration is corrected.

Time to Say "Good-bye" to Animal Milk

There are no advantages of animal milk except that it provides vitamin B_{12} and calcium especially in vegetarians. In fact there are many disadvantages of animal milk, like:

- It can result in milk protein allergy.
- Micro-hemorrhages or GIT bleeds increases prevalence and severity of iron deficiency anemia.
- It can result in constipation.

Hence, an episode of diarrhea is probably the right time to say "good-bye" to animal milk. In place of milk, curd or

Table 113.1: Feeding during acute diarrhea

State of hydration and feeding pattern	*Recommended schedule of feeding*
During rehydration phase	
• Breast-fed infants	• Continue breastfeeding
• Non-breastfed infants	• Should be preferably given only ORS till rehydrated. Animal milk/food should be offered if rehydration takes longer than 4 hours
• Severely malnourished children	• Offer some food as soon as possible along with ORS (ReSoMal)
After rehydration phase	
• Breast-fed infants	• Breastfeed more frequently
• Non-breastfed infants	• Offer undiluted animal milk/formula as before
• Older children	• In addition to breastfeeds, give energy rich foods (thick preparations of staple food with extra vegetable oil/animal fats), foods rich in potassium (legumes, banana) and carotene (dark green leafy vegetables, carrots, pumpkin)

butter milk may be used which has many advantages like:

a. Curd may be more palatable and acceptable to the children especially in form of 'lassi'.
b. It can be used in cases of lactose intolerance and other cases of diarrhea.
c. It provides the advantage of lactobacillus i.e. probiotics.
d. It avoids the use of bottle (a potent "baby killer instrument" in any developing country), which can lead to development of "bottle baby disease" (diarrhea, dehydration and malnutrition which is the result of unsafe bottle feeding).

III. Older Infants and Children

Infants more than 6 months of age who are receiving solid or semisolid complementary foods in addition to breast milk and/or animal milk have a low load of lactose in their diet. They are less affected with the transient lactose intolerance than the young infants. They often derive a large part of their calorie intake through non-milk diet. Whatever slight amount of lactose is present in such mixed diet, is shown to be well-tolerated even by known lactose intolerant children. In a randomized controlled trial of 87 children between 5 to 36 months of age, such mixed diet was proven to have a clinical outcome which is even better than that seen with the artificial lactose-free soy-protein isolate formula available commercially, both in terms of duration of diarrhea as well as the stool output on the first day of diarrhea. Further, during an episode of acute diarrhea, as much as 80-95% of carbohydrates, 70% of fats, and 75% of nitrogen has been shown to be actually absorbed from mixed diets based on common foods, and hence, a significant nutritional advantage is obtained from continued feeding.

For these reasons, routine lactose-free feeding is not required in acute diarrhea even when reducing substances are detected in stools because lactose malabsorption needing dietary modification is very uncommon in acute diarrhea. In very rare circumstances, this may be needed where the diarrhea persists beyond 8-10 days with progressive weight loss and more than 1% reducing substances are found in stools.

In all other circumstances, routine complementary foods without any dietary modifications are recommended. The general principles while choosing, preparing and feeding the complementary foods during diarrhea remains the same as in any other child.

- If a child more than 6 months of age has not yet started receiving complementary foods, instead of waiting for the diarrheal episode to get cured, the opportunity should be grabbed to start quality complementary food.
- *Amount and frequency of feeding* should be tailor-made to the age of the child. The following recommendations from the Government of India's Integrated Management of Neonatal and Childhood Illness (IMNCI) program (modified from UNICEF's IMCI program) can be used for approximating the minimum amount of serving at each feeding and frequency of feeding in a day. If a child wants more, it should never be denied. Breastfeeding must be continued in addition.
  - Age 6 months upto 12 months:
    - ✦ At least 3 times a day if breastfed and at least 5 times a day if not.
    - ✦ At least one katori serving at a time.
  - Age 12 months upto 2 years:
    - ✦ At least 5 times a day whether breastfed or not.
    - ✦ At least one and a half katori serving at a time.
  - Age 2 years and beyond:
    - ✦ At least 3 meals and at least 2 snacks in between the meals per day.
- *Common foods* that can be given during diarrhea include the following:
  - Cooked rice, milk and sugar (Kheer).
  - At least one and a half katori serving at a time. Cooked rice and lentils (Daal rice/Khichri).
  - Ground rice, milk and sugar (Phirni).
  - Ground rice and black gram (Idli).
  - Broken wheat, milk and sugar (Dalia).
  - Wheat flour, Bengal gram flour and sugar (Panjiri).
  - Wheat roti (Chapati)/ Bread mixed in thick dal/milk/ gravy.
  - Semolina, milk and sugar (Suji kheer).
  - Semolina, Bengal gram flour and vegetables (Uppuma).

It may be remembered that this list can very well be modified according to the local availability, acceptability and affordability issues. Also, wherever possible, initial roasting in oil/ghee or adding extra oil/ghee/sugar improves the calorie content. Cooked vegetables and fresh fruits should be added wherever possible to improve the micro-nutrient intake.

Use of Fruits

Use of fruits provides some amount of minerals and vitamins. There is also social and customary acceptance to fruits in any society. A locally available, culturally acceptable, cheap, low fiber containing seasonal fruit may be added to the diet of the child. Fruits like banana also act as binding agent and, hence, may be useful, especially in persistent and non-infective diarrhea.

Nutritional Management in Persistent Diarrhea

Dietary therapy is the cornerstone of treatment of persistent diarrhea as it is the most important, feasible and cost-effective method of treating a persistent diarrhea. Breastfeeding must be continued. As many as 70% cases, of persistent diarrhea can be adequately managed at home. However, if after few days of domiciliary therapy, there is no improvement, the child should be hospitalized. Other indications where hospitalization should be considered from the beginning are:

- Age less than 4 months and not breastfed.
- Presence of dehydration.
- Severe malnutrition.
- Proven or suspected systemic infection.

Various feeding recommendations for dietary management of persistent diarrhea can be described separately according to the age of the child.

I. Feeding in Infants Aged Less than 6 Months

Persistent diarrhea is quite rare in breastfed infants below 6 months. Hence, exclusive breastfeeding must be recommended and continued in all infants. The child should be given more frequent, longer breastfeeds, in day as well as in night time. If the mother doesn't have enough milk, she should be helped to *re-establish lactation*. In spite of all efforts towards exclusive breastfeeding, if animal milk has to be given, it should be replaced with yogurt (curds or Dahi) or a lactose free formula. Curds contain less amount of lactose than milk as: Lactobacillus and other bacteria convert some amount of lactose from the milk to lactic acid due to the fermentation. If required, the disaccharide content of the milk/curds/lactose free formula can be further reduced by adding cooked rice. Very rarely, the young infants who don't show any improvement with these measure, may require to be put on the equivalent of diet C of the stepwise dietary algorithm (vide infra).

II. Feeding in Infants Aged More than 6 Months (Older Infants) and Young Children

Breastfeeding must be continued, especially in children less than 2 years of age.

A. At Home

- If the child is still breastfeeding, then as described earlier, he/she should be given more frequent, longer breastfeeds, in day as well as in nighttime.
- If the child is receiving some other milk:
  - Replace it with increased breastfeeding.
    OR
  - Replace it with fermented milk product e.g. curds.
    OR
  - Replace half the amount of animal milk the child usually receives with nutrient rich semisolid food.
  - Add cereals (e.g. rice, wheat, semolina) to milk.
- Give other complementary foods (see above: *Common foods*) in amounts and frequency according to the child's age (See above: *amount and frequency of feeding*).
- If the child improves on suggested dietary therapy at home, same foods should be continued for about a week and then the usual diet should be slowly reintroduced over some days. If there is no improvement or the child develops any of the indications for hospitalizations as discussed above, he should be admitted.

B. At Hospital

A large study of 592 children with persistent diarrhea over a period of 1 year, showed that most of the children whose persistent diarrhea did not respond to domiciliary treatment, responded satisfactorily to a reduced lactose or a lactose free diet. This algorithmic approach from a "reduction in lactose load" to "complete elimination of lactose load" to "complete elimination of all di- and polysaccharides" is found to be very effective. The patients are treated in a stepwise manner and a patient not responding to the first step is put on the second step and so on. The steps are enumerated in Table 113.2.

1. **Step 1: The Initial Diet A** is a **Reduced Lactose Diet (Table 113.2)**
   - The rationale is that total elimination of milk is neither desired nor necessary at this stage. Hence, the daily intake of milk is restricted to 50-60 ml/kg. For this, instead of diluting milk with water, it is mixed with cereals and oil.
   - Such milk-cereal mixtures, when compared to the milk free diets (Diet B and C) are highly palatable, can be consumed in large quantities, provide quality proteins and micronutrients and result in faster weight gain. Hence every child with a persistent diarrhea must be first given a trial of Diet A before moving on to Diet B or C.
   - The Diet A can be started in 6-7 feeds per day at a calorie intake of *minimum* 100-120 Cal/kg/d. This should be slowly increased to 150 Cal/kg/d if weight gain is needed. In case of poor oral acceptance, as it is likely to be in case of systemic infections, nasogastric feeding can be initially used.
2. **Step 2:** 30-35% children do not improve on *Diet A* and require *Diet B*, which is a *lactose free, reduced starch diet (Table 113.2)*
   - For children from vegetarian families, cooked moong daal can replace egg white.
   - The rationale is that the children who don't respond to Diet A may have impaired digestion of starch and other non-lactose disaccharides. For this, lactose is completely eliminated, starch is reduced, and carbohydrates are provided partially by the reduced amount of starch present in this diet and also partially by the added glucose. Proteins (which are primarily provided by milk in Diet A) are provided by the egg white. Complete substitution of starch by glucose is

Table 113.2: Stepwise diets recommended for treatment of persistent diarrhea

The Initial Diet A (Reduced Lactose)			*The Second Diet B (Lactose Free, Reduced Starch)*			*The Third Diet C (Starch Free, Monosaccharide Based)*		
Ingredients	*Measures*	*Weight/Volume*	*Ingredients*	*Measures*	*Weight/Volume*	*Ingredients*	*Measures*	*Weight/Volume*
Milk	1/3 katori	50 ml	Egg white	10 tsp	1/2 egg white	Chicken puree	5 tsp	15 g
Puffed rice powder*	2 tsp	6 g	Puffed rice powder*	3 tsp	9 g	OR Egg white	10 tsp	1/2 egg white
Sugar	1-1/2 tsp	7 g	Glucose	1-1/2 tsp	7 g	Glucose	1-1/2 tsp	7 g
Oil	1 tsp	4.5 g	Oil	1-1/2 tsp	7 g	Oil	1-1/2 tsp	7 g
Water	2/3 katori	100 ml	Water	3/4 katori	120 ml	Water	1 katori	150 ml
Calories/ 100 g	85 Cal		Calories/ 100 g	90 Cal		Calories/ 100 g	67 Cal	
Proteins/ 100 g	2.0 g		Proteins/ 100 g	2.4 g		Proteins/ 100 g	3 g	

* It can be substituted by cooked rice.
Note: The weights and volumes shown are approximations.

avoided as it increases osmolarity tremendously and may lead to osmotic diarrhea.

3. **Step 3:** A total of about 15-20% children may not be benefited by even Diet B and require Diet C, which is a starch free, monosaccharides based diet (Table 113.2).
   - For children from vegetarian families, instead of chicken puree or egg white, soya or milk protein (casein) hydrolysate can be used.
   - The rationale is that these children don't tolerate even the reduced quantity of starch in the Diet B. Therefore, starch is completely replaced with glucose and oil is added for building up the energy intake.

MONITORING THE RESPONSE AND FOLLOW UP

While following this stepwise dietary algorithm, each diet should at least be tried for 7 days. *Successful treatment* is characterized by following signs:

- Decreased frequency of diarrheal stools (≤ 2 liquid stools/day for 2 consecutive days.
- Adequate food intake.
- A steady weight gain after an initial weight loss for 1-2 days.

Such a child with a successful treatment may be discharged after giving required supplements. If the child was discharged on Diet B, then at home, small amounts of milk can be introduced as a part of a mixed diet after about 10 days. If there are no signs of lactose intolerance viz. diarrhea, vomiting, abdominal pain, abdominal distension, excessive flatulence, the amount of milk can be gradually increased and an age-appropriate normal diet can be resumed after about a week. Such children should be followed up closely for continuing weight gain and compliance with the feeding advice.

Treatment failure is defined as presence of one of the following signs:

- No weight gain by day 7. OR
- Signs of dehydration returning any time after starting the diet. OR
- A marked increase in stool frequency any time after the initial 48 hours, after starting a particular diet.

If treatment failure is diagnosed, the child must be examined and/or investigated for any evidence of an infection. If there are no initial or hospital acquired infections, then diet should be changed to the next diet in the order according to the stepwise dietary algorithm.

SUPPLEMENTAL VITAMINS AND MINERALS

Vitamin A: Persistent diarrhea is known to precipitate frank vitamin A deficiency even weeks to months after the diarrheal episode especially in children who already have a preclinical vitamin A deficiency. On the other hand, vitamin A deficiency leads to transient immune compromise and ineffective mucosal repair, thus perpetuating the persistent diarrhea. Hence, a child with persistent diarrhea should be given carotene rich foods (Table 113.1) and foods rich in preformed vitamin A.

In persistent diarrhea, a single dose of 2,00,000 IU and 1,00,000 IU of vitamin A should be given orally to children older than 12 months and aged 6 to 12 months respectively if it has not already been given in last 30 days. If weight of the child is less than 8 kg, then irrespective of the age, only 1,00,000 IU should be given. In addition to this, the IMNCI guidelines also recommend a single dose of 50,000 IU of vitamin A in a child less than 6 months of age having persistent diarrhea.

Zinc: Zinc deficiency can occur in diarrhea due to reduced dietary intake compounded with the increased zinc losses in the diarrheal stools, more so in case of an invasive diarrhea. Zinc is thought to improve absorption of water and electrolytes by helping in early regeneration of intestinal mucosa, restoration of enteric enzymes and enhancing humoral and cellular immunity.

Various studies have shown decreased plasma levels of zinc after recovery from diarrheal episodes and significant reduction in the duration of clinical recovery in malnourished children and significant increase in the gain in weight and height in the follow up. A systematic analysis of various randomized trials has shown that children with acute diarrhea who are given zinc supplements have a 15% lower probability of continuing diarrhea on a given day compared to those who are not whereas the children with persistent diarrhea have a 24% lower probability of continuing diarrhea and a 42% lower rate of treatment failure or death if given zinc supplements. Stool output, one of the most objective marker of severity and a surrogate for dehydration risk, is also shown to be reduced by 31% in zinc supplemented children with acute diarrhea than in the placebo group.

The IAP National Task Force for use of zinc in diarrhea recommends a uniform dose of 20 mg of elemental zinc per day during the period of *acute diarrhea* and for 7 days after cessation of diarrhea to all children older than 3 months. The IMNCI guidelines of Government of India recommend 20 mg elemental zinc daily for 14 days for all children from age 2 months upto 5 years who have *persistent diarrhea*.

Others: Supplemental multivitamins and minerals should be given in the dose of twice the RDA for 2-4 weeks to all children with persistent diarrhea. Iron supplements should never be started in the acute phase of diarrhea.

Special Situations: If along with persistent diarrhea, there is associated *severe PEM, magnesium* sulfate (0.2 ml/kg of 50% solution given intramuscular twice a day for 3 days) and *potassium* (5-6 mEq/kg/d orally or as intravenous infusion) should especially be supplemented. Children on *milk free diet* should receive *calcium* supplements.

Probiotics

Probiotics are defined as live bacteria, microbial cell preparations or components of microbial cells that survive the passage through the gastrointestinal tract and have a beneficial effect on the health and well-being of the host. Thus these are the preparations containing the "good" or "health promoting" bacteria or their components. The most commonly agents include *Lactobacillus GG, Lactobacillus reuteri, Lactobacillus rhamnosus, Lactobacillus acidophilus, Bifidobacterium bifidum, Bifidobacterium lactis, Enterococcus faecium*, and *Saccharomyces boulardii*. Of these, *Lactobacillus GG* showed the most consistent effect; although other probiotic strains may also be effective. These bacteria are helpful in diarrhea in many different ways.

- After ingestion, the activity of the lactic acid bacteria modifies the intestinal flora in a positive manner. They also physically replenish the good bacteria lost from the gastrointestinal tract through vomiting, diarrhea etc.
- Lactobacilli digest lactose, thus helping in the transient lactose malabsorption seen in diarrhea.
- They help to absorb certain minerals by producing an acidic medium.
- Studies have shown that there is some amount of immuno-modulation and the probiotics also increase the antibody response and other gut related immune functions.
- Some probiotics help in production of vitamins, increase resistance to bacterial infections, and increase body's supply of gamma interferon, which is helpful in preventing viral infections.

In general, in pediatric populations, the effect of probiotic agents appears to be most significant against acute infections, mainly viral (rotaviral), diarrhea. Studies documenting effects in other types of diarrheal diseases in children are limited, although some preliminary results are promising. Even the beneficial effects in acute infectious diarrhea are significant only in watery diarrhea and viral gastroenteritis, but virtually non-existent in invasive, bacterial diarrhea. The evidence provided on the prevention of community-acquired diarrhea, though statistically significant, but is of questionable clinical importance. Almost all these studies are from developed countries where gut microbial colonization is different. No study has specifically evaluated the probiotic species available in Indian market. Hence the IAP National Task Force for Use of Probiotics in Diarrhea has concluded that there is presently insufficient evidence to recommend probiotics in Indian setting.

NUTRITIONAL MANAGEMENT DURING RECOVERY

During recovery, the body tries to catch up with all the nutrients lost during the episode of the acute or persistent diarrhea. Hence, in this period, a calorie intake of at least 125% of normal RDA should be planned. This should continue at least till the child regains the pre-illness weight and ideally till he achieves normal nutritional status as evidenced by a normal weight for height or weight for age. This will sure take several weeks or even longer depending on the degree of deficit. For this catch up growth, addition of one extra meal at least for 2 weeks after each episode of acute diarrhea, and for 1 month after persistent diarrhea is helpful in the nutritional rehabilitation of the child.

KEY LEARNING POINTS

- Diarrhea and malnutrition form a dreaded combination, one perpetuating to the other and thus setting up a vicious cycle.
- Mainstay of nutritional management in acute diarrhea is continuing breastfeeding plus routine complementary foods.
- In case of a hospitalized child with persistent diarrhea, stepwise treatment with Diet A (reduced lactose diet), Diet B (lactose free, reduced sucrose diet) and Diet C (starch-free monosaccharide-based diet).
- Supplementation with vitamin A, other vitamins,

zinc, etc. is beneficial in persistent diarrhea in particular.
- Role of probiotics remains controversial.
- During recovery, energy intake of at least 125% of normal RDA is recommended.

FURTHER READINGS

1. Bhatnagar S, Bahl R, Sharma PK, Kumar GK, Saxena SK, Bhan MK. Zinc treatment with oral rehydration therapy reduces stool output and duration of diarrhea in hospitalized children: A randomized controlled trial. *J Pediatr Gastroenterol Nutr* 2004;38:34-40.
2. Bhatnagar S, Bhandari N, Mouli UC, Bhan MK. Consensus Statement of IAP National Task Force: Status Report on Management of Acute Diarrhea. *Indian Pediatr* 2004;41:335-347.
3. Government of India and UNICEF. *Integrated Management of Neonatal and Childhood Illness Module 5: Assess and Classify the Sick Child Age 2 months upto 5 years.* New Delhi: Ministry of Health and Family Welfare, Government of India and UNICEF 2005:10-17.
4. Government of India and UNICEF. *Integrated Management of Neonatal and Childhood Illness: Physician Chart Booklet.* New Delhi: Ministry of Health and Family Welfare, Government of India and UNICEF 2005:21-24.
5. Government of India and UNICEF. *Integrated Management of Neonatal and Childhood Illness Module 7: Treat the Child.* New Delhi: Ministry of Health and Family Welfare, Government of India and UNICEF 2005:3-10.
6. Government of India and UNICEF. *Integrated Management of Neonatal and Childhood Illness: Physician Chart Booklet.* New Delhi: Ministry of Health and Family Welfare, Government of India and UNICEF 2005:18-19.
7. Government of India. *National Child Survival and Safe Motherhood Program.* New Delhi: MCH Division, Department of Family Welfare, Ministry of Health and Family Welfare 1994.
8. Hambidge M. Human zinc deficiency. *J Nutr* 2000;130:1344S-1349S.
9. Jelliffe DB, Jelliffe EFP. *Dietary Management of Young Children with Acute Diarrhea,* 2nd Edn. Geneva: World Health Organization 1991:3-26.
10. Park K. *Park's Textbook of Preventive and Social Medicine,* 17th Ed, Jabalpur: Banarasidas Bhanot 2002:175-178.
11. Patwari AK. Nutritional management of diarrhea. *Indian J Pract Pediatr* 1998;6:329-338.
12. Persistent Diarrhea in Children in Developing Countries. Memorandum from a WHO meeting. *Bull WHO* 1988;66:707-717.
13. Saavedra J. Probiotics and infectious diarrhea. *Am J Gastroenterol* 2000;95(1 Suppl):S16-18.
14. Sheth M, Parnami S, Gurudasani R. Diet in diarrhea. In: Gupte S (ed): *Textbook of Pediatric Nutrition.* New Delhi: Peepee 2006:399-404.
15. Szajewska H, Mrukowicz JZ. Probiotics in the treatment and prevention of acute infectious diarrhea in infants and children: A systematic review of published randomized, double-blind, placebo-controlled trials. *J Pediatr Gastroenterol Nutr* 2001;33 Suppl 2:S17-25.
16. Szajewska H, Mrukowicz JZ. Use of probiotics in children with acute diarrhea. *Pediatr Drugs* 2005;7(2):111-122.
17. World Health Organization. *Program for Control of Diarrheal Diseases.* Geneva: World Health Organization 1994.
18. World Health Organization. *The Management and Prevention of Diarrhea: Practical Guidelines,* 3rd Edn. Geneva: World Health Organization, 1993.
19. Zinc Investigators Collaborative Group. Therapeutic effect of oral zinc in acute and persistent diarrhea in children in developing countries: Pooled analysis of randomized controlled trials. *Am J Clin Nutr* 2000;72:1516-1522.

114 Nutritional Support in Celiac Disease

• Karoly Horvath

INTRODUCTION

Celiac disease (CD) is a chronic small intestinal disease that occurs in genetically predisposed individuals. It is characterized by severe, immune-mediated damage of the small intestine when exposed to gluten, the storage protein in wheat, barley and rye. Based on recent epidemiological studies CD affects 1:100-300 people worldwide.

The humoral and cell-mediated immune response to gluten peptides found in wheat, barley, and rye occur primarily in individuals who carry a certain human leukocyte antigen (HLA) type, DQ2, or in some populations, DQ8. The humoral immune response leads to the production of antibodies to gliadin and the tissue transglutaminase (tTG) enzyme. The cell-mediated inflammatory response injures the mucosa that leads to a defective ability to digest and absorb both macro and micronutrients.

Historically, classic presentation of CD included diarrhea, abdominal distention, and failure to thrive. Now, with the availability of serological screening, a variety of other clinical manifestations exist. Atypical presentations may include vomiting, constipation, short stature, delayed puberty, iron and folate deficiency with anemia, recurrent abdominal pain, dental enamel defects, neurologic abnormalities, oral ulcerations, infertility, elevated liver enzymes, osteopenia, or premature osteoporosis. Based on a large epidemiological study, only one out of seven children presents with classical symptoms.

Serological markers are most often used to evaluate patients with suspected CD. Due to their higher sensitivity and specificity, the best available tests include IgA anti-endomysial antibodies (EMA) and IgA tissue transglutaminase antibodies (tTG). Positive antibody tests warrant a small intestinal biopsy to confirm the diagnosis of CD.

This chapter will focus on the nutritional management of children with CD.

NUTRITIONAL MANAGEMENT

The management of celiac disease includes dietary/nutritional and medical components.

The nutritional management is a continuous process and includes the initial assessment, diet counselling, and follow-up visits (Table 114.1).

Table 114.1: Nutrition assessment for celiac disease

Initial Assessment	*Counseling*	*Follow-up*
Growth parameters	Definition of gluten	Growth parameters
Diet history	Gluten-containing products	Diet compliance
Nutritional deficiencies	Hidden sources of gluten	Support systems
Nutritional requirements	Cross contamination	Nutritional adequacy
Supplementation	Gluten-free resources and product information	
	Importance of strict compliance	
	Support systems	

Initial Assessment

Once the diagnosis of CD has been made, it is recommended that the parents and the child meet with a physician and nutritionist with expertise in CD.

The growth parameters (height, weight, body mass index) are usually obtained during the first visit of the child before the diagnosis is made. These should serve as baseline data for the continuous management of the child.

Upon diagnosis, the nutritionist should evaluate the usual intake of the child, including the role of gluten-containing grains in the diet of the family. The gluten-free (GF) diet often requires a radical change in the diet of the entire family. Obtaining a thorough diet history is important to identify commonly eaten foods, where meals are eaten, who purchases and prepares meals, and convenience food consumption.

The initial visit should include a thorough nutrition assessment. The nutritionist should review all the lab tests performed prior to or after the intestinal biopsy that usually include tests for nutritional deficiencies. Nutritional deficiencies of iron, folate, calcium and fat-soluble vitamins can be present. Temporary or long-term supplementations may be required to correct these deficiencies. Diet instruction can then be tailored to meet the needs of the child.

The classical celiac cases present with growth failure or weight loss. They require additional calorie intake for catch-up growth and weight gain. Liberal use of butters, oils, nuts, yogurts, cheeses, milk, cream, and gluten-free sauces and dressings can be used to achieve increased calorie needs. Commercially available high calorie, gluten-free supplements may also be used to promote weight gain.

Gluten-free Diet Counseling

Treatment for celiac disease requires complete omission of gluten from the diet. Gluten is the general term for prolamins found in wheat (gliadin), rye (secalin), and barley (hordein). There are multiple other grains that are derived from these three and have toxic prolamins. They have various names in different parts of the world. Table 114.2 includes a list of gluten-containing grains. Gluten may also be found as a hidden ingredient in foods such as thickeners in commercial products and as an additive in medications. Table 114.3 lists examples of gluten: containing ingredients and ingredients which may contain gluten.

Table 114.2: Gluten: Containing grains

Wheat	*Barley*	*Rye*	*Durum*	*Seitan*
Farina	Bran	Bulgar	Graham flour	Udon
Einkorn wheat	Emmer wheat	Farro	Triticale	Wheat bran
Kamut	Malt	Couscous	Matzo flour/meal	Wheat germ
Rye	Semolina	Spelt	Panko	Wheat starch

Table 114.3: Gluten: Containing ingredients and ingredients to question

Gluten containing ingredients	*Ingredients to question*
Cereal binding	Seasonings
Filler	Flavorings
Malt extract	Flavorings
Malt flavoring	Modified food starch
Malt syrup	Dextrin

Minimum Gluten Allowed

Currently, there is a lack of scientific evidence that has established a daily minimum amount of gluten that can safely be ingested. Several countries have established their own minimum levels of safe gluten intake. Codex Alimentarius, a Geneva-based organization jointly run by the World Health Organization (WHO) and the Food and Agriculture Organization (FAO) of the United Nations, defines gluten-free as an ingredient that contains less than 20 ppm (<20 mg/kg) of gluten.

Cross Contamination

Cross contamination can occur when grains are milled, harvested, stored and manufactured with wheat, barley and rye or their gluten-containing derivatives. Although oats have traditionally been considered as toxic for celiac patients, a body of literature suggests that moderate amounts of oats (50-70 grams per day) may safely be consumed. Careful investigation is needed to ensure that the oats are not harvested, milled, stored or transported with wheat sources. Oats that can be contaminated with gluten should be avoided.

Gluten contamination can also happen in the home. Utensils and pans should be washed properly to avoid contamination. Countertops and food preparation surfaces should be cleaned frequently to remove gluten-containing crumbs. Deep frying foods in oils or fats that are also used for gluten-containing products may also be a source of contamination. *Cross contamination* may happen in stores where grains are available from open bins.

Eating out can present a challenge on the GF diet but it is possible with careful planning. Individuals may contact a restaurant's cook or chef regarding their restrictions ahead of time. Often, they will be able to accommodate GF requests. Informing the restaurant server of GF restrictions is also helpful. Many children prefer to bring their own GF foods to restaurants, social events, and school to prevent cross contamination risk.

Gluten-Free Foods

The GF diet can be well balanced and include a variety of foods. Most fresh fruits and vegetables, plain meats, dairy products, potatoes, and rice are considered gluten-free if they are not prepared with gluten-containing ingredients. Some stores may also carry commercially available gluten-free products such as bread, pasta and baked goods.

Gluten-Free Grains

Amaranth: Known for its nutty flavor, amaranth seeds can be milled into flour and used to make bread products or pasta. It is a good source of fiber, protein, iron, zinc, magnesium, calcium and B vitamins.

Buckwheat: Buckwheat seeds can be used as a side dish, in soups or cereals, or ground into flour for baking. Roasted buckwheat is known as kasha. Buckwheat provides a good source of protein, magnesium, B_6, fiber, iron, niacin, thiamin and zinc.

Millet: Millet's mild sweetness can be enjoyed as a cereal, side dish, polenta, or soup. Millet is high in protein and fiber.

Quinoa: This nutrient-dense grain is often prepared as a side dish. Quinoa is an excellent source of protein, iron, magnesium, B vitamins and calcium.

Teff: This sticky grain is often prepared as porridge or polenta or ground into flour for bread. Teff is high in protein, calcium, iron and B vitamins.

Wild rice: Wild rice is a grass that varies in taste, aroma, and size. Wild rice is often consumed as a side dish or in soups. It is high in fiber, protein, potassium, and zinc.

Follow-up Visits

After the initial nutritional assessment and GF counseling, a return visit should be scheduled within 3 months to assess the child's growth, symptomatic improvement, parents' and the child's knowledge, acceptance, and compliance to the GF diet. Weight gain is expected in children with classical symptoms in response to gluten withdrawal. Based on the child's progress, the nutritional status should be reevaluated, including energy needs, vitamin and mineral adequacy. Because of the restriction of grains on the GF diet, patients with CD may be particularly vulnerable to insufficient intake of iron and fiber.

Support Systems

Adherence to a GF diet is a lifelong requirement. In families preparing their own foods from basic ingredients, the diet does not present as a challenge once they have learned the basics of GF diet. However, as more and more families rely on commercial products, continual education and awareness on the part of the individual with CD as well as their families and friends is necessary.

Celiac support groups can offer an avenue for new information for the parents and comfort and encouragement for children when they are among others that also have CD. Local support groups can often also provide information on GF restaurants and vendors in the area.

MEDICAL MANAGEMENT

Lactose Malabsorption

Lactose malabsorption is common at the time of diagnosis of CD due to damage of the brush border membranes of the intestinal epithelial cells. Table 114.4 shows the prevalence of disaccharidase deficiencies measured in the initial intestinal biopsies in our patients.

The lactase enzyme, which breaks down lactose to glucose and galactose, is located on the surface of the small intestinal epithelial cells. Symptoms of lactose malabsorption include abdominal distention, pain, bloating, flatulence, and diarrhea. Reduction or elimination of lactose containing foods or supplementation with a lactase enzyme may be warranted at diagnosis for individuals with lactose malabsorption. Lactose malabsorption usually is a temporary problem and resolves on GF diet within a few weeks once the intestinal epithelium recovers and the villus surface increases.

Table 114.4: Prevalence of disaccharidase deficiencies (<3 percentile of normal) in celiac children (n=74)

Lactase	*Maltase*	*Sucrose*	*Palatinase*
89%	76%	77%	70%

Other Disaccharidase Deficiencies

In addition to low lactase activity, other disaccharidase deficiencies may also be present when CD is diagnosed. The inability to break down lactose, maltose, and sucrose into monosaccharides can cause osmotic diarrhea and abdominal distention. However, the maltase, palatinase and sucrase deficiencies rarely represent a clinical problem and resolve shortly after the GF diet starts. A low lactose diet is the most often prescribed diet for disaccharidase deficiencies.

Iron Supplementation

Anemia is diagnosed concurrently with CD in upto 84% of children. Iron absorption occurs in the proximal small intestine, where the villi damage is the most severe. Initiation of GF diet and ferrous iron supplementation is recommended to correct iron deficiency anemia.

Repeat Serology Tests

Serology tests can be used to assess initial response to a gluten-free diet. Antigliadin antibodies and antitissue transglutaminase antibodies typically return to normal within 6 to 12 months on the GF diet. Patients with elevated antibodies that have been following a gluten-free diet greater than 12 months warrant a thorough assessment of diet to assess for accidental gluten intake. Serological tests do not, however, detect slight dietary errors.

KEY LEARNING POINTS

- Celiac disease is an autoimmune enteropathy that affects the proximal small intestine when gluten is ingested in genetically susceptible individuals.
- Dietary sources of gluten include wheat, barley, rye and related grains.
- CD is treated by a lifelong exclusion of gluten from the diet.
- A complete nutritional assessment and diet instruction is recommended at diagnosis of CD.
- Gluten-free diet instruction and additional nutritional advice should be tailored to meet the needs of the patient.
- Ongoing medical follow-ups and support systems are key for lifelong dietary compliance.

FURTHER READINGS

1. American Gastroenterological Association. American Gastroenterological Association medical position statement: Celiac sprue. *Gastroenterology* 2001; 120:636-651.

2. Barera G, Mora S, Brambilla P, *et al.* Body composition in children with celiac disease and the effects of a gluten-free diet: A prospective case-control study. *Am J Clin Nutr* 2000; 72: 71-75.
3. Bonamico M, Vania A, Monti S, *et al.* Iron deficiency in children with celiac disease. *J Pediatr Gastroenterol Nutr* 1987; 6:702-706.
4. Case S. *Gluten-Free Diet: A Comprehensive Resource Guide.* Regina, Saskatchewan: Case Nutrition Consulting 2001.
5. Farrell R, Kelly C. Current concepts: Celiac sprue. *N Engl J Med* 2002; 346:180-188.
6. Fasano A, Catassi C. Current approaches to diagnosis and treatment of celiac disease: An evolving spectrum. *Gastroenterology* 2001; 121:1527-1528.
7. Green P, Jones R. Celiac Disease: A Hidden Epidemic. New York: Harper Collins 2006.
8. Grehn S, Fridell K, Lilliecreutz M, Hallert C. Dietary habits of Swedish adult celiac patients treated by a gluten-free diet for 10 years. *Scand J Nutr* 2001; 45:178-182.
9. Horvath K, Mehta D. Celiac Disease—A worldwide problem. *Indian J of Pediatr* 2000; 67:757-762.
10. Janatuinen E, Kemppainen T, Julkunen R, *et al.* No harm from five-year ingestion of oats in celiac disease. *Gut* 2002;50:332-335.
11. Murray J. The widening spectrum of celiac disease. *Am J Clin Nutr* 1999;69:354-365.
12. Picarelli A, Di Tola M. Sabbatella L, *et al.* Immunologic evidence of no harmful effect of oats in celiac disease. *Am J Clin Nutr* 2001;74:137-140.
13. Thompson T. Folate, iron and dietary fiber contents of the gluten-free diet. *J Am Diet Assoc* 2000; 100: 1389-1396.
14. Thompson T. Gluten contamination of commercial oat products in the United States. *N Engl J Med* 2004;351:2021-2022.
15. Thompson T. Oats and the gluten-free diet. *J Am Diet Assoc* 2003;103: 376-380.
16. Troncone R, Mayer M, Spagnuolo F, Maiuri L, Greco L. Endomysial antibodies as unreliable markers for slight dietary transgressions in adolescents with celiac disease. *J Pediatr Gastroenterol Nutr* 1995; 21:69-72.
17. Van Heel D, West J. Recent advances in celiac disease. *Gut* 2006; 55:1037-1046.

115 Nutritional Support in Cystic Fibrosis

KE Elizabeth

INTRODUCTION

Cystic fibrosis (CF), one of the most common autosomal recessive diseases, especially among the whites, is characterized by maldigestion, malabsorption, intestinal obstruction, chronic airway disease, superadded infections and, sometimes, endocrine pancreatic dysfunction like diabetes.

Nutritional support plays a key role in the management of CF. Various workers have demonstrated positive association of nutritional support with survival and improvement in both weight and height.

NUTRITIONAL SUPPORT

It is very important in view of the increased energy expenditure on one side and malabsorption on the other. Energy, protein and fluid should be given liberally as per the RDA. Fat should be given as per tolerance and with enzyme replacement.

Factors that are considered in planning nutritional support are listed in Table 115.1.

Table 115.1: Important factors in planning nutritional support

- Age at diagnosis
- Nutritional status at diagnosis
- Degree of pancreatic involvement
- Respiratory involvement
- Hypoalbuminemia
- Anemia
- Fat soluble vitamin deficiency and EFA deficiency
- Electrolyte depletion
- Degree of stool energy losses
- Degree of anorexia.

1. Type of Feed

Breast milk or whey-based formulas are suitable for young infants. In those with growth failure, energy supplementation with protein hydrolysate or nasogastric feeding may be needed. In those with short bowel disease following surgery for meconium ileus, a pre-digested protein hydrolysate preparations like Pregestimil or Peptijunior are beneficial.

Breastfeeding

Breast milk is optimum for most babies. The advantages of breast milk include:

1. The lipase and amylase present in it partially compensating for the pancreatic insufficiency.
2. Optimal fatty acid profile.
3. Optimal amino acid profile including taurine, which is needed for bile salt synthesis and fat absorption.
4. Immunological properties including immunoglobulins, lysozymes, lactoferrin, epidermal growth factors, secretory IgA etc., that offer protection against infection and development of cow's milk allergy.
5. Bioavailability of micronutrients like iron, calcium, phosphorus etc.
6. Hormonal factors.
7. Psychological benefit.

In spite of all these well-known benefits of human milk, only a small proportion of CF babies are breastfed upto 6 months of age. The discrepancy between those who are capable and those who succeed may pinpoint weakness amongst those who support them rather than the women themselves. Breastfeeding is a hormonally controlled supply and demand process. The more the infant suckles, the more milk will be produced. Slow weight gain among the breastfed can be corrected by increasing the feeding frequency.

Artificial Feeding

Many babies need artificial feeding due to various reasons. A whey-based formula is recommended. Those with persistent symptoms even after enzyme therapy may be having cow's milk allergy. In such cases, protein hydrolysate formula is better in view of additional soya intolerance.

Age of Weaning

Weaning can be introduced at 6 months of age. There is no

advantage of early weaning. Weaning on to low energy pureed rice, fruits and vegetables may slow weight gain. Milk based feeds should be given throughout to promote weight gain. Introduction of solids and cow's milk based formula require an increase in pancreatin therapy.

Sodium Supplementation

This is especially important in hot countries. The normal requirements is 2-4 mmol/kg. Na content of breast milk low and standard infant formulae, 200 ml/kg supply 1.6 mmol/kg. Protein hydrolysate, and 200 ml/kg supply 2.8 mmol/kg. Supplementation is required in growth failure and negative sodium balance on monitoring. 600 mg sodium chloride = 10 mmol Na.

Medium Chain Triglycerides (MCT)

MCT supplementation in formula and addition of MCT oil like coconut oil and cottonseed oil may be useful. MCT will be directly absorbed into portal vein even during fat malabsorption and promote weight gain. Upto 10% of the energy intake can be given as visible MCT oil.

2. Oral Supplements

Some may need oral supplements in addition to usual diet. The examples are energy/calorie only (Duocal, Maxijul, Polycal), protein-calorie (Scandishake), fruit-based (Enlive, Fortijuice), milk-based nutritionally complete (Ensure Plus, Entera, Fortisip), etc.

3. Micronutrients

Vitamin A

Vitamin A deficiency is anticipated in CF. It may be multifactorial and not simply due to malabsorption. There may be faecal loss of vitamin A unrelated to the degree of fat loss. Vitamin A status correlates with plasma retinal binding protein (RBP) rather than plasma retinal level. The latter is dependent on the former and the retinal level may be depressed in acute infections. Five to ten times the requirement i.e. about 5000-10,000 IU/ day, may be given. Loading doses of vitamin A may cause hypervitaminosis.

Vitamin D

Even though clinical evidence of vitamin D deficiency is uncommon, reduced plasma levels of 25-Dihydroxy cholecalciferol have been documented in CF. Reduced bone mineral density (BMD) and increased fragility of bones may occur in CF. Almost 10 times the requirement, 400-800 IU of vitamin D is required to maintain normal blood level of 25-Dihydroxy vitamin D in most cases. Hypervitaminosis D has not been reported in CF.

Vitamin E

Symptomatic vitamin E deficiency has been noted in CF. Vitamin E is very important in slowing the lung disease and in offering protection against free radical disease, erythrocyte survival and nerve conduction. Vitamin E level correlates better with erythrocyte vitamin E level rather than plasma level. Large doses, 10-200 mg/day may be needed. Adverse effects are not usually seen, except the possibility of necrotizing enterocolitis especially in very young infants.

Vitamin K

Vitamin K deficiency as evidenced by protein induced in vitamin K absence (PIVKA) is the rule in CF. Deficiency is due to fat malabsorption, bile salt deficiency, liver disease and antibiotic therapy. Overt bleeding is rare, but osteopenia and osteoporosis due to decreased formation of osteocalcin may occur. Various workers recommend daily or at least weekly supplementation. Hypervitaminosis K has not been reported in CF. The suggested dose is 1 mg/year to a maximum of 10 mg/dose. The natural kenadione preparation may be better than synthetic menadione preparation.

Water Soluble Vitamins

Routine supplementation is needed if the intake is poor. Vitamin B_{12} injections are needed in children with short bowel disease following intestinal surgery for obstruction.

4. Pancreatic Enzyme Replacement Therapy (PERT)

PERT is needed when there is fat malabsorption. Obvious symptoms include fatty stools and weight loss between birth and diagnosis or poor weight gain. Steatorrhoea should be confirmed by direct microscopy for fat globules. Indirect pancreatic function tests like fecal Pancreatic elastase–1 (PE-1) measurement and chymotrypsin are also useful. A concentration PE-1 less than 100 mcg/g is indicative of severe pancreatic insufficiency. Most babies develop significant insufficiency by one year of age. As approximately 50% of the energy in infants is through fat, PERT is absolutely beneficial in them.

Principles of PERT

1. Use microsphere or mini-microsphere enzyme preparations that are acid resistant especially in infants.
2. The dose should be adjusted upto lipase 10,000 IU/kg/day.
3. Pancreatin should be mixed with only small quantity of food or drink immediately before feeding.
4. As PERT enhances vitamin absorption, vitamins may be given along with meals and pancreatin.

The various enzyme preparations are given in Table 115.1.

The microsphere and microtablets contain porcine pancreatin coated with a thin layer of acid resisting phthalate. The initial dose can be 1/4-1/3 Creon 10000 (2500-3333 IU lipase) for infants, 1/2 scoop Creon for children (2500

IU lipase) or 1/3-1/2 Pancreas (1666-2500 IU lipase) per fed. These doses equate to approximately 400-800 IU lipase/g fat. Mix enzymes with formula/expressed breast milk or fruit puree and give from a spoon directly at the beginning of the feed. The dose can be gradually increased according to objective assessment of absorption, growth and clinical symptoms. Enzyme dose should be varied according to the fat content of the weaning food. Because of the multiple factors affecting enzyme efficacy dose requirements can vary between 500-4000 IU/g fat.

Powdered enzyme preparations e.g. Pancrex V Forte. This can be mixed with a small amount of feed or water and given by mouth or syringe down tube. Over 90% activity may be destroyed by gastric acid. If this is used, give acid suppression, preferably a proton pump inhibitor.

Advantages

1. Highly water soluble.
2. Rapid release of lipases.
3. Absorption through gastric mucosa in neonates.
4. Bile salts not required for absorption.

Table 115.2: The various pancreatic enzyme preparations

Product	*Manufacturer*	*Lipase*	*Protease*	*Amylase*
Enteric-coated Microsphere				
Nutrizym GR	Merck	10,000	650	10,000
Pancrease	Jassen Cilag	5,000	330	2,900
Enteric-coated Minimicrosphere				
Creon	Solvay	10,000	600	8,000
Enteric-coated Microtablets				
Nutrizym 10	Merck	10,000	500	9000
Pancrease HL	Jassen Cilag	25,000	1250	22,500
Cotazym S	Organon	8,000	30,000	30,000
Others Enteric-coated tablets				
Pancrex V	Paine and Byrne	1900	110	1700
Enzox Plus	Tidal	4800	305	4600
Festal N	Aventis	6000	300	4500
Farizym Forte	Organon	6000	350	4000
Pankreoflat	Duphar	6500	400	5500
Capsules	Paine and Byrne	8000	430	9000
Pancrex V				
Buff powder	Paine and Byrne	25,000	1400	30,000
Pancrex V				
Coated granule	Paine and Byrne	5000	300	4000

5. Carnitine Independent Passage

The disadvantages include incomplete oxidation, thermogenic effect, ketogenic effect and poor deposition in adipose tissue. Gastro-oesophageal reflux disease (GERD) and failure to thrive (FTT) are common associated problems. GERD has increased incidence in CF. It compounds poor weight gain, aggravates respiratory symptoms. Treatment includes antacids, PPIs, motility stimulants and feed thickeners. Failure to thrive can be tackled by energy supplementation via high-energy formula and enteral or parenteral nutrition. Is dense formula that supply 1Kcal/1ml is well tolerated.

Enteral Tube Feeding

Intermittent or overnight continuous infusions should be tried in those less than 2 years with—FTT despite oral supplements. In 2-18 years enteral feeding is needed in those with either % weight/height <85 or weight falling below 2 major centile positions or no weight gain for 6 months. In those >18 years, this may be useful in those with BMI <18.5 kg/m^2 or >5% weight loss over <2 months.

Upto 150% of the RDA of energy requirement may be given and also upto 200 ml/kg of fluid can be given under supervision. The choices are normal milk based feed with 1.5-2.0 Kcal/ml and enzymes given at the beginning and at the end of feeding. Overnight continuous infusions are the most beneficial and convenient.

Short-term benefits are increase in weight, body fat, and lean body mass and muscle mass. Long-term benefits are increase in weight and height, improved well-being and slower progression in respiratory function. Younger patients have a more successful outcome. Those with a positive outlook to feeding have a better outcome.

Routes of Feeding

The preferred routes are via nasogastric (NG) tubes or gastrostomies that are sited operatively or percutaneously by endoscopic placement (PEG). These are well suitable for long-term nutritional support. Polyvinyl chloride (PVC) NG tubes are used in short-term cases and they need to be changed every week. Polyurethane or silicone tubes are used for long-term cases and may remain for a month. Intermittent bolus gravity assisted feeding mimics physiological conditions, but may induce vomiting by reverse peristalsis, whereas continuous feeds do not evoke vomiting. No. 6 French gauge pediatric incubator tubes or 8 French gauge fine bore feeding tubes are suitable for feeding. Blocked tubes can be flushed with 20 ml water with or without ¼ tsp sodabicarb or pancreatic enzyme powder.

Percutaneous endoscopic gastrostomies (PEGs) may be retained for 2 years without replacement. Newer style balloon buttons called the Mickey's gastrostomy buttons can be inserted into a ready formed track and changed by pulling the existing PEG and simply inserting the button. The complications of gastrostomies are pain following insertion and rarely peritonitis.

Type of Feeds

Elemental/semi-elemental feeds include MCT and Pepdite ranges. Polymeric feeds include Fortini, Nutrini, Pediasure, Novasource Junor and so on. The requirement of enzymes with elemental dirt is not fully settled. Some may need special feeds such as Pulmocare (Abbott) in those with severe pulmonary disease and Generaid in those with hepatic disease. Timing of feeding can be adjusted as per the lifestyle of the patient.

Parenteral Nutrition

It is an option for short-term nutritional support especially following abdominal surgery. Proper fluid and electrolyte balance and monitoring, supervised by the TPN team, is essential for success of such interventions.

6. CF-Related Diabetes Mellitus (CFRD)

As the survival in CF has improved, CFRD is becoming increasingly common. It may also be precipitated by steroid therapy and may need short term insulin therapy. Conflicts between CF and DM diet should be resolved in favour of the CF diet. High-energy diet based on complex starch with modifications like avoidance of refined sugars and drinks that cause rapid rise in blood sugar is advisable.

7. Nutritional Complications

- Distal intestinal obstruction syndrome (DIOS), an equivalent of meconium ileus.
- Fibrosing colonopathy with proximal colon strictures.
- Pancreatitis.
- Growth faltering; and
- Multiple deficiencies are some of the complications of nutritional support in CF.

8. Associated Celiac Disease

Occasionally, celiac disease may complicate CF. High index of suspicion and rapid diagnosis and timely treatment with withdrawal of gluten-containing foodstuffs is important in such children.

9. Behavioral Problems

More than 70% of parents of children with CF identified mealtimes as problematic. Mealtimes were the most frequently cited management problem for parents of pre-school children with CF.

Solutions

1. Set rules and expectations at mealtimes as with healthy children.
2. Limit mealtimes to 30 minutes.
3. Make food attractive.
4. Encourage positive and discourage negative statements about eating.
5. Decide on a goal and split it into manageable tasks.
6. Implement reward systems for "good" eating behaviour. These should be consistent and immediate. Bad behaviour should be ignored.
7. Avoid empty threats, unless threatened punishment is carried out discipline is meaningless.
8. Give parents information about child's developmental abilities so that they can focus on the child to increase their responsibility.
9. Dietary supplements should be taken in addition to diet to improve total energy intake and improve weight gain rather than blame the child.

10. Growth Monitoring

Growth monitoring with appropriate weight, height, weight for height and BMI charts form the cornerstone in the follow-up of children with CF. The minimum goals of therapy are:

1. Weight and height above 5th centile.
2. Weight for age >80%.
3. Height for age >90% and weight for height >85%.

KEY LEARNING POINTS

- Our understanding of the treatment of the nutritional needs of patients with CF continues to evolve.
- Early nutritional intervention to prevent or resolve malnutrition is most effective.
- Meticulous attention to both the quantitative and qualitative aspects of the diet is essential for improving survival and quality of survival in cystic fibrosis.
- Pancreatic enzyme replacement thereby is the lifeline of nutritional support in CF.

FURTHER READINGS

1. Cade A, Walters MP, Mc Ginley N *et al.* Evaluation of fecal pancreatic elastase-1 as a measure of pancreatic exocrine function in children with cystic fibrosis. *Pediatr Pulmomol* 2000; 29: 172-176.
2. Griffiths M. Single stage percutaneous gastrostomy button insertion—A leap forward. *J Parenter Enter Nutr* 1996; 20: 237-239.
3. Gupte S, Anderson RA. Pediatric gastroenterology. In: Gupte S (ed): *The Short Textbook of Pediatrics*, 11th edn. New Delhi: Jaypee 2008 (In press).
4. Lai HC, Kosorok MR, Sondel SA, *et al.* Growth status in children with cystic fibrosis based on the National CF patient registry data: Evaluation of certain criteria used to identify malnutrition. *J Pediatr* 1998; 132: 478-485.
5. Lester LA, Rothberg RM, Dawson G *et al.* Supplemental parenteral nutrition in cystic fibrosis. *J Parenter Enter Nutr* 1986;10:280-295.
6. Sharma M, Singh M. Nutritional management of children with cystic fibrosis. *Indian Pediatr* 2003;40:1055-1063.
7. UK Cystic Fibrosis Trust Nutrition Working Group. *Nutritional Management of Cystic Fibrosis.* London: CF Trust 2002.
8. Wilson DC, Kalnins D, Stewart C, *et al.* Challenges in the dietary treatment of cystic fibrosis related diabetes. *Clin Nutr* 2000; 19: 87-93.

116 Nutritional Support in Diabetes Mellitus

Kara Feigenbaum

INTRODUCTION

Approximately 10% of the diabetic population belongs to type 1 which is usually caused by an autoimmune destruction of the beta cell resulting in insulin deficiency. Decreased tissue sensitivity to insulin and inadequate beta cell function characterize type 2 diabetes, which accounts for 90% of diabetes cases.

Type 1 is primarily diagnosed in childhood and adolescence. It is one of the most common and increasingly prevalent chronic diseases in the pediatric population. Progressively more problematic, however, is the rapidly growing number of children developing type 2 diabetes worldwide.

Consistent diet and lifestyle modification is key for both type 1 and type 2 diabetes in prevention of such long-term complications as neuropathy, retinopathy, nephropathy, peripheral vascular disease, hyperlipidemia, hypertension, atherosclerosis, and coronary artery disease. A multidisciplinary team approach to diabetes education and treatment is recommended. Ideally, this would include a physician, diabetes educator, social worker, psychologist and dietitian trained in the care of children with diabetes. With support and involvement from family and diabetes team, children and adolescents can improve and maintain metabolic control through self-management. Consideration of the patient's age, eating patterns and food preferences, physical activity, past medical history, school or work schedule, home environment, personality, and cultural factors should all be integrated into education process.

NUTRITIONAL GOALS

Box 116.1 summarizes the goals of diet in diabetes mellitus.

Box 116.1: Nutrition goals for diabetes management

- Achieve normal growth and development.
- Maintain healthy weight.
- Maintain optimal blood pressure, blood glucose and lipid levels to help prevent/delay both short- and long-term medical problems and complications.

Energy

The diet for diabetes focuses on providing adequate energy to achieve or maintain a healthy and realistic body weight and support growth. Caloric requirements are personalized, based on weight, height, ideal body weight, activity level, and average energy allowance. Several predictive equations are available to calculate calorie needs in children. Indirect calorimetry may also be helpful in the obese population.

Carbohydrates

Carbohydrates are the primary energy fuel source for the body. They make up approximately 50-60% of caloric intake and supply 4 calories per gram. Types of carbohydrates include sugar, starch and fiber. Carbo-hydrates have the greatest influence on blood glucose levels. Glycemic response most closely reflects the total amount of carbohydrates consumed. Although dietary carbohydrate increases postprandial blood glucose levels, eliminating carbohydrates from the diet in diabetes will not maintain blood glucose levels in the normal range, since glucose will be produced by the body from protein and fat if dietary carbohydrate intake is restricted. The brain and central nervous system and several other body organs depend on a steady supply of glucose for fuel. Carbohydrate-containing foods are also the most important dietary source of fiber and water-soluble vitamins and minerals. Restricting total carbohydrate intake to <130 grams is not recommended.

Protein

Protein provides about 10-20% of total calories in the diabetic diet. One gram of protein supplies 4 calories. Adequate intake is needed for growth, development, maintenance of lean body mass, and cell function and metabolism. Although protein is not the primary stimulus for insulin release, it does augment insulin release when ingested with a carbohydrate, increasing glucose clearance from blood in type 2 diabetics.

Fat and Cholesterol

Fat makes up approximately 30% of total calories and provides 9 calories per gram. Of the 30%, no more than 10% should come from saturated and trans fats, upto 10% should come from polyunsaturated sources, and 10-15% from monounsaturated fat. Dietary fat is needed to supply energy and essential fatty acids, and for absorption of fat-soluble vitamins. In diabetes management, fat affects blood glucose response by delaying the glucose peak when ingesting a mixed fat and carbohydrate meal. Because of the increased risk of cardiovascular disease in diabetes, it is recommended that cholesterol and triglyceride levels be maintained as near to normal range as possible. Dietary fat goals should focus on decreasing intake of saturated and trans fats by limiting fast foods and convenience foods and choosing lean protein sources. Use of monounsaturated fats such as peanut, olive, and canola oils are encouraged to replace saturated and trans fats in the diet. Overall fat restriction may be necessary to decrease total caloric intake when weight loss is needed. National Cholesterol Education Program (NCEP) guidelines recommend restriction of saturated fat to <7% of total calories and cholesterol intake <200 mg/dl for treatment of elevated LDL cholesterol levels (Box 116.2).

Box 116.2: Consensus guidelines for diagnosis of dyslipidemia in children

Total Cholesterol	Borderline ≥170 mg/dL
	Abnormal ≥200 mg/dL
LDL Cholesterol	Borderline ≥100 mg/dL
	Abnormal ≥130 mg/dL
HDL Cholesterol	Abnormal <40 mg/dL
Triglycerides	Abnormal ≥200 mg/dL

Fiber

Fiber is an important dietary component in blood glucose and cholesterol control. Fiber is a category of carbohydrates that are not fully digested or absorbed. There are two types of fiber, soluble and insoluble. Gum, mucilage, and pectin comprise soluble fiber, which bind to fatty substances in the gut and are excreted through the stool. Consuming soluble fiber has been proven to lower cholesterol and LDL levels. Insoluble fiber, including cellulose, hemicellulose, and lignan, add bulk to foods, which may help with satiety for weight management. Insoluble fiber also plays a key role in bowel regularity. Recommended fiber intake for children over age 2 is (age in years + 5 grams) however individualized recommendations are warranted for children who are at high risk of or already have diseases or conditions that may require adjustments in dietary fiber intake.

Non-Nutritive Sweeteners (Sugar Substitutes, Artificial Sweetners)

The non-nutritive sweeteners provide a sweet taste to foods with little or no effect on blood sugar levels. Common non-nutritive sweeteners include saccharin, aspartame, acesulfame potassium (or acesulfame K), sucralose, and neotame. Both children and adults can safely enjoy a range of nutritive and non-nutritive sweeteners when consumed in a diet that is guided by current federal nutrition recommendations as well as individual health goals.

In addition to its minimal effect on blood glucose levels, non-nutritive sweeteners also provide little to no calories. As part of a healthy, low fat diet, replacement of concentrated sugar beverages with those containing non-nutritive sweeteners are recommended for diabetic and obese children.

Sugar alcohols, or polyols, are another form of low calorie sweetener. Sugar alcohols include sorbitol, mannitol, xylitol, erythritol, lactitol, maltitol, isomalt, maltitol syrup, and hydrogenated starch hydrolysates. Most sugar alcohols provide approximately 2 calories per gram and should be counted as providing half the calories by weight of other carbohydrates. Sugar alcohols are absorbed slowly and incompletely from the intestine by passive diffusion. Therefore, amounts greater than 50 grams of sorbitol and or 20 grams of mannitol should be avoided in children due to its laxative effect.

ASSESSMENT OF FOOD NEEDS

Glycemic Index

The glycemic index (GI) is a concept that assesses foods based on postprandial blood glucose response. It is defined as the area under the glucose response curve after consumption of a 50 gram carbohydrate containing test food divided by the area under the curve after consumption of 50 grams of carbohydrate from a control food (white bread or glucose). Factors determining the glycemic index of a food include carbohydrate type and fiber, protein, fat and method of preparation and storage. The usefulness of glycemic index in the treatment of diabetes has been controversial. A low GI diet improves blood glucose control and decreases total cholesterol and triglycerides in subjects with type 2 diabetes.

Carbohydrate Counting

Carbohydrate counting is a flexible and effective way to allow a variety of foods to fit into the meal plan of children with diabetes. When counting carbohydrates, it is important to look at the portion size and total grams of carbohydrate in the product. Use of measuring cups and spoons are recommended to ensure accurate portion size. Reference books and food labels are used to obtain number of grams in a specific food or beverage.

Table 116.1: Determining insulin dose using insulin: Carbohydrate ratio and correction formula

Sample meal	*Grams (g) of carbohydrate*	
8 oz juice	27 g	Premeal blood sugar: 320
Bagel	60 g	Sample insulin to carb ratio: 1:15
1 tbsp butter	0 g	Sample correction formula:
4 oz milk	6 g	Blood sugar–120/50
8 oz coffee	0 g	
Total carbs consumed:	93 g	
Units of insulin to cover blood sugar: 320 – 120/50 = 4 units		
Units of insulin to cover meal: 93/15 = 6.2 units		
Total insulin dose: 4 + 5.2 = 10.2 or 10 units		

TREATMENT STRATEGIES FOR TYPE 1 DIABETES

Meal planning for children with type 1 diabetes is highly individualized, based on lifestyle and insulin regimen. Use of rapid acting insulin with meals and long acting background insulin is a popular and effective treatment option in the pediatric population. Also referred to as a multiple daily injection (MDI) regimen, children are allowed more flexibility in the number of carbohydrates consumed and the timing of consumption than with traditional diabetes management plans. A dose of rapid acting insulin is given with each meal, calculated using a personalized insulin to carbohydrate ratio, along with a correction formula, or sliding scale, to cover premeal hyperglycemia. Children on this regimen are required to check blood sugar before each meal and at bedtime. Use of a correction formula and insulin to carbohydrate ratio (Table 116.1) are also used for continuous subcutaneous insulin infusion (CSII) regimens. For those children who wish to initiate MDI and CSII therapy they or their caregiver must be able to accurately count carbohydrates and measure and weigh portions, demonstrate adequate math skills for calculating insulin dose, and be willing to keep a blood sugar log to assess trends.

Plasma blood glucose and A1C goals for type 1 diabetes by age group are given in Table 116.2.

For children whose diabetes is being managed according to a more traditional regimen, such as twice-daily injections of a combination of intermediate- and rapid-acting insulins, consistent carbohydrate intake is stressed to maintain normoglycemia. These children work with a dietitian to develop daily carbohydrate goals based on calorie requirements. The total number of carbohydrates suggested is then distributed throughout the day for meals and snacks.

TREATMENT STRATEGIES FOR TYPE 2 DIABETES

There is a direct correlation between the increasing incidence of obesity and type 2 diabetes in children and adolescents. Impaired glucose tolerance associated with insulin resistance is common. Children who are obese are more likely to become obese adults and parental obesity more than doubles the risk of adult obesity among both obese and nonobese children under 10 years of age. Strategies for prevention and treatment of obesity and type 2 diabetes focus on lifelong healthy food choices, portion control, and physical activity. Education should be aimed at both child and family, rather than child alone.

When evaluating patients with type 2 diabetes, a thorough diet history should be obtained. It is important to assess the child's usual food intake, eating behaviors, and family eating habits.

Treatment strategies are personalized, based on diet and pharmacological therapies. Children are often instructed on how to count carbohydrates and maintain a consistent carbohydrate intake throughout the day. Portion control should be stressed, focusing on appropriate portion sizes for age. Calorie restriction may be needed to attain and maintain a healthy weight. An improved glycemic response and decreased glycosylated hemoglobin levels follows a lower carbohydrate, higher protein diet by type 2 diabetics. No significant change in renal function is noted. A carbohydrate to protein to fat ratio of 40:30:30 may be favorable.

Table 116.2: Plasma blood glucose and A1C goals for type 1 diabetes by age group

	Plasma blood glucose goal range (mg/dl)		
Values by age	*Before meals*	*After meals*	*A1C(%)*
Toddlers and Preschoolers (<6 years)	100-180	110-200	<8.5 (but >7.5)
School age	90-180	100-180	<8 (6-12 years)
Adolescents	90-130	90-150	<7.5 (or <7.0 if achieved without excessive hypoglycemia)

Physical activity, in conjunction with diet modification, is essential for type 2 diabetes management to achieve a healthful weight and increase insulin sensitivity.

SUMMARY AND CONCLUSIONS

The diet for diabetes parallels a healthy diet for all people in amounts and types of nutrients consumed. Intake of fruits, vegetables, whole grains, low fat and non-fat dairy products, beans, fish, and lean meat is recommended. Saturated and transfats should be replaced with monounsaturated sources whenever possible. Non-nutritive sweeteners are most beneficial when used to replace calorie-dense and nutrient-diluted products such as soda and fruit flavored beverages. Convenience foods should be limited and portion control is stressed to avoid excessive weight gain and achieve normal linear growth. Teaching strategies for nutrition are individualized based on each patient's treatment goals and desired outcomes. The education process should include both child and caregiver.

KEY LEARNING POINTS

- Consistent diet and lifestyle modification is the key to prevention of complications in both type 1 and type 2 diabetes mellitus.
- Intake of fruits, vegetables, whole grains, low fat and nonfat dairy products, beans, fish and lean meat is beneficial.
- Saturated and transfat should be replaced with unsaturated fats.
- Non-nutritive sweeteners as replacement for calorie-dense and nutrient-diluted products like soft drinks and fruit-flavored beverages.
- Convenience foods need restriction.
- Education on diet needs to be addressed to both the child and the careproviders, usually parents.

FURTHER READINGS

1. Alemzadeh R, Ellis J, Holzum M, Parton E, Wyatt D. Beneficial effects of continuous subcutaneous insulin infusion and flexible multiple daily insulin regimen using insulin glargine in type 1 diabetes. *Pediatrics* 2004;114: e91-e95.
2. American Diabetes Association: Standards of Medical Care in Diabetes. *Diabetes Care* 2005; 28(Suppl 1): S4-S36.
3. American Dietetic Association Position Statement. Use of nutritive and non-nutritive sweeteners. *J Am Dietet Assoc* 2004;104: 255-275.
4. Anderson B, Ho J, Brackett J, Finkelstein D, Laffel L. Parental involvement in diabetes management tasks: Relationships to blood glucose monitoring adherence and metabolic control in young adolescents with insulin dependent diabetes mellitus. *J Pediatr* 2005;130: 257-265.
5. Garnier-Sagne I, Leblanc J, Verger P. Calculation of the intake of three intense sweeteners in young insulin-dependent diabetics. *Food Chem Toxicol* 2001;39:745-749.
6. Fagot-Campagna A. Emergence of type 2 diabetes mellitus in children. *J Pediatr Endocrinol Metab* 2000;13(Suppl 6):1395-1402.
7. Fisher J, Rolls B, Birch L. Children's bite size and intake of an entrée are greater with large portions than with age-appropriate or self-selected portions. *Am J of Clin Nutr* 2003;77: 1164.
8. Gannon M, Nuttall F, Saeed A, Jordan K, Hoover H. An increase in dietary protein improves the blood glucose response in persons with type 2 diabetes. *Am J Clin Nutr* 2003;78: 734-741.
9. Gannon M, Nuttall F. Effect of a high protein, low carbohydrate diet on blood glucose control in people with type 2 diabetes. *Diabetes* 2004;53: 2375-2382.
10. Kavey R, Daniels S, Lauer R, Atkins D, Hayman L, Taubert K. American Heart Association. American heart association guidelines for primary prevention of atherosclerotic cardiovascular disease beginning in childhood. *Circulation* 2003; 107: 1562-1566.
11. Nemet D, Barkan S, Epstein Y, Friedland O, Kowen G, Eliakim A. Short and long term beneficial effects of a combined dietary-behavioral-physical activity interventin for the treatment of childhood obesity. *Pediatrics* 2005;115: e443-e449.
12. Opperman A, Venter C, Oosthuizen W, Thompson R, Vorster H. Meta-analysis of the health effects of using the glycemic index in meal planning. *Br J Nutr* 2004;92: 367-381.
13. Sinha R, Fisch G, Teague B, Tamborlan W, *et al.* Prevalence of impaired glucose tolerance among children and adolescents with marked obesity. *N Engl J Med* 2004;346: 802-810.
14. Gidding S, Dennison B, Birch L, *et al.* Dietary recommendations for children and adolescents. *Circulation* 2005;112: 2061-2075.
15. Wolfsdorf J. Improving Diabetes control in adolescents. *Diabet Care* 2005;22: 1767-1768.

117 Nutritional Support in Inflammatory Bowel Disease

Sabeena Farhath • Millie Boettcher • Karoly Hoarvath

INTRODUCTION

Inflammatory bowel disease (IBD), a non-specific, chronic inflammation that includes two diseases, Crohn's disease (CD) and ulcerative colitis (UC), is the result of an inappropriate response by the gut-associated immune system to bacterial and nutritional factors though the trigger of this reaction is unknown.

ETIOLOGIC ASPECTS

While CD can occur in any part of the digestive tract from the mouth to the anus and characterized by patchy, *transmural* inflammation with skip areas interspersed between actively diseased segments, UC involves only the superficial layers of the *mucosa* with continuous lesions starting in the rectum and it is limited to the colon (Figs. 117.1 and 117.2).

Factors playing significant role in pathogenesis of IBD are listed in Table 117.1.

Table 117.1: Factors significantly contributing to the pathogenesis of IBD

- Mucosal immune system
- Bacterial flora
- Diet
- Genetic background

Immune System

The immune dysregulation in IBD involves both the innate and adaptive immunity. The defect in innate immunity is the result of the damage in the epithelial barrier, which is the first line of defense against pathogenic organisms. The exaggerated host response to luminal antigens leads to chronic inflammation and increased secretion of pro-inflammatory cytokines. Antigen presenting cells and macrophages play an important role in this process.

Bacterial Flora

The distal ileum and colon contain high concentrations of bacteria (>10^{12} organisms/g). These may include pathogens and bacterial factors that could be directly responsible for initiating IBD. The role of bacterial flora in the pathogenesis is supported by indirect data, such as beneficial response to antibiotics (Cipro, metronidazole) and the positive effect of probiotics in cases with CD. There are no specific bacteria identified as the trigger of abnormal immune response.

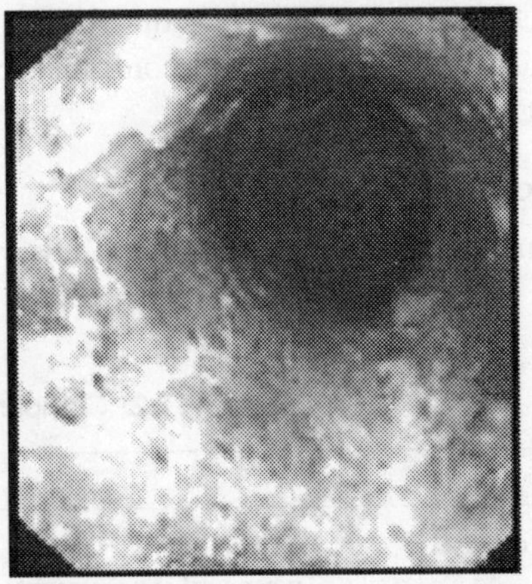

Fig.117.1: Endoscopic pictures of ulcerative colitis. Note the diffuse involvement of the colon

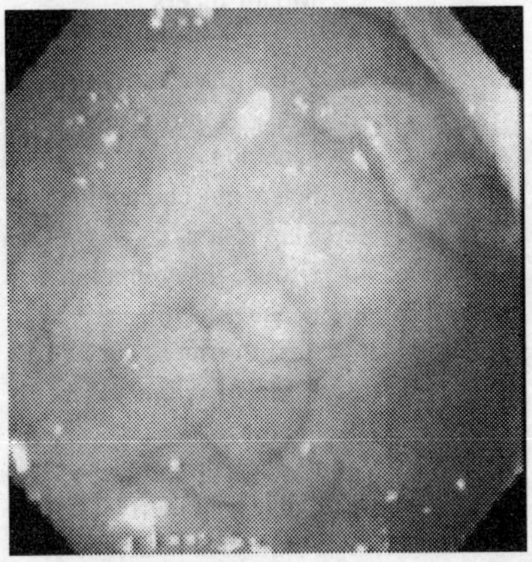

Fig. 117.2: Endoscopic picture of Crohn's disease. Note the typical ulceration and skip area

Diet

Dietary antigens represent a daily challenge to the gut-associated immune system; therefore diet is logically implicated in the pathogenesis of IBD. However, there are no specific dietary antigens identified as etiologic factors in either UC or CD. Differences in diet might explain the significant geographical differences in the prevalence of IBD. A study conducted in Sweden found that the incidence of UC and CD were higher in urban than in rural areas. Another study examining the association between diet and IBD found that the relative risk associated with consumption of fast foods at least two times a week was estimated at 3.4 (95% confidence interval=1.3-9.3) for CD and 3.9 (95% confidence interval=1.4-10.6) for UC. A Japanese study reported that the combined consumption of Western foods (bread for breakfast, butter, margarine, cheese, meats, and ham and sausage) was associated with an increased risk of UC (p=0.04). Among individual foods, consumption of margarine was positively associated with UC (p=0.005). A recent study reported from England identified meat, especially red meat consumption as a factor in the increased relapse in UC patients.However, the results of these epidemiological studies have to be confirmed by further investigations.

Genetic Background

Most of the evidence for genetic background in inflammatory bowel disease is derived from family and twin studies. The concordance rate for monozygotic twins for CD and UC are approximately 58.3% and 18.2% respectively, while the rates for dizygotic twins are 0% and 4.5% respectively. On genetic analysis of families with high incidence of CD specific chromosomal regions with significant degrees of genetic linkage have been identified. One of them is the CARD15/NOD2 gene.

The typical management of children with IBD includes the use of steroids, anti-inflammatory medications (5-ASA preparations), immunosuppressants (mercaptopurine, azathioprine, methotrexate), biological agents (anti-TNF) and nutritional therapy.

GROWTH OF CHILDREN WITH IBD

Generally, children with CD have growth failure, vitamin and mineral deficiencies, delayed bone age and decreased bone density then those with UC. This is due to the differences between these two diseases (Table 117.2).

Growth Failure

It had been described decades ago that growth failure is one of the main initial manifestations of IBD. It is much more prevalent in children with CD. The prevalence varies from 10 to 50% in the reported studies partially due to the different criteria used. Short stature may develop years before the manifestations of digestive symptoms.

Table 117.2: Comparison of Crohn's disease and ulcerative colitis

		Crohn's Disease	*Ulcerative Colitis*
Extent of the disease	Localization	From mouth to anus	Colon
	Transmural involvement	Common	Unusual
	Ileum involvement	Frequent	Absent (only blackwash ileitis)
	Rectal involvement	Occasional	Universal
Extraintestinal involvement	Fistula/stricture	Common	Absent
	Intraabdominal/ perianal abscess	Common	Absent
	Mouth ulcers	Common	Rare
	Erythema nodosum	Common	Less common
	Pyoderma gangrenosum	Less frequent	More frequent
	Iritis, iridocyclitis	More frequent	Less common
	Clubbing	Common	Less frequent
	Sclerosing cholangitis	Less frequent	More frequent
Endoscopic finding	Skip lesions	Common	Absent
	Diffuse inflammation	Less common	More common
Histology	Granuloma	30-50%	Unusual
	Crypt abscess	Less common	Common
Bleeding/ diarrhea	Rectal bleeding	Less common	Common
	Diarrhea	Less common	Always present
Growth/ nutrition	Growth failure	Common	Less frequent
	Delayed puberty	Common	Less common
	Nutritional deficiencies	Common	Less frequent
	Osteopenia	Common	Less frequent

As one of the peak ages when IBD manifests is the teenage period a delay in sexual maturation (delayed puberty) is an important feature of the CD in children.

Failure to gain weight is also an initial symptom while weight loss becomes a significant feature at the time of diagnosis. Bone age can be delayed by more than 2 years of the actual chronological age at presentation of CD.

The etiology of growth failure associated with IBD is multifactorial. It includes inadequate intake, increased loss, malabsorption and increased energy requirement.

Malnutrition and inflammation can change the insulin-like growth factor-1 (IGF-1) blood level. GF-1 is produced by the liver in response to growth hormone (GH) stimulation and it mediates the effects of growth hormone on the growth plate of bones. The association between impaired growth in CD and low IGF-1 levels has been reported two decades ago. The factors influencing IGF-1 levels are malnutrition, direct cytokine effects and chronic corticosteroid therapy (Fig. 117.3).

Nutrient deficiency may result in altered cellular immunity with increased risk of infection and delayed wound healing.

Box 117.1: Factors affecting the nutritional status in IBD

- **Decreased nutrient intake**
  - Anorexia
  - Fear of eating due to nausea, vomiting or crampy pain
  - Feeling of early fullness (early satiety)
  - Difficulty in swallowing
  - Side-effects of medications
  - Oral aphthous ulcerations
  - Diminished taste acuity (zinc deficiency)
- **Increased nutrient loss**
  - Vomiting
  - Diarrhea
  - Protein losses from the inflamed, ulcerated mucosa
  - Bleeding
- **Malabsorption/Maldigestion**
  - Extensive small bowel disease
  - Small bowel bacterial overgrowth
  - Bile salt-losing enteropathy
  - Surgical resection/short gut syndrome
  - Fat and fat soluble vitamin malabsorption
- **Increased calorie/nutrient requirements**
  - Increased calorie need for catch-up growth
  - Increased vitamin and mineral needs
  - Fever, stress
  - Abscess, fistula
  - Repletion of losses.

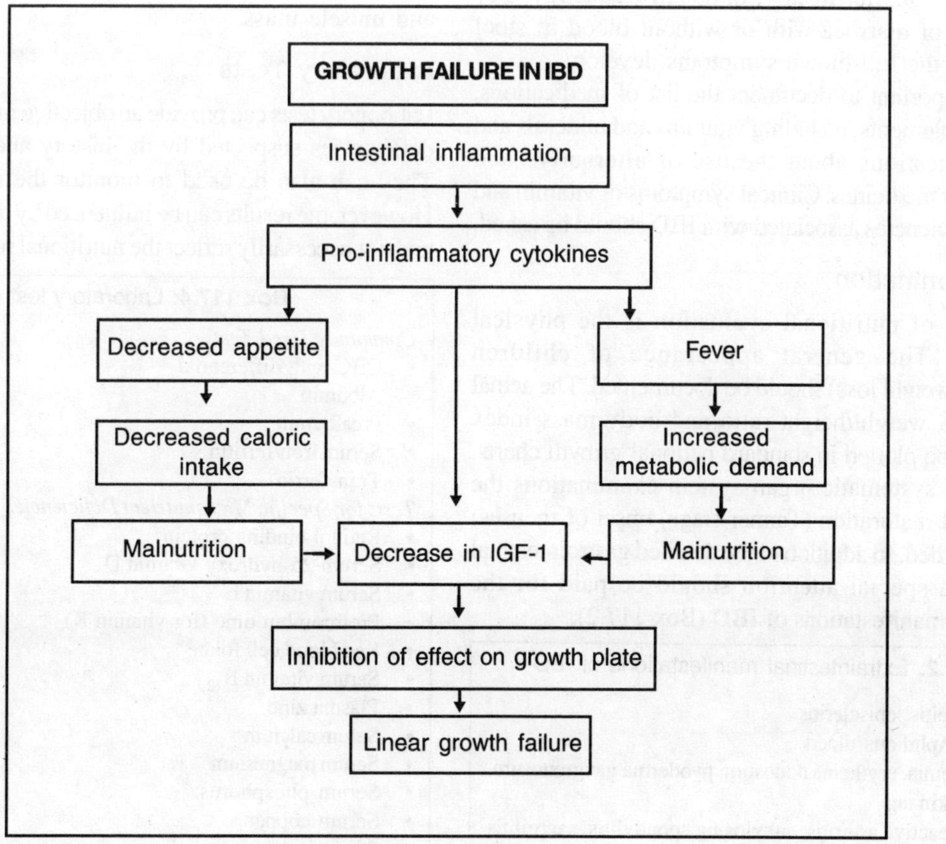

Fig. 117.3: Pathogenesis of linear growth failure in children with CD

Assessment of Nutritional Status

A good history and physical examination are the best clinical tools to assess the nutritional status of a patient. Although malabsorption is less prevalent in UC due to the absence of small intestinal involvement the nutritional status is affected in this disease as well. Assessment of nutritional status includes:

- History.
- Physical examination.
- Laboratory testing.
- Imaging studies.

History

It is very important to obtain growth charts showing the weight, height, and growth velocity in the previous years, especially in children suspected of having CD. The history should include questions related to appetite, diet and eating habits. Early fullness, eating small meals, pain during or after eating, and taste sensation changes are all associated with CD. A 24-hour dietary history, which is analyzed by a clinical nutritionist or a registered dietitian, can provide useful and more objective information. CD can start as a silent disease with gradual growth failure and may take years to develop gastrointestinal symptoms. Patients with UC typically have a shorter history, although frequently they have episodes of diarrhea with or without blood in stool months before the full-blown symptoms develop.

It is also important to document the list of medications, nutritional supplements, including vitamins and minerals and also to ask questions about the use of alternative and complementary medicines. Clinical symptoms of vitamin and nutritional deficiencies associated with IBD should be asked.

Physical Examination

The next part of nutritional evaluation is the physical examination. The general appearance of children (malnutrition, weight loss) should be documented. The actual weight, height, weight/height ratio and body mass index (BMI) should be plotted in standard national growth charts. As part of the systematic organ system examinations the stage of sexual maturation (Tanner stage, onset of menses) should be recorded. In addition to the detailed gastrointestinal examination a special attention should be paid for the extraintestinal manifestations of IBD (Box 117.2).

Box 117.2: Extraintestinal manifestations of IBD

- **Eyes:** Uveitis, episcleritis
- **Mouth:** Aphthous ulcers
- **Skin:** Anemia, erythema nodosum, pyoderma gangrenosum, perianal skin tag
- **Joints:** Reactive arthritis, ankylosing spondylitis, sacroilitis
- **Extremities:** Clubbing
- **Liver:** Cholelithiasis (RUQ tenderness), primary sclerosing cholangitis (jaundice)
- **Renal:** Nephrolithiasis

Many nutritional deficiencies are characterized clinically in changes involving the skin, eyes, oral cavity, skeletal system and neuromuscular system. Nutritional deficiencies of vitamins and minerals have specific clinical symptoms and signs.

Box 117.3: Manifestations of vitamin and mineral deficiencies

• Vitamin A:	Keratomalacia, night blindness, xerophthalmia
• Vitamin D:	Rickets, osteomalacia, bone pain, muscle weakness, tetany
• Thiamine (B_1):	Anorexia, confusion, edema, cardiac failure
• Riboflavin:	Cheilosis, glossitis, photophobia, angular stomatitis
• Folic acid:	Sore mouth, glossitis, forgetfulness
• Vitamin B_{12}:	Megaloblastic anemia, paresthesias, ataxia
• Iron:	Microcytic anemia, fatigue
• Calcium:	Osteopenia, osteoporosis, tetany
• Magnesium:	Tremor, muscle weakness, arrhythmias, confusion, seizures
• Zinc:	Growth failure, acrodermatitis, diarrhea, hair loss, hypogeusia

Simple measures such as triceps skinfold thickness and mid-arm circumference can be used to estimate body fat and muscle mass.

Laboratory Tests

Laboratory tests can provide an objective measure of nutritional deficiencies suspected by the history and physical findings. They can also be used to monitor the nutritional therapy. However, the results can be influenced by the underlying illness and not necessarily reflect the nutritional reserve of the patient.

Box 117.4: Laboratory test in IBD

Commonly Used Tests

- CBC with differential
- Albumin
- Prealbumin
- Serum iron/ferritin
- Transferrin

Tests for Specific Micronutrient Deficiencies

- Retinol binding protein
- Serum 25-hydroxy vitamin D
- Serum vitamin E
- Prothrombin time (for vitamin K)
- Red blood cell folate
- Serum vitamin B_{12}
- Plasma zinc
- Serum calcium
- Serum magnesium
- Serum phosphorus
- Serum copper
- Plasma selenium

Imaging Studies

Studies of bone age and bone density are useful in the evaluation of children with IBD.

Bone Age: An X-ray of the left hand and wrist to evaluate bone age may be obtained to assess skeletal maturation, and may be repeated over time if needed. It provides information about the relationship between chronologic age and skeletal maturation.

Bone Mineral Density: IBD patients, especially those with CD require Dual Energy X-ray Absorptiometry (DEXA) to assess bone mineral density. Bone demineralization, accelerated bone loss and osteopenia are a significant problem in patients with CD.

Factors contributing to the bone abnormalities are inadequate nutrition (vitamin D and calcium deficiency), poor absorption, reduced physical activity and the use of corticosteroids. Recent studies suggested that circulating pro-inflammatory cytokines produced in the inflamed bowel can effect the bone metabolism, particularly bone resorption.

The reasons for hypovitaminosis include inadequate intake, small intestinal involvement, chronic steroid therapy and limited exposure to sunlight. Corticosteroids affect bone mineralization by inhibiting osteoblasts, impairing intestinal calcium absorption and antagonizing the biological activity of growth hormone.

NUTRITIONAL MANAGEMENTS IN IBD

Nutritional support should be an integral part of the management of all children with IBD. The nutritional management starts with a nutritional assessment as described above. Nutritional therapy should be individualized to each patient depending on the nutritional status at the time of diagnosis. Management goals should include:

- Achieve a catch-up growth.
- Correction of nutritional deficits.
- Continuous monitoring of growth and nutritional parameters.

The nutritional management is more challenging in the newly diagnosed then in the established patients. Evidently malnutrition, characterized by weight loss, growth failure and micronutrient depletion are the main problems in the newly diagnosed children. Good control of intestinal inflammation and appropriate nutritional support are important for the enhancement of linear growth and achieve a catch-up weight gain. Children with CD generally have greater nutrient needs, based on age, gender, and weight, than do children with UC.

Nutritional intervention not only improves the body mass but it potentially improves the inflammation through the modulation of pro-and anti-inflammatory cytokine profiles.These changes preceded any significant changes in nutritional parameters.

Nutrition in patients with IBD has been used as primary therapy and as supplemental therapy.

Nutrition as Primary Therapy

Patients stop eating regular foods and receive all calories either as elemental or polymeric formula by mouth, through nasogastric or gastric tube or in the form of total parenteral nutrition. Enteral nutrition costs less than parenteral nutrition, maintains gut integrity, stimulates immunocompetence, and helps to control symptoms and overall disease activity.

Enteral Nutrition (EN)

EN has been used successfully as primary therapy in children. It has been hypothesized that enteral formulas decrease the stimulation of the gut-associated immune system. Over the past two decades, a number of studies supported that EN as primary therapy able to induce remission and control disease activity in patients with CD. Various forms of EN have been evaluated, including elemental, hypoallergenic and polymeric formulas based on their protein content. The elemental diets contain amino acids, semi elemental diet has oligopeptides and polymeric diet consists of whole proteins. Studies in children supports that elementary formulas do not have advantage over polymeric ones, in fact a multicenter randomized controlled trial reported that children with CD ingesting polymeric formula gained more weight. It seems that the type of formula used did not make difference in response as both elemental and polymeric diets were associated with improved disease activity scores, histologic healing, and down-regulation of pro-inflammatory cytokines. Clinical indications of enteral nutrition are given in Box 117.5.

Box 117.5: Indications of EN in IBD

Proven indications
- Reversing growth failure by avoiding steroid use
- Steroid resistant
- Steroid dependent

Potential indications
- Postoperatively developed fistula
- Perianal disease
- Intestinal stricture
- Maintenance of remission

Meta-analysis published in the mid-1990s concluded that enteral nutrition as primary therapy for CD is less effective than corticosteroids to induce clinical remission. A recent meta-analysis of four trials that included 130 patients treated with enteral nutrition and 123 treated with steroids yielded a pooled OR (odds ratio) of 0.30 favoring steroid therapy (95% CI: 0.17, 0.52).

However, pediatric studies support the concept that EN is equal to steroid therapy. The choice between EN and steroid therapy for a child with newly diagnosed CD is straightforward from medical point of view. Because both therapies have a similar efficacy, but EN has no side-effect, has beneficial effects on growth, leads to a rapid nutritional restitution; therefore most pediatricians have no difficulty to recommend it. Due to the poor palatability of elemental solutions they have to be given via feeding tube as continuous night time feeding. It requires either the passage of the feeding tube every evening or long-term placement of feeding tube. However, the permanent presence of tube makes it socially unacceptable especially for teenagers. Although polymeric diet is easier to digest, many families and children do not like opting for it.

Feeding through gastrostomy tube is an option. There is no risk of fistula formation based on a retrospective study on 25 patients with CD who underwent surgical or endoscopic gastrostomy tube placement. A study conducted in children confirmed the safety of PEG tubes and indicated that they were more tolerable than nasogastric tubes. Gastric tube placement can be considered in children with severe malnutrition whose compliance with an EN is poor.

There are special formulas developed for patients with IBD. Transforming growth factor beta (TGF-α) is a polypeptide that modulates intestinal epithelial cell growth and development and has anti-inflammatory effects. In a trial with polymeric diet with added TGF-α2 (Modulen, Nestle) 79% of patients achieved remission within 8 weeks.

Total Parenteral Nutrition (TPN)

Enteral route should be the preferred method of nutrition whenever possible. It has significantly less complications and costs much less than TPN. TPN is justified in severely malnourished CD patients who are unable to tolerate enteral feeding or in whom enteral feeding is contraindicated (Box 117.6).

Box 117.6: TPN as primary therapy in IBD

- Enteral route cannot be used
- Enteral route is ineffective in maintaining nutritional support
- Extensive small bowel disease
- In children before and after surgery
- Severely undernourished children with short bowel syndrome
- Toxic megacolon
- Intestinal obstruction
- Perforation
- Severe perianal disease
- Fistulizing disease.

Both bowel rest and TPN reduce intestinal inflammation and decrease disease activity in selected patients with CD. However, in UC it does not have any advantage over EN with polymeric formula.

TPN has some effect on the closure of intestinal fistula(s) in patients with CD. The initial closure rate was 44% and of these only 37% remains closed for an extended period of time.

Nutrition as Supplemental Therapy

Calorie Intake

Children with CD have greater nutrient needs, based on age, gender, and weight, than children with UC. The excess caloric needs depend on the disease activity. Resting energy expenditure (REE) in well-nourished children with CD is not different from values obtained in healthy children. The apparent increase in REE in children with CD is a result of their lower fat-free mass. These changes in REE are reversible and sustainable with aggressive enteral feeding. An expert panel of NASPGHAN recommends that the energy needs may be increased above recommended dietary intakes by 5% to 35% in children with CD depending on their nutritional status and the degree of inflammatory disease activity.

In some children with active CD, who are unable to increase their enteral intake night time continuous feeding is needed to provide adequate amount of calories for a catch-up growth. Foods and formulas can be enriched with medium-chain-triglyceride (MCT) oils that have a better absorption. However, a care should be taken not to exceed the threshold dose. MCT oil upto 50 g/day mixed with foods or formula can be introduced gradually into the diet.

Protein Intake

There is an increase in the protein turnover especially with systemic inflammation and infections due to losses from inflammation of the intestinal tract, and increased catabolism. It requires additional protein supplementation above the normal daily requirement. There is no clear recommendations for protein intake, so it should be individualized. A glutamine-enriched enteral nutrition formula diet did not offer advantage over a low-glutamine diet in children with CD in a double-blind randomized controlled trial.

Nutritional Supplements

A recent placebo controlled randomized study in adults reported decreased steroid use ($p<0.01$) in patients with UC who received 18 oz of the oral supplement enriched with fish oil, fructooligosaccharides, gum arabic, vitamin E, vitamin C, and selenium compared with those who received a carbohydrate-based placebo formula each day for 6 months. The following paragraph describes various nutritional supplements and they effect on the disease activity in IBD.

Folic acid/B_{12}: Medications used to treat IBD, such as methotrexate, a folate antagonist, and sulphasalazine, which interferes with folic acid absorption, may result in deficiency. Typically 1mg/day of folic acid supplementation is given to children with IBD. The best indicator of folic acid status is red blood cell folate content. Some past studies showed decreased relapse rate in patients receiving folate supplementation. Hyperhomocysteinemia is significantly more common in patients with IBD compared to healthy controls and is associated with lower levels of vitamin B_{12} and folate. Increased levels are inversely proportionate to folate levels (and to a lesser degree with B_{12} levels). While the clinical significance is uncertain, elevated homocysteine levels have been associated with a hypercoagulable state, thus possibly contributing to the hypercoagulability that has been observed in patients with IBD. There is an association between hyperhomocysteinemia and osteoporosis, which also support the practice of folic acid supplementation.

Vitamin B_{12} deficiency can be due to decreased factor production, inflammation or resection of the terminal ileum, which is the site of absorption. It occurs upto one third of the patients. Serum methylmalonic acid is a more sensitive indicator of cobalamin deficiency than serum vitamin B_{12}. A nasal gel form of B_{12} is now available but it is much more expensive compared with monthly IM administration.

Multivitamins with Minerals: Vitamin and mineral deficiencies have been well documented in IBD. The list of the reported deficiencies are: vitamin A, D, E, thiamine, riboflavin, folate, vitamin B_{12}; iron; calcium; magnesium; potassium and zinc. Fat soluble vitamin deficiency (vitamins A, D, E and K) can occur secondary to decreased bile acid pool and fat malabsorption in patients with CD. Patients with IBD are advised to take multivitamin supplements, although there are no controlled trials to support this practice. The multivitamin/mineral preparations have all water and fat-soluble vitamins and minerals such as iron, zinc, magnesium, calcium, selenium etc.

Calcium: Risk factors for low body calcium include corticosteroids, vitamin D deficiency, malabsorption, and systemic inflammation. Assessment of adequate calcium and vitamin D intake is important in all patients with IBD and supplementation is needed if the diet is found deficient. Osteoporosis is present in approximately 30% of children with CD. DEXA scan is recommended to evaluate bone density. In adolescent 1200-1500 mg of calcium and a multivitamin containing 400 IU of vitamin D is recommended per day. Given, the lack of data on biphosphonates use in children, this therapy is not recommended at the present time. Osteopenic patients should undergo monitoring of vitamin D and calcium status and bone density.

Iron: Iron deficiency results from excessive iron loss due to chronic, occult, or gross bleeding and from proximal intestinal disease leading to malabsorption of iron.

Upto 66 percent of patients with ulcerative colitis and 25 to 40 percent of those with CD are iron-deficient. Concerns about intolerance, lack of efficacy, or worsening of disease state due to supplemental iron therapy among patients with IBD have not been substantiated in clinical studies.

***Zinc*:** Patients with IBD can have excessive stool losses and urine excretion of zinc. Clinical signs of deficiency include acrodermatitis, peeling of palms and soles of feet. Serum measurement is less reliable indicator of zinc status then e.g. measurement from hair samples. A deficient state is often reflected by a decreased serum alkaline phosphatase concentration, as it is a zinc metalloenzyme. Excessive losses of zinc may be observed in patients with ostomies, fistulas, and profuse diarrhea.

Magnesium: Magnesium deficiency in patients with IBD may result from decreased oral intake, malabsorption, and increased intestinal losses, and may contribute to osteopenia. Oral supplementation with magnesium can lead to diarrhea. If magnesium supplementation is needed magnesium gluconate has a higher degree of solubility, making it a better choice for intestinal supplementation.

Selenium: Selenium occurs naturally in meats, cereals and fish. It is an essential part of the antioxidant glutathione peroxidase. Selenium concentration in whole blood and glutathione peroxidase activity can be decreased in patients with IBD. Selenium deficiency may result in a potentially fatal but reversible cardiomyopathy.

***Fish oil*:** Fish oil contains n-3-PUFA (poly-unsaturated fatty acid), which inhibits production of proinflammatory cytokines and has some benefit in the treatment of CD. Fish oils have been used as complementary nutritional therapy in IBD. In addition their known beneficial effect on vascular epithelium they influence the leukotriene balance by shifting LTB4 production to LTB5, which much less pro-inflammatory. Fish oil have anti-inflammatory effects exerted through several potential mechanisms: (1) reduced production of leukotriene B4 and thromboxane-A2, (2) inhibition of inflammatory cytokines such as interleukin-1 and tumor necrosis factor, and (3) scavenging of free radicals. A double-blinded, placebo controlled one-year study in adult patients receiving 2.7 g of n-3 fatty acids per day reported decreased relapse rate compared with the placebo group (28% vs. 69%).

A reduction in disease activity and a corticosteroid sparing effect was noted in patients with UC, but not CD when they received treatment with omega-3 long chain fatty acids. However, in other study there was no difference in relapse rates between the treatment and placebo groups.

Nutritional Modification of Intestinal Bacterial Flora

***Prebiotics*:** Prebiotics are oligosaccharides that cannot be hydrolyzed by human digestive enzymes. Therefore, they reach the colon and are metabolized by bacteria. The two main groups of prebiotics are fructooligosaccharides (FOS), such as inulin, lactulose and galactooligosaccharides (GOS). They are naturally present in our foods including onions, garlic, asparagus, leeks, bananas, artichokes and chicory root. The quantity of prebiotics cannot be high as studies showed that ingestion of prebiotics over 10 grams per day can cause increased diarrhea and cramping. Recently enteral tube feeding formulas are available that containing FOS (Peptamen with FOS, Jevity Plus and Nepro).

In the next few years, important advances are expected in understanding the interactions between prebiotics, intestinal flora and the colonic mucosa in health and diseases, which may lead to improvement of therapy and nutritional management of susceptible individuals.

There are increasing evidences suggesting that some components of the enteric flora play role the pathogenesis of IBD. Probiotics are living organisms that favorably modify the bacterial flora in the colon. They help re-establishing the normal intestinal flora by creating an environment that is unfavorable to potential pathogenic bacteria and maintain the integrity of the gut mucosal barrier. The mechanism of these actions is not fully understood, but may include direct effect on bacteria, changes in the colonic pH and stimulation of the intestinal immune system by enhancing macrophage and natural killer activities and proliferation of lymphocytes. Lactobacillus strains and bifidobacterium are the most frequently used probiotics.

Clinical trials on patients with CD and postoperative pouchitis demonstrated a significantly benefit of probiotic therapy compared to the control groups. The three trials involving patients with UC found no significant difference in relapses.

There are yoghurts with live cultures that have high concentration of probiotics and can be used as alternative to probiotic capsules or tablets. In addition they provide extra calories.

Dietary Restrictions in IBD

Dietary restrictions should be avoided unless intestinal obstruction or specific abnormalities of digestion or absorption exist.

Dietary lactose only restricted if patients have symptoms associated with dietary intake or has a positive breath hydrogen test. Since dairy products are excellent source of calcium the use of lactase enzyme supplement is recommended rather than a full elimination of milk. The prevalence of lactose malabsorption in IBD patients is estimated to be between 10% and 20%. Lactose restrictions should only be employed in patients exhibiting symptoms, such as crampy pain, gas and diarrhea after consuming dairy products.

Ad libitum diets are equally as effective as *low residue diets* in maintaining remission in adults with CD. Soluble fiber metabolized to short chain fatty acids like butyrate is the preferred fuel for colonocytes. The diet of IBD should be a balanced diet with appropriate fiber content. The typical daily fiber in a balanced diet is approx. 0.5g/kg/day. There is often confusion between low fiber and low residue diets. Low fiber diet reduces fiber intake while a low residue diets limit fiber as well as any other food known to leave a residue in the GI tract (such as milk products, prune juice, etc). "Diet as tolerated" is still remains the recommendation to patients with IBD.

In patients with *strictures* it may be prudent to avoid such fiber containing food as broccoli, raw carrot, grapes, nuts, seeds, mushrooms, popcorn, celery and all fruits with skins as they are potentially able to cause obstruction. It is important to warn patients to chew their foods well if strictures are present. Some patients may need to rely on liquids as the sole source of nutrition if strictures or narrowing do not allow passage of normal foods, however, in these cases surgical management should be considered. Fig. 117.4 shows the barium study of a child with CD who developed stricture in the ascending colon and required resection and ileostomy.

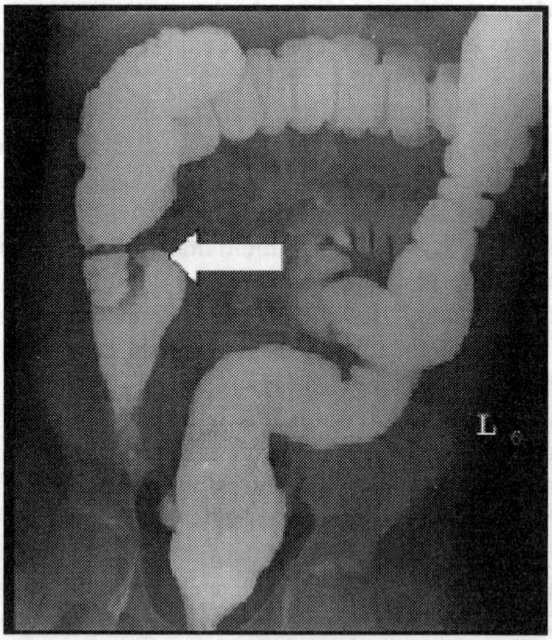

Fig. 117.4: Barium enema study of a child with CD who developed a stricture in the ascending colon and required surgical resection and temporary ileostomy

Patients with new *ileostomies* represent a special category. They are instructed to avoid the high fiber foods listed above for a period of 2-4 weeks to allow post-operative swelling to subside. Fiber-containing foods typically are added back slowly beginning with water-soluble fibers (e.g. oatmeal, banana, rice and apple sauce) followed by insoluble fibers (wheat, bran, corn or nuts) as tolerated. However, this practice is not based on research data.

Patients with ileostomies may require additional fluid and electrolytes due to losses.

Low oxalate diet is required in patients with terminal ileum resection or with significant fat malabsorption, because these patients have the propensity for oxalate kidney stones.

IBD AND PREGNANCY

Since an increasing proportion of teenagers are getting pregnant, a word on IBD and pregnancy should be in order.

Fertility is reduced in patients with CD compared to UC. Women are naturally concerned about the effects of IBD on fertility, pregnancy and fetus and how pregnancy may affect their disease activity. UC and CD behave in a similar manner with a relapse rate of approximately 30-35% during gestation. Most pregnant women are concerned about the risks of drugs to the fetus. There are controversies regarding medical therapy in pregnant IBD patients. Nutritional support is an important adjunct during the pregnancy in IBD patients. Drug therapies and the disease by itself may lead to vitamin deficiency states. It is very important that folate supplementation be reinforced as it has a protective effect on neural tube defects.

KEY LEARNING POINTS

- Pathogenesis of growth failure and malnutrition in IBD includes reduced nutrient intake, malabsorption, increased energy expenditure, and enteral losses.
- Nutritional management is essential for the care of children with IBD, as it can help prevent growth failure and improves mucosal healing. It should include the assessment of dietary intake, body composition, determination of bone age, and routine laboratory studies, including specific testing for micronutrient deficiencies.
- Nutritional support should be an integral part of the management of children with IBD. Growth failure is frequent in newly diagnosed children and it requires additional enteral supplementation for a catch-up growth. Adequate nutrition results in an improvement in the well-being, nutritional status, and growth and also leads to a reduction in the biochemical and histologic markers of disease activity and potentially reduces corticosteroid use, particularly in CD.
- Enteral diets alone are effective to induce remission in children with active CD. There is no advantage in using the more expensive elemental formulas because polymeric ones are also effective. Fish oils that are rich in omega-3 long-chain fatty acids are able to reduce disease activity and corticosteroid use.
- Periodic nutritional assessment of children with IBD and appropriate nutritional therapy provides an effective complementary therapy in inflammatory bowel diseases.

FURTHER READINGS

1. Bannerjee K, Camacho-Hubner C, Babinska K, Dryhurst KM, Edwards R, Savage MO, *et al.* Anti-inflammatory and growth-stimulating effects precede nutritional restitution during enteral feeding in Crohn disease. *J Pediat Gastroenterol Nutr* 2004;38:270-275.
2. Duerr RH. Update on the genetics of inflammatory bowel disease. *J Clin Gastroenterol* 2003;37:358-367.
3. Ekbom A, Montgomery SM. Environmental risk factors (excluding tobacco and microorganisms): Critical analysis of old and new hypotheses. *Best Pract Res Clin Gastroenterol* 2004;18:497-508.
4. Fernandez-Banares F, Cabre E, Esteve-Comas M, Gassull MA. How effective is enteral nutrition in inducing clinical remission in active Crohn's disease? A meta-analysis of the randomized clinical trials. *JPEN J Parenter Enteral Nutr* 1995;19:356-364.
5. Griffiths AM. Inflammatory bowel disease. *Nutrition* 1998;14:788-791.
6. Hyams JS, Wyzga N, Kreutzer DL, Justinich CJ, Gronowicz GA. Alterations in bone metabolism in children with inflammatory bowel disease: An in vitro study. *J Pediatr Gastroenterol Nutr* 1997;24:289-295.
7. Kirschner BS, Sutton MM. Use of ulcerative colitis: A prospective cohort study. *Gut* 2004;53:1479-1484.
8. Somatomedin-C levels in growth-impaired children and adolescents with chronic inflammatory bowel disease. *Gastroenterology* 1986;91:830-836.
9. Ludvigsson JF, Krantz M, Bodin L, Stenhammar L, Lindquist B. Elemental versus polymeric enteral nutrition in paediatric Crohn's disease: A multicentre randomized controlled trial. *Acta Paediatr* 2004;93:327-335.
10. Persson PG, Ahlbom A, Hellers G. Diet and inflammatory bowel disease: A case-control study. *Epidemiology* 1992;3:47-52.
11. Strober W, Fuss IJ, Ehrhardt RO, Neurath M, Boirivant M, Ludviksson BR. Mucosal immunoregulation and inflammatory bowel disease: New insights from murine models of inflammation. *Scand J Immunol* 1998;48:453-458.
12. Zachos M, Tondeur M, Griffiths AM. Enteral nutritional therapy for inducing remission of Crohn's disease. *Cochrane Database Syst Rev* 2001:CD000542.

118 Nutritional Support in Renal Diseases

Maria Puangco-Curcio • Anupama Chawla

INTRODUCTION

Nutritional challenges vary with the stage of renal insufficiency and according to the patient's ongoing therapy. This chapter addresses nutrition support in specific renal insufficiency scenarios such as chronic renal insufficiency with and without dialysis as well as acute renal failure.

CHRONIC RENAL INSUFFICIENCY (CRI)

Nutritional and Metabolic Consequences of Chronic Renal Failure

The consequences of chronic renal failure and the medical therapies necessary to treat the symptoms complicate provision of adequate medical nutrition therapy. Consequences of the disease such as fluid overload, azotemia, metabolic acidosis, hypertension and renal osteodystrophy among others will compromise the growth of the child if they are inadequately treated. Symptoms of uremia such as nausea, growth retardation and edema respond favorably to medical nutrition therapy.

Other complications of chronic renal insufficiency (CRI) such as altered gastrointestinal absorption that could decrease absorption of calcium and iron and affect nitrogen metabolism can be treated to prevent or halt the progression of renal osteodystrophy or anemia, respectively. Hyperphosphatemia and secondary hyperparathyroidism as an adaptive mechanism in response to uremia can be avoided with proper medical and diet therapies. Cachexia due to factors such as low dietary intake, decreased appetite, catabolic illness, dialysis and blood loss can be prevented with proper medical therapies and dietary modifications. The potential metabolic complications of renal failure are summarized in Table 118.1. The goal of all therapies is to optimize growth, minimize uremic toxicity and other metabolic derangements and to retard the progression of renal failure.

The National Kidney Foundation Kidney Disease Outcome Quality Initiative Clinical Practice Guidelines (NKF K/DOQI) have been widely adopted in the United States to improve the quality and consistency of clinical care provided to individuals with chronic renal disease throughout the country. These recommendations have focused primarily on the adult population. More recently guidelines have been

Table 118.1: Metabolic complications of renal failure

Metabolic alterations
Glucose
Insulin resistance
Hyperglycemia
Lipids
Hypercholesterolemia
Hypertriglyceridemia
Protein and amino acid abnormalities
Decreased protein and amino acid synthesis
Increased protein catabolism
Azotemia
Fluid and electrolyte
Volume expansion and contraction
Hypo- or hypernatremia
Hypo- or hyperkalemia
Hypo- or hyperphosphatemia
Hypocalcemia
Metabolic acidosis
Gastrointestinal
Nausea and vomiting
Altered taste acuity
Gastroenteritis
Peptic ulceration
Ascites
Endocrine
Renal osteodystrophy
Secondary hyperparathyroidism
Amenorrhea
Infertility
Cardiac
Hypertension
Hyperlipidemia
Atherosclerosis
Nutritional
Anorexia
Anemia
Vitamin deficiencies

developed addressing the clinical needs of the pediatric population with chronic renal disease who are receiving maintenance dialysis only (Table 118.2). However, the guidelines developed are both evidence and opinion outcomes-based. The availability of the former is limited.

Table 118.2: NKF K/DOQI clinical practice guidelines/ nutrition of chronic renal failure American Society of Pediatric Nephrology

1. Patient evaluation of protein-energy nutritional status
2. Management of acid-base status
3. Urea kinetic modelling
4. Interval measurements
5. Energy intake for children treated with maintenance dialysis
6. Protein intake for children treated with maintenance dialysis
7. Vitamin and mineral requirements
8. Nutrition management
9. Nutritional supplementation for children treated with maintenance dialysis
10. Recommendations for the use of recombinant human growth hormone for children treated with maintenance dialysis

However, there is general agreement among practitioners that early recognition in this population to maximize growth potential and to minimize complications is essential to treating CRI. Several studies have demonstrated impaired linear growth and weight patterns in mild stages of CRI. The North American Pediatric Renal Transplant Cooperative showed average decreased growth rates at GFR <75 ml/min/1.73 m^2. On average this data showed -1.5 SDS for height and -0.6 SDS for weight.

Principles of Medical Nutrition Therapy CRI

The goal of medical nutrition therapy is to maintain nutrition status and to optimize growth and development. Currently the NKF K/DOQI Clinical Guidelines for routine evaluation apply to adults. However, in the pediatric population evaluation of nutritional status every 6 to 12 months when GFR < 60 mL/min/1.73 m^2 is prudent. When GFR <30 ml/min/1.73m^2 or when malnutrition is evident assessment of nutrition status every 1 to 3 months has been recommended.

Optimizing growth and development through early recognition and treatment of factors that can compromise growth is fundamental to treating CRF. As stated previously impaired linear growth and weight patterns in mild stages of CRI have been shown. Other contributing factors that can contribute to short stature result from metabolic acidosis, altered growth hormone, insulin-like growth factor, or delayed sexual maturation due to renal insufficiency. The recommendations for monitoring growth and nutrition status in children with CRI is summarized in Table 118.3.

Table 118.3: Nutrition assessment and monitoring in renal failure

- Diet history
- Diet recall
  - 7-day diet journal
- Anthropometrics
  - Height for age
  - Weight for age
  - Weight for height
  - Body mass index
  - Head circumference
  - Tricep skinfold
  - Midarm circumference
  - Midarm muscle circumference
- Nitrogen status
  - Protein equivalent of nitrogen appearance (PNA)
  - BUN
  - Creatinine
  - Creatinine clearance
- Laboratory measures
  - Electrolytes
    - Sodium
    - Potassium
    - Chloride
    - Bicarbonate
  - Minerals
    - Calcium
    - Phosphorus
    - Magnesium
    - Parathyroid hormone
  - Glucose
  - Triglyceride
  - Cholesterol
  - Albumin
  - Transferrin

Monitoring

Growth

Growth should be assessed at the intervals recommended by NKF K/DOQI Clinical Guidelines. These parameters should include height for age, weight for age, weight for height and body mass index. Other useful anthropometric measures of nutrition status include the tricep skinfold, mid arm circumference, mid arm muscle circumference and head circumference. NKF K/DOQI Clinical Guidelines also recommend using the SDS or Z score when interpreting height velocity. Evaluation of the adequacy of the patient's diet is best obtained by a diet history. It is controversial as to which is the best method. Studies indicate that 7-day histories account best for the variation in a child's appetite in the course of a week. The underreporting of oral intake has been found to be a common occurrence in older American children and adolescents.

Electrolytes and Minerals

Routine monitoring of electrolytes is essential to prevent

metabolic imbalances that can be prevented with diet modification and medication if necessary.

Fluid Intake

A child's urine output and insensible losses determine prescribed total fluid.

Sodium

A reduced GFR has been associated with decreased tolerance to dietary sodium. Factors that may require sodium restriction include hypertension, fluid retention and daily steroid therapy. Increasing sodium may be necessary with increased urine losses.

Potassium

Maintaining potassium homeostasis is feasible; exceptions to this include post-obstructive renal damage, severe reflux nephropathy and CRF due to interstitial nephritis. Decreasing endogenous potassium may be necessary when GFR falls to <5% or when hyperkalemia occurs. Diuretic therapy may require that oral potassium be increased.

Acid-Base Balance

Regular monitoring of acid-base balance can prevent growth impairment. Growth turnover is associated with mineralization of bone that increases hydrogen production. Subsequently infants and young children usually have larger hydrogen ion load than adults. Persistent metabolic acidosis is common and associated with failure to thrive in this population. Decreased re-absorption of bicarbonate associated with CRI limits the effectiveness of base therapy in correcting the acidosis.

Calcium, Phosphorus and Magnesium

Routine monitoring of calcium, phosphorus, and magnesium is important to achieve and maintain calcium and phosphorus homeostasis. This promotes adequate bone mineralization and may prevent elevations in parathyroid hormone (PTH) and subsequent renal osteodystrophy. It has been proposed that hyperphosphatemia has been associated with a reduced rate of conversion of 25-OH to 1,25 OH vitamin D. This decreases serum ionized calcium and thus increases levels of PTH. Deficiency of calcium occurs due to resistance to vitamin D's effect on calcium absorption.

Laboratory Monitoring

Regular monitoring of ammonia and urea nitrogen are essential for treatment of chronic renal disease. More controversial are laboratory indices of nutrition status. Low prealbumin and albumin levels have been linked to increased mortality in patients with chronic renal failure. Currently prealbumin is recommended for use in adults but there is insufficient data to recommend its routine use in the pediatric population. Hypoalbuminemia is common in CRI. It is not a marker of acute changes in nutrition status because of its long half life. However, caution is recommended when interpreting it as an indices of visceral protein status as the result is influenced by fluid balance. Excessively low albumin levels can also be seen as a consequence of marked fluid overload.

Transferrin and serum iron are useful indices of iron deficiency. This is most common in children when creatinine clearance values <40 ml per minute per 1.73 m. Causes of iron deficiency anemia include blood loss in dialysis, inadequate iron intake, Fe malabsorption and blood loss due to bleeding diathesis associated with uremia.

There is insufficient evidence to recommend protein equivalent of total nitrogen appearance (PNA) for routine use in pediatrics. However, estimates can be calculated by measuring urea in 24-hour urine collection.

Medical Nutrition Treatment of CRI

Calories and Protein

Patients who receive at least 80% calories of the Dietary Reference Intakes (DRI) or greater for height age have improved nitrogen balance without compromised renal function. No added benefit to renal function has been shown when protein and calories are restricted further. Using height for age to determine energy and protein needs is a more practical and reliable because it is not influenced by fluid shifts. Also, it can be measured reliably. Calorie recommendations for infants with CRI is 6-11.9 calories/cm/d and protein 0.15 g/cm height or less with adequate calories. In adults with GFR <25 ml/min, low protein diet 0.6 g/kg/d of high biologic value protein is recommended by NKF K/DOQI guidelines. In the pediatric population children with a creatinine clearance <50% who consume 8% of total calories as protein and 100% of calorie requirements remain well below 12-15% of protein calories consumed in the average American diet. In general it is recommended that in children with CRI to limit protein to DRI for height age. Studies have shown this ratio of calories to protein resulted in the best nitrogen retention while preserving remaining renal function. Potential obstacles to provision of this nutrition therapy are fluid restriction and gastroesophageal reflux in infants. In addressing these issues it may be necessary to concentrate formula upto 60 calories per ounce. Figure 118.1 illustrates a method how this can be accomplished using a combination of formula and carbohydrate, fat and protein supplements. When concentrating formula it is important to keep in mind the calorie and protein recommendations for height previously mentioned.

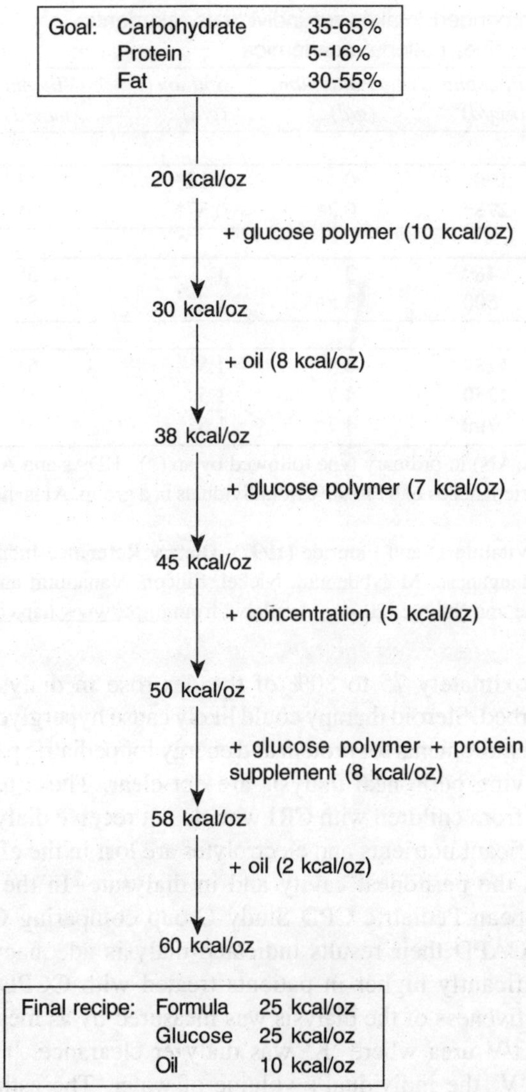

Fig. 118.1: Method of concentrating formula upto 60 calories per ounce

Electrolytes and Minerals

A sodium restriction may be prescribed in the presence of hypertension, fluid retention and/or daily steroid therapy. Diuretic therapy may require that potassium from food be increased or a potassium supplement prescribed.

Reduced phosphorus intake may be necessary to prevent elevation in parathyroid hormone and renal osteodystrophy. Usually a reduction in protein intake especially meats also decreases phosphorus intake. Other foods that are high in phosphorus include dairy, chocolate, nuts and colas (Table 118.4). Soy formulas are lower phosphorus substitutes for cow-milk based formulas. It may be necessary to use medication to treat hyperphosphatemia. Traditionally non-aluminum and non-magnesium-containing phosphate binders are recommended.

Occasionally calcium supplementation may be required due to vitamin D resistance or decreased gastrointestinal absorption associated with renal insufficiency. Supplementation with calcium may also help bind intestinal phosphorus. Effective supplement forms include calcium carbonate, lactate, citrate or gluconate supplementation. Dosage is prescribed in milligrams for DRI age (Table 118.5).

Nutrition Supplements

When a child is not growing or if the diet is analyzed for apparent nutrient deficiencies, supplementation may be necessary. Most of the studies investigating the use of nutrition supplements in chronic renal failure to date have been in the adult population. The results of those studies to date have been mixed regarding the beneficial effect of nutrition supplements. One study showed a significant improvement in height SDS in children with mild and moderate CRI. This same study showed children receiving supplementation also exceeded 80% of DRI for energy.

Vitamins

Multivitamin supplementation is recommended due to multiple restrictions of the diet. Supplementation with vitamin D as 1,25 OH or analogue, a-hydroxy vitamin D and dihydrotachysterol have been shown to enhance calcium transport. Folic acid amounts of 0.5-1 mg per day may be necessary. Iron supplementation may be necessary only when serum iron and/or transferrin levels are low. When patients are receiving erythropoietin or ferritin, iron supplementation is usually required. Regular monitoring of iron status is necessary as iron toxicity is possible due to multiple blood transfusions.

CRF with Dialysis

Peritoneal dialysis is recommended for infants and small children and hemodialysis (HD) and peritoneal dialysis (PD) for older children. Nutritional management depends on the

Table 118.4: Phosphorus content of foods

High phosphorus	*Lower phosphorus substitutions*
Dairy foods (milk, cheese, yogurt)	Liquid non-dairy creamer
Beans (baked, kidney, lima, pinto)	Soy
Processed meats (hot dogs, canned meat)	Soy
Colas, canned iced teas, lemonades	Water, seltzer, powdered tea and lemonade mixes, apple and cranberry juice
Bran cereal	Corn and rice cereals
Egg yolks	Rice, pasta

Table 118.5: Dietary reference intakes (DRIs): Recommended intakes for individuals, elements food and nutrition board, institute of medicine, national academies

Life stage group	*Calcium (mg/d)*	*Iron (mg/d)*	*Magnesium (mg/d)*	*Phosphorus (mg/d)*	*Potassium (g/d)*	*Sodium (g/d)*	*Vitamin D (mcg/d)*
Infants							
0-6 mo	210*	0.27*	**30***	**100***	0.4*	0.12*	5*
7-12 mo	270*	**11**	**75***	**275***	0.7*	0.37*	5*
Children							
1-3 years	500*	**7**	**80**	**460**	3	1	5*
4-8 years	800*	**10**	**130**	**500**	3.8	1.2	5*
Males/Females							
9-13 years	1300*	**8**	**240**	**1250**	4.5	1.5	5*
14-18 years	1300*	**11**	**410**	**1250**	4.7	1.5	5*
19-30 years	1000*	**8**	**400**	**700**	4.7	1.5	5*

Recommended Dietary Allowances (RDA) in bold type and Adequate Intakes (AIs) in ordinary type followed by an (*). RDAs and AIs may both be used as goals for individual intake. RDAs are determined to meet to nutrient needs of 97 to 98% of individuals in a group. AI is the mean intake.

Sources: Dietary Reference Intakes for Calcium, Phosphorus, Magnesium, Vitamin D and Fluoride (1997); Dietary Reference Intakes for Vitamin A, Vitamin K, Arsenic, Boron, Chromium, Copper, Iodine, Iron, Manganese, Molybdenum, Nickel, Silicon, Vanadium and Zinc (2001); and Dietary Reference Intakes for Water, Potassium, Sodium, Chloride and Sulfate (2004). Available from http://www.nap.edu.

type of dialysis. However, the nutrition goals and monitoring indices (see CRI without dialysis) are the same as for conservative management of CRI. Anthropometric parameters monitored are the same as in the pediatric population not receiving dialysis. Data from the Mid-European Pediatric CPD Study Group (MPCS), 1999 suggests that patients receiving continuous cycling peritoneal dialysis (CCPD) may have better growth than those patients receiving continuous ambulatory peritoneal dialysis (CAPD). The authors suggest an association between small solute clearances and growth.

Calories and Protein

As stated previously determining calorie and protein requirements is more reliably assessed using height for age.

For those receiving hemodialysis 10 calories per centimeter per day has been recommended. Another study evaluating protein intake in dialyzed children showed that with protein intake at 0.3 grams per centimeter per day and energy intakes of 10 calories per centimeter per day produced positive nitrogen balance without a need for additional dialysis. For those receiving HD, DRI for chronological age plus an additional increment 0.4 g/kg/d of protein has been recommended. Children receiving PD should have their initial dietary protein intake based on DRI for chronological age plus an additional increment based on anticipated peritoneal losses. The maximum amount of protein depends on the type of dialysis as protein losses in peritoneal dialysis vary from 5 to 24 g/d. Dextrose absorption from peritoneal dialysate should be considered in determining calorie intake. The amount absorbed depends on the volume infused, dwell time and dextrose concentration. Reported dextrose absorption is 25 to 50% after dwell times of 2 and 4 hours, respectively. In 6 hours approximately 75 to 80% of the dextrose in dialysate is absorbed. Steroid therapy could likely cause hyperglycemia.

Requirements for protein and energy for pediatric patients receiving peritoneal dialysis are not clear. These tend to vary from children with CRI who do not receive dialysis as significant nutrients and electrolytes are lost in the effluent from the peritoneal cavity and in dialysate. In the Mid-European Pediatric CPD Study Group comparing CCPD and CAPD their results indicated dialysis adequacy was significantly higher in patients treated with CCPD. The effectiveness of the dialysis was measured by as measured by Kt/V urea where 'K' was dialyzer clearance, 't' time and 'V' the individual's volume of water. The estimated protein catabolic rate (PCR) was significantly higher in the CCPD group (1.39 ± 0.6 g/kg/d) compared to the CAPD patients (1.08 ± 0.48 g/kg/d). Because nutritional requirements per kilogram of body weight are higher in children than in adults, it is of the opinion of the Peritoneal Dialysis Adequacy Work Group that protein doses in children and infants receiving PD are higher than doses in adults. Protein recommendations have been made as follows: upto age 5 years 3 g/kg/d, 5 years to puberty 2.5 g/kg/d, puberty 2 g/kg/d and post puberty 1.5 g/kg/d. Periodic calculations of urinary and dialysate urea nitrogen, dialysate protein and amino acids and nitrogen losses are recommended. The NKF K/DOQI clinical practice guidelines recommend for pediatric PD patients that nutrition status be assessed every 6 months using the protein equivalent of nitrogen appearance (PNA) and other standard nutritional assessments. The PNA equation is as follows: PNA (g/d) = [6.49*UNA]+ [0.295*V] + protein losses (g/d) where urea nitrogen assessment equals UNA and patient's total body water is represented by 'V'.

Lipids and fats are a critical and calorie dense source. However, hypertriglyceridemia due to decreased hepatic lipase activity occurs. A diet restricted in fat and carnitine supplementation remains controversial and usually not recommended.

Fluid and Electrolytes

The prescribed fluid depends on the child's urine output. A child's intake of sodium and potassium intake depends on the child's residual renal function and the type and effectiveness of dialysis. Restriction of foods containing large quantities of sodium such as those cured, canned and pickled are usually necessary. Food high in potassium may also be restricted (Table 118.6). Severe restriction of these electrolytes except in acute instances of elevated levels is not generally recommended as diet adherence is usually poor due to acceptance of a strictly restricted and unpalatable diet.

Minerals

Restrictions to the diet and treatment are the same as for individuals with CRI. PTH concentrations have shown a significant increase with both moderate and severe CRI.

Vitamins

Vitamin supplementation in patients receiving dialysis is similar to those not receiving dialysis. Because of the diet restriction a multivitamin is recommended. In addition, water soluble vitamins that include folate 1 mg per day, vitamin B_6 5-10 mg per day and upto 100 mg vitamin C per day are recommended.

Laboratory Data

Low prealbumin and albumin levels have also been linked to increased mortality. Hypoalbuminemia is common in patients with CRI on dialysis. Currently monitoring prealbumin is recommended for use in adults but there is insufficient data to recommend its routine use in the pediatric population.

Table 118.6: Potassium content of foods

High potassium	*Lower potassium substitutions*
Oranges, orange juice	Apples, apple juice
Melons	Cranberry juice
Apricots	Canned fruit
Banana	Strawberries, blueberries, raspberries
Kiwi	Plums, pineapple
Potatoes	Rice, pasta
Tomatoes	
Sweet potatoes	Cauliflower
Cooked spinach	Mustard, turnip greens
Beans (baked, kidney, lima, pinto)	Broccoli

Transferrin and serum iron levels should be monitored routinely. Supplementation should be given in response to low levels, however, this population is at risk for iron overload due to multiple blood transfusions.

Despite current evidence indicating a possible correlation between PNA and nitrogen balance, urea kinetic modeling as a tool to calculate PNA in patients receiving dialysis is not currently recommended for routine use in the pediatric population.

NUTRITION SUPPORT OF ACUTE RENAL FAILURE

The mortality rates from acute renal failure (ARF) are high. The data are limited as to the optimal provision of medical nutrition therapy for the pediatric patient with ARF. However, it is known that ARF causes changes in substrate utilization. Treatment of the disease and its metabolic derangements can interfere with providing adequate nutrition therapy. These include fluid restriction, poor oral intake due to anorexia secondary to uremia and/or underlying illness, poor gastrointestinal absorption and loss of nutrients in dialysate especially continuous veno-venous hemodialysis (CVVHD) or veno-venous hemofiltration (CVVHF).

Calories and Protein

In the absence of sepsis, recommended energy is based on calories for centimeter of age height. Factors that could affect energy requirement are the degree of renal dysfunction, continuous renal replacement therapy (CRRT), the presence of multisystem organ failure and the underlying disease. The dialysis process has been reported to raise energy requirements. It has been reported that CRRT can reduce oxygen consumption due to significant heat losses thus theoretically raising energy consumption. Utilization of adequate calories could be compromised by insulin resistance.

The causes of hypercatabolism are multifactorial. Insulin resistance could decrease glucose uptake by upto 50%. The dextrose in dialyate should be considered when determining energy intake. The presence of insulin resistance and uremia could impair amino acid transport into the cell. Hepatic gluconeogenesis even in the presence of adequate nutrition could lead to muscle wasting and loss of lean body mass.

A study in which patients were treated with at least 1.5 g/kg/d and upto 2 g/kg/d of protein achieved positive nitrogen balance. These investigators found that positive nitrogen balance increased the probability of survival by 21%. Another study demonstrated that as protein intake was increased and energy requirements was decreased the protein sparing was improved. Varying the amino acid combinations does not affect nitrogen balance.

Impaired lipolysis due to inhibition of peripheral lipoprotein lipase and hepatic triglyceride lipase could lead to increased TG, VLDL-C, LDL-C and decreased HDL-C and total cholesterol.

Micronutrients

Hyperkalemia is commonly associated with ARF. This is due mainly to either impaired renal excretion or to increased release of potassium from cells during catabolism. Hypokalemia occurs most often due to refeeding syndrome or in unusual instances potassium restriction.

Phosphorus abnormalities may occur due to impaired renal excretion and increased cellular release during catabolism and increased mobilization from bone leading to hyperphosphatemia. Supplementation of phosphorus may be necessary when hypophosphatemia occurs from hemodialysis dialyzers that affectively remove phosphorus.

Calcium excretion is decreased in ARF. Impaired activation of 1,25 dihydroxycholecalciferol can lead to decreased intestinal calcium absorption. Skeletal resistance to PTH is another cause of hypocalcemia and hyperphosphatemia. CRRT has been associated with hypercalcemia. Other factors include immobilization, calcium concentration in dialysate solutions, malignancy and high PTH levels.

Causes of abnormalities in magnesium levels have been associated with increased intake or infusion leading to hypermagnesemia. Medications such as cyclosporine and cisplatin are associated with magnesium wasting. CRRT raises magnesium requirements due to increased losses in dialysate.

Vitamins

Water soluble multivitamin is recommended due to the dietary restrictions. Additional thiamine and pyridoxine may be necessary to improve energy metabolism. Fat soluble vitamins except vitamin K are generally recommended due to decreased renal hydroxylation of active forms of these vitamins.

Renal failure is associated with metabolic derangements and electrolyte abnormalities. Often the treatments such as diuretics, fluid restriction and dialysis contribute to the challenge of providing adequate nutrition support for children with either chronic renal insufficiency or acute renal failure. Further studies are needed on what are useful tools for nutrition assessment, optimal protein requirements and calcium therapy especially in the pediatric population with the compounded demands of growth.

With considerable attention to close monitoring of electrolytes and macro- and micronutrients the nutritional outcome has improved considerably over the past couple of decades. However, meeting the nutritional needs of the patient as determined by the achievement of near normal growth and development still remains suboptimal.

KEY LEARNING POINTS

Chronic Renal Insufficiency (CRI)

- Subjects should receive at least 80% calories of the DRI for improved nitrogen balance without compromising renal function.
- In terms of height for age, calorie recommendation is 6 to 11.9 calories/cm/d and protein 0.15 g/cm height.
- Multivitamin supplementation is recommended.

Acute Renal Failure (ARF)

- Data regarding optimal provision of nutrition therapy in pediatric ARF are limited.

Supplematation with multivitamin and macro and micronutrients is recommended.

FURTHER READINGS

1. Bandini LG, Cyr H, Must A, Dietz WH. Validity of reported energy intake in preadolescent girls. *Am J Clin Nutr* 1997;65:1138S-1141S.
2. Blumenkrantz MJ, Gahl GM, Kopple JD, Grodstein GP, Coburn JW. Protein loss during peritoneal dialysis. *Kidney Int* 1981;19:593-602.
3. Boydstun II. Chronic kidney disease in adolescents. *Adolesc Med* 2005;185-199.
4. Druml W. Metabolic aspects of continuous renal replacement therapies. *Kidney Intl Suppl* 1999:72;S56-S61.
5. Druml W. Nutritional management of acute renal failure. *Am J Kidney Dis* 2001;37:S89-S94.
6. Fivush BA, Jabs KA, Neu AM, Sullivan EK, Feld L, Kohaut E, *et al.* Chronic renal insufficiency in children and adolescent: The 1996 annual report of NAPRTCS. *Pediatr Nephrol* 1998 12:328-337.
7. Foster BJ and Leonard MB. Measuring nutritional status in children with chronic kidney disease. *Am J Clin Nutr* 2004;80:801-14.
8. Gonzalez-Espinoza L, Gutierrez-Chavez J, Martin del Campo F, Martinez-Ramirez HR, Cortez-Sanabria L, Rojas-Campos S, *et al.* Randomized, open label, controlled clinical trial of oral administration of an egg albumin-based protein supplement to patients on continuous ambulatory peritoneal dialysis. *Pert Dial Int* 2005;25:173-180.
9. Grupe WE, Harmon WE, Spinozzi NS. Protein and energy requirements in children receiving chronic hemodialysis. *Kidney Int Suppl* 1983 15:S6-S10.
10. Hellerstein S, Holliday MA, Grupe WE, Fine RN, Fennell RS, Chesney RW, *et al.* Nutritional management of children with chronic renal failure. Summary of the task force on nutritional management of children with chronic renal failure. *Pediatr Nephrol* 1987;1:195-211.
11. Ikizler TA, Wingard RL, Sun M, Harvell J, Parker RA, Hakim RM. Increased energy expenditure in hemodialysis patients. *J Am Soc Nephrol* 1996;7:2646-2653.
12. Kapadia FN, Bhojani K, Shah B. Special issues in the patient with renal failure. *Crit Care Clin* 2003 19:233-251.

13. Kist-van Holthe tot Echten JE, Nauta J, Hop WCJ, deJong MC, Reitsma-Bierens WC, Ploos van Amstel SL, Martinez-Ramirez HR, Cortez-Sanabria L, Rojas-Campos S, *et al.* Protein restriction in chronic renal failure. *Arch Dis Child* 1993;68;371-375.
14. Kopple JD. NKF K/DOQI Clinical Practice Guidelines for nutrition in chronic renal failure. *Am J Kidney Dis* 2001;37:66-70.
15. Livingstone MB, Robson PJ. Measurement of dietary intake in children. *Proc Nutr Soc* 2000;59:279-293.
16. Neyra R, Chen KY, Sun M, Shyr Y, Hakim RM, Ikizler TA. Increased resting energy expenditure in patients with end-stage renal disease. *J Paren Enterl Nutr* 2003;27:36-42.
17. NKF K/DOQI Clinical Practice Guidelines 2000. II. Pediatric Guidelines, Urea Kinetic Modeling 2000 Available on www. http://kidney.org/professionals/KDOQI/guidelines_updates. Accessed on 9 June 2006.
18. NKF K/DOQI Clinical Practice Guidelines for nutrition in chronic renal failure. Available from http://www.aspeneph.com/guidelines.html. Accessed on 31 May, 2006.
19. Norman LJ, Coleman JE, Macdonald IA, Tomsett AM, Watson AR. Nutrition and growth in relation to severity of renal disease in children. *Pediatr Nephrol* 2000; 15:259-265.
20. Norman LJ, Macdonald IA, Watson AR. Optimising nutrition in chronic renal insufficiency—progression of disease. *Pediatr Nephrol* 2004 19:1245-1252.
21. Radtke HW, Claussner A, Erbes PM, Scheuremann EH, Schoeppe W, Koch KM. Serum erythropoietin concentration in chronic renal failure: Relationship to degree of anemia and excretory renal function. *Blood* 1979 54:877-884.
22. Schaefer F, Klaus G, Mehls O: Peritoneal transport properties and dialysis dose affect growth and nutritional status in children on chronic peritoneal dialysis. Mid-European Pediatric Peritoneal Dialysis Study Group. *J Am Soc Nephrol* 10:1786-1792, 1999.
23. Schaefer F, Wolf S, Klaus G, Mehls O: Higher KT/V urea associated with greater protein catabolic rate and dietary protein intake in children treated with CCPD compared to CAPD. Mid-European Pediatric CPD Study Group (MPCS). *Adv Perit Dial* 10:310-314, 1994.
24. Scheinkestel CD, Karl L, Marshall K, Bailey M, Davies A, Nyulsai I, *et al.* Prospective randomized trial to assess caloric and protein needs of critically ill, anuric, ventilated patients requiring continuous renal replacement therapy. *Nutrition* 2003;19:909-916.
25. Seikaly MG, Salhab N, Gipson D, Yiu V, Stablein D. Stature in children with chronic kidney disease: Analysis of NAPRTCS database. *Pediatr Nephrol* 2006; 21:793-799.
26. Spinozzi NS, Grupe WE. Nutritional implications of renal disease. *J Am Diet Assoc* 1977;70:493-497.
27. Strejc JM. Considerations in the nutritional management of patients with acute renal failure. *Hemodial Internat* 2005;9:135-142.
28. Teixido-Planas J, Ortiz A, Coronel F, Montenengro J, Lopez-Menchero R, Ortiz R. Oral protein-energy supplements in peritoneal dialysis: A multicenter study. *Perit Dial Int* 2005; 25:163-172.
29. Wideroe TE, Smeby LC, Berg KJ, Jorstad S, Svartas TM. Intraperitoneal (125I) insulin absorption during intermittent and continuous peritoneal dialysis. *Kidney Int* 1983;23:22-28.
30. Wingen AM, Fabian-Bach C, Schaefer F, Mehls O. Randomised multicentre study of a low-protein diet on the progression of chronic renal failure in children. *Lancet* 349:1117-1124.

119 Nutritional Support in HIV/AIDS

Swati Kolpuru • Karoly Horvath

INTRODUCTION

It was recognized at the beginning of the HIV epidemic that malnutrition is a common and one of the earliest complications of HIV/AIDS. It was further appreciated that malnutrition plays a significant and independent role in the morbidity and mortality of HIV infection. During the last two decades, in keeping with the significant improvement in our scientific knowledge in virology, antiretroviral therapies, management of chronic psychosocial problems and multisystem disorders related to human immunodeficiency virus (HIV) infection, the nutritional management of HIV infection has demonstrated a significant progress.

PATHOGENESIS OF MALNUTRITION IN HIV

According to the World Health Organization (WHO), malnutrition is *"the cellular imbalance between supply of nutrients and energy and the body's demand for them to ensure growth, maintenance, and specific functions"*.

Malnutrition is associated with adverse consequences, irrespective of the level of immune status. The pathogenic mechanisms of malnutrition in HIV are multifactorial (Table 119.1).

Table 119.1: Modus operandi of developmnt of malnutrition in HIV infection

- Decreased calorie and nutrient intake.
- Poor appetite.
- Malabsorption.
- Diarrhea.
- Opportunistic infection with increased requirement.
- Metabolic disturbances.
- Psychosocial factors.

The nutritional implications of HIV infection for children are more devastating because children have additional nutritional demands for growth and development. Periods of rapid growth increase the demands of muscle and other organs. If the supply of any essential nutrient does not meet the demand, growth retardation and other functional deficits may occur. Poor weight gain, failure to thrive and short stature are common in children with untreated HIV infection and AIDS.

It has been reported that nutrition by either enteral nutrition (tube feeding) or parenteral nutrition improves the immunity (CD_4 count) and intestinal function in HIV-infected children. This underlines the importance of proper nutrition in immune function. The clinical and biochemical association between malnutrition and altered immune function is well established.

Recent advances in antiretroviral therapy have decreased the prevalence of opportunistic infections and malnutrition. However, the introduction of highly active antiretroviral therapy (HAART) results in body fat redistribution problems in a substantial proportion of HIV-infected children.

GROWTH FAILURE IN HIV-INFECTED CHILDREN

The CDC-defined wasting in HIV-infected children based on their age:

- <13 years of age a weight loss of more than 10% of baseline.
- A decline of at least 2 percentile lines on the weight-for-age chart in a child aged 1 year or older; or
- Less than the 5th percentile on the weight-for-height chart on two consecutive measurements at least 30 days apart.
- Plus chronic diarrhea or documented fever for at least 30 days, whether intermittent or constant.

A change in body composition, particularly a decline in body cell mass (loss of cells) should raise the suspicion of HIV-related wasting in the absence of other explanations for weight loss. HIV-infected children experience wasting of lean body mass over time without significant change in fat mass. The identification and treatment of wasting is critical to ensure long-term survival and quality of life in children with HIV infection. The consequences of malnutrition are the following:

- **Shortened survival:** Death from wasting in AIDS is related to the degree of tissue depletion. Progressive depletion of body cell mass occurs in patients near death.
- **Decreased quality of life**: Weight loss is significantly

associated with a decline in functioning and quality of life.

- **Immune dysfunction**: Malnutrition is associated with a rapid decrease in CD_4 cell numbers. Nutritional intervention may be able to improve intestinal absorption and result in increase in the CD_4 cell numbers.
- **Increase in opportunistic infections**: Weight loss can increase the risk of opportunistic infections by as much as 61% to 176%.

With the introduction of HAART, there have been dramatic declines in AIDS-related morbidity and mortality in populations that have access to these new treatments.

NUTRITIONAL ASSESSMENT OF A PATIENT WITH HIV

Every child who is infected with HIV should receive a complete baseline nutritional assessment within 3 months of diagnosis in order to assess the need for early nutritional intervention. Follow-up assessment should be conducted every 1 to 6 months, depending on the child's age and nutritional status.

History and Physical Examination

All children with HIV should first have a comprehensive history and physical examination. Clothing often masks subtle signs of wasting, such as abdominal, gluteal, and limb atrophy. Therefore, the patient should be completely undressed for the examination The triage of these patients should include:

- Weight, height, weight for height, body mass index (BMI) percentile in children 11 to 17 years old.
- Head circumference in children from birth to 3 years.
- Midarm circumference and triceps skinfold in children older than 1 year.

Previous growth data are very useful. A gradually declining weight growth velocity, followed by a gradually declining height growth velocity, reflects chronic undernutrition or malabsorption. In case abnormalities in height growth velocity precede weight changes, it may reflect altered endocrine function (probably growth hormone deficiency).

During the medical history taking, special attention should be given to such details as listed in Table 119.2.

Table 119.2: Special details during medical history taking

- Caloric intake
- Alterations in body weight and body shape
- Changes in appetite, eating behaviors, feeding skills
- Eating habits
- Food availability and storage
- Gastrointestinal function
  - Number and characteristics of stools, symptoms
  - Difficulties with chewing or swallowing
  - Abdominal pain
- Presence of underlying infection

Contd.

Contd.

- Other medical problems
- Functional status (including physical activity)
- Perceived levels of weakness, fatigue
- Medications
- Use of nutritional supplements: vitamin and mineral supplements, and herbs
- Use of complementary treatments
- Social history

Table 119.3: Laboratory and clinical tests

- Plasma HIV RNA
- CD4:CD8 ratio
- CBC with differential
- Serum iron, total iron-binding capacity
- Serum glucose
- Fasting cholesterol, and triglycerides (especially on HAART)
- Liver function tests
- Serum vitamin A and E
- Serum zinc
- Thyroid function tests if clinically warranted
- Stool examination for opportunistic pathogens in patients with diarrhea
- Blood cultures in case of fever
- Chest radiography
- Pulse oximetry if there is breathing problem
- Barium radiography
- Upper gastrointestinal endoscopy and colonoscopy with biopsy
- A 24-hour recall or diet record should be obtained and compared with estimated needs to assess adequacy of intake

Estimation of Body Fat Content

The collection of various body composition measurements is critical to establish the diagnosis of HIV-associated wasting. Basic data include the patient's age, height, weight, ideal body weight and BMI.

Body Weight (BW)

BW is the most common body composition measurement taken in the clinical setting.

Advantage

Useful in monitoring the HIV infected children's growth compared with the normal growth curves.

Disadvantage

- Fluid overload or deficits decreases its accuracy.
- Cannot distinguish between fat, lean mass and water.

Body Mass Index (BMI)

BMI represents an individual's weight for height as an index number.

Advantage

It most accurately reflects a person's body fat content.

Disadvantage

BMI cannot differentiate between lean tissue and either fat or extracellular water. Clinicians therefore, should not rely solely on BMI as their only measurement technique.

Skinfold Measurements

It provides estimates of fat and fat-free mass only. Measuring skinfold thickness is the most widely used technique for estimating fat mass.

Advantages

- Useful in identifying individuals with HIV associated fat redistribution.
- Readily available and inexpensive.

Disadvantages

- Observer error is possible.
- There may also be errors because of inter-individual variability in fat redistribution.
- Hard to standardize.
- Not efficient for small changes.

Cross-sectional Imaging

Advantage

Magnetic resonance imaging (MRI) and computed tomography are the most precise of the available measures that allow differentiation of subcutaneous adipose tissue and visceral adipose tissue and can measure changes in these compartments.

Disadvantage

It needs expensive equipments and experienced technicians.

Dual-Energy X-ray Absorptiometry (DEXA)

Reflects regional body composition, especially in the limbs.

Advantages

- Very accurate.
- Brief scanning time.
- Safe radiation level.

Disadvantages

- High equipment cost.
- Not portable.
- Hydration status affects results.

Bioelectrical Impedance Analysis (BIA)

BIA uses the electrical impedance of body tissues to estimate body composition. It provides an estimate of the total body water by measuring changes in a low electrical current passed between electrodes placed on the upper and lower extremities. The sizes of other body compartments (including body cell mass) are then calculated using equations based on assumptions about the relationships between different body compartments and total body water. The validity and reliability of the results depend on the correct placement of the electrodes, room temperature, patient exercising, hydration status and the equations used to estimate body cell mass.

Loss of body cell mass, as measured by BIA, occurs early in the course of HIV infection, even in patients who are otherwise asymptomatic and is an independent adverse prognostic marker of clinical progression and survival.

Advantages

- Rapid and easy to perform.
- Portable and therefore can be used in clinical settings and hospitals.

COMPLEX NUTRITIONAL MANAGEMENT OF CHILDREN WITH HIV INFECTION

Because HIV can be transmitted through breast milk, the CDC recommends that HIV antibody-positive women in the United States avoid breastfeeding and use commercially available formulas for their child.

Children with HIV infection may be at increased nutritional risk because of the energy and micronutrient demands necessary to compensate for infection as well as support growth and development. The management should focus on not only the compliance to medications and nutrition but also address additional measures (Table 119.4). The patients who are compliant with HAART are less likely develop opportunistic infection and wasting.

Table 119.4: Important aspects of nutritional management of HIV infected children

• Implementation of nutritional support • Drug therapy • Oral care • Nutritional aspects of highly active antiretroviral therapy (HAART) • Follow up assessments

Implementation of Nutritional Support

Nutrition plays an essential role in supporting the health and quality of life of children with HIV disease. Nutrition intervention should begin soon after diagnosis. For optimal care, a nutritionist should perform an initial nutrition evaluation and periodic follow-ups.

For many children, nutritional status is often directly related to their socio-economic status and it is an important determinant of overall nutritional status and growth.

Oropharyngeal and esophageal abnormalities associated with AIDS should be addressed before any nutritional intervention. If children have any signs of oral candidiasis, aphthous ulcers, gingivitis, poor dentition, leukoplakia, herpetic lesions they need to be treated. In such cases, high-calorie, smooth, nonirritating foods should be offered frequently throughout the day to maintain adequate total caloric intake.

Upto 75% of HIV-infected children have mild to severe developmental delay. HIV-associated encephalopathy not only results in delayed acquisition or loss of developmental milestones but also may affect oral motor skills. If poor feeding skills are suspected, the oral motor and self-feeding skills should be observed at the clinic and referral to an occupational therapist for evaluation should be made. If the possibility of aspiration is raised videofluoroscopic swallowing study should be ordered.

Several medications commonly used in the treatment of HIV disease, especially antiretroviral agents, macrolide antibiotics and chemotherapy, may cause anorexia, nausea or vomiting. In addition, drug interactions can increase serum levels of offending medications, exacerbating the problem.

Antiretroviral medications, especially the protease inhibitors, are unpalatable and difficult to administer to younger children. It is recommended adding the medication to a small amount of cold food (ice cream, shakes, fruit juices) or thick, sweet foods (honey, jellies, frozen juice concentrate) or small amounts of peanut butter, pudding, applesauce, or yogurt can make it palatable. These medications should be added to small quantities of food in order to be completely swallowed and the full dose be taken. In infants the placement of medication into a full bottle of formula should be avoided because the infant may not ingest the whole formula.

There is a great variation of nutritional requirements and feeding modes in HIV infection. There is a high prevalence of malabsorptive disorders in untreated HIV-infected children. In case of suspected or proven malabsorptive disorders, protein hydrolysate and elemental formulas are better tolerated. All children with HIV and AIDS require high-energy, high-protein, nutrient-dense diets. The protein intake should be between 100% and 150% of the recommended daily allowance (RDA) in order to support the immune system and avoid muscle wasting. Caloric and protein needs should be adjusted for fever, infections, viral load, catch-up growth, and activity level.

The first step should be a trial with dietary manipulation. The caregivers should be counseled on food choices, frequency of meals and snacks, and methods of increasing caloric density. Commercially available nutritional supplements, high calorie drinks are cheaper than special high calorie formulas and still provide high-nutrient addition to the diet.

If the oral route fails to provide enough calorie and nutrients, supplemental enteral nutrition (EN) should be the next step. Enteral supplementation can improve weight and fat mass in HIV-infected children when other oral supplements fail. EN improves not only weight, but also triceps skinfold thickness and decreases the number of hospital admission days.

A trial of nasogastric (NG) feeding is easily available and it may prove that a child is able to gain weight. The disadvantages of NG-tube feeding are complications such as sinusitis, worsening esophageal candidiasis. Additional limitations include the inability of the caregiver to maintain the NG feeding or a non-cooperative child.

The next step can be the endoscopic or surgical placement of a gastrostomy feeding tube. It has been reported that a low weight for height at the initiation of gastrostomy tube feedings predicts a good response to enteral supplementation. An additional benefit of a gastrostomy tube in HIV infected young children is that it eases administration of unpalatable antiviral liquid medications.

Nutritional deficiencies should be addressed. Commonly deficient nutrients include thiamine mononitrate (vitamin B_1), riboflavin (vitamin B_2), pyridoxine hydrochloride (vitamin B_6), cyanocobalamin (vitamin B_{12}), folate, ascorbic acid (vitamin C), tocopherol (vitamin E), vitamin A, selenium, and zinc.

Adolescents and young adults often have lifestyle and eating habits that lead to poor-quality diets. Obesity is a common nutrition problem for both HIV-infected and uninfected teenagers. In addition, HIV-infected teenagers are at increased risk of developing metabolic abnormalities and micronutrient deficiencies, and at highest risk of being deficient in vitamins A and E and zinc. It was reported that supplemental vitamin A and zinc can decrease the frequency of respiratory and diarrheal illnesses. Experimental studies have suggested that high serum levels of vitamin E may be associated with slower disease progression.

Micronutrients play important roles in maintaining immune function and neutralizing the reactive oxygen intermediates produced by activated macrophages and neutrophils in their response to microorganisms. Micronutrient status reflects the efficiency of the body's cellular functions. Insufficient dietary intake, malabsorption, diarrhea, and impaired storage and altered metabolism of micronutrients can contribute to the development of micronutrient deficiencies. In addition, infection and its evolution likely lead to an increased requirement for nutritional micronutrients, especially antioxidants.

Although the mechanisms are not known, micronutrient deficiencies may exacerbate the oxidative stress induced by HIV. Because young children have difficulty taking pills or capsules, a single complete multivitamin and mineral supplement in liquid or powdered form is ideal for them.

Drug Therapy

Appetite Stimulants

If diet with supplements does not lead to the desired weight gain, appetite stimulants can be considered as a short-term approach to reversing malnutrition. *Megestrol acetate,* an agent used for the treatment of metastatic breast cancer, is associated with appetite stimulation and weight gain. It has been shown in anorectic patients to improve appetite, quality of life and total body weight. Megestrol acetate-induced weight gain is primarily the result of an increase in body mass. It is a relatively non-toxic drug with a low incidence of side effects. A dose of 20 to 40 mg of megestrol acetate daily may improve weight gain in children. The adult dose is up to 800 mg/day.

Disadvantages

- No survival benefit or decrease in morbidity has been seen.
- Therapy is costly.
- May cause loss of lean body mass in some patients.
- Decreases serum testosterone levels.

Anabolic Agents

Androgen deficiency is a common endocrine abnormality among adult men and women with HIV infection. Low testosterone concentrations are associated with lower CD_4 cell count, advanced stage of illness, medication use, and weight loss. Androgens—particularly oxandrolone (Oxandrin), nandrolone (DecaDurabolin), oxymetholone (Anadrol-50) and testosterone have been used to increase body cell mass in patients with wasting syndrome. However, there are no accepted standards for indications, dosages and duration of therapy. In addition to its effects on body composition, testosterone treatment results in improved mood and libido in HIV-infected women and increased bone mineral density in HIV-infected men. Anabolic agents have not been studied in children infected with HIV but has been studied in children with severe burns, which showed that long-term administration of oxandrolone safely improves lean body mass, bone mineral content, and bone mineral density.

Recombinant Human Growth Hormone (rhGH)

Body shape abnormalities are the side effect of highly active antiretroviral therapy (HAART), therefore has been great interest in potential interventions. Recombinant human growth hormone therapy is approved by the US Food and Drug Administration (FDA) and it is highly effective therapy for increasing lean body mass. rhGH treatment may enable patients with wasting to perform activities of daily living that would be exhausting. However, the safety and efficacy of long-term rhGH therapy and its impact on survival are unknown. At this stage the use of rhGH is reserved for patients who are undergoing unexplained significant weight loss, have not responded to other therapies or require short-term treatment to maintain body cell mass during acute infection.

Oral Care

Studies have estimated that majority of persons with HIV infection will have at least one oral manifestation at some time during the course of their disease. Over 30 different oral manifestations of HIV disease have been reported since the beginning of the AIDS epidemic, which include infections, tumors, conditions caused by direct HIV activity, as well as adverse side-affects of antiretroviral and other antimicrobial drugs.

Patients with HIV infection may not have dental care. Patients should be examined for oral diseases and be treated. The medical staff plays an important role in educating the patient about good oral hygiene and the prevention and treatment of these conditions.

Nutritional Aspects of Highly Active Antiretroviral Therapy (HAART)

The presentation of the nutritional problems of HIV-infected children has changed since the implementation of the HAART. While the early reports on HIV infection mainly discussed the problems of malnutrition and wasting, the introduction HAART therapy in developed countries has added two additional nutritional problems, which are truncal obesity and insulin resistance, to the management of HIV-infected children. Miller *et al.* reported that protease inhibitor therapy improves weight, weight for height, and muscle mass of HIV-infected children, independent of the concurrent decrease in HIV-1 viral load and improved CD_4 T-lymphocyte counts.

Body Morphology Changes and Lipid Abnormalities

Lipodystrophy (LD) is a general term used to describe varying degrees of fat redistribution, including fat loss or lipoatrophy and fat accumulation or lipohypertrophy, fat accumulation includes dorsocervical fat accumulation ("buffalo hump"), visceral adiposity, and breast enlargement. Fat loss includes facial-fat and limb-fat loss. Though LD was observed in persons with HIV infection before highly active treatment regimens were developed, the prevalence of LD has increased drastically with the widespread use of more active therapies. It has been reported mostly in adult but there is report in children.

Clinical fat redistribution is significantly associated with older age, duration of antiretroviral treatment and highly active antiretroviral therapy and hypertriglyceridaemia. The clinical importance of these is demonstrated by the increased prevalence of cardiovascular disease and diabetes in adult

HIV infected persons. Many studies have suggested a link between the use of protease inhibitors (PI) and nucleoside analogues and LD.

There is ongoing research to diminish the clinical and biochemical features of fat redistribution syndrome. Therapeutically, oral hypoglycemic agents, such as metformin and troglitazone, and exercise training have been tried.

Follow-up Assessments

Reassessment of nutritional status is part of the management of HIV infected children. The extent of nutritional evaluation during follow-up visits in addition to the routine developmental measures depends on the progress of a child.

Development and Body Mass Assessments

Weight and height growth velocities should be monitored every 3 to 6 months. Head circumference reflects brain growth and it should be monitored monthly for the first 3 years of life. A deviation from that normal growth warrants further investigation. Chronic malnutrition will eventually compromise brain growth and cognitive development.

Body composition measurements provide a more accurate assessment of nutritional status than weight and weight changes alone. In HIV-positive adults, bioelectric impedance analysis (BIA) is the method often used to assess lean body mass, adipose tissue, and fluid changes, however, there are no generally accepted BIA standards for children. It is more difficult due to changes in fluid status and lean body mass distribution in growing children.

Routine subscapular skinfolds compared with triceps skinfolds or routine abdominal girth may help identify children with changes in body shape or emerging lipodystrophy. Serial measurement of mid-arm circumference and skinfold can be an indicator of nutritional status if serially measured in the same children by the same person. Mid-arm circumference, triceps and subscapular skinfolds, and a calculated arm muscle area should be measured at a child's initial assessment and at least every 6 months.

Laboratory Tests

In addition to the routine blood and immunological tests, markers of nutritional status should be periodically measured during follow-up visits. Serum prealbumin or transferrin are sensitive markers of nutritional change and it is recommended to monitor them serially.

Because deficiency of numerous micronutrients have been identified in patients with HIV infection, folate, zinc selenium, iron, and vitamins A, C, B_6, and B_{12} may need to be monitored in selected patients, especially in children who refuse or avoid one or more food groups.

Children on antiretroviral and nucleoside analogue therapies need fasting serum glucose and lipids monitoring routinely in order to detect possible antiretroviral-induced changes.

KEY LEARNING POINTS

- Optimal nutritional status is very important for the welfare of HIV infected children as it supports immune function and improves the quality of life.
- Initial nutritional assessment followed by regular clinical nutritional reassessment should be an integral part of the management of these children.
- The dietary treatment is often challenging due to HIV related diseases, medication side effects, psychosocial factors and age related nutritional problems in children.
- The goal of nutritional management is to optimize the child's growth, prolong survival and improve the quality of life.

FURTHER READINGS

1. Arpadi SM, Cuff PA, Horlick M, Wang J, Kotler DP. Lipodystrophy in HIV-infected children is associated withhigh viral load and low CD4+ -lymphocyte count and CD4+ -lymphocyte percentage at baseline and use of protease inhibitors and stavudine. *J Acquir Immune Defic Syndr* 2001;27:30-34.
2. Bhutta ZA, Bang P, Karlsson E, Hagenas L, Nizami SQ, Soder O. Insulin-like growth factor I response during nutritional rehabilitation of persistent diarrhoea. *Arch Dis Child* 1999;80:438-442.
3. Gadewar S, Horvath K. Enteral nutrition. *In: Gupte S (ed) Recent Advances in Pediatrics* 2005;14:1-26.
4. Guarino A, Spagnuolo MI, Giacomet V, Canani RB, Bruzzese E, Giaquinto C, *et al.* Effects of nutritional rehabilitation on intestinal function and on CD4 cell number in children with HIV. *J Pediatr Gastroenterol Nutr* 2002;34:366-371.
5. Heller LS. Nutritional Support for Children With HIV/AIDS. *AIDS Read* 2000;10:109-114.
6. Hadigan C, Corcoran C, Basgoz N, Davis B, Sax P, Grinspoon S. Metformin in the treatment of HIV lipodystrophy syndrome: A randomized controlled trial. *JAMA* 2000;284:472-477.
7. Kruzich L, Marquis G, Wilson C, Stephensen C. HIV-infected US youth are at high risk of obesity and poor diet quality: A challenge for improving short- and long-term health outcomes. *J Am Diet Assoc* 2004;104(10):1554-1560.
8. Marquis G, Carriquiry A, Wilson C, Stephensen C. US youths in the early stages of HIV disease have low intakes of some micronutrients important for optimal immune function. *J Am Diet Assoc* 2004;104:1095-1101.
9. Miller T, Mawn B, Orav E, Wilk D, Weinberg G, Nicchitta J, *et al.* The effect of protease inhibitor therapy on growth and body composition in human immunodeficiency virus type 1-infected children. *Pediatrics* 2001;107:E77.
10. Palella FJ, Jr., Delaney KM, Moorman AC, Loveless MO, Fuhrer J, Satten GA, *et al.* Declining morbidity and mortality among patients with advanced human immunodeficiency virus infection. HIV Outpatient Study Investigators. *N Engl J Med* 1998;338:853-860.
11. Schwenk A, Beisenherz A, Romer K, Kremer G, Salzberger B,

Elia M. Phase angle from bioelectrical impedance analysis remains an independent predictive marker in HIV-infected patients in the era of highly active antiretroviral treatment. *Am J Clin Nutr* 2000;72:496-501.

12. Wilson IB, Cleary PD. Clinical predictors of declines in physical functioning in persons with AIDS: results of a longitudinal study. *J Acquir Immune Defic Syndr Hum Retrovirol* 1997;16:343-349.
13. Wheeler DA. Weight loss and disease progression in HIV infection. *AIDS Read* 1999;9:347-353.

Part D

Pediatric Investigations

120 Laboratory Tests

Karoly Horvath • Jeremy King

This chapter outlines the interpretation of commonly used tests in pediatric gastroenterology. It is not intended to be a complete list. Specific and unique tests are discussed in the chapters dealing with the diseases.

The gastroenterology tests can be divided as blood tests, stool tests, breath tests, tests on body fluids, tissue tests and genetic tests.

BLOOD TESTS

ALBUMIN

Albumin is synthesized exclusively in the liver and constitutes 60% of total protein in the blood. Albumin is synthesized in the hepatocytes at the rate of 150 mg/kg/day. The synthetic capacity of liver is limited and it can increase albumin synthesis only two-fold. The half-life of albumin is approximately 17 days.

The main physiological role of albumin is that it exerts significant osmotic effect. Therefore, it is important in the tissue circulation. In addition, it serves as transporter for both endogenous and exogenous substances (e.g., thyroxine, bilirubin, calcium, magnesium, heme, penicillin, cortisol, estrogen, free fatty acids, etc.). Measurements of albumin concentrations is important in the interpretation of calcium and magnesium levels because these ions are bound to albumin. So decreases of albumin are directly responsible for depression of their concentrations.

The reasons of a *decrease in serum albumin* (Table 120.1) can be diminished synthesis in the liver (cirrhosis, chronic liver disease) or increased loss through the skin (burns, exudative skin disease), urine (nephrotic syndrome) or gastrointestinal tract (mucosal inflammations in the stomach, intestine, colon and pancreas; lymphangiectasia, etc.).

Table 120.1: Causes of low serum albumin

Intestine	*Kidney*	*Liver*	*Skin*
Malabsorption/ IBD	Nephrotic syndromes	Cirrhosis	Burns
Protein-losing enteropathy		Chronic liver disease	Exudative skin disease

Other reasons for decreased albumin are malignancy, rapid rehydration and overhydration.

Elevation in serum albumin level may occur in dehydration or in case of sample collection or handling problems, such as prolonged tourniquet use during blood drawing or in case of specimen evaporation. Typically hemoglobin and hematocrit are also increased in these patients.

Evidently, serum albumin measurement is not specific for any disease. However, combined with other tests, it can be useful to monitor the progress of various diseases.

ALKALINE PHOSPHATASE (AP)

Alkaline phosphatase catalyzes the hydrolysis of phosphate esters at alkaline pH. It is present in the *liver, biliary tree, bone, placenta, intestine and kidney.* In the clinical practice, elevation in alkaline phosphatase is usually considered of hepatobiliary or bone origin.

Mild elevation in AP can be seen during accelerated growth such as infancy and the adolescent period. There are *other factors influencing the serum level of AP*:

- In patients with blood groups of B and O it remains increased upto 30 U/L after meals that lasts upto 12 hours.
- It is higher in patients with increased body mass index (BMI).
- It can be lower in patients with hemolysis.
- Smoking and contraceptives increase the levels by 10-30%.
- It is higher by 10-15% in African American people.

Pathological Conditions with Elevated AP (Table 120.2)

Liver disease is suspected if other liver function tests are abnormal. Isolated elevation of AP poses a problem to

Table 120.2: Causes of alkaline phosphatase elevation

Liver	*Bone*	*Other*
Cholestasis: Biliary atresia, Alagille's syndrome,	Rickets Fractures	Hypervitaminosis D Hyperthyroidism
Total parenteral nutrition; sepsis, drugs, biliary stones, AIDS cholangiopathy, primary sclerosing	Bone growth (childhood and adolescence)	AIDS
cholangitis, benign recurrent intrahepatic cholestasis	Paget's disease	Renal malignancy/ infarction
Parenchymal Disease		
Hepatitis (infectious, autoimmune),	Osteomalacia	Mastocytosis
cirrhosis, congestion/ ischemia, steatosis,	Osteitis fibrosa cystica	Pulmonary infarct
drugs, hemochromatosis, α-1-antitrypsin deficiency	Osteoblastic bone tumors	Acromegaly

differentiate between hepatobiliary and bone disease as the etiology. In this situation the measurement of 5' nucleotidase, which is specific for the hepatobiliary tree, is very helpful. If it is not available then GGT (gamma-glutamyltranspeptidase) should be ordered. However, although GGT is sensitive for biliary tract disease, it is not specific (See GGT later).

Marked increase in AP levels raises the suspicion of extrahepatic biliary obstruction, primary biliary cirrhosis, drug-induced cholestasis, primary sclerosing cholangitis or infiltrative process in the liver.

Pathological Conditions with Decreased AP

AP can be abnormally low in diseases with decreased serum zinc such as Crohn's disease, hypothyroidism, hypophosphatasia, pernicious anemia, etc. Serum AP activity is usually low in Wilson's disease, particularly during acute presentation. There are medications decreasing AP level, such as *alendronate, clofibrate, theophylline etc.*

ALPHA-1-ANTITRYPSIN

Alpha-1-antitrypsin (A1-AT) is an anti-protease that inactivates circulating proteases (trypsin, elastase etc.). A1-AT deficiency is the most common genetic metabolic disease of the liver with a prevalence of 1:2000 in the US. Serum measurement is important in any child with unclear liver disease, chronic hepatitis and cirrhosis. The gold standard of diagnosis is A1-AT phenotyping that can be detected by gel electrophoresis. This is called the protease inhibitor system (Pi), and the phenotype PiZZ is the only one clearly associated with the development of neonatal hepatitis and cirrhosis due to abnormal A1-AT hepatocyte storage.

As A1-AT is resistant to digestion by intestinal bacteria, it also can be used as a marker of protein-losing enteropathy. A single stool sample measurement is usually appropriate in the clinical practice. Calculation of the clearance is possible by simultaneous stool and blood level measurements.

A1-AT is an acute phase reactant. Its level may increase in inflammatory diseases. However, such elevations lack clinical specificity.

ALPHA FETOPROTEIN (AFP)

Elevation in serum α-fetoprotein is sensitive and specific for hepatocellular carcinoma and hepatoblastoma. There is a strong correlation between the presence of hepatocellular cancer and AFP levels of >500 ng/mL, especially in the presence of a liver mass. AFP is elevated in >90% of patients with hepatocellular cancer. AFP measurement is useful in monitoring response to treatment. The levels will fall with successful treatment of hepatocellular cancer.

It may also be mildly elevated in acute liver disease, chronic liver disease, cirrhosis, and hepatic metastasis. In patients with cirrhosis, serial measurements of the AFP level are useful as an increase should prompt the clinician to consider the possibility of hepatocellular cancer.

AMMONIA

Ammonia is the end product of amino acid and nucleic acid metabolism. Ammonia is produced mostly by the large intestine. The liver clears about 80% of portal vein ammonia in a single pass. The liver is the only organ that detoxifies ammonia by converting it into urea. Ammonia level are used for the laboratory diagnosis of hepatic encephalopathy. However, a normal ammonia level does not exclude this diagnosis. Hepatic encephalopathy is a clinical diagnosis, which is based on the presence of neurological signs and symptoms consistent with hepatic encephalopathy in children with known liver disease. Conditions with ammonia elevations are listed in Table 120.3.

The blood sample for ammonia level should be obtained and handled properly in order to avoid false elevation. Ammonia level is higher in the arterial than in the venous blood. Furthermore, arterial level has a better correlation

Table 120.3: Causes of elevated serum ammonia level

Excessive GI bleeding	*Excessive dietary protein intake*	*Blood transfusion*
Hemodialysis	Alkalosis	Renal insufficiency
Hepatocellular dysfunction	Porto-systemic venous shunt	Acute leukemia
Reye syndrome, Urea cycle defects		
Medications (valproic acid, glycine,etc.)	Asparaginase therapy	

with the liver function. Use of tourniquet and clenching fist increases venous ammonia levels. Exercise may increase ammonia levels by 2-3 folds. It is higher in men then in women. Delay in sample processing results in an increase in ammonia levels because of metabolism by red blood cells: 20% in 1 hour and 100% by 2 hours. The blood collecting tube should be on ice water and the blood should be centrifuged as soon as possible. The ammonia concentration remains constant for at least 24 hours if the sample is frozen at –20°C.

AMYLASE

Serum amylase level is widely used to diagnose acute pancreatitis. Amylase increases in the serum 2-12 hours after the symptoms start. It has a peak between 12-72 hours and returns to normal within 5 days. It is most useful in the first 24-36 hours.

It is not specific for the pancreas as it is produced by the salivary gland, too. In patients with kidney disease and impaired clearance the amylase can be elevated but usually less than three times of the upper limit. Amylase can bind to immunoglobulins forming macroamylase that has a much longer renal clearance.

Differential diagnosis of amylase elevation includes pancreatic disease, salivary gland disease, acute abdomen (perforation, ischemia, obstruction, appendicitis, cholecystitis, abdominal trauma), gynecological disease (cysts, ruptured ectopic pregnancy), malignancies (myeloma, pheochromocytoma), diabetic ketoacidosis, burns and medications.

ASPARTATE AMINOTRANSFERASE/ALANINE AMINOTRANSFERASE (AST/ALT)

Aspartate aminotransferase (AST; SGOT) and alanine aminotransferase (ALT; SGPT) are enzymes found in the hepatocytes. These two enzymes transfer amino groups from aspartate and alanine to α-ketoglutarate that result in the formation of oxaloacetic acid and pyruvic acid.

Any damage involving hepatocytes may raise the serum levels of these enzymes. However, the enzymes are not specific for liver disease; especially AST is present in many other organs, including heart, skeletal muscle (Table 120.4).

ALT content is highest in the liver and kidney but smaller amounts are present in heart and skeletal muscle. ALT elevation is more specific for liver disease then AST.

AST and ALT are not sensitive marker of chronic liver diseases. Patients with cirrhosis may have normal enzyme levels if there is no ongoing tissue injury. Children with hepatitis C infection may not have elevated enzymes. Neonates with hemochromatosis have normal enzymes while there is a severe liver synthetic function defect.

Table 120.4: Organs/tissues with high AST content (in descending order)

1. Liver	4. Pancreas	7. Lung
2. Heart	5. Kidney	8. White blood cell
3. Skeletal muscle	6. Brain	9. Red blood cell

There are other *factors influencing the serum levels* of these enzymes:

- There is a day-to-day variation which is upto 10% in AST and upto 30% in ALT.
- It is in average 15% higher level in African-American men.
- There is a direct relationship between body weight and AST/ALT and it can be upto 40-50% higher in children with high body mass index.
- Strenuous exercise increases AST level in men upto three times.
- Muscle injury increases AST level more significantly then that of ALT and the elevation goes parallel with the elevation of creatine phosphokinase (CPK).
- ALT/AST elevation without evidence of liver disease in young children should prompt investigations for muscular dystrophies, especially if the CPK is elevated.
- Hemolysis results in increase in the AST level.
- AST can form complex with serum IgG (macro-AST), which results in long-lasting elevation due to the slow clearance.

Degree of Transaminase Elevation

In clinical practice, a 2-3 times elevation in AST/ALT levels is considered as mild, 2-20 times elevation as moderate and over 20 times increase is a severe elevation.

Severe transaminase elevation (>1000 units/L) occurs in acute viral hepatitis, autoimmune hepatitis, acute biliary obstruction, ischemic (poor perfusion) hepatitis and drug (e.g. acetaminophen) or toxin induced hepatitis. The elevation is more sustained in viral or autoimmune hepatitis while the ischemic elevation usually returns to normal within a week. Ischemic hepatitis is also associated with a significant elevation in LDH. Transaminase elevation may occur within hours after a biliary obstruction and decreases over 1-3 days. It seems that the degree of transaminase elevation does not correlate with the extent of hepatocellular damage. Therefore, the degree of the transaminase elevation does not predict the patient's prognosis.

Decreased AST/ALT Levels

The coenzyme for both AST and ALT is pyridoxal phosphate (B_6). In case of vitamin B_6 deficiency, abnormally low measured serum levels of the enzymes (particularly ALT) may be reported. Uremia also may cause a spuriously low level of AST.

BILIRUBIN

Bilirubin is the end product of the catabolism of the red

blood cells and other hemoproteins (i.e., cytochrome P_{450}). The heme is initially converted to biliverdin by heme oxygenase and the biliverdin reductase will convert it to bilirubin. The bilirubin is reversibly bound to albumin and transported into hepatocytes. The next step is a conjugation by the UDP-glucuronyl transferase. The rate-limiting step is the canalicular secretion. The excreted bilirubin is transferred into the duodenum through the biliary tree. The bacteria in the terminal ileum and colon will reduce it to urobilinogen. Part of the urobilinogen is passed through the stool, but another part is reabsorbed and it is either excreted in urine (the urobilinogen that is reported in the urinalysis) or in bile (enterohepatic circulation).

Conjugated vs. Unconjugated Hyperbilirubinemia

The causes of hyperbilirubinemia can be prehepatic, hepatic and posthepatic. The first step is to determine that whether the hyperbilirubinemia is conjugated or unconjugated. The conjugated bilirubin is water-soluble.

While the unconjugated bilirubin is typically seen in prehepatic causes, conjugated hyperbilirubinemia indicates liver or posthepatic problems and associated with other liver function test abnormalities. A predominantly conjugated hyperbilirubinemia is when 30% or more of the serum bilirubin is in the conjugated form. The conjugated form can be bilirubin monoglucuronide and diglucuronide (Table 120.5).

A fourth form occurs in the serum with conjugated bilirubinemia when it becomes bound to albumin and it is called delta (δ)-bilirubin. Due to the much longer half-life of albumin the proportion of δ-bilirubin tends to be increased

Table 120.5: Causes of conjugated hyperbilirubinemia

Hepatocellular	*Cholestasis*	
	Intrahepatic	*Extrahepatic*
Viral hepatitis	Biliary atresia/ malformation	Viral hepatitis
Hepatic vein thrombosis	Choledocholithiasis	
Autoimmune hepatitis	Pancreatitis	Systemic infection
Drug-induced	Primary sclerosing cholangitis	Drug-induced
Hepatotoxins	Cholangio-carcinoma	Total parenteral nutrition
Ischemia	AIDS cholangiopathy	Benign recurrent intrahepatic cholestasis
α-1-antitrypsin deficiency	Tumors	Primary biliary cirrhosis
Wilson's disease		Cholestasis of pregnancy
Rotor's syndrome		
Dubin-Johnson syndrome		

as the total bilirubin concentration decreases during recovery from an obstructive hepatobiliary disorder.

Overproduction of Bilirubin

Overproduction of bilirubin occurs with hemolysis, resorption of large hematoma and increased erythropoesis.

Hereditary Disorders of Bilirubin Metabolism

Gilbert's Syndrome is a benign disease with mild elevation (3-4 mg/dL) of unconjugated bilirubin that occurs mostly in older children after fasting, illness, stress, exercise, or lack of sleep. The etiology may be multifactorial with increased hemolysis, decreased uptake, and decreased conjugation all may playing a role.

Crigler-Najjar Syndrome Type 1 is due to the absence of the glucuronyl transferase that results in severe neonatal jaundice (kernicterus).

Crigler-Najjar Syndrome Type 2 is associated with low glucuronyl transferase and can be managed with phenobarbital.

Dubin-Johnson Syndrome (DJS) is a chronic idiopathic jaundice due to point mutation in MRP2 (canalicular multispecific organic ion transporter) leading to impaired excretion of conjugated bilirubin with direct and indirect bilirubin elevation in the serum. It is a benign, autosomal disorder. The typical finding is dark pigment in liver cells, melanin-like or epinephrine polymers.

Rotor Syndrome is similar to DJS, except that there is no dark pigment in liver cells.

CERULOPLASMIN

Ceruloplasmin is the major copper binging protein that is synthesized by the liver. Its level is depressed markedly in patients who are homozygotes for Wilson's disease. Some patients with Wilson's disease may have normal to only slightly decreased levels. In these cases a 24-hour urine collection for copper excretion can be helpful in making a diagnosis.

C-REACTIVE PROTEIN

It is an acute phase reactants produced by the liver that present in low concentration in healthy individuals. It increases within 6 to 12 hours after the inflammatory or infectious process started. It decreases more rapidly than ESR.

Like ESR it is not a disease-specific test. The CRP test is used in patients with inflammatory bowel disease and autoimmune diseases to assess the disease activity and to monitor the treatment.

ERYTHROCYTE SEDIMENTATION RATE (ESR)

ESR is the measure of the distance of the RBC sedimentation in millimeters within an hour in a specific tube.

ESR is high in acute and chronic inflammations, infections and tissue necrosis or injury. It is not specific for any particular disease. Furthermore, normal ESR does not rule out the possibility of inflammatory disease.

It is a useful marker of disease activity in children diagnosed with inflammatory bowel disease, sclerosing cholangitis, autoimmune hepatitis, etc.

The RBC number and morphology influences the result. It is decreased in sickle cell disease, polycythemia, corticosteroids, spherocytosis, anisocytosis, hypofibrinogenemia, and increased serum viscosity.

FERRITIN

Ferritin is a major circulating iron storage protein that reflects the body iron reserve. It is mostly distributed in human tissues, with a small amount in the serum. Ferritin can be elevated secondary to inflammation or other iron overload conditions. It is useful for the detection of neonatal and idiopathic hemochromatosis.

GAMMA GLUTAMYL TRANSFERASE *(GGT)*

It is a microsomal enzyme found in the epithelium of small bile ductules and hepatocytes and catalyzes the transfer of α-glutamyl groups between peptides or to an amino acid residue.

GGT is not specific for liver disease because an elevated GGT may reflect disease in other organs including the *kidney, pancreas, intestine, spleen, brain, heart, lung and placenta*. It has higher level in the proximal tubules of kidneys then in the liver.

There are non-disease factors influencing GGT level, such as race (higher in African-Americans), BMI (higher over >30), meal (decreases after meal, increases with fasting), smoking, alcohol and pregnancy.

Many drugs can cause elevation in GGT level e.g. carbamazepine cimetidine, furosemide, heparin, isotretinoin, methotrexate, oral contraceptives, phenobarbital, phenytoin and valproic acid

GGT is found to be elevated in 80% to 95% of patients with acute hepatitis, independent of the cause. GGT levels increase in many liver diseases. Therefore, its use in differentiating different types of liver diseases is limited. However, in case of isolated elevation of the alkaline phosphatase, an elevated GGT level supports hepatobiliary disease as the etiology of the elevated alkaline phosphatase. A normal GGT level strongly argues against the presence of hepatobiliary disease. The highest levels of GGT are found in biliary obstruction. Extremely high levels are also found in intrahepatic cholestatic disorders such as Alagille's syndrome.

The newborn may have very high levels of GGT, upto five to eight times the upper limit of normal for adults. While GGT levels decline rapidly in full-term infants, in the premature infants the decline may take 6-9 months.

LACTATE DEHYDROGENASE (LDH)

LDH measurement usually provides no additional information to the routinely used AST, ALT, albumin, bilirubin, and alkaline phosphatase levels in the diagnosis of liver disorders. There are specific situations in which an LDH level may be helpful:

- LDH levels may rise in acute viral hepatitis and ischemic hepatitis.
- In ischemic hepatitis, there may be such a significant elevation in the LDH level that typically not seen in patients with acute viral hepatitis.
- Prolonged LDH elevation along with an increased alkaline phosphatase level may be seen in malignancy infiltrating the liver.

LIPASE

Serum lipase increases 4-8 hours after the onset of symptoms of pancreatitis. It peaks by 24 hours and returns to normal within 8-14 days. After the first 24-36 hours of pancreatitis the sensitivity of lipase is higher than those of amylase. However, there is no correlation between the level of elevation and the severity of pancreatitis.

Similarly to amylase the decline is slower in patients with chronic kidney disease. Lipase can form macrolipase with immunoglobulins that slows down its elimination from the serum.

Lipase is present in the stomach and the tongue, called gastric and lingual lipase. It is unusual to have higher elevation than three times of the normal upper level from these sources.

5' NUCLEOTIDASE

5' nucleotidase is located in the sinusoidal and canalicular membranes of the liver and the most specific enzyme for the detection of biliary tract disorders. It is not a routinely used assay. An isolated increase in alkaline phosphatase is the main indication for the measurement of a 5' nucleotidase. 5' nucleotidase has a higher predictive value than GGT and alkaline phosphatase in the detection of hepatobiliary disease. It also has a lower false positivity than GGT and alkaline phosphatase. 5' nucleotidase is particularly helpful in detecting liver disease during childhood, adolescence, and pregnancy when alkaline phosphatase is physiologically elevated.

PREALBUMIN (TRANSTHYRETIN)

The term prealbumin is a misnomer because the prefix "pre" suggests that it is a precursor of albumin, which is not the case. The name was given because it migrates faster than albumin in acidic starch gel.

The correct biochemical name is transthyretin because it binds thyroxine and retinol. Transthyretin consists of 127 amino acids and plays a significant role in the metabolism of vitamin A by forming a complex with the retinol-binding protein (RBP). Because RBP is a small protein it would be rapidly filtrated through the kidney if it were not bind to the larger prealbumin.

Prealbumin is produced by the choroid plexus, pancreatic islet cells in the embryonic yolk sac, and by enterochromaffin cells in the gastrointestinal mucosa, but the liver is quantitatively the most important source.

Prealbumin has a relatively short biological half-life (~2 days) and smaller serum pool makes it a better indicator of protein status than albumin or transferrin. Therefore, the preferred marker for protein malnutrition is prealbumin.

Like albumin, prealbumin is a negative acute-phase reactant. This limits its use as a screening tool for malnutrition because low levels could result from either inadequate nutrition or inflammatory stress.

It is not a real diagnostic tool. Rather, it should be used as an indicator of how well nutritional interventions are working. The very short half-life and small serum pool allows small changes in nutritional status to be identified in a short time frame.

Prealbumin levels can be drawn once or twice per week.

This assay is not influenced by the hydration status like albumin; however, elevated prealbumin levels may be seen in patients taking corticosteroids and in patients with Hodgkin disease.

PROTHROMBIN TIME (PT) AND PARTIAL THROMBOPLASTIN TIME (PTT)

Except factors VIII and von Willebrand, all other factors are synthesized in hepatocytes.

PT: It measures the rate of conversion of prothrombin to thrombin in the presence of tissue extract (thromboplastin), calcium ions, and activated clotting factors V, VII and X. Because of the shorter half-lives of coagulation factors, PT is more useful to detect acute liver failure than albumin. At least 80% of the liver synthetic capacity is compromised before there is a prolongation in PT. Prolongation of greater than 2 seconds is considered pathologic; values greater than 3 seconds above control indicate a risk for bleeding. Another important cause is vitamin K deficiency. Parenteral administration of vitamin K results in a 30% decrease in PT within 6-24 hours in vitamin K deficiency, while there is no or minimal change in liver disease. Because Factor VIII is synthesized in non-hepatic sites, mostly vascular endothelium, its activity is usually normal or even elevated in all forms of liver disease unless it is being consumed in disseminated intravascular coagulation (DIC).

PTT: The activated PTT is sensitive to deficiency or inhibition of factors in the intrinsic pathway. These include the contact factors; high molecular weight kininogen (HMWK), prekallikrein and factor XII along with procoagulant factors VIII, IX, X, XI, V, prothrombin and fibrinogen. False elevation occurs if the blood is coagulated, contaminated with heparin or mixed with IV fluid, in polycythemia or if the sample stored for long period of time before testing. Real prolongation occurs in factor VIII, IX, XI, XII deficiencies and von Willebrand's disease. Presence of lupus anticoagulant in various diseases also may lead to PTT prolongation without or with PT prolongation.

It is important to know that PTT is prolonged in premature infants (Table 120.6). Many of the clotting factors, including the vitamin K-dependent Factors II, VII, IX and X, are demonstrated to be less than 70% of adult levels in both the full-term and preterm newborn (Table 120.6).

Table 120.6: Postnatal changes in PT and PTT in healthy premature (30-36 weeks gestational age)

Postnatal age	*PT(s)*	*Activated PTT(s)*
Day 1	13.0 (10.6-16.2)	53.6 (27.5-79.4)
Day 5	12.5 (10.0-15.3)	50.5 (26.9-74.1)
Day 30	11.8 (10.0-13.6)	44.7 (26.9-62.5)
Day 90	12.3 (10.0-14.6)	39.5 (28.3-50.7)
Day 180	12.5 (10.0-15.0)	37.5 (21.7-53.3)
Adult	12.4 (10.8-13.9)	33.5 (26.6-40.3)

SERUM IRON

Iron deficiency anemia is present in children with malabsorptions or chronic gastrointestinal bleeding. The typical pattern of microcytic hypochromic anemia shows:

- Low serum iron.
- Increase total iron binding capacity.
- Decreased transferring saturation (<15%).
- Decreased serum ferritin (<10 ng/ml).
- Increased serum soluble transferrin receptor.
- Decreased mean corpuscular volume of RBCs (<80fL).

FERRITIN

Ferritin is a circulating iron binding protein that reflects the body iron storage. It is a useful marker of iron deficiency. Low serum ferritin level (<10 ng/ml) is diagnostic for iron deficiency.

However, ferritin is an acute phase reactant and its level increases in iron deficient children with concomitant inflammation.

High serum ferritin is one of the markers elevated in neonatal hemochromatosis while there are severe coagulation defect and normal transaminases. Serum ferritin is elevated in children with sickle cell disease receiving transfusions.

ZINC

Zinc is an essential cofactor for over two hundreds of enzymes including those controlling DNA synthesis, wound healing, growth, brain development, behavior, reproduction, membrane stability and bone formation. Zinc deficiency produces growth retardation, alterations of taste, anorexia and delayed sexual maturation.

It is the second most abundant trace element in the human body. The average amount of zinc in the adult body is about 1.4 to 2.3 g with 63% in the muscle and 28% in the bones. Only 1% is in the extracellular fluid. The plasma zinc concentration is between 70 and 120µg/dL. Most of zinc is bound to albumin.

The recommended daily zinc requirements are 3-5 mg for infants and 10 to 15 mg for adults. The main food sources are meat, daily products, shell-fish (oysters, mussels), nuts, legumes, and whole grains. Approximately 20% to 40% of the dietary zinc is absorbed. Zinc induces the production of metallothionein, a metal-binding protein that binds to zinc in the gut mucosal cells. The intracellular metallothionein-zinc is lost with the normal sloughing of the enterocytes that prevent the absorption of excessive amounts of zinc. The daily loss of zinc thorough intestinal secretions and cell sloughing is approximately 2-5 mg and there is additional loss in the urine and sweat.

The best detection is atomic absorption spectrometry. It is important to prevent contamination during blood draw. Plasma levels of zinc can be affected by its binding affinity to albumin, exogenous steroid administration, and hemolysis. Although the plasma measurement is the easiest and generally used first test, it is not a reliable marker of the body zinc status. Measurement of both plasma zinc and plasma metallothionine may differentiate dietary zinc deficiency from other causes such as stress, infection, or other metabolic conditions.

Causes of zinc deficiency are decreased intake, decreased absorption (celiac disease, Crohn's disease), increased excretion in hypoalbuminemia, catabolic states (burns, trauma, infections, malignancies) and acrodermatitis enteropathica.

Zinc toxicity occurs with oral ingestion and manifests with gastrointestinal irritation with fever, vomiting, nausea, diarrhea, abdominal pain and a metallic taste.

VITAMINS

Vitamin D

It is either produced by skin after sun exposure (ultraviolet irradiation) or enters the body by ingestion. Vitamin D deficiency develops if the intake is decreased, in malabsorption (celiac disease, pancreatic insufficiency, biliary atresia, cystic fibrosis, short gut etc.), in the absence of sunlight, increased loss, decreased production (liver and kidney diseases) or medication (anticonvulsants) effects.

Vitamin K

Carboxylation of the glutamic acid residues is important for the proper functioning of factors II, VII, IX, X and protein C and S. Vitamin K deficiency may be the result of malnutrition, malabsorption and antibiotic use. It can lead to prolongation in PT.

WHITE BLOOD CELLS

Eosinophilia: It is defined as a count over 0.5×10^6/ml. There is a diurnal variation in eosinophils with the peak between midnight and 4 A.M. and falls to the lower value morning. Therefore, if repeat test is needed it is important to obtain at the same time of the day. Table 120.7 shows a few causes of eosinophilia.

Typically infestations with helminths results in significant eosinophilia, while among parasites *Dientamoeba fragilis* and *Isosopra belli* are associated with peripheral eosinophilia. Drug-induced eosinophilia may occur in patients taking penicillins, cephalosporins, phenytoin or sulphonamides.

Table 120.7: Diseases and conditions with eosinophilia

Infections	*Autoimmune disorders*	*Asthma/ Atopic disorders*	*Skin disorders*	*Miscellaneous*
Parasites	Eosinophilic gastroenteritis	Seasonal allergy	Bullous pemphigoid	Drug induced
Aspergillosis	IBD	Chronic	Episodic angioedema	Adrenal insufficiency
Coccidio-mycosis	Rheumatoid	Urticaria		ALL
Tuberculosis	Arthritis	Atopic dermatitis		Hodgkin's lymphoma
Scarlet fever				

SEROLOGICAL TESTS

Antibody production against specific target antigens are found in many gastrointestinal disorders (Table 120.8).

Celiac disease: The most sensitive and specific test for celiac disease is the endomysium antibody test (EMA) that is an immunofluorescent test performed on monkey esophagus or umbilical cord slides incubated with dilutions of the patients' sera. The antigen for EMA test was identified as the tissue transglutaminase enzyme. The ELISA based anti-tissue transglutaminase test is sensitive but less specific then the EMA test. The antigliadin IgG and IgA antibody tests are much less sensitive and specific (Table 120.9).

Helicobacter pylori: Chronic infection results in antibody production. The IgG antibody test has a sensitivity of 90% and specificity of 70-80%.

Liver Serologies

Anti-mitochondrial Antibody: Positive in primary biliary cirrhosis (85-90%), chronic active hepatitis (25-30%), cryptogenic cirrhosis (25-30%).

Table 120.8: Autoantibodies in gastrointestinal disorders

Disease	*Target*	*Substrate*
GIT		
Atrophic gastritis	Gastric parietal cell	Mouse stomach/ kidney
Pernicious anemia	Intrinsic factor	Radioactive vitamin B_{12} binding assay
	Salivary duct cells	Unfixed human salivary gland
	Gastric parietal cell	Human, monkey, mouse, or rat gastric mucosa substrate
Ulcerative colitis	Colon; lipopolysaccharide; p-ANCA associated	Human or rat colon; Ethanol-fixed neutrophils
Crohn's disease	Reticulin	Mouse kidney
	ASCA	Saccharomyces cerevisiae
Celiac disease	Tissue transglutaminase	Tissue transglutaminase (ELISA)
	IgA endomysial	Monkey esophagus
	Gliadin	Gliadin (ELISA)
	Reticulin	Mouse kidney
LIVER		
Autoimmune hepatitis	Smooth muscle	Mouse stomach/ kidney
	Liver-kidney microsomal	Mouse stomach/ kidney; ELISA
	ANA	Hep-2 cells
Primary biliary cirrhosis	Mitochondrial (M2)	Mouse stomach/ kidney; ELISA
Primary sclerosing cholangitis	p-ANCA	Ethanol-fixed neutrophils

Table 120.9: Value of the celiac serology tests in children

Test	*Sensitivity (%)*	*Specificity (%)*
Antigliadin IgA	90-100	86-100
Antigliadin IgG	91-100	67-100
Endomysium antibody	100-100	100-100
Tissue transglutaminase	95-98	94-95

Smooth Muscle Antibody: Positive (>1:80) in chronic active hepatitis and autoimmune hepatitis; Lower titer (<1:80), primary biliary cirrhosis, Epstein Barr Virus (EBV), Cytomegalovirus (CMV)

IBD Serologies (Table 120.10)

p-ANCA: Antineutrophyl cytoplasmic antibody (ANCA) reacts with neutrophil cell antigens. p-ANCA is characterized by staining of the perinuclear area and probably histon H1 is the antigen, but it cross reacts with bacterial antigens, e.g. recognizes an outer membrane porin, OmpC, normally found in the cell wall of *E. coli.* p-ANCAs have been reported in about 75% to 80% of patients with active ulcerative colitis (UC) or primary sclerosing cholangitis,

Table 120.10: Prevalence of serological markers in patients with Crohn's disease (CrD) and ulcerative colitis (UC)

Antibody	*Antigen*	*Non-IBD (%)*	*CrD (%)*	*UC (%)*
ASCA	Anti-*Saccharomyces cerevisiae*	5%	50-70%	6-14%
DNase-sensitive pANCA	Histone H, bacterial antigen?	<5%	10-20%	50-80%
Anti-OmpC	*Escherichia coli*	<5%	38-50%	2%

about 75% of patients with chronic active hepatitis, about 30% of patients with primary biliary cirrhosis and 20% of patients with Crohn's disease (CrD).

ASCA: Anti-saccharomyces cerevisiae antibody (ASCA) refers to antibody against the baker's yeast Saccharomyces cerevisiae. ASCA recognizes proteoglycans (phosphopeptidomannans) in the yeast cell wall. ASCA is found in 50 to 70% of patients with CD and only 6 to 14% of patients with UC. There is a subset of patients with Crohn's disease expressing distinct OmpC antibodies but this subgroup is different than the p-ANCA-positive patients.

STOOL TESTS

Inspection of stool: The presence of mucus in a stool specimen is abnormal. Mucus associated with pus and blood is found in stools of patients with ulcerative colitis, bacillary dysentery, and intestinal tuberculosis.

Fecal fat: Fat malabsorption is an important cause of poor growth in infancy and childhood. A simple screening test for detection of steatorrhea includes microscopic examination of feces for *fat globules*. Typically if 60 or more stained droplets of neutral fats per high-power field are seen, it is a strong indicator of steatorrhea. The definitive test for steatorrhea is the fecal fat determination.

The *72-hour balance study* is a considered the gold standard for fat malabsorption in infants and adults. It requires the calculation of the dietary fat intake and measures the excreted amount of fat in the stool.

The acid steatocrit is a rapid method to estimate the amount of fat excretion. It is similar to the capillary hematocrit and is considerably more convenient than a conventional 72- hour stool analysis. The homogenized stool is centrifuged in a hematocrit tube. The lipid and liquid phases and stool residues separate, with the lipid phase on top of the liquid phase and the stool residue. Studies in infants and children suggested good correlations between steatocrit values and fecal fat content.

In a smaller adult study a sensitivity rate of 100% and a specificity rate of 95% for detecting steatorrhea were found when compared with the 72-hour quantitative fecal fat measurements. It can be used to monitor a patient's response to therapy.

Steatorrhea is defined as a fecal fat output in excess of 7% of ingested fat in patients over 6 months of age and in excess of 15% in patients under 6 months of age.

Fecal leukocytes: It is a simple stool examination under light microscope. A small drop of liquid stool is placed on a glass microscopic slide and two drops of Loffler methylene blue are added and mixed thoroughly. A cover slip is placed on the mixture, and after two to three minutes of nuclear staining the average number of leukocytes and erythrocytes can be counted per high power field.

Occult blood in stool: The most frequently used, rapid, inexpensive qualitative test is the guaiac based test (Hemoccult). Compounds with peroxidase activity or oxidants are able to turn the colorless guaiac to blue. The hem has pseudoperoxidase activity therefore induces color change if it is present in the stool. The qualitative immunochemical test uses antibodies against the human hemoglobin. It is more expensive and needs laboratory processing and detects intact hemoglobin. The third method is the heme-porphyrin test that is quantitative and based on spectrofluorometric detection of hemoglobin. It needs lab processing and the most expensive among the three tests.

Non-human hemoglobin (red meat) can cause false positive guaiac and immunochemical tests. Peroxidase in food produces blue reaction in the guaiac test. Iron does not influence these tests but vitamin C may cause false negative guaiac test (Table 120.11). For an accurate test it is recommended to stop vitamin C, aspirin and NSAIDs a week before the guaiac testing.

Table 120.11: Factors influencing the result of the guaiac tests

False positive	*False negative*
Uncooked, peroxidase containing vegetables and fruits (Radishes, cantaloupes, bean sprouts, cauliflower, broccoli and grapes)	Vitamin C Bacterial degradation of heme by colonic bacteria Delayed card development
Red meats	
Aspirin, NSAIDs: can cause bleeding	
Rehydration of stool	

Reducing substance test: Sugar malabsorption can be easily detected from the stool by the Clinitest tablet (Bayer Diagnostics, Australia). The reducing sugars are glucose, fructose, galactose and the disaccharidases maltose and lactose. They contain both ketone and aldehyde groups. Sucrose is not a reducing carbohydrate. In order to detect sucrose, the stool sample should be mixed 1:2 with 1 N HCl and boiled. In patients with sugar intolerance the amount of total reducing substances in the stool usually exceeds 0.25 g/dL feces. Stools can be analyzed for sugars by chromatography.

Electrolytes: Measurement of the stool sodium and potassium content allows the distinction between osmotic and secretory diarrheas.

Osmotic gap= 290 mOsmol/L-2 (Stool $Na^+ + K^+$)

A gap of <50 is suggestive of secretory diarrhea, while a low sodium (<60 mmol/L) and osmotic gap >125 is indicative of osmotic diarrhea. In osmotic diarrhea the diarrhea improves if the patient is fasted.

Fecal elastase: The pancreatic elastase stool test is an EIA method that quantifies elastase in stool. It allows the diagnosis or exclusion of pancreatic exocrine insufficiency (chronic pancreatitis, cystic fibrosis, pancreatic tumor). There is no agreement its specificity and sensitivity in mild-moderate cases of pancreatic hypofunction. It seems superior to the fecal chymotrypsin determination. The gold standard for pancreatic function testing remains the secretin and cholecystokinin stimulation test.

Clostridium difficile: The test is indicated in acute diarrhea especially if there was antibiotic exposure in the last 3 months. However, it can occur without previous antibiotic treatment. Fresh stool sample is preferable. There are different methods. The tissue cytotoxic assay considered as gold standard (Table 120.12).

Table 120.12: Value of tests used in Cl. difficile toxin detection

Assay	*Sensitivity*	*Specificity*
Cytotoxic assay	67-100%	85-100%
ELISA (Toxin A and B)	63-99%	93-100%
Latex agglutination test	LOW	LOW

Ova and parasite (O and P) tests: Due to the intermittent excretion of parasites in the stool, three sequential stool specimens are necessary for reliable detection. Examination of a first stool specimen detects parasites and/or ova in 58% of patients; examination of a second specimen identifies an additional 21% and examination of a third specimen yields another 21% of previously undetected patients.

Routine O and P examinations do not include acid-fast stains important for the detection of *Cyclospora* infection and *Cryptosporidium,* therefore a special request must be made.

Stool specimens must be free from foreign materials such as barium, bismuth and non-absorbable antidiarrheal agents or mineral oil. Fresh specimens are required to detect live trophozoites and larvae, because many parasites deteriorate rapidly outside the bowel lumen. Fecal samples preserved in 10% buffered formalin are employed for wet mounts. Polyvinyl alcohol-fixed specimens are useful for trichrome-staining.

Giardia lamblia tests: Giardia can be detected with regular ova/parasite test. However, it is less reliable and investigator dependent. The intermittent patterns of excretion of cysts and trophozoites (variable shedding) or the low levels of excretion probably may cause false negative results. It is recommended collecting 3 specimens in different days for O and P examination. The maximum detection increases from ~70% with one examination to ~85% for examinations of 3 stools.

The detection of antigens by ELISA or immunofluorescence from the stool improves diagnostic yield, shorten turnaround time and decrease labor costs.

Examination of the freshly collected duodenal juice is possible during endoscopic procedures. Light or stereo-electronmicroscopy of duodenal biopsy is an alternative method.

Helicobacter pylori: The stool is accurate for the diagnosis of H. pylori infection as it reaches a sensitivity of 95-98% and specificity of 92-95%. It confirms the eradication at 7 days or later after a triple therapy. The rule is the same then for other H. pylori tests. Patients should stop proton pump inhibitors, antibiotics and bismuth compounds (e.g. Pepto-Bismol) two weeks prior to the test.

BREATH TESTS

Breath tests are noninvasive and well-tolerated in children. The two major gases in expired air are carbon dioxide (CO_2) and hydrogen (H_2). Methane (CH_4), is also used as marker in breath tests.

Breath tests can use non-labeled substrates, radioactive and natural isotope (^{13}C) substrates. The substrates are fermented by normal ileocolonic intestinal flora, abnormal flora (e.g. bacterial overgrowth, Helicobacter pylori) or metabolized in the body.

An accurate test requires continuous collection techniques; however, for clinical purposes interval sample collections seem to be adequate. For the tests the correlation between the intestinal gas production and the concentration in the expired air is established. Approximately 21% of the intestinal gas is excreted through the lungs. Because a few percents of the population do not have methane producing flora the simultaneous measurement of H_2 and CH_4 helps overcoming this problem. Table 120.13 lists the most frequently used carbohydrate breath tests.

Table 120.13: Carbohydrate breath tests

Clinical condition	*Substrate*	*Dose/ concentration*	*Max g*	*Interval/ duration*
Lactose malabsorption	Lactose	2 g/kg (20%)	50	Every 30 minutes for 3 hours
Sucrose malabsorption	Sucrose	2 g/kg (20%)	50	
Glucose malabsorption	Glucose	1 g/kg; (20%)	50	
Fructose malabsorption	Fructose	0.3-0.5 g/kg; (20%)	20	
Bacterial overgrowth	Glucose	1g/kg (20%)	20	Every 15 min for first hour; then every 30 min for 3 hours

The sensitivity rates of glucose and lactulose breath tests for detecting bacterial overgrowth was 62% and 68% and specificity rates of 83% and 44%, respectively, when compared with culture. Duodenal aspiration and culture remains the gold standard for diagnosing bacterial overgrowth.

Urea breath test: The test is based on the fact that *Helicobacter pylori has* significant urease activity. The substrate is urea with either radiolabeled carbon (^{14}C) or natural carbon isotope (^{13}C). After fermentation in the stomach the labeled CO_2 absorbs into the blood and is excreted through the lungs and captured in the expired air. It is measured with either beta-counter (^{14}C) or mass spectrograph (^{13}C). The test can be used for both the diagnosis and for the assessment of eradication. Because antibiotic treatment, pepto-bismol and proton pump inhibitors reduce the number of bacteria and may cause false negative results it is recommended not to take them for at least 10 days before the diagnostic test. It is better to check the eradication at approx 4 weeks after the eradication therapy.

TESTS OF BODY FLUIDS

Tests on Pancreatic Juice

Pancreatic juice can be collected with double lumen tube (one for gastric juice removal) or during endoscopy and can be used for cultures to rule out bacterial or fungal overgrowth. The freshly collected juice examined under microscope can be used to diagnose Giardia infestation. The juice collected after secretin and/or cholescystokinin stimulation is used to measure the activities of pancreatic enzymes (amylase, lipase, trypsin, chymotrypsin, elastase, carboxypeptidases).

Urobilinogen

Urobilinogen is formed from the excreted conjugated bilirubin by intestinal bacteria. Approximately 20% of it reabsorb and enter the portal circulation. In children with hepatic dysfunction more urobilinogen escapes the hepatic uptake and thus appears in the urine. In the case of *complete biliary obstruction*, the urinary urobilinogen decreases to almost zero. The excretion of urinary urobilinogen has some diurnal variation, with peak urinary output in early afternoon (between 12:00 and 16:00 hours). The urinary excretion of urobilinogen depends strongly on the *urinary pH*; tubular re-absorption increases and urobilinogen stability decreases as pH decreases. *Antibiotic therapy* decreases intestinal production therefore urinary excretion also less. *Diarrhea* also decreases the production of urobilinogen.

Sweat Test

Pilocarpine is introduced into the skin by iontophoresis to stimulate locally increased sweat gland secretion. The chloride can be measured directly using 20 µL samples with a chloride analyzer. Sweat chloride test is the initial screening for cystic fibrosis. Values over 60 mmol/L are pathologic. It is recommended repeating the test if value is over 40 mmol/L.

TISSUE TESTS

The most commonly used tissue tests are histological examinations on biopsy tissues obtained from the digestive canal and from the liver.

Intestinal Biopsy: Disaccharidase Assays

Disaccharide absorption is diminished either due to congenital disaccharidase deficiencies (sucrase-isomaltase deficiency, lactase deficiency, primary alactasia, primary trehalase deficiency) or secondary disaccharidase deficiencies (celiac disease, tropical sprue, acute vital gastroenteritis, or drugs such as orally administered neomycin, kanamycin and methotrexate). The secondary disaccharidase deficiencies are usually temporary and involve more than one enzyme. The third form is the adult hypolactasia when the lactase activity is present at birth and diminishes later in life. About 10% of Caucasians, 70% to 80% of African-Americans, and an even greater percentage of Asians have some degree of lactose intolerance. Definitive diagnosis of disaccharidase deficiencies is the measurement of the specific enzyme activities in intestinal biopsy tissue after homogenization and incubation with the substrate.

Gastric Biopsy: CLO-Test

The principle of this test is based on the high urease activity of *H. pylori*. Urea is mixed in gel that contains a pH indicator. If *H. pylori* present it hydrolyses the urea to CO_2 and ammonia. The pH becomes alkaline due to the ammonia production of H. pylori and the color of the gel changes from yellow to magenta. This can happen from 20 minutes to 24 hours in the sample kept at 37 ºC. The CLO-test can turn positive in 75% of H. pylori positive patients in 20 minutes, within an hour 85% of positive patients will be detected, and within 3 hours 90% are detected. If the gel remains yellow at 24 hours the test is negative.

GENETIC TESTS

In the last decade, there is a significant progress in the understanding the genetic basis of disorders. The etiology of both inherited and acquired gastrointestinal (GI) diseases is now understood at the DNA level. The new genetic methods have resulted in remarkable changes in disease screening, susceptibility testing, diagnostics, and therapeutics. Physician must understand the impact of genetic testing on medical management, future health, insurance, employment, and psychosocial issues. Some examples of the effect of genetic tests on the management of patients are given below.

Gene technology helps identifying subgroup of patients as it was demonstrated in Crohn's disease (CrD). The first gene identified as CrD susceptibility gene is the CARD 15/NOD2 gene. Patients with CrD who carry CARD 15/NOD2 are more likely to develop ileal strictures. Patients with CrD frequently carry a polymorphism in the multidrug resistance gene 1 (MDR1) resulting in decreased activity of the gene.

Table 120.14: Genetics of familial gastrointestinal cancers

Disorder	*Associated tumours*	*Gene*	*Chromosome Location*	*Gene product*
	Tumor suppressor genes (autosomal dominant)			
Familial adenomatous polyposis?	Colorectal, duodenal carcinoma	*APC*	5q21	APC
Familial gastric cancer?	Gastric carcinoma	*CDH1*	16q22	Cadherin 1
Multiple endocrine neoplasia type 1	Pancreatic islet cell, pituitary, parathyroid tumors	*MEN1*	11q13	Menin
Peutz-Jeghers syndrome?	Gastrointestinal tumors	*STK11*	19p13	STK11
	Oncogenes (autosomal dominant)			
Multiple endocrine neoplasia type 2	Medullary thyroid carcinoma, pheochromocytoma, parathyroid hyperplasia/adenoma	*RET*	10q12	RET
	DNA repair genes (autosomal dominant)			
Hereditary nonpolyposis colon cancer (HNPCC)	Colorectal, endometrial carcinoma	*MSH2*	2p16	MSH2
		MLH1	3p21	MLH1
		PMS1	2q32	PMS1
		PMS2	7p22	PMS2
		MSH6	2p16	MSH6

MDR1 knockout mice develop spontaneous IBD that may be related to their inability to export bacterial products from their intestinal epithelium. This gene may contribute to the known differences in pharmacogenetics in patients with CrD.

There are inherited diseases with known genetic defect. This knowledge allows the detection of these markers in the next generation (Table 120.14).

KEY LEARNING POINTS

- Blood tests include albumin, AP, A1-AT, AFP, ammonia, amylase, AST/ALT, bilirubin, CRP, ESR, ferritin, LDH, GGT, lipase, 5' nucleotidase, prealbumin, PT and PTT, vitamins, micronutrients and serology for celiac disease, IBD, *H. pylori*, liver disease, etc.
- Stool tests include fecal fat, leukocytes, occult blood, reducing substances, elastase, *C. difficile*, *H. pylori* and ova and cysts.
- Breath tests include urea breath test and carbohydrate breath tests.
- Tests on body fluids include sweat test, pancreatic juice and urobilinogen.
- Intestinal biopsy and gastric biopsy are the most commonly used tissue tests.
- New genetic tests have resulted in a remarkable improvement in disease screening, susceptibility diagnostics and therapeutics.

FURTHER READINGS

1. Abreu MT, Taylor KD, Lin YC, Hang T, Gaiennie J, Landers CJ, *et al.* Mutations in NOD2 are associated with fibrostenosing disease in patients with Crohn's disease. *Gastroenterology* 2002;123:679-688.
2. Amann ST, Josephson SA, Toskes PP. Acid steatocrit: A simple, rapid gravimetric method to determine steatorrhea. *Am J Gastroenterol* 1997;92:2280-2284.
3. Batres L, Maller E. Laboratory assessment of liver function and injury in children. *In: Suchi F.J, Sokol* RJ, Balistreri WF (eds): *Liver Disease in Children.* Philadelphia. Lippincott, Williams and Wilkins 2001:155-170.
4. Beaven S, Abreu M. Biomarkers in inflammatory bowel disease. *Curr Opin Gastroenterology* 2004;20:318-327.
5. Brant SR, Panhuysen CI, Nicolae D, Reddy DM, Bonen DK, Karaliukas R, *et al.* MDR1 Ala893 polymorphism is associated with inflammatory bowel disease. *Am J Hum Genet* 2003;73:1282-1292.
6. Cohen GA, Goffinet JA, Donabedian RK, Conn HO. Observations on decreased serum glutamic oxalacetic transaminase (SGOT) activity in azotemic patients. *Ann Intern Med* 1976:275-280.
7. Connelly MS, Kennedy HJ, Dawson CM, Howe GD, Tickner TR. Innocent elevation of aspartate aminotransferase. *Lancet* 1989;1:847.
8. Corazza GR, Menozzi MG, Strocchi A, Rasciti L, Vaira D, Lecchini R, *et al.* The diagnosis of small bowel bacterial overgrowth. Reliability of jejunal culture and inadequacy of breath hydrogen testing. *Gastroenterology* 1990;98(2):302-09.
9. Desai SP, Isa-Pratt S. Clinician's Gurde to Laboratory Medicino: A Practical Approching: Hudson, Cleveland Lexi-comp Inc 2002.
10. Desai SP, Isa-Pratt S. Clinician's Guide to Laboratory Medicine. A Practical Approach. Hudson, Cleveland, Lexi-Comp Inc. 2002.
11. Diehl AM, Potter J, Boitnott J, Van Duyn MA, Herlong HF, Mezey E. Relationship between pyridoxal 5'-phosphate deficiency and aminotransferase levels in alcoholic hepatitis. *Gastroenterology* 1984;86:632-636.
12. Dufour DR, Lott JA, Nolte FS, Gretch DR, Koff RS, Seeff LB. Diagnosis and monitoring of hepatic injury. I. Performance characteristics of laboratory tests. *Clin Chem* 2000;46:2027-2049.
13. Guarino A, Tarallo L, Greco L, Cesarano L, Guandalini S, Rubino A. Reference values of the steatocrit and its modifications in diarrheal diseases. *J Pediatr Gastroenterol Nutr* 1992;1:268-1274.
14. Hill RE, Hercz A, Corey ML, Gilday DL, Hamilton JR. Fecal clearance of alpha 1-antitrypsin: A reliable measure of enteric protein loss in children. *J Pediatr* 1981;99:416-418.
15. Iacono G, Carroccio A, Montalto G, Cavataio F, Gioeli RA, Di Dato AM, *et al.* Steatocrit test: Normal range and physiological variations in preterm and low-birth-weight full-term newborns. *Acta Paediatr* 1992;81:933-934.
16. Jennette JC, Falk RJ. Antineutrophil cytoplasmic autoantibodies in inflammatory bowel disease. *Am J Clin Pathol* 1993;99:221-223.
17. Katz DE, Taylor DN. Parasitic infections of the gastrointestinal tract. *Gastroenterol Clin North Am* 2001;30:797-815.
18. King JC. Assessment of zinc status. *J Nutr* 1990;120 Suppl 11:1474-1479.
19. Mulder AH, Horst G, Haagsma EB, Kleibeuker JH, Kallenberg CG. Anti-neutrophil cytoplasmic antibodies (ANCA) in autoimmune liver disease. *Adv Exp Med Biol* 1993;336:545-549.
20. Oudkerk Pool M, Ellerbroek PM, Ridwan BU, Goldschmeding R, von Blomberg BM, Pena AS, *et al.* Serum antineutrophil cytoplasmic autoantibodies in inflammatory bowel disease are mainly associated with ulcerative colitis. A correlation study between perinuclear antineutrophil cytoplasmic autoantibodies and clinical parameters, medical and surgical treatment. *Gut* 1993;34:46-50.
21. Tormey WP, O'Brien PA. Clinical associations of an increased transthyretin band in routine serum and urine protein electrophoresis. *Ann Clin Biochem* 1993;30 :550-554.
22. Warnock LG, Stone WJ, Wagner C. Decreased aspartate aminotransferase ("SGOT") activity in serum of uremic patients. *Clin Chem* 1974;20:1213-1216.

121 Pathological Examinations

Robert Garola

ESOPHAGUS

Developmental Disorders

Atresia and fistulas

- Rare.
- Etiology and embryologic mechanism are unknown.
- Usually found after birth.
- Some are incompatible with life.
- Frequently associated with other congenital malformations.
- Atresia:
  - Anatomically consists of a non-canalized cord with blind pouches in either side (more details in small and large intestine).
- Fistula:
  - Occurs in 80-90% of the cases of atresia.
  - Anatomically consists of a communication of one of the pouches with the main airway (tracheoesophageal fistula) (Fig. 121.1).

Neuroenteric remnants

- They result from the failure of separation of the endoderm from ectoderm at early stages of development.
- In addition of the esophagus, they may be located at any level of the gastrointestinal tract.

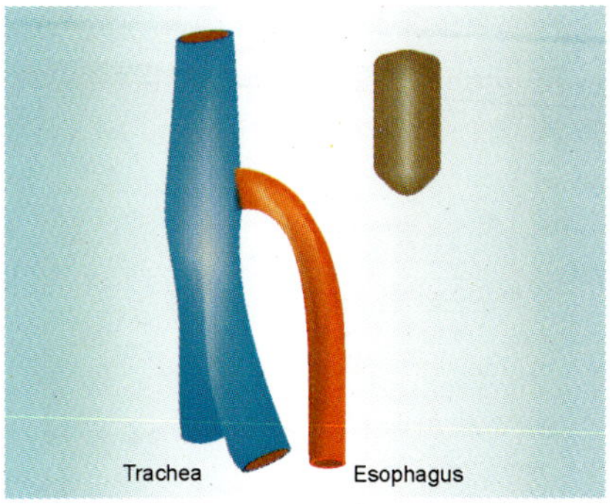

Fig. 121.1: Esophageal atresia; draw of most common type of esophageal atresia with tracheoesophageal fistula

- Originate from the dorsal midline of the gastrointestinal tract and attach or pass through the vertebral column to the skin of the dorsum acquiring the forms depicted in Fig. 121.2.

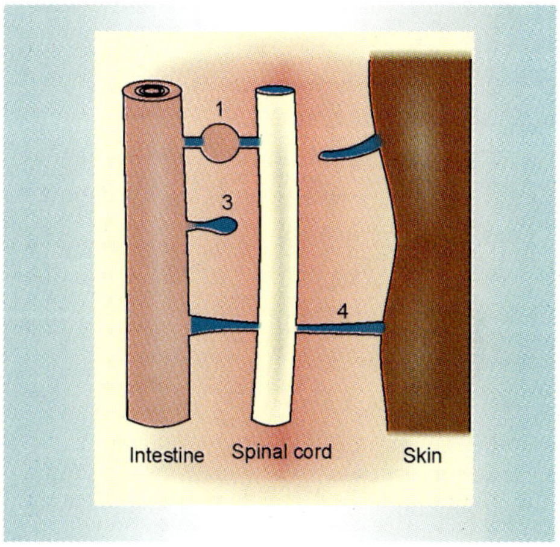

Fig. 121.2: Neuroenteric remnants; (1) Dorsal enteric cyst (located dorsal to the tract and anterior to the vertebral column). (2) Dorsal enteric sinus (deep invagination of the epidermis in the dorsum). (3) Dorsal enteric diverticulum (enteric pouch). (4) Dorsal enteric fistula (from the gastrointestinal tract to the skin of the dorsum passing through the vertebral column).

Inflammatory Diseases

The biopsy is crucial to diagnose (endoscopic negative) inflammatory diseases of the esophagus.

Esophagitis

- The two most common pediatric diseases seen in the esophagus are:
  - Reflux and eosinophilic esophagitis.
  - Both diseases have similar pathologic characteristics but different pathogenesis.

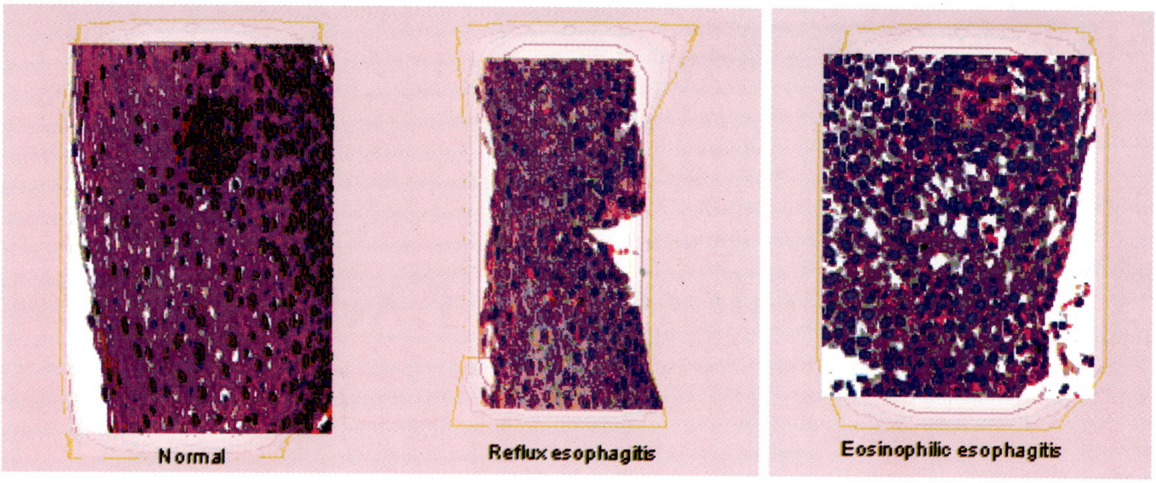

Fig. 121.3: Reflux (RE) and eosinophilic esophagitis (EE); notice marked intraepithelial eosinophilia in EE compared to less dense eosinophilic infiltrate in RE. In addition, there is marked intercellular edema and greater reactive cellular changes throughout the epithelial wall in EE (H & E stain)

Reflux Esophagitis (RE)

- Reflux to the esophagus of gastric contents is the most common cause of esophagitis in children:
  - Anatomic characteristics:
    - □ Intraepithelial inflammatory cells (Fig. 121.3):
      - ✓ Eosinophils, neutrophils and lymphocytes:
        - ➢ Eosinophils usually less than 5 per high power field (HPF).
        - ➢ Increased lymphocytes.
    - □ Epithelial basal layer hyperplasia;
      - ✓ More than 1/5 of the full thickness of the squamous epithelium.
    - □ Elongation of the of lamina propria papillae, usually with capillary congestion:
      - ✓ More than 2/3 of the full thickness of the squamous epithelium.
    - □ Involves the distal segment of the esophagus (see Table 121.1).
    - □ Several biopsies are recommended for better diagnostic yield.

Eosinophilic Esophagitis (EE)

- Characterized by severe eosinophilic infiltration of the esophageal epithelium:
  - Patients do not respond to antireflux therapy.
  - Though attributed to food allergy, the etiology is unclear.
  - May be isolated or be part eosinophilic gastroenteritis.
  - Peripheral eosinophilia is seen in 20 to 60% of the cases.
  - Frequent individual or family history of allergy including asthma, eczema and rhinitis.
  - The definitive diagnosis of EE is made by mucosal esophageal biopsy.
  - Anatomic characteristics:
    - □ Intraepithelial eosinophilia:
      - ✓ Involves the distal and mid segments of the esophagus.
      - ✓ Aggregation and superficial mucosal location of eosinophils.
      - ✓ Most patients with EE have 20 or more intraepithelial eosinophils per HPF (Fig. 121.3).
      - ✓ Prominent epithelial hyperplasia and intercellular edema.

Table 121.1: Esophagitis (EE) and gastroesophageal reflux disease (GERD)

	EE	*GERD*
Distal Esophagus	> 20 per hpf*	< 5 per hpf
Mid Esophagus	> 20 per hpf	1 or none per hpf

*hpf = light microcopy high power field

Infectious Esophagitis

- Inflammation in the esophagus caused by infectious agents:
  - Relatively uncommon.
  - Most cases affect immunocompromised children.
  - Most common infectious agents include:
    - □ ***Fungus:***
      - ✓ Candida species.
      - ✓ Torulopsis glabrata.
    - □ ***Virus:***
      - ✓ Herpes simplex.
      - ✓ Cytomegalovirus.
      - ✓ Varicella zoster.
    - □ ***Bacteria:***
      - ✓ Diphtheria (toxin of Corynebacterium diphtheriae).
      - ✓ Mycobacterium tuberculosis.

- ***Candida Esophagitis:***
  - Commonly is associated with oropharyngeal infection.
  - May occur in immunocompetent and immunocompromised children.
  - Anatomic characteristics:
    - □ Acute inflammation, superficial necrosis and ulceration associated with granulation tissue, eventual fibrosis and stricture (common to all infectious esophagitis).
    - □ Gray-white pseudo-membranes embedding fungal elements.
    - □ Organisms can be highlighted by the use of fungal stains such as Gomori Methenamine Silver (GMS) or Periodic acid of Schiff (PAS).
    - □ Diagnosis of invasive disease requires that pseudohyphae and yeasts be found within the mucosal tissue (Fig. 121.4).

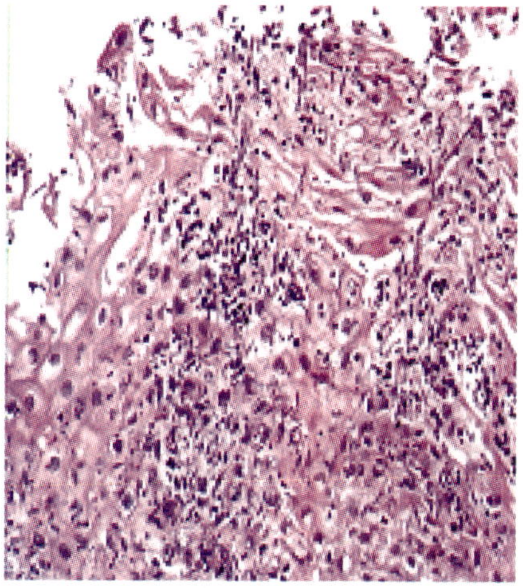

Fig. 121.4: Candida esophagitis; yeast, pseudohyphae and cell debris invading the squamous epithelium of the esophagus (H&E stain). *From Johns Hopkins Pathology Surgical Pathology Unknown conference*

- ***Herpes simplex esophagitis:***
  - Most of the cases seen in immunocompromised patients.
  - Anatomic characteristics (Fig. 121.5):
    - □ Coalescent ulcers surrounded by normal looking mucosa.
    - □ Microscopic diagnostic criteria include:
      - ✓ Nuclear inclusions.
      - ✓ Ground glass nuclei.
      - ✓ Nuclear molding.
      - ✓ Multinucleated giant cells.
      - ✓ Ballooning changes in the degenerating infected epithelial cells.
      - ✓ Involves squamous cells.
      - ✓ Specific antigen immunohistochemistry confirms the diagnosis.

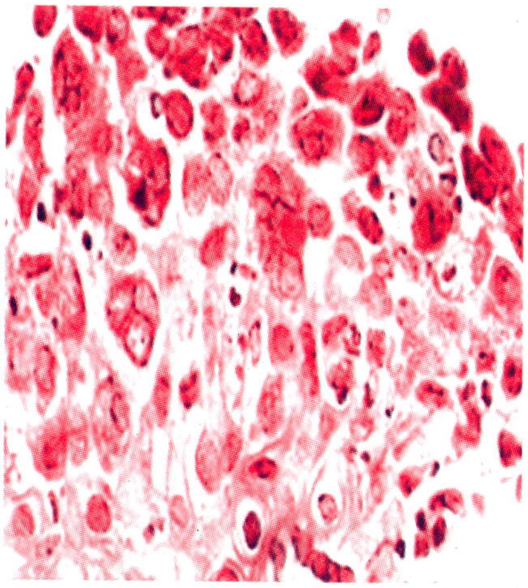

Fig. 121.5: Herpes esophagitis; epithelial cells with characteristic herpes cytopathic inclusions including giant cells and eosinophilic nuclear inclusions (H and E stain)

- ***Cytomegalovirus (CMV) esophagitis:***
  - Most of the cases seen in immunocompromised patients.
  - Anatomic characteristics:
    - □ Multiple ulcers.
    - □ Nuclear and cytoplasmic inclusions involving endothelial cells and inflammatory fibroblasts in ulcer bed.
    - □ Specific antigen immunohistochemistry confirms the diagnosis.
- ***Bacterial esophagitis:***
  - Very rare in children.
  - Most cases associated with bacteremia.
- ***Other forms of esophagitis:***
  - Systemic graft-versus-host disease (GVHD).
  - Autoimmune diseases.
  - Epidermolysis bullosa.
  - Crohn's disease.

Neoplastic Diseases

- Tumors of the esophagus are rare in children.
- ***Squamous papilloma:***
  - Is the most common tumor of the esophagus in children:
    - □ Benign.
    - □ Anatomic characteristics:
      - ✓ Stromal core covered by benign squamous epithelium.
  - Half of the cases show human papilloma virus genetic material.

STOMACH

Developmental Disorders

Malformations of the stomach are rare.

Congenital Hypertrophic Pyloric Stenosis

- This is the most common developmental abnormality of the stomach.
- Etiology is unknown.
- It consists of:
  - Dilated stomach.
  - Elongated and thickened (twice the normal) of the pylorus due to (Fig. 121.6):
    - □ Hyperplasia and hypertrophy of the circular layer of the visceral muscle.
  - Degeneration of the myenteric plexuses.

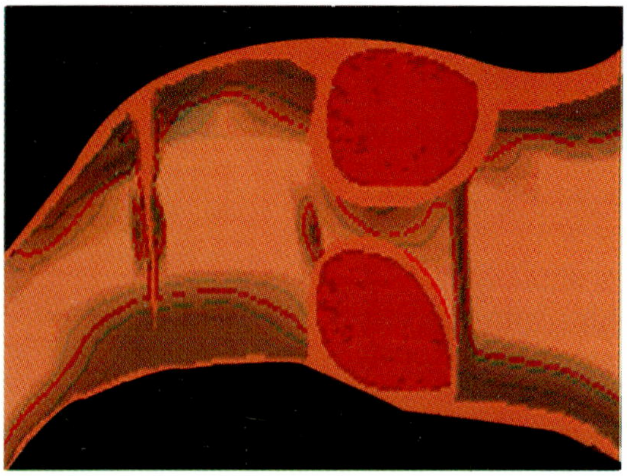

Fig. 121.6: Congenital hypertrophic pyloric stenosis; draw showing pyloris stenosis due to muscle hypertrophy of the pyloric sphincter

Inflammatory Diseases

Gastritis:

- Spectrum of inflammatory changes in the gastric mucosa with well recognized and characterized architectural patterns of tissue response to different factors (Table 121.2).
- Two third of the gastritis found in the pediatric population are:
  - Helicobacter pylori related and chronic nonspecific.
- The remaining third, includes diseases that frequently involves other segments of the gastrointestinal tract.

Helicobacter pylori gastritis:

- Occurs worldwide.
- This is the most common bacterial infection in humans.
- Its prevalence is highest in developing countries.
- The infection is acquired by oral ingestion of the organism.
- In the stomach, because its ability to produce urease (hydrolyzes urea into CO_2 and ammonia), survives the acidity of the stomach and attach to the surface of the mucosa to cause continuous gastric inflammation.
- The diagnosis is suggested by noninvasive methods:
  - Urea breath test.
  - Serologic tests.
  - Stool antigens.
- The diagnosis is confirmed by endoscopic biopsy.
  - Anatomic characteristics:
    - □ Antral location.
    - □ Acute stage:
      - ✓ Erythematous mucosa infiltrated by lymphocytes, neutrophils and eosinophils in the lamina propria and invading the epithelium.
      - ✓ Reactive epithelial changes including nuclear hyperchromasia and mucin depletion.
    - □ Chronic stage.
    - □ Nodular mucosa due to lymphoid hyperplasia with follicular formation.

Table 121.2: Major causes of bacterial enterocolitis

Organism	*Pathogenic mechanism*	*Source*
Escherichia coli		
*ETEC	Cholera-like toxin, no invasion	Food, water
*EHEC	Shiga-like toxin, no invasion	Undercooked beef products
*EPEC	Attachment, enterocyte effacement, no invasion	Weaning foods, water
*EIEC	Invasion, local spread	Cheese, water, person-to-person
Salmonella	*Invasion, translocation, lymphoid inflammation, dissemination*	*Milk, beef, eggs, poultry*
Shigella	Invasion, local spread	Person-to-person, low-inoculum
Campylobacter	*Toxins, Invasion*	*Milk, poultry, animal contact*
Yersinia enterocolitica	Invasion, translocation, lymphoid inflammation, dissemination	Milk, pork
Vibrio cholerae, other vibrios	Enterotoxin, no invasion	Water, shellfish, person-to-person spread
Clostridium difficile	Cytotoxin, local invasion	Nosocomial environmental spread
Clostridium perfringens	Enterotoxin, no invasion	Meat, poultry, fish
Mycobacterium tuberculosis	Invasion, mural inflammatory, foci with necrosis and scarring	Contaminated milk, swallowing of coughed-up organisms

*ETEC, *enterotoxigenic E. coli;* EHEC, *enterohemorrhagic E. coli;* EPEC, *enteropathogenic E. coli*; EIEC, *enteroinvasive E. coli*

- □ In both stages the organism is seen on the mucosal epithelium:
  - ✓ H pylori are not invasive.
  - ✓ The organism is small, curved and easy to identify in hematoxylin and eosin stained tissue sections.
  - ✓ Special stains such as silver and giemsa can make the organisms obvious (Fig. 121.7).

Cytomegalovirus gastritis

- May occur in immunocompromised children.
- Anatomic characteristics:
  - – Mucosal redness and erosion (endoscopy).
  - – Non-specific inflammatory infiltrate:
    - □ Mucosal edema.
    - □ Classical CMV inclusions.
    - □ An unusual presentation is:
      - ✓ Foveolar hyperplasia mimicking Ménétrièr's disease* believed to be a consequence of over expression of transforming growth factor.

Lymphocytic gastritis

- Associated with celiac disease and occasionally seen in H pylori gastritis.
- Anatomic characteristics:
  - – Increased intraepithelial lymphocytes.

Autoimmune gastritis

- Very rare in children.
- Characterized by:
  - – Mucosal atrophy.
  - – Serum gastric autoantibodies against parietal cell antigens.

Idiopathic inflammatory gastrointestinal disease

- Crohn's disease (CD) and rarely ulcerative colitis (UC) may be associated with gastritis.
- In CD the two morphologic patterns of gastritis include:
  - – Granulomatous inflammation (*Granulomas in the gastric mucosa may also be seen in chronic granulomatous disease and tuberculosis infection).*
  - – Non-specific chronic inflammation.
- In UC morphologic changes include:
  - – Focal nonspecific gastritis (Fig. 121.7).

Chronic nonspecific gastritis

- This is the most common form of anatomic gastritis in the USA being, its prevalence is unknown in developing countries.
- Its cause is unknown.
- Anatomic characteristics:
  - – Antral location.
  - – Focal chronic inflammation with predominance of lymphocytes and plasma cells (Fig. 121.7).

Neoplastic Diseases

Gastric pediatric tumors are extremely rare. The most common is juvenile polyp (to be discussed later).

SMALL AND LARGE INTESTINES

Developmental Disorders

Stenosis and Atresia of the Intestine

- Stenosis is narrowing of the intestinal lumen.
- Atresia is complete obstruction of the intestinal lumen.
- The majority of these abnormalities are believed to occur

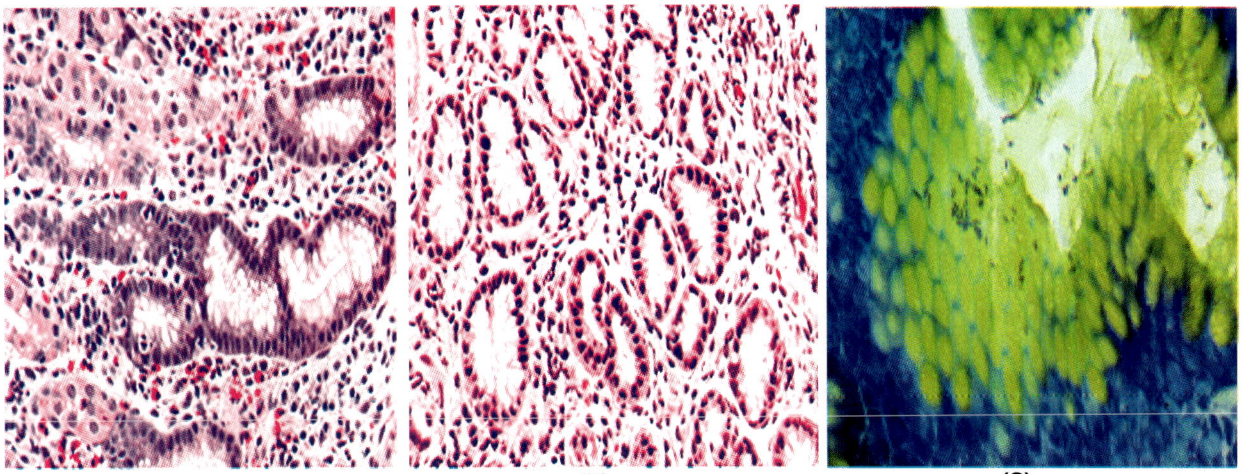

(A) (B) (C)

Fig. 121.7: Helicobacter pylori (HP) and chronic nonspecifc gastritis; (A) Acute stage of HP gastritis, notices a mixed inflammatory infiltrate of the gastric mucosa with epithelial cell mucin depletion, and nuclear hyperchromasia (H&E stain) (B) Helicobacter pylori bacteria seen on the mucosal surface (Giemsa stain, methilene blue counterstain) (C) Chronic nonspecific gastritis, notices a mild inflammatory infiltrate and epithelial changes of mucosal injury. This pattern of gastritis can also be seen with HP infection though finding the organisms differentiate both (H&E stain)

*Giant hypertrophic gastritis after the name of French Physician, Pierre Menetrier (1859-1935).

by infarction of the fetal bowel secondary to vascular accidents of unclear nature.

- The anatomic defect may have one the characteristics illustrated in Fig. 121.8.

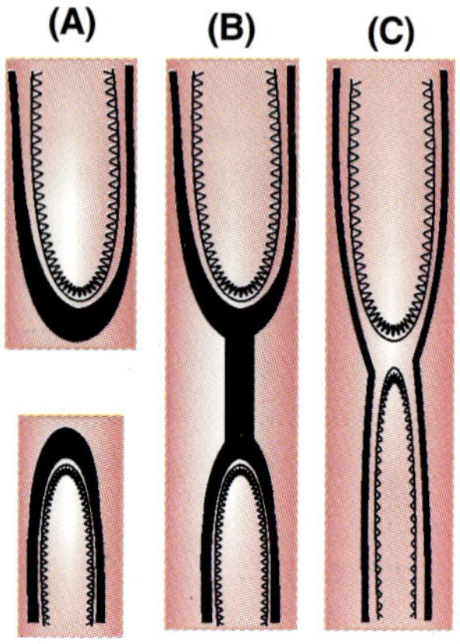

Fig. 121.8: Anatomic types of atresia; (A) Unconnected blind ends (B) A fibrous cord connect the blind ends (C) A membrane formed by fused muscularis propria lined on both sides by mucosa

Duplication Cysts

- May occur at any level of the GI tract.
- Most are cystic (adherent to the adjacent bowel, covered by mesentery) or less frequently tubular with the appearance of a giant diverticulum seating along the bowel.
- The wall of the duplications is muscular and the mucosa lined by the same epithelium of the bowel associated with it (Figs. 121.9 and 121.10).

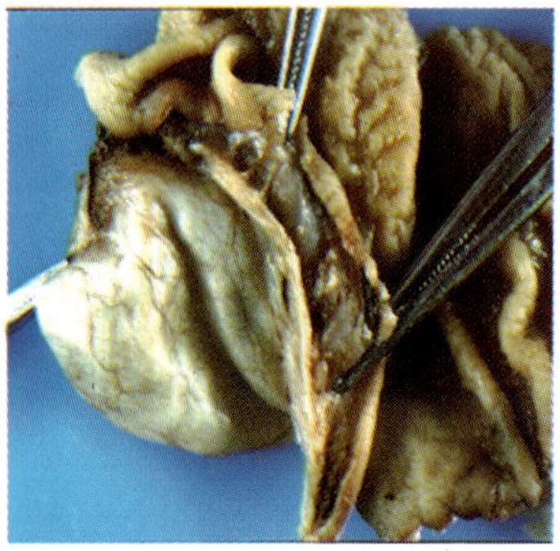

Fig. 121.9: Gastric duplication: Figure shows duplicated, red arrow, gastric chamber

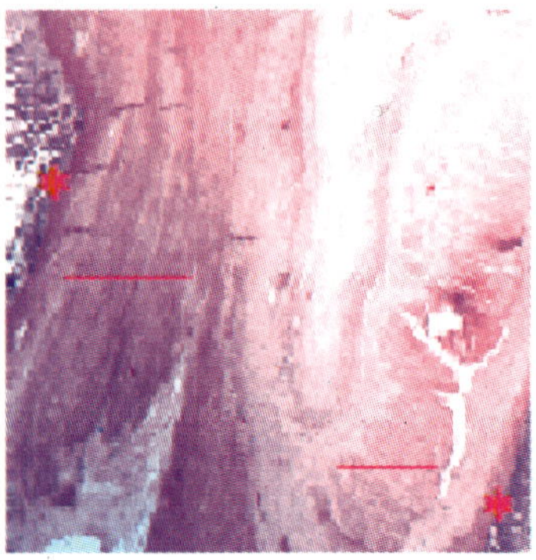

Fig. 121.10: Histological changes of ileal duplication: Picture shows common wall of duplicated intestine with double mucosa and double layer of muscularis propria (H&E stain)

Omphalocele

- Failure of the intestine to return to the abdominal cavity during development.
- The failure produces a sac that contains abdominal viscera covered by peritoneum and the epithelium of the umbilical cord (derivate of the amnion).

Gastroschisis

- Abnormal linear closing of the abdominal wall with extrusion of the abdominal viscera into the amniotic cavity without involving the umbilical cord.
  - Most of the cases occur on the right side of the abdomen (Fig. 121.11).

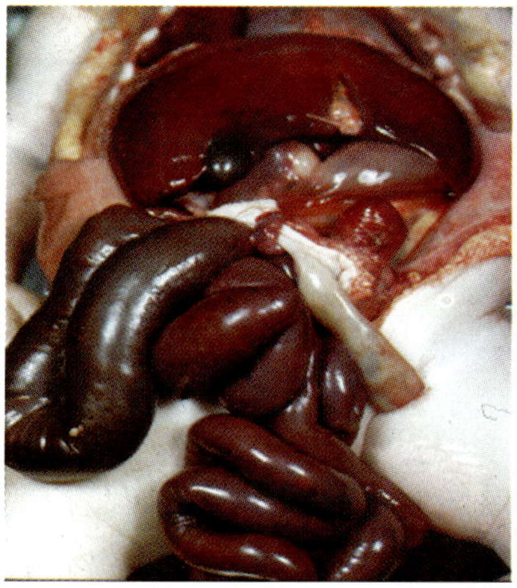

Fig. 121.11: Illustration of gatroschisis; uncovered extrusion of abdominal organs without involvement of the umbilical cord

Non-Rotation of the Intestine

- The entire colon is on the left side of the abdomen (Fig. 121.12).
- The intestine may twist to cause obstruction of the superior mesenteric artery with consequent ischemic necrosis of the intestine.

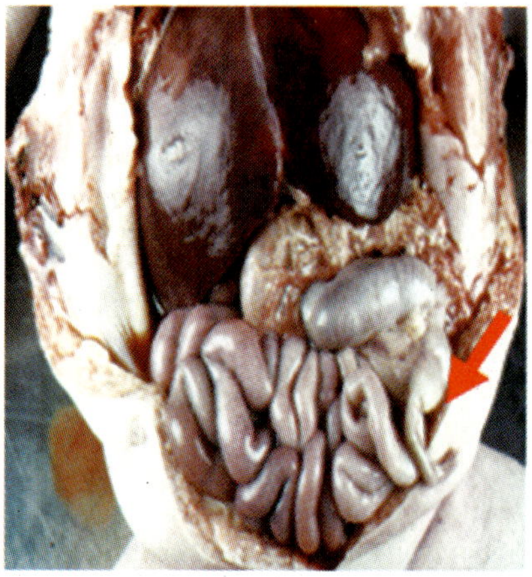

Fig. 121.12: Example of non-rotation of intestine; the entire colon is on the left side (red arrow) of the abdominal cavity

Mixed Rotation of the Midgut

- Is the most common form of malrotation seen clinically.
- It is the result of an incomplete final 90-degree rotation of the midgut.
- The cecum is located inferior to the pylorus and is fixed to the posterior abdominal wall by a fibrous band that passes over the duodenum usually causing duodenal obstruction.

Yolk Sac Remnants

- The entire or a segment of the omphalomesenteric duct may remain patent or may persist as fibrous cord between the umbilicus and the ileum (Fig. 121.13).
- Meckel's diverticulum:
  - Remnant of the proximal portion of the omphalomesenteric duct.
  - It occurs in 2-4% of the people.
  - When inflamed, causes appendicitis-like symptoms.

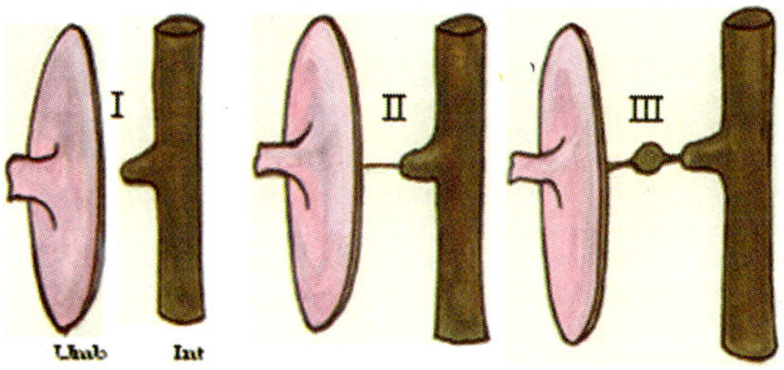

Fig. 121.13: Draw of yolk sac remants; (I) Meckel's diverticulum, (II) Meckel's diverticulum attached to the umbilicus by fibrous cord, (III) Vitelline cyst attached to intestine and umbilicus by fibrous cord. Umb=umbilicus, Int=intestine

  - Its walls, in addition of being formed by ileal tissue, may contain small areas of gastric mucosa and pancreatic tissue.
  - When there is gastric mucosa, ulceration, acute and chronic hemorrhage (edema) may occur.
  - It appears as a finger-like pouch arising from the antimesenteric border of the wall located at 40-50 cm from the ileo-cecal valve (Fig. 121.14).

Anorectal Malformations

- Group of anomalies that result from abnormal development of the urorectal septum, classified as indicated in Table 121.3.

Meconium Ileus

- Complication of cystic fibrosis caused by meconial inspissation and subsequent intestinal obstruction.
- The intestine distal to the obstruction becomes hypoplastic because lack of function.
- Anatomic characteristics:
  - Thick meconium with abundant mucin and distension of the ileum.
- If the ileum perforates in uterus meconium peritonitis occurs.

Table 121.3: Anal rectal malformations

Low
Anal agenesis Anal stenosis Membranous anal atresia
High
Anal rectal agenesis (most common) Rectal atresia

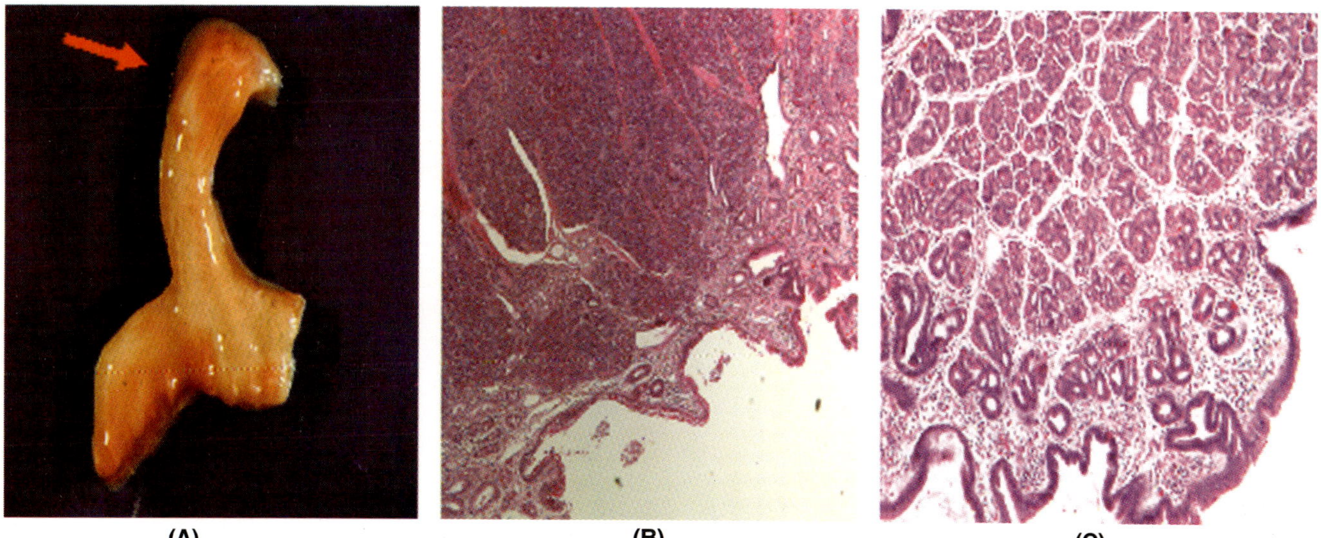

Fig. 121.14: Meckel's diverticulum. (A) Finger-like pouch that originates in the ileum. Pancreatic tissue (B) and gastric mucosa (C) as part of the wall of the diverticulum (H&E stain)

Congenital Aganglionic Megacolon or Hirschsprung's Disease

- Disease of the enteric nervous system characterized by a dilatation of a portion of the intestine due to the absence of autonomic ganglion cells in the myenteric and sub-mucosal plexuses of the intestinal wall distal to the dilated segment.
- Worldwide frequency of HD is approximately 1/1500 to 1/7000 newborns and 80-90% of the cases are diagnosed during the neonatal period.
- Considered to be the result of the lack of migration of neuroblasts into the distal plexuses of the gastrointestinal tract.
- Deletion of the RET proto-oncogene were found associated with some familial forms of Hirschsprung's disease:
  - Deletion of the RET proto-oncogene were found associated with some familial forms of Hirschsprung's disease.
  - This gene appears to play an important role in regulating the development of the intestinal nervous system.
- Recent research also demonstrated absence of NCAM (neural cell adhesion molecule) in aganglionic segments of intestine.
- Approximately 20% of the cases will have one or multiple developmental anomalies involving the central nervous, cardiovascular, urogenital and gastrointestinal systems.
- May be associated with Down's syndrome and multiple endocrine neoplasia type II.
- The length of the aganglionic segment of bowel is variable:
  - Confined to recto sigmoid in 75%.
  - Sigmoid, splenic flexure and transverse colon in 17%.
  - Total colon along with a short segment of ileum in 8%.
- Definitive diagnosis of HD is made by rectal biopsy:
  - Suction rectal biopsy is the most accurate test, having a mean 93% sensitivity and mean 98% specificity:
    - □ Tissue should be from at least 2.5 cm above dentate (the segment below this line is normally aganglionic).
    - □ The biopsy, to be adequate for diagnosis, should demonstrate mucosal and sub-mucosal tissue in a 1:1 proportion.
    - □ The histopathology consists of absence of ganglion cells in the myenteric and submucosal plexus and hypertrophied nerve trunks that can also be demonstrated with acetylcholinesterase stain.

Inflammatory Diseases

Infectious Enterocolitis

- Infections of the gastrointestinal tract are prevalent in children of developing countries.
- Caused by viruses, bacteria and parasites.
- Mechanism of bacterial enterocolitis include:
  - Ingestion of toxins formed by the organisms.
  - Infection by toxigenic organisms that proliferate in the intestinal lumen and produce enterotoxins.
  - Infection by enteroinvasive organisms that invade and destroy mucosal cells.
- ***Bacterial enterocolitis*** is consequence of:
  - Bacterial adhesion to the mucosal epithelium related to adhesive molecules on the bacterial surface.
  - Bacterial toxins:
    - □ Polypeptides, secretagogues, that stimulate fluid secretion (cholera toxin).

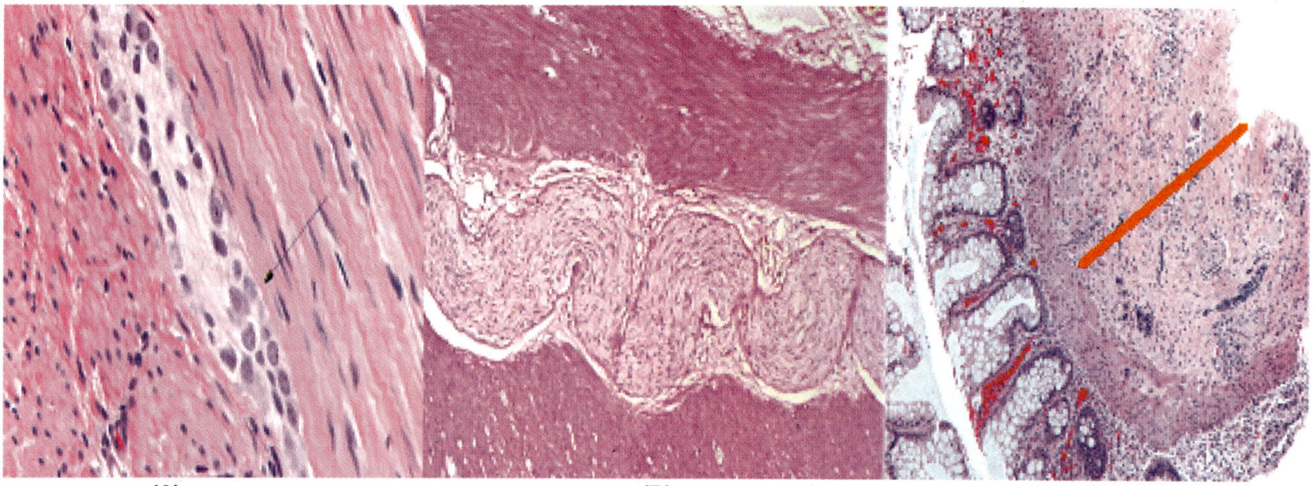

(A) (B) (C)

Fig. 121.15: Aganglionosis; (A) Normal myenteric plexus with ganglion cells associated with nerve trunk. (B) Aganglionic myenteric plexus with nerve hypertrophy as seen in Hirschsprung's disease. (C) Adequate suction rectal biopsy to show the amount of submucosal tissue required for assessment of ganglion cells (H and E stain)

  - Cytotoxins (e.g. shiga toxin) that cause direct epithelial cell necrosis.
- Bacterial invasion by stimulation of endocytosis, intracellular proliferation and cytolysis with spread of the organism to circulation (e.g. salmonella, E. coli).
- Anatomic changes of *bacterial enterocolitis* include:
  - Non-specific:
    - ✓ Damage of the surface epithelium.
    - ✓ Increased epithelial cell mitosis.
    - ✓ Congestion and edema of the lamina propria.
    - ✓ Neutrophilic infiltrate of lamina propria and epithelium.
  - Characteristic:
    - ✓ *Clostridium perfringens:*
      - ➢ Mild necrotizing enterocolitis.
    - ✓ *Shigella, Campylobacter SP and enteroinvasive E. coli:*
      - ➢ Mucosal erosion and exudation.
    - ✓ *V. Cholera and enterotoxigenic E. coli.*
      - ➢ No significant mucosal changes.
    - ✓ *Yersinia, enterocolitica and pseudotuberculosis*:
      - ➢ Involves ileum, appendix, colon and lymph nodes.
      - ➢ Necrotizing granulomas.
- Morphologic changes of ***viral enterocolitis*** in the small intestine include:
  - Villi shortening.
  - Inflammation of the lamina propria.
  - Injury of the superficial epithelial mucosal cells.

- ***Parasites*** and ***protozoa*** are highly prevalent in large part of the world population and most common organisms include:
  - Nematodes, strongyloides, ascaris, hookworms.
  - Flatworms; tapeworms and flukes.
  - Protozoa; entamoeba histolytica and giardia lamblia.
  - Anatomic characteristics:
    - Reactive inflammation.
    - Mucosal injury associated with the infective parasite or protozoa.
    - The diagnosis is made by direct examination and identification of the parasite in tissue and/or stool.

Necrotizing Enterocolitis

- Inflammation of the small and large intestine that mostly affects premature babies.
- The etiology is unknown, but several theories exist:
  - Weakening of the gut because intestinal ischemia and subsequent bacterial invasion.
  - Abnormal intestinal flora.
  - Functional immaturity.
- Anatomic characteristics:
  - Mucosal to full-thickness necrosis.
  - Mucosal edema.
  - Hemorrhage.
  - Mucosal inflammation.
  - Pneumatosis (Fig. 121.16).

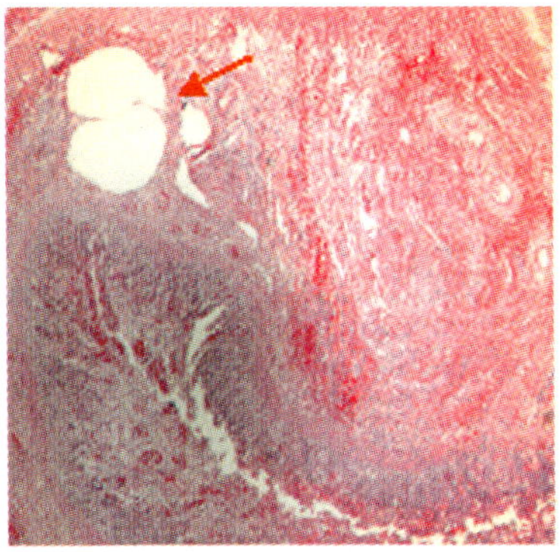

Fig. 121.16: Intestine in a case of necrotizing enterocolitis to show air (pneumatosis) in the wall (H&E stain)

Pseudomembranous Colitis

- Acute mucosal lesion with epithelial damage underlying an adherent inflammatory membrane.
- Mostly caused by toxins of clostridium difficile in patients treated with antibiotics.
- May also be secondary to ischemia or infection.
- Anatomic characteristics:
  - Plaque-like adherent membrane formed by fibrino-purulent necrotic debris and mucus overlying mucosal cell necrosis (Fig. 121.17).
- The diagnosis of the antibiotic related form is made by detection C. difficile toxin in feces.

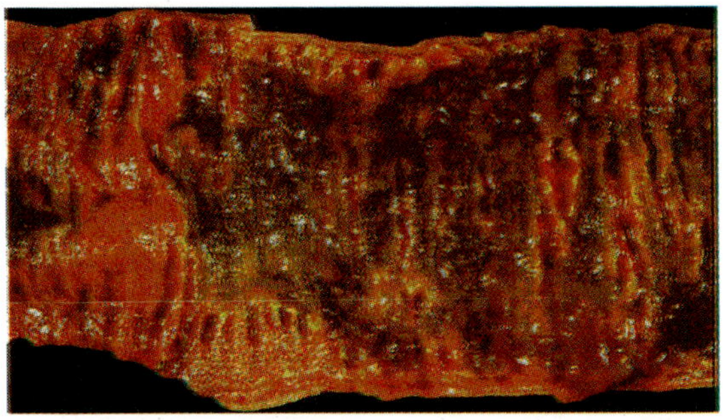

Fig. 121.17: Pseudomembranous colitis; notice brown and yellow layer of exudative and necrotic material seating on the intestinal mucosa

Malabsorption Syndrome (Table 121.4)

Intestinal Defective or Inadequate Absorption of Nutrients

Celiac Disease

- Intestinal lesion due to intolerance to proteins of the gluten.

Table 121.4: Causes of malabsorption in children

In developed countries	*In developing countries*
• Celiac disease • Food allergy • Cystic fibrosis • Giardiasis • Post infectious enteritis • Specific digestive enzyme deficiency (e.g. lactase) • Immune deficiency • Crohn's disease • Chronic bacterial enteritis • Abetalipoproteinemia (rare) • Microvillous inclusion disease (rare)	• Infections • Celiac disease • Lactose intolerance • Tropical sprue • Chronic pancreatitis • Immunoproliferative small intestinal disease

- The mechanism is T-lymphocyte mediated inflammation caused by intolerance to gluten.
- The majority of the patients with the disease have histocompatibility complex class II or HLA-DQ8 haplotype.
- A diet restricted in gluten revert the inflammatory changes in most cases.
- Anatomic characteristics:
  - Marked villous atrophy.
  - Increase intraepithelial lymphocytes.
  - Elongated and hyperplastic crypt elongation.
  - Mixed inflammatory infiltrate in the lamina propria.
  - Changes are nonspecific. Involves chiefly the duodenum and can be seen in other diseases involving the small bowel.

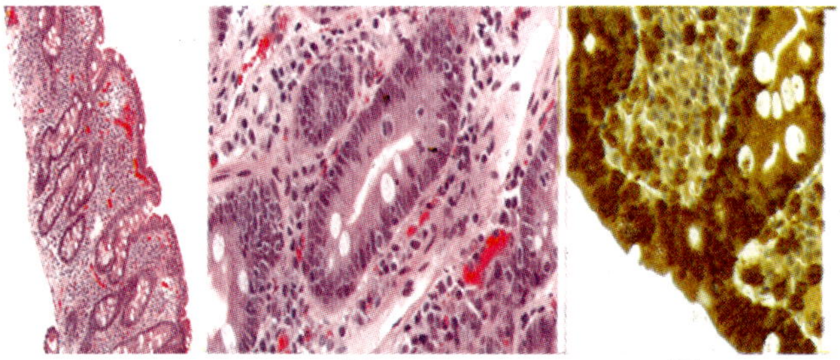

(A) (B) (C)

Fig. 121.18: Celiac disease: Duodenal biopsy from a child with malabsorption. (A) The tissue shows villous atrophy, expansion of the lamina propria by inflammatory cells and crypt hyperplasia. (B) A close up that shows frequent mitosis of epithelial cells (H&E stain). (C) Numerous intraepithelial T- lymphocytes brown stain highlighted by CD3 immunohistochemistry

Tropical Sprue

- Inflammatory condition morphologically similar to celiac disease but involving the whole small intestine.
- It is common in the Caribbean, except Jamaica, central and southern Africa, India and South East Asia, and part of Central and South America.
- The etiology is unknown, bacterial overgrowth by enterogenic bacteria has been implicated.
- Morphologic changes include:
  - In addition to the changes seen in celiac disease, nuclear enlargement due to Folate/Vitamin B_{12} deficiency.

Intolerance to Food Proteins

- Cow's milk, soya, chicken and fish proteins can generate intestinal intolerance.
- Morphologic changes include:
  - Patchy villous atrophy, less intense than celiac disease.
  - Increased eosinophils and mast cells in the inflammatory infiltrate.

Acquired Lactase Deficiency

- Common disorder associated with intestinal bacterial/ viral infections or other intestinal disorders.
- There are no anatomic changes associated with lactase deficiency.

Eosinophilic Gastroenteritis

- Intestinal abnormality that involves different segment of the gastrointestinal tract.
- The changes in the small intestine are mild, less intense than those seen in the esophagus, stomach and recto-sigmoid.
- Attributed to allergy though less than 20% of the cases have history of allergies.
- Morphologic changes, non-specific, include:
  - Mucosal eosinophilia involving the epithelium and lamina propria (Fig. 121.19).
  - Villous changes are rare.
  - Occasionally might be villous destruction with changes similar to those of celiac disease.

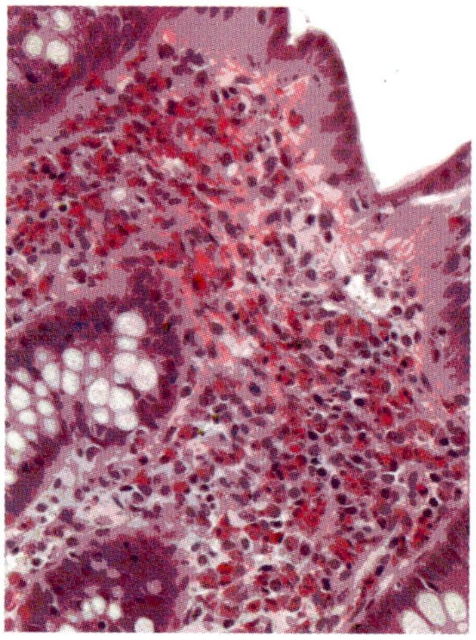

Fig. 121.19: Numerous eosinophils in the colonic mucosa of a patient with eosinophilic gastroenteritis (H and E)

Infectious Diseases that Cause Malabsorption

- Self-limited malabsorption may be caused by:
  - Viral and common bacterial infections.
  - Giardiasis, strongyloidiasis and tuberculosis are very common infectious causes of malabsorption in developing countries.

Giardiasis

- The most prevalent protozoan-related gut disorder worldwide.
- Morphologic changes include:
  - Blunting of villi.
  - Decreased villous-crypt ratio.
  - Mixed inflammatory infiltrate of the lamina propria.
- Infection cause block of absorption.
- The diagnosis of giardiasis is made direct microscopic examination of the stools, serology or detection of giardia antigen in stool by immunoassay.

Strongyloidosis

- Intestinal changes are related to the presence of parasitic females embedded in the mucosa of small intestine.
- Cause malabsorption due to organism-related mucosal destructive changes and poor nutrition.
- A definitive diagnosis is made by detection of the larvae in the stool.

Tuberculosis

- Relatively common in developing countries.
  - Morphologic changes include:
    - □ Most affected areas are the jejunoileum and ileocecum.
    - □ Associated with lymphoid tissue.

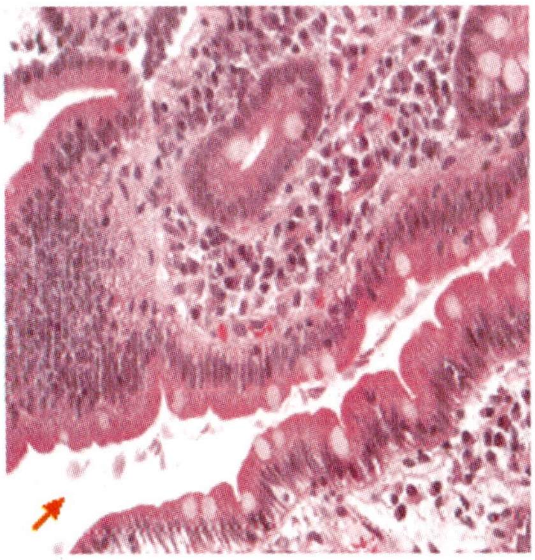

Fig. 121.20: Duodenal biopsy of a child with diarrhea. Trophozoites of giardia lamblia on the mucosal surface. The inflammatory changes in the mucosa are minimal (H and E)

    - □ Annular ulcers occasionally with stricture.
    - □ Local lymph nodes involved with caseating granuloma.
    - □ Intestinal granulomas with caseating foci surrounded by multinucleated giant cells, lymphocytes and fibrosis in Payer's patches.
- The diagnosis is based on the identification of mycobacterium tuberculosis:
  - 0.5-2 microns curved bacillus that can be visualized by acid-fast stain.
  - Microbial culture.
  - Polymerase chain reaction analysis.

Idiopathic Inflammatory Bowel Disease

- Inappropriate activation of the mucosal immune system triggered by normal intestinal flora.
- Probably consequence of defects in the barrier functions of the intestinal epithelium and the mucosal immune system.
- Multiple etiologic factors considered:
  - □ Genetic.
  - □ Infectious.
  - □ Noninfectious antigens.
- Two clinical-anatomic forms: (Fig. 121.21)

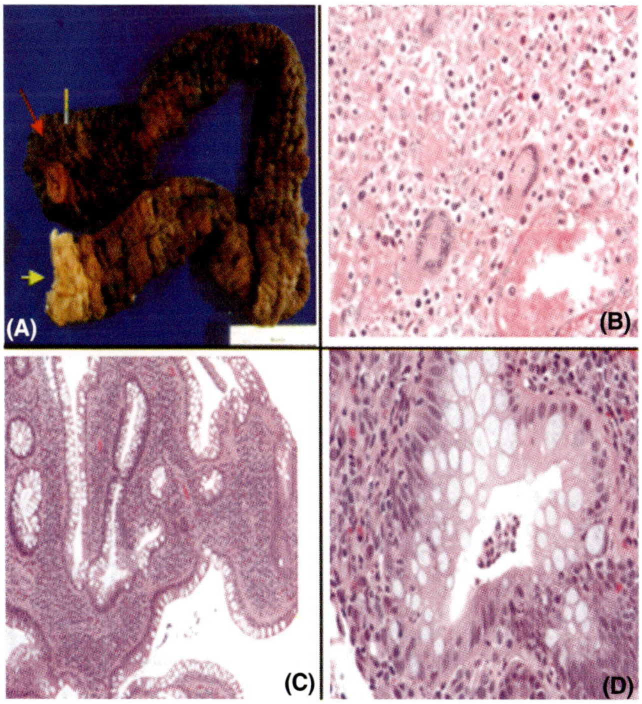

Fig. 121. 21: Inflammatory bowel disease: In (A) a colectomy specimen from an adolescence with ulcerative colitis. Though the specimen was previously fixed, the nodularity and redness of the mucosa can be appreciated. In (B) colonic wall that shows granulomatous inflammation, notice the multinucleated giant cells. In (C) glandular architectural distortion; branching and loss of the glandular symmetry. In (D) acute inflammatory cells in the lumen of a crypt (crypt abscess)

  - ***Crohn's disease***
    - □ Granulomatous inflammation that involves any

segment of the gastrointestinal tract, most commonly ileum and colon.
  - In children is more common than ulcerative colitis.
  - About 20% of Crohn's disease are first diagnosed before 20 years of age.
- *Ulcerative colitis*
  - Mucosal colonic nongranulomatous inflammatory disease.
  - Rare in children.

The main differences between Crohn's disease and ulcerative colitis are listed in Table 121.5.

Acute Appendicitis

- Is the most common form of acute surgical emergency in children above one year of age.
- Result from luminal obstruction by fecalith, tumor, worms (Oxyuris vermicularis) (Fig. 121.22) that leads to increased intraluminal pressure, ischemic injury and bacterial invasion of the wall.
- Early histologic changes include:
  - Few acute inflammatory cells distributed throughout the wall, associated with edema and congestion (Fig. 121.23).
  - Late histological changes include; prominent exudative inflammation, involving the lumen and serosa, and necrosis, in some cases with rupture of the wall.
- Most common complications are: perforation, thrombosis of portal venous drainage, liver abscess and bacteremia.

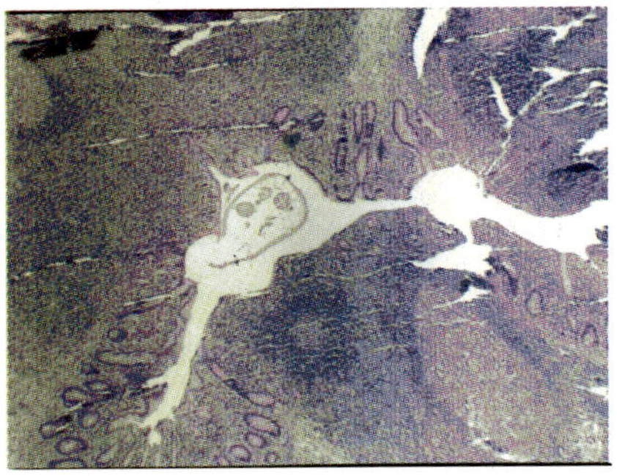

Fig. 121.22: Vermiform appendix with oxyurus vermicularis in the lumen

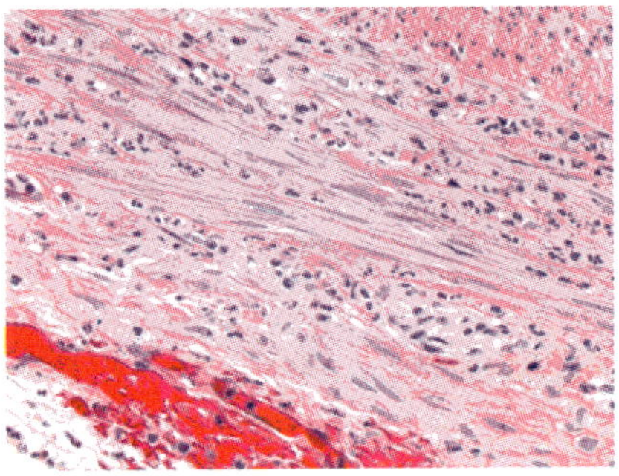

Fig. 121.23: Case of acute appendicitis that shows acute neutrophils infiltrating the musculari propria of the vermiform appendix

Intussusception

- The telescoping of variable length of intestine into a more distal segment.
- It is characterized by:
  - Mostly spontaneous and reversible.
  - Is more common in boys.
  - Majority occurs under one year of the age apparently due to hyperactivity of the intestine and prominence of the lymphoid tissue.

Table121.5: Distinctive features of Crohn's disease and ulcerative colitis

Feature	*CD, SI*	*CD,C*	*UC*
Gross anatomy:			
• *Involved segment*	Ileum +/- colon	Colon +/- ileum	Colon
• *Distribution*	Segmental	Segmental	Diffuse
• *Stricture*	Early	Variable	Rare
• *Wall*	Thickened	Thin	Thin
• *Dilatation*	No	Yes	Yes
Histology:			
• *Inflammatory polyps*	Rare	Frequent	Frequent
• *Ulcers*	Deep and linear	Deep and linear	Superficial
• *Lymphoid aggregation*	Prominent	Prominent	Mild
• *Fibrosis*	Prominent	Moderate	Mild
• *Serositis*	Prominent	Variable	Mild
• *Granulomas*	Yes, most cases	Yes, most cases	No
• *Fistulas or sinuses*	Yes	Yes, most cases	No
Clinical:			
• *Malabsorption*	Yes	Yes, if ileum	No
• *Malignant potential*	Yes	Yes	Yes
• *Response to therapy*	Poor	Variable	Good

CD, SI=Crohn's disease involving small intestine
CD, C=Crohn's disease involving colon
UC=ulcerative colitis
Table adapted from Ref 28

- Many cases are related to viral infection with subsequent lymphoid hyperplasia.
- Rarely in children, the point of traction is a tumor, e.g. ileal lymphoma, polyps or Meckel's diverticulum.
- 95% occurs in the ileocecal region.
- The clinical presentation is intestinal obstruction (Fig. 121.24).

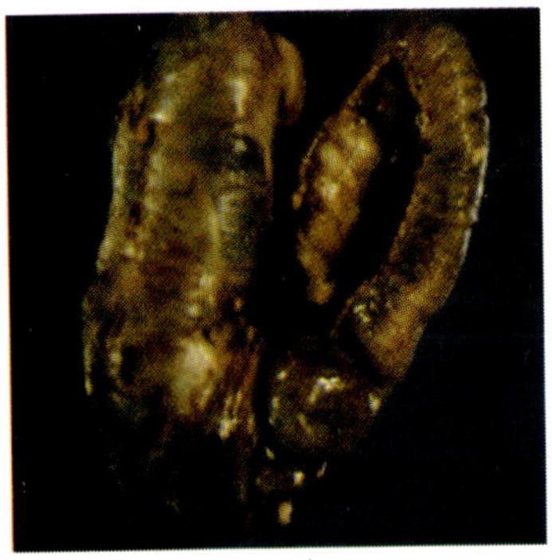

(A)

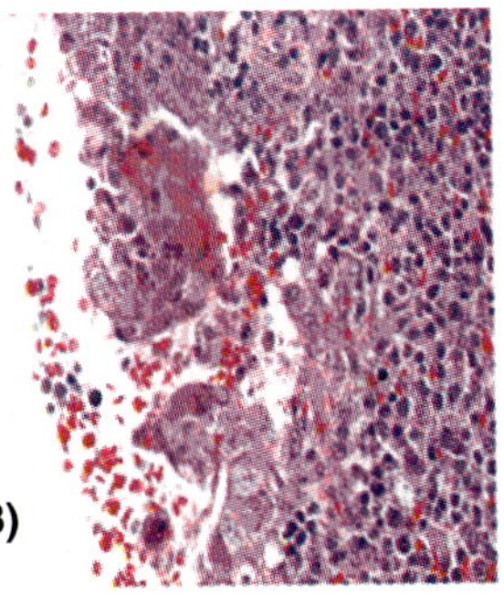

(B)

Fig. 121.24: Ileocecal intussusception; (A) The ileum is penetrating into the colon. (B) Inclusions of adenovirus found in the bowel of the patient (H and E).

Non-neoplastic and Neoplastic Polyps

Most of the intestinal tumors affecting children are benign polyps.

- Polyp is a mass that protrudes into the intestinal lumen.
- Can be ***non-neoplastic*** and ***neoplastic:***
  - Pedunculated: with stalk.
  - Sessile: without stalk.

Non-neoplastic Polyp

- Originate from mucosal tissue with abnormal maturation driven by inflammation and abnormalities of differentiation.
- In general, do not have malignant potential.
- The various types include:
  - *Juvenile polyps:*
    - □ Most common polyp in children.
    - □ Most commonly present with rectal bleeding or passing per rectum following autoamputation.
    - □ Considered to be non-neoplastic.
    - □ Often: multiple, involving rectosigmoid.
    - □ Anatomic characteristics:
      - ✓ Granular red external surface.
      - ✓ Its cut section shows irregular, small "cystic" cavities.
      - ✓ Histology shows:
        - ➢ Superficial ulceration covered by granulation tissue.
        - ➢ Cystically dilated crypts filled with mucus and separated by inflamed stroma.
        - ➢ Occasional epithelial hyperplasia, foci of dysplasia and adenomatous changes (Fig. 121.25).

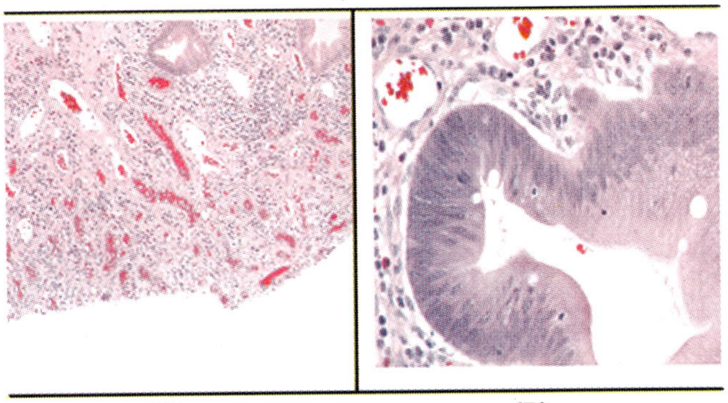

(A) (B)

Fig. 121.25: Juvenile polyp; (A) Low power view of the changes seen in juvenile polyp; dilated colonic glands, angiogenesis at the periphery and erosion of the surface. (B) Mild dysplasia in a juvenile polyp (H and E)

  - ***Juvenile polyposis syndrome***
    - □ Is rare.
    - □ Autosomal dominance inheritance.
    - □ Numerous polyps, and increased risk of adenomatous changes with progression to adenocarcinoma.
  - ***Cronkite-Canada syndrome*** (Table 121.6).

Table 121.6: Cronkite-Canada syndrome

• Nonhereditary
• Multiple juvenile colorectal polyps
• Associated ectodermal changes:
– Alopecia
– Nail atrophy
– Hyperpigmentation
• Colorectal carcinoma may develop

  - ***Hamartomatous polyps:***
    - □ Usually component of Peutz-Jeghers syndrome.
    - □ Often sporadic.
    - □ Large, pedunculated and lobulated external surface.
    - □ Histologic changes include:
      - ✓ Glands, formed by several different types of cells (columnar, goblet cells, endocrine and Paneth cells), supported by broad bands of smooth muscle fibers (Fig. 121.26).
  - ***Peutz-Jeghers syndrome*** (Table 121.7).
  - ***Hyperplastic polyps:***
    - □ Stomach is the more common location in children, otherwise rare.

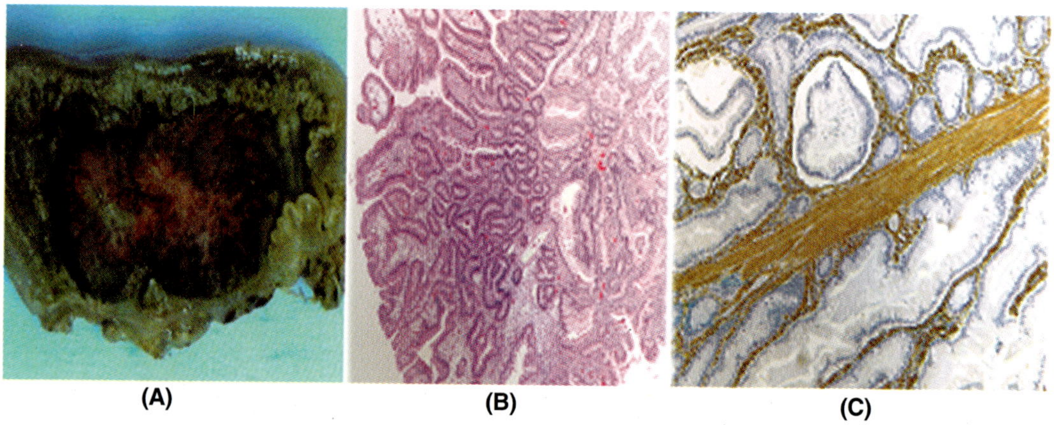

Fig. 121.26: Hamartomatous polyp; (A) Cut surface of a partially necrotic hamartomatous polyp in the intestinal cavity. (B) Delicate arborization characteristic of hamartomatous polyp. (C) Stroma with thick bundles of smooth muscle highlighted by smooth muscle actin

- ☐ Do not become malignant.
- ☐ Usually small and sessile.
- ☐ Result from delayed shedding of surface epithelial cells.
- ☐ Histologic changes include:
  - ✓ Well-formed mature, elongated glands and scant lamina propria.

Table 121.7: Peutz-Jeghers syndrome

• Hamartomatous polyps of the small and large intestine
• Melanotic pigmentation of mucosal and skin surfaces
• Increased risk of carcinomas (ovary, pancreas, breast, lung, uterus)

Neoplastic Polyps

- Originate from dysplastic mucosal tissue, called adenomas.
- They have malignant potential:
  - *Adenomatous polyps:*
    - ☐ Are very rare in children except in familial adenomatosis.
    - ☐ Can be detected early in high-risk patients by endoscopy.
    - ☐ Single or multiple.
    - ☐ Most common location is the colon, they might also occur in stomach and small intestine.
    - ☐ Morphologic changes include:
      - ✓ Usually small.
      - ✓ May be sessile or pedunculated.
      - ✓ Histology includes:
        - ➢ Glandular hyperplasia with disorderly arranged epithelial cells characterized with cigar shaped hyperchromatic nuclei and increased mitosis (Fig. 121.27).
    - ☐ Epithelial cells show persistence of DNA synthesis, elevated ornithine decarboxylase and K-ras mutation in 25% of the polyps.

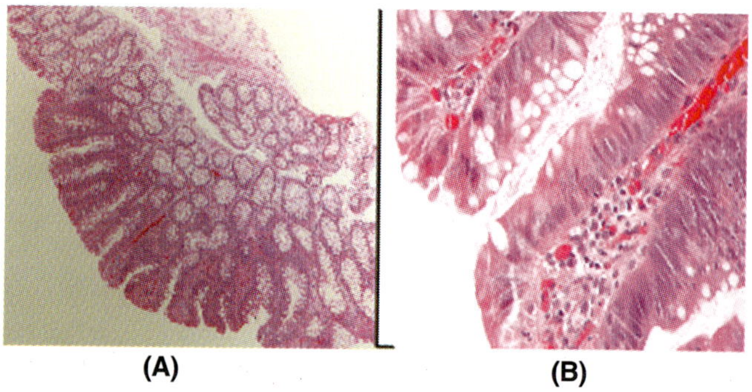

Fig. 121.27: (A) (B) Adenomatous changes in a patient with FAP. Non-transformed mucosa is seen in part A (H and E)

  - ***Familial adenomatous polyposis*** (Table 121.8).
    - ☐ Average age of onset is teens.
    - ☐ May be associated with carcinoma in other organs.
    - ☐ Most of the cases evolve to adenocarcinoma.
    - ☐ Ulceration or fixations to deeper tissue are signs of malignization.
    - ☐ Intestinal mucosa is dotted by thousands of small mucosal elevations with adenomatous changes:
      - ✓ Minimum of 100 polyps required for diagnosis.
    - ☐ Prophylactic colectomy is curative.
    - ☐ Diagnosis is made by PCR of APC gene mutation.

Table 121.8: Familial adenomatous polyposis

• Average age of onset is teens
• May be associated with carcinoma in other organs
• In most of the cases leads to adenocarcinoma
• Ulceration or fixation to deeper tissue are signs of malignization
• Intestinal mucosa is dotted by thousands of small mucosal elevations with adenomatous changes. Minimun of 100 polyps required for diagnosis
• Prophylactic colectomy is curative
• Diagnosis is made by PCR of APC gene mutation

  - ***Gardner's syndrome*** (Table 121.9).
  - ***Other polyps:***
    - ☐ Mucosal lymphoid aggregates (normal).

Table 121.9: Gardner's syndrome

Adenomatous polyps associated with one or more of:
• Multiple osteomas of skull and mandible
• Multiple keratinous cysts of the skin
• Soft tissue neoplasms, commonly fibromatosis
• Potential for development of intestinal carcinoma

- ◻ Inflammatory, mostly secondary to inflammatory bowel disease.

Malignant Neoplasms

- Rare in children.
- Approximately 80% occur in the small and large intestine.
- Lymphomas are the most common followed by carcinoid and adenocarcinoma.
- ***Lymphomas:***
  - Most common malignant tumors involving the gastrointestinal tract.
  - Mostly located in the small intestine.
  - ***Burkitt's lymphoma:***
    - ◻ Most common type of lymphoma in children.
    - ◻ Is a B-cell malignancy that occurs in two varieties:
      - ✓ ***Endemic:***
        - ➢ Childhood lymphoma (5-10-year olds).
        - ➢ Prevalent in equatorial Africa.
        - ➢ Intimately associated with both Epstein-Barr Virus (EBV) infections.
        - ➢ Characterized by translocation of the c-myc gene (a gene involved in cellular proliferation).
      - ✓ ***Sporadic*:**
        - ➢ A world-wide lymphoma.
        - ➢ Affects slightly older childhood patients.
        - ➢ Associated with c-myc changes but less so with EBV infection.
      - ✓ Histological characteristics include:
        - ➢ Diffuse proliferation of intermediate cells with round nuclei and coarse chromatin.
        - ➢ Multiple nucleoli.
        - ➢ Moderate amount of amphophilic cytoplasm.
        - ➢ High mitotic index and cell death.
        - ➢ Starry-sky appearance (Fig. 121.28).
      - ✓ Genetic features include translocation of the c-myc gene with chromosome 8.
    - ◻ Involvement of the gastrointestinal tract is less common in endemic than sporadic cases.
- ***Adenocarcinoma:***
  - Extremely rare in children.
  - The majority occurs in association with juvenile adenomatous polyposis and hereditary non-polyposis colorectal cancer syndrome.
  - Pathologic characteristics include:
    - ◻ Fungating or annular, encircling mass formed by neoplastic glands, with variable differentiation, that invades the submucosa and muscularis propria.

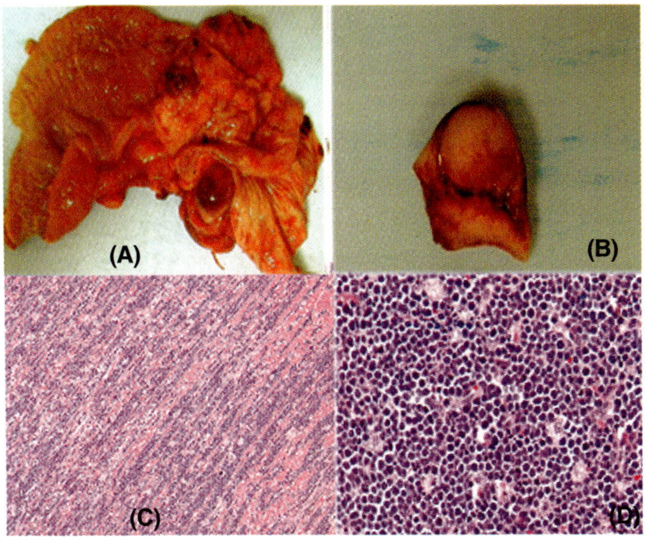

Fig. 121.28: A case of Burkitt's lymphoma in a child that presented with intussusception. (A) Fresh specimen to show a mass growing from the wall into the lumen. Regional involved lymph nodes (red arrow) are seen in the picture. (B) Shows the relationship between the wall and the mass. (C) Muscularis propria infiltrated by lymphoma cells. (D) Characteristic starry sky pattern (H and E)

- ***Carcinoid:***
  - Originate from gut endocrine cells:
    - ◻ Rare in children.
    - ◻ Most common location in the gastrointestinal tract is the appendix.
    - ◻ Benign biology when located in the appendix and rectum.
    - ◻ Most synthesize bioamines.
    - ◻ Pathologic features include:
      - ✓ Yellow mass growing in the gut wall.
      - ✓ Islands of gland, trabeculae, or sheets of monotonous cells with scant granular cytoplasm and round nuclei separated by stroma (Fig. 121.29).

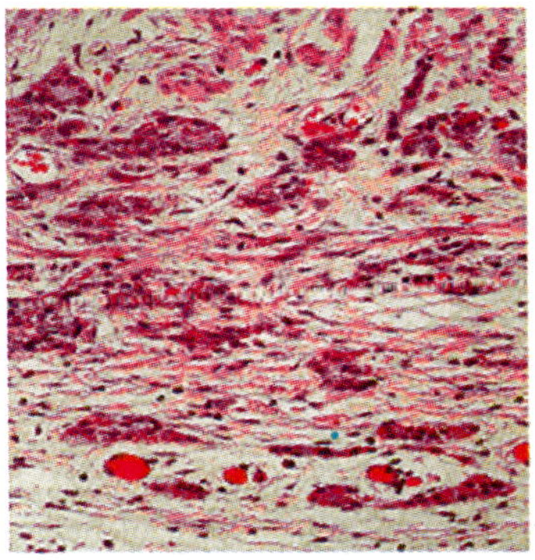

Fig. 121.29: Wall of the vermiform appendix infiltrated by carcinoid cells stained red with antibodies (immunohistochemistry) for chromogranin

LIVER AND BILIARY TRACT

Pediatric liver diseases are the consequence of developmental, metabolic, toxic, microbial, circulatory and neoplastic injuries.

Developmental Disorders of Liver and Biliary Tract

- ***Liver agenesis*;** rare, incompatible with life and in most cases associated with other anomalies.
- ***Single lobe agenesis*;** more common than complete agenesis and usually involves the tight lobe.
- ***Heterotopic liver tissue;*** have been reported in other abdominal and thoracic organs.
- ***Heterotopic tissue in the liver;*** incidentally found, includes pancreas, adrenal and thyroid.
- ***Absence of the portal vein*;** rarely reported in association with other anomalies.
- ***Biliary tract agenesis, duplication and abnormalities of position;*** in most cases without clinical significance in children.

Ductal Plate Malformation (DPM)

- The ductal plate formation is the consequence of development of intrahepatic bile ducts from bipotential liver progenitor cells in contact with the mesenchyme of the portal vein.
- The ductal plates are remodelled into mature tubular ducts.
- Lack of remodelling cause ductal plate malformation (DPM).
- All congenital disease of the intrahepatic bile ducts are examples of DPM including:
  - Extrahepatic biliary atresia.
  - Congenital hepatic fibrosis.
  - Autosomal recessive polycystic kidney disease.
  - Caroli's disease.
  - Biliary hamartoma.
  - Mesenchymal hamartoma.

Congenital Hepatic Fibrosis

- Hereditary recessive disease that presents with hepatomegaly in childhood and adolescence.
- Anatomic characteristics:
  - Thick bands of biliary fibrosis with occasional trapping of liver cells.
  - Anastomosis of prominent bile ducts and cholangiolar proliferation often containing bile duct plugs.
  - Minimal portal inflammation sometimes associated with acute cholangitis and cholestasis.
  - Paucity of portal veins and portal venous radicles.
  - Increase in copper-binding protein in the liver parenchyma.
  - Occasionally complicated by duct rupture with formation of microabscesses (Fig. 121.30).

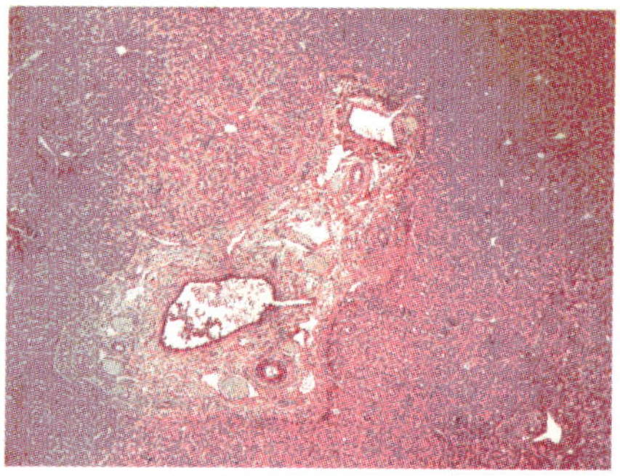

Fig. 121.30: Prominent ecstatic bile ducts embedded in expanded fibrotic portal tract in a case of congenital hepatic fibrosis (H and E)

DISEASES OF LIVER AND BILIARY TREE ASSOCIATED WITH CHOLESTASIS

Cholestasis represents an important group of disorders that affect neonates and infants.

Cholestasis

- Retention of bilirubin, bile solutes and cholesterol.
- May be the result of hepatocytic dysfunction or biliary obstruction.
- Elevation of alkaline phosphatase.
- Anatomic changes include:
  - Accumulation of bile pigments within the hepatic tissue with dilatation of bile canaliculi and degeneration of hepatic cells.
  - With obstruction:
    - □ Portal tract distension.
    - □ Bile duct proliferation.
    - □ Periductular neutrophils.
    - □ Edema in the portal tract (Fig. 121.31).

Neonatal Cholestasis

- Occurs in the first 3 months of life.
- Seventy percent of the cases are due to neonatal hepatitis and extrahepatic biliary atresia.
- The most common causes in the neonatal period are listed in Table 121.10.

Extrahepatic Biliary Atresia

Obliterative disorder of the bile ducts that cause obstructive jaundice in neonates:

- Occurs in about 1 in 10000 live births.
- This is the most common cause of neonatal cholestasis requiring corrective surgery and liver transplantation.

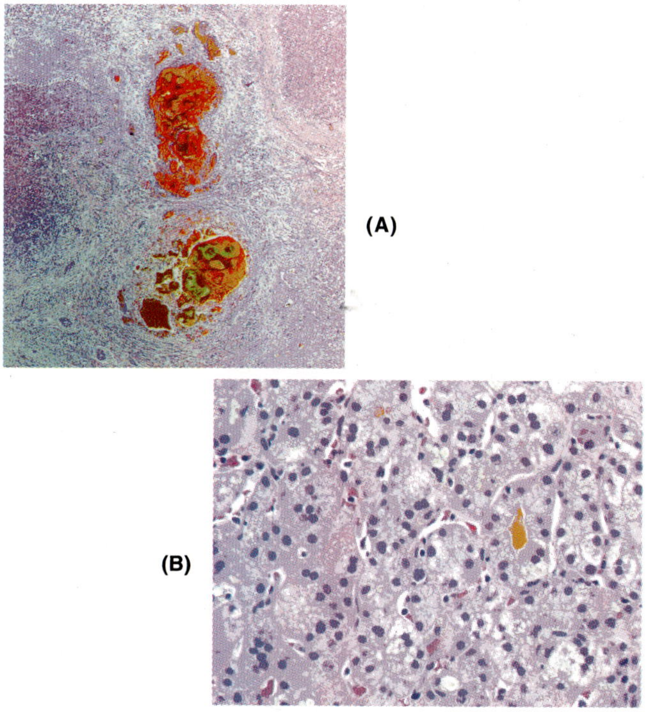

(A)

(B)

Fig. 121.31: Hepatic changes of cholestasis; (A) Bile lakes chiefly located in the central liver (B) Intracellular and intracanalicular accumulation of bile (H and E)

Table 121.10: Most common causes of neonatal cholestasis

- Bile duct obstruction
  - Biliary atresia
  - Choledocal cyst
  - Bile duct paucity
    - □ Syndromic
    - □ Non syndromic
- Neonatal infection
  - Cytomegalovirus
  - Bacterial sepsis
  - Urinary tract infection
  - Syphilis
- Toxic
  - Parenteral nutrition
  - Drugs
- Metabolic diseases
  - Tyrosinemia
  - Niemann-Pick disease
  - Galactosemia
  - Alpha 1 antitrypsin deficiency
  - Cystic fibrosis
- Hypoperfusion
- Indian childhood cirrhosis
- Idiopathic neonatal hepatitis

- If not corrected, the disease leads to complete biliary obstruction and cirrhosis.
- Different possible causative factors have been suggested:
  - Infectious (viral), toxic.
  - Genetically induced abnormal development.
  - Ischemia/hypoxia.
  - Immunologic dysfunction.
- Anatomic changes include:
  - Extrahepatic:
    - □ Inflammation and fibrosing with stricture of the extrahepatic, progressing to the intrahepatic, biliary tree (Fig. 121.32).

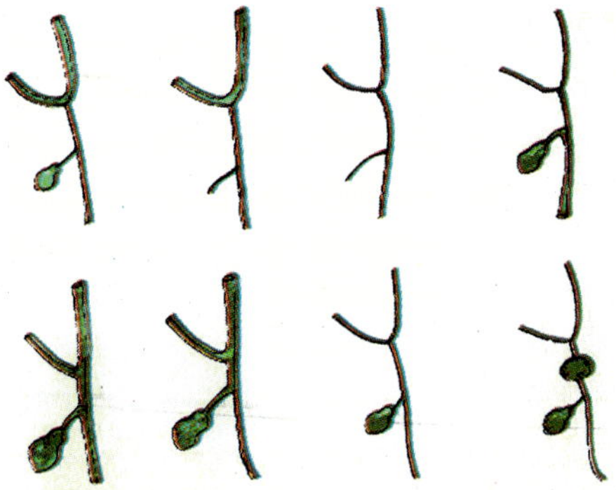

Fig. 121.32: Different anatomic variants of extrahepatic biliary atresia. With and without atresia of the hepatic bile ducts combined with segmental atresia of the common bile duct and cystic duct. Occasionally atresia is associated with cystic changes in the biliary tree

  - Intrahepatic:
    - □ Bile ductular proliferation.
    - □ Portal tract edema and variable inflammation.
    - □ Fibrosis progressing to cirrhosis within 4 to 6 months (Fig. 121.33).

Primary Sclerosing Cholangitis

Chronic progressive disease characterized by inflammation and obliterative fibrosis with segmental dilatation of the intra- and extrahepatic bile ducts:

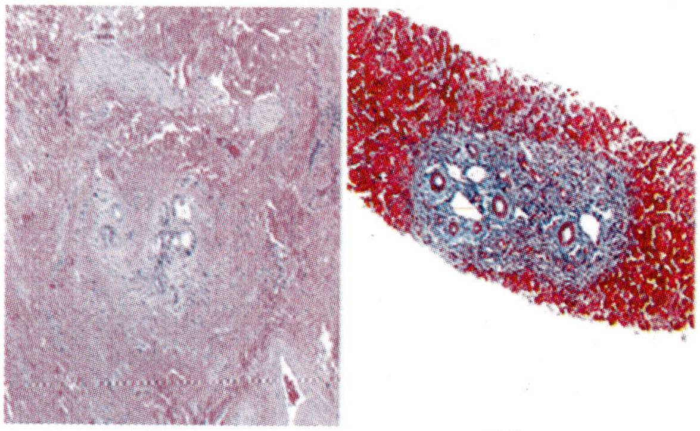

(A) (B)

Fig. 121.33: Histological changes of extrahepatic biliary atresia (EHBA). (A) Section of extrahepatic biliary tree that shows small clusters of bile ducts remnants embedded in fibrous tissue. On the right upper corner the epithelial cells of the remnant are stained with Keratin AE1/AE3 antibodies by immunohistochemistry (B) Expanded portal tract and bile duct proliferation (arrows) in the liver of a patient with EHBA (H and E)

- Pathogenesis is unknown.
- Strongly associated with ulcerative colitis and in minor degree with pancreatic, bronchiectasis and autoimmune diseases.
- Anatomic changes include:
  - Inflammation and concentric fibrosis around bile ducts.
  - Atrophy and proliferation of the bile duct lumen.
  - Portal fibrosis progressing to cirrhosis.

Most common causes of secondary sclerosing cholangitis are listed in Table 121.11.

Table 121.11: Most common causes of pediatric secondary sclerosing cholangitis

• Langerhans cell histiocytosis
• AIDS-related cholangiopathy
• Cryptosporidiasis in immune-compromised patients
• Cholelithiasis
• Cystic fibrosis
• Hodgkin's disease
• Mechanical (surgery-related) injury
• Ischemia

Intrahepatic Biliary Atresia (Bile Duct Paucity)

An anatomic observation that consists of a reduction in number of interlobular bile ducts, the diagnosis is based on the examination and quantification of terminal bile ducts in a liver biopsy with adequate number of portal tracts:

- Causes of bile duct paucity are divided in:
  - ***Syndromic*** (Alagille syndrome).
  - ***Non-syndromic*** (causes listed in Table 121.12).

Table 121.12: Pediatric non-syndromic causes of bile duct paucity

• Metabolic and genetic
– Alpha-1 antitrypsin deficiency
– Cystic fibrosis
– Down's syndrome
• Congenital infections
• Inflammatory and immune disorder
– Graft vs host disease
– Chronic allograft rejection
– Sclerosing cholangitis
• Drug-related vanishing of bile ducts
• Idiopathic

- Alagille syndrome:
  - Autosomal dominant disorder caused by mutations of the JAG1 gene, characterized by developmental abnormalities of the liver, heart, skeleton, eye and face.
- Histologic changes of both, ***syndromic*** and ***non-syndromic,*** include:
  - Absence of interlobular bile ducts (Fig. 121.34).
  - Giant cell transformation of hepatocytes.
  - Extramedullary hematopoiesis.
  - Mild lymphocytic infiltration in portal tracts.
  - Does not progress to cirrhosis (syndromic).
  - Diffuse interstitial fibrosis and cirrhosis may occur (non-syndromic).

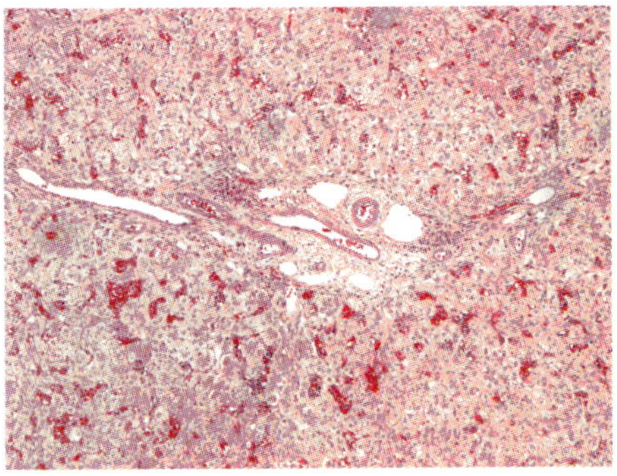

Fig. 121.34: Bile duct paucity; portal tract devoid of interlobular bile ducts (H and E)

Choledochal Cysts

Congenital dilatation of the common bile ducts:

- Etiology is obscure.
- Frequency is about 1: 150000 live births in western countries though the incidence is higher in Asian countries.
- Two third of the patients have elevated gamma glutamyl-transferase (Figs. 121.35 and 121.36).

Progressive Familial Intrahepatic Cholestases

Group of inherited disorders with progressive, severe cholestasis occurring in infants and characterized by:

- Normal serum levels of cholesterol and gamma-glutamyl transpeptidase.
- Genetically heterogeneous with mutations in chromosomes 2 and 18.
- Anatomic changes include:
  - Perivenular cholestasis, rosette formation and giant cell transformation.
  - Bile duct proliferation, early, evolving to bile duct paucity.
  - May progress to cirrhosis.
  - Increase of copper and copper binding protein in periportal and paraseptal hepatocytes.

Total Parenteral Nutrition

Children receiving total parenteral nutrition may develop:

- Hyperbilirubinemia occurs between the first and sixth weeks after the onset of TPN.
- Cholestasis develop in more than 80% of the children if treatment lasts more than 8 weeks.
- Liver histological changes include:
  - Intracellular and intracanalicular cholestasis, preferentially perivenular.
  - Mild lobular inflammation.

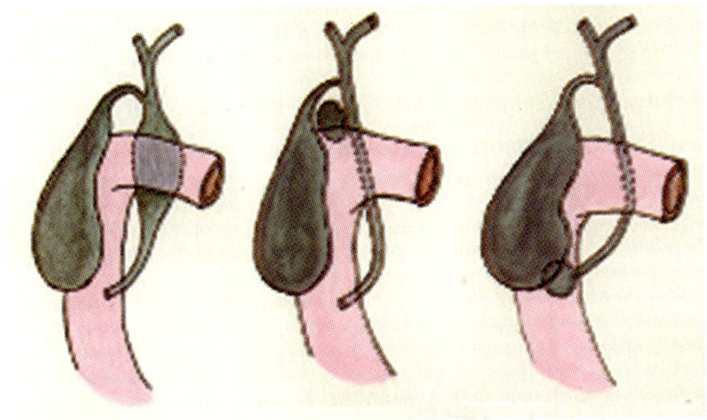

Fig. 121.35: Types of choledocal cysts; From left to right, dilatation of the common bile duct, pouch in common bile duct (center) and cystic dilatation extending to the duodenum

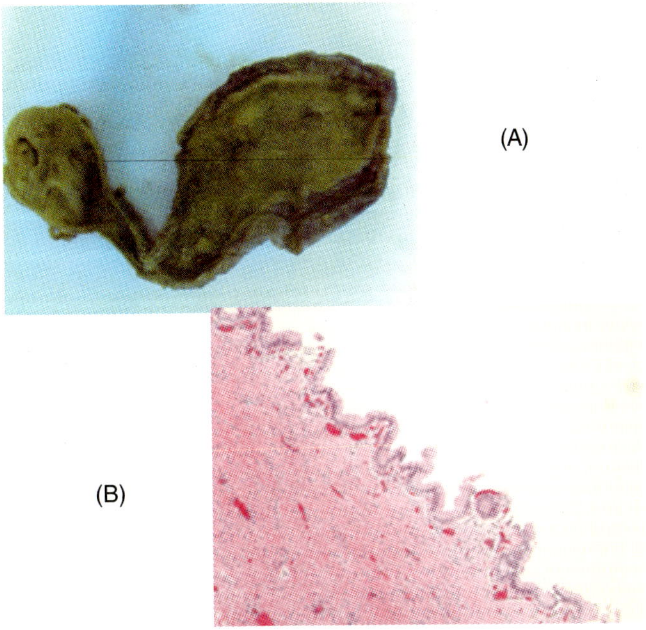

Fig. 121.36: (A) Choledocal cyst in the common bile duct . The largest structure in the specimen is gallbladder. (B) Section of the wall of choledocal cyst, notice the biliary type epithelium lining the mildly fibrous wall of the cyst (H and E)

- Rosettes of liver cells.
- Giant cell transformation.
- Sinusoidal fibrosis.
- Portal inflammation including neutrophils.
- Biliary fibrosis evolving to cirrhosis may occur if treatment is prolonged.

Idiopathic Neonatal Hepatitis

Idiopathic neonatal hepatitis is characterized by cholestasis presenting in the neonate associated with liver enlargement and variable hepatic dysfunction:

- Anatomic changes include:
  - Diffuse presence of giant cell transformation.
  - Occasional presence of neutrophils associated with giant cells.
  - Cholestasis and lobular mononuclear inflammation.
  - Variable sinusoidal fibrosis.
  - Portal mononuclear inflammation.
  - Extramedullary hematopoiesis may be present (Fig. 121.37).

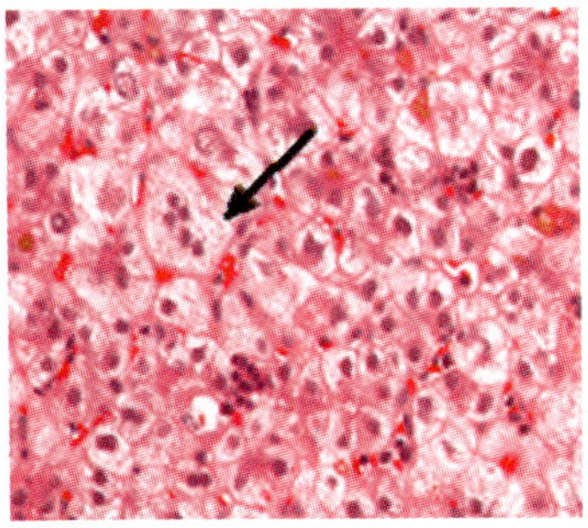

Fig. 121.37: Liver section that shows characteristic changes of neonatal hepatitis including giant cell transformation and cholestasis (H and E)

- Definitive diagnosis require ruling out congenital infections, biliary obstruction and metabolic diseases.
- Frequent favorable outcome.

Congenital Infections

- Acquired during pregnancy and at birth.
- Viruses are the most common infectious agents causing congenital hepatitis.

Cytomegalovirus

- The most common perinatal infection.
- Intrapartum infection is less severe than intrauterine infection.
- Neonates present with hepatosplenomegaly, jaundice and thrombocytopenia.
- It may be associated with chorioretinitis.
- Histopathology includes:
  - Variable cholestasis, prominent hematopoiesis, giant cell transformation and characteristics viral inclusions.

Herpes Simplex Virus

- Involves the liver when the infection is disseminated (multiorgan involvement).
- Histological changes include: zonal necrosis without collapse of the reticulin network, scanty inflammatory infiltrate and viral cytopathic changes (Fig. 121.38).
- The diagnosis is usually clinical.

Rubella, echovirus, coxsackie B virus, parvovirus and hepatitis A, B and C virus may also cause congenital hepatitis.

- The most common bacteria that cause congenital hepatitis are:
  - ***Listeria monocytogenes***:
    - ✓ Usually systemic, associated with meningitis in most cases.

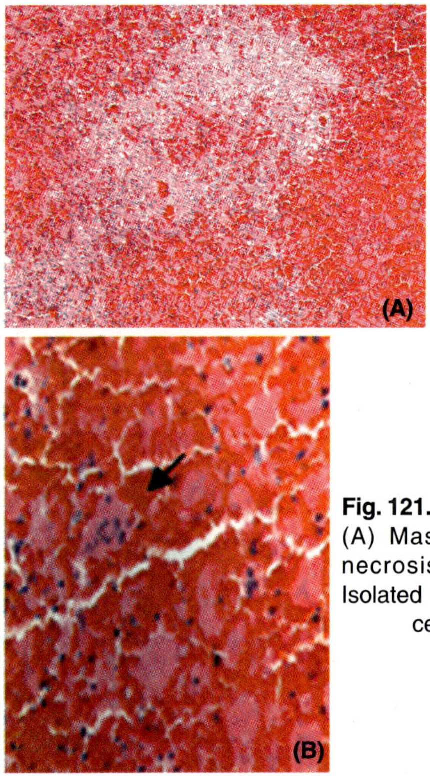

Fig. 121.38: Herpes hepatitis: (A) Massive hemorrhagic necrosis of the liver (B) Isolated multinucleated giant cells (H and E)

✓ Liver involvement includes: hepatomegaly with microabscesses, granulomatous, inflammation and bacteria within the lesions.

– *Syphilis*:
  - ☐ Caused by the treponema pallidum, an obligate anaerobe spirochete.
  - ☐ The infection is acquired from mothers contracting the infection during the third trimester of pregnancy.
  - ☐ Clinically presents with cholestasis, hepatosplenomegaly, elevated liver enzymes, skin rash, anemia and neurologic abnormalities.
  - ☐ Histological features include:
    - ✓ Giant cell transformation, associated with necrosis and numerous spirochetes visualized by the Warthin-Starry reaction.
    - ✓ Small granulomas.
    - ✓ Portal and interstitial fibrosis in the late stages of the disease.

– *Toxoplasma:*
  - ☐ Caused by ingesting merozoites in uncooked or raw meats of the parasite Toxoplasma gondii.
  - ☐ Histological changes are similar to those seen in idiopathic neonatal hepatitis.

Chronic Hepatitis

Clinically persistent hepatitis for at least 6 months after acute onset of the disease.

- The two most common causes in children are ***viral*** and ***autoimmune***.
- The diagnosis is based on clinical, serologic and anatomic changes.
- Morphologic changes are non-specific:
  - Necroinflammatory changes.
  - Fibrosis.
  - Involve the portal, interface and lobular components of the liver tissue (Fig. 121.39).

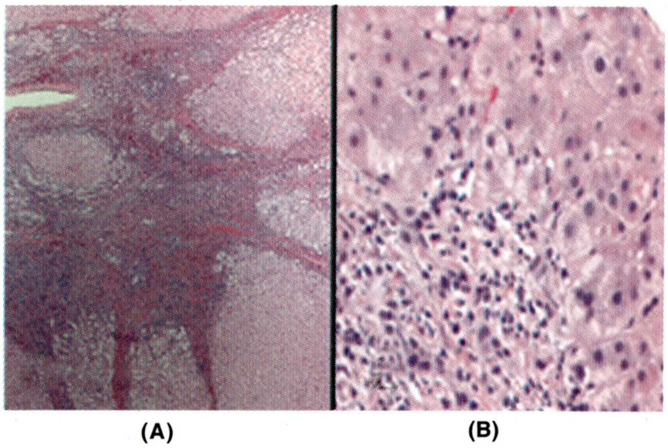

Fig. 121.39: Histological changes of chronic hepatitis; (A) Portal and incomplete septal fibrosis. (B) Close up of portal/parenchymal interface that show parenchymal inflammatory invasion with degenerative changes of the hepatocytes contacting the inflammatory cells (H and E)

- Histological differences of viral and autoimmune hepatitis are as follows:
  - Hepatitis B:
    - ☐ Ground glass hepatocytes.
    - ☐ Immunohistochemistry for virus B antigens.
  - Hepatitis C:
    - ☐ Fatty change.
    - ☐ Lymphoid follicles.
    - ☐ Damage of bile ducts.
  - Autoimmune hepatitis:
    - ☐ Necroinflammatory changes.
    - ☐ Plasma cells infiltrate.
- Chronic hepatitis in variable proportion progress to cirrhosis.

Cirrhosis

Liver cirrhosis is the consequence of chronic liver disease characterized by replacement of liver tissue by fibrosis and regenerative nodules, leading to progressive loss of liver function.

- Cirrhosis is defined by 3 morphologic characteristics:
  - Septal fibrosis.
  - Nodular regeneration.
  - Disruption of the parenchymal architecture of the liver (Fig. 121.40).

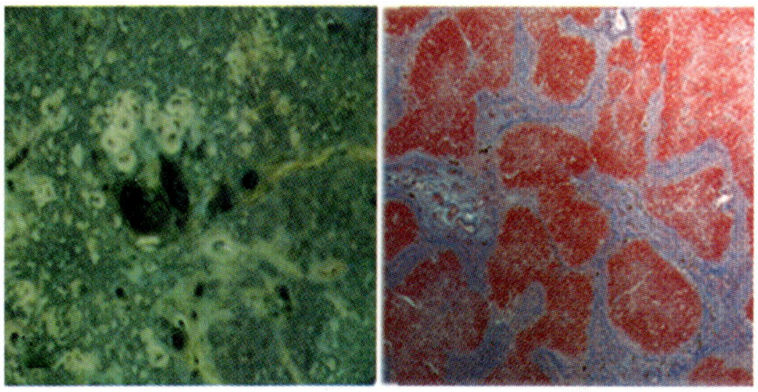

Fig. 121.40: Biliary cirrhosis: (A) Cut surface of liver is green with large dilated bile ducts that contains bile and small nodules associated with thickened wall bile ducts (B) Nodules of regenerated liver tissue separated by broad septa of fibrosis (Trichrome)

- Most common causes of cirrhosis in children include:
  - Bile obstruction:
    - ☐ Biliary atresia.
    - ☐ Choledochal cyst.
  - Toxic:
    - ☐ Total parenteral nutrition.
    - ☐ Drug.
  - Metabolic:
    - ☐ Alpha-1-antitrypsin deficiency.
    - ☐ Cystic fibrosis.
    - ☐ Galactosemia.
    - ☐ Glycogen storage disease.
    - ☐ Gaucher's disease.
    - ☐ Hemochromatosis.
  - Inflammatory and immune dysfunction:
    - ☐ Chronic viral hepatitis.
    - ☐ Autoimmune hepatitis.
    - ☐ Neonatal hepatitis.
    - ☐ Graft versus host disease.
    - ☐ Chronic allograft rejection.
    - ☐ Chronic granulomatous disease.
  - Others:
    - ☐ Idiopathic.
    - ☐ Indian childhood cirrhosis.

Liver Disease in Inborn Errors of the Metabolism

- Single gene defects result in abnormalities in the synthesis or catabolism of proteins, carbohydrates, or fats.
- Most are due to a defect in an enzyme or transport protein, which results in a block in a metabolic pathway.
- Effects are due to toxic accumulations of substrates before the block, intermediates from alternative metabolic pathways, defects in energy production and use caused by a deficiency of products beyond the block, or a combination of these metabolic deviations.
- Nearly every metabolic disease has several forms that vary in age of onset, clinical severity, and often, mode of inheritance.
- Major inborn errors of the metabolism associated with neonatal liver disease includes:
- ***Galactosemia***
  - Accumulation of galactose in the lens due to deficiency of liver galactose-1-phosphate uridyltransferase.
  - Early histologic changes include fatty change, cholangiolar proliferation and cholestasis.
  - Giant cell transformation, hemosiderosis and extramedullary hematopoiesis.
  - Late histologic changes include bile duct dilation often containing eosinophilic material and fibrosis leading to cirrhosis.
- ***Tyrosinemia***
  - Accumulation of tyrosine and its metabolites due to deficiency of fumarylacetoacetase, enzyme acting in the metabolic pathway of phenylalanine and tyrosine:
    - ☐ Histological changes include:
      - ✓ Intracanalicular cholestasis in cases associated with pseudoacinar transformation of hepatocytes.
      - ✓ Liver cell dysplasia.
      - ✓ Extramedullary hematopoiesis may be present.
      - ✓ Variable intrasinusoidal fibrosis.
      - ✓ Macrovesicular fatty change.
      - ✓ Hemosiderosis.
      - ✓ Cirrhosis.
      - ✓ Hepatocellular carcinoma complication can occur.
    - ☐ Laboratory studies include; plasma quantitative amino-acids, urine succinylacetone.
- ***Alpha-1-antitrypsin deficiency:***
  - Autosomal recessive disorder characterizes by low serum levels of protease inhibitor (PI) that leads to emphysema in the lung and cholestasis or cirrhosis in the liver.
  - The gene that controls the synthesis of PI is in chromosome 14.
  - Most common allele is PiM.
  - Homozygotes for the PiZ allele have very low circulating levels of alpha-1-antitrypsin, due to the production of a molecularly abnormal protein that accumulates in the endoplasmic reticulum of liver cells.
  - The accumulation of the abnormal product cause the following morphologic changes:
    - ☐ Neonatal hepatitis picture with characteristics PAS-diastase resistant intracytoplasmic globules (Fig. 121.41).
    - ☐ Cirrhosis in the adult.
  - Laboratory studies include; quantitative serum alpha-1-antitrypsin, PI typing.

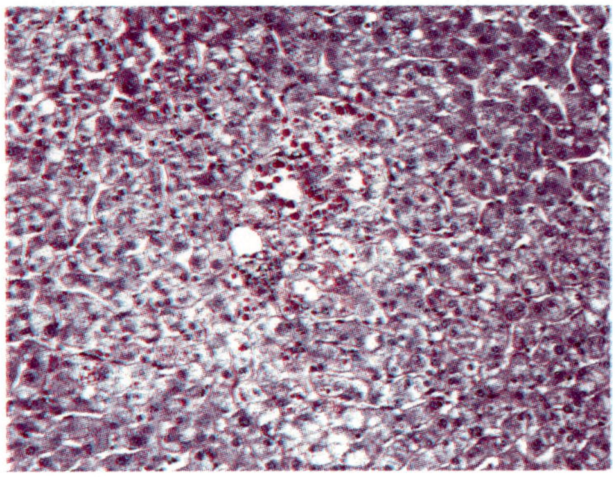

Fig. 121.41: Intrahepatocytic globules of PAS positive diastase resistant inclusions of alpha-1-antitrypsin (PAS)

- ***Hereditary hemochromatosis***
  - A homozygous recessive genetic disorder caused by a mutation (C282Y and H63D) of the HFE gene located in the chromosome 6.
  - It is characterized by excessive accumulation of iron in parenchymal cells of various organs including the liver.
  - Morphologic changes include:
    - □ Accumulation of hemosiderin in periportal hepatocytes and eventually diffusely throughout the liver parenchyma (Fig. 121.42).

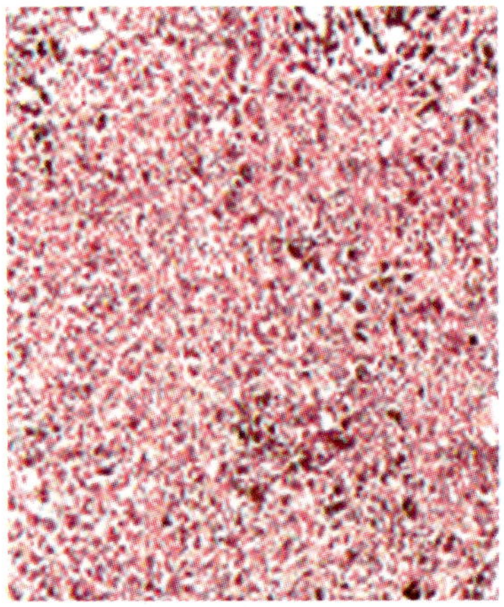

Fig. 121.42: Granules of iron in hepatocytes of a patient with hemochromatosis

    - □ Hemosiderin in the bile duct epithelium.
    - □ Rarely Kupffer cells contain hemosiderin.
    - □ Neonatal hepatis pattern of lesion can be seen.
  - The standard for quantitating liver iron is chemical measurement of hepatic iron in fresh liver tissue.
  - Laboratory studies include: serum ferritin and liver biopsy.
- ***Zellweger syndrome***
  - Characterized by absence of functional peroxisomes.
  - Morphologic changes include:
    - □ Sinusoidal fibrosis.
    - □ Cholestasis and focal necrosis.
    - □ Hemosiderin present in Kupffer cells.
    - □ Biled duct paucity.
    - □ Rarely cirrhosis.
  - Laboratory studies include: plasma very long-chain fatty acids.
- ***Niemann-Pick disease, type C***
  - Characterized by lysosomal accumulation of sphingomyelin due to deficiency of sphingomyelinase.
  - Morphologic changes include:
    - □ Large, vacuolated to foamy Kupffer cells and porta macrophages that are positive with fat stains.
    - □ Neonates can present with changes of neonatal hepatitis.
    - □ Intra sinusoidal fibrosis.
    - □ Paucity of bile ducts.
  - *Laboratory studies include:* Skin biopsy for fibroblasts culture and studied of cholesterol esterification and accumulation.
- ***Glycogen Storage Disease***
  - Group of autosomal recessive disorders caused by defects in the synthesis or catabolism of glycogen.
  - Type IV cause neonatal liver disease.
  - Anatomic characteristics include:
    - □ Enlarged liver.
    - □ Hydropic vacuolated liver cells with central nuclei and high cytoplasmic content of glycogen.
    - □ Type I, II and VI: prominent fatty change.
    - □ Type IX, X; thin fibroid septa without cirrhosis.
    - □ Type IA; multifocal liver cell adenoma, hepatocellular carcinoma, Mallory bodies.
    - □ Type I, III, VI: glycogenated nuclei.
    - □ Type IV; eosinophilic cytoplasmic PAS-diastase resistant inclusions in liver cells, predominantly periportal.
  - Laboratory studies include: liver biopsy and biochemical analysis or skin biopsy with assay of enzymes related to the metabolization of glycogen.
- ***Cystic Fibrosis***
  - The consequence of disruption of chloride resorption secondary to mutations of a gene in chromosome 7 that encodes the protein Cystic Fibrosis Transmembrane Conductance Regulator (CFTR). It causes inspissation of secretion.
  - In the neonatal period present with cholestasis.
  - Liver disease in children and young adults is generally asymptomatic.
  - Morphologic changes include:
    - □ Feature of neonatal hepatitis.
    - □ Fatty change.

- ☐ Hemosiderin deposition in periportal hepatocytes.
- ☐ Sinusoidal fibrosis.
- ☐ Variable cholangiolar proliferation, early.
- ☐ Bile duct paucity, late.
- ☐ Marked cholestasis with acute and chronic inflammatory cell in the periportal zones.
- ☐ Mucinous material in extrahepatic, and rarely intrahepatic bile ducts.
- ☐ Biliary fibrosis, late.

– Laboratory test include; sweet chloride concentration.

Liver Tumors

- The majority of the large liver tumors in the pediatric population are malignant.
- Only 30% of them are benign and in most cases of vascular origin.
- Hepatoblastoma is the most common malignant tumor followed by hepatocellular carcinoma.

Hepatoblastoma

Rapidly progressive malignancy responsible for approximately 40% of all tumors in pediatric patients upto 2 years of age:

- Serum alpha-fetoprotein (AFP) is elevated in upto 90% of the cases:
  - It should be considered that AFP is normally elevated at birth to rapidly decrease to normal values by 1 year of age (from 10000-14000 to 5-10 ng/ml).
  - Associated conditions include: osteopenia, precocious puberty and adenomatous polyposis coli gene mutation.
- Hepatic angiography and CT scans most valuable preoperative assessment of tumor location and extent.
- Morphologic changes include:
  - Large (upto 25 cm) brown-green occasionally cystic and patchily calcified mass.
  - Two histologic presentation:
    - ☐ Epithelial, 2/3 of the cases.
    - ☐ Mixed epithelial mesenchymal, 1/3 of the cases.
      - ✓ Epithelial component consists of 3 variants:
        - ➢ *Fetal:* Polygonal small cells with round nuclei, large single nucleoli and granular cytoplasm arranged forming cords and sinusoids with bile ducts that occasionally contain bile. Hematopoiesis is common (Fig. 121.43).
        - ➢ *Embryonal:* Small round to spindle cells with scanty cytoplasm and small nuclei that form rosettes, cords and ribbons.
        - ➢ *Anaplastic:* Solid proliferation of poorly cohesive small-undifferentiated cells.
      - ✓ Mesenchymal component includes: Immature spindle cells and might contain osteoid, chondroid, rhabdomyoblastic, teratoid differentiation.
  - Frequent venous invasion with thrombosis.
  - Positive immunohistochemical markers:

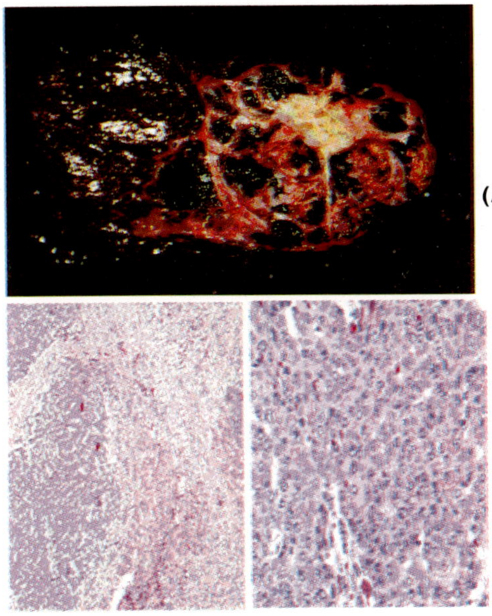

Fig. 121.43: Hepatoblastoma: (A) Large hepatic mass with variegated surface, hemorrhage and necrosis. (B) (C) Lobules formed by neoplastic polygonal small cells

    - ☐ AFP.
    - ☐ HepPar1.
    - ☐ CEA-p.

Hepatocellular Carcinoma

Malignant tumor with hepatocyte differentiation:

- Though more common in adults, in children may present in infancy with a second peak of incidence around puberty and adolescence (some cases are second malignancies in successfully treated Wilms' tumor patients).
- Strong association with hepatotropic viral infections (HBV and HCV) and cirrhosis.
- High incidence in Africa and Southeast Asia.
- Males > females, especially when associated with cirrhosis.
- Usual presentation:
  - Abdominal pain.
  - Ascites.
  - Liver enlargement.
- Elevated serum AFP.
- Morphologic changes include: (Fig. 121.44)
  - Single pink/yellow or green mass or multiple nodules (when associated with cirrhosis).
  - Well differentiated:
    - ☐ Tubules or trabecula formed by well-differentiated hepatocytoid cells.
  - Anaplastic:
    - ☐ Pleomorphic giant cells, small undifferentiated cells, spindle cells or completely anaplastic cells
  - Positive immunohistochemical markers:

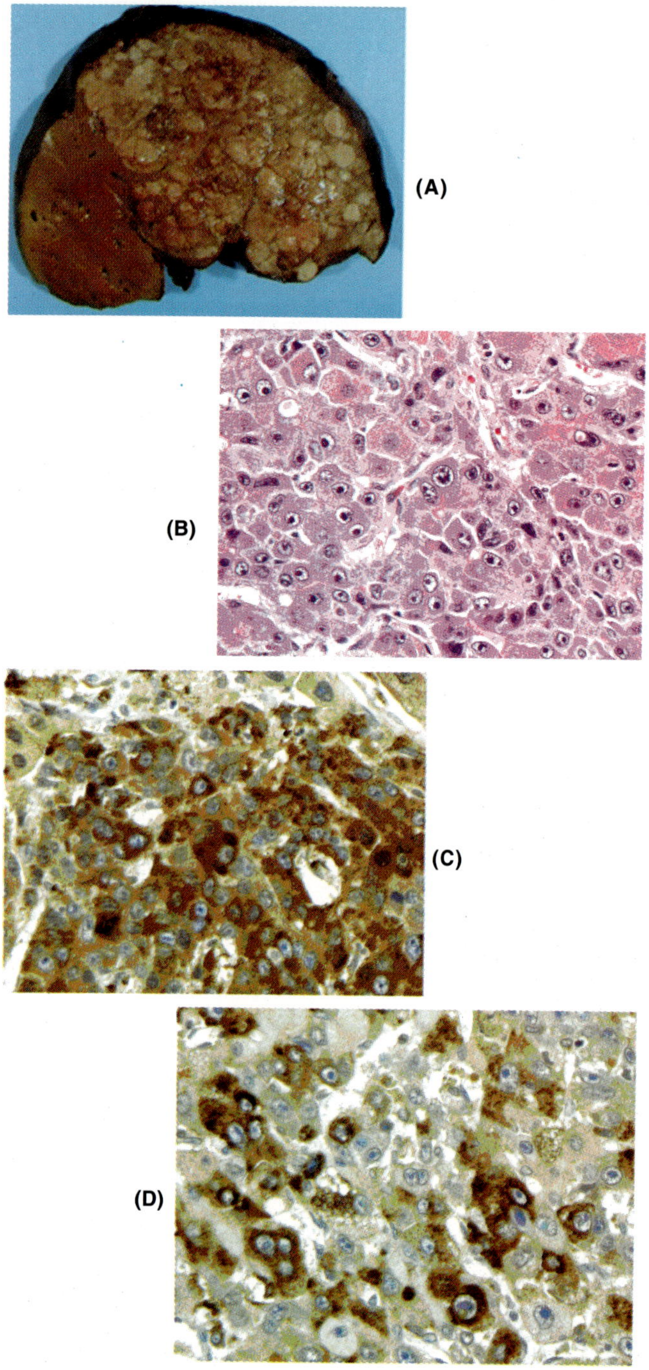

Fig. 121.44: Hepatocellular carcinoma (HCC): (A) Cut section of liver with a large mass characterized by nodularity and homogeneous color, lighter than the normal liver, (B) Micrograph that shows malignant neoplasm formed by large polygonal cells with poor hepatocytic differentiation, abundant cytoplasm, large nuclei with prominent nucleoli. HepPar-1, (C) Alpha-1 antitrypsin, and (D) Immunohistochemistry in HCC

- ☐ AFP.
- ☐ HepPar1.
- ☐ CEA-P.
- ☐ CD10.

- Poor prognosis.

Infantile Hemangioendothelioma

Well-differentiated vascular tumor:

- Account for approximately 10% of liver tumors of the childhood.
- The majority detected in infancy.
- Hepatomegaly and congestive cardiac failure, from arterious-venous shunts is seen in ¼ of the cases.
- Occasional spontaneous regression.
- Malignant transformation with metastasis may rarely occur.
- Morphologic changes:
  - Red brown multinodular or diffuse spongy tumor.
  - Two histologic patterns seen:
    - ☐ Type 1:
      - ✓ Vascular cavities lined by a single layer of well-differentiated endothelial cells (Fig. 121.45).
      - ✓ Central cavernous spaces with thrombosis and infarction.
      - ✓ Small bile ductules throughout the lesion.
      - ✓ Occasional hematopoiesis.

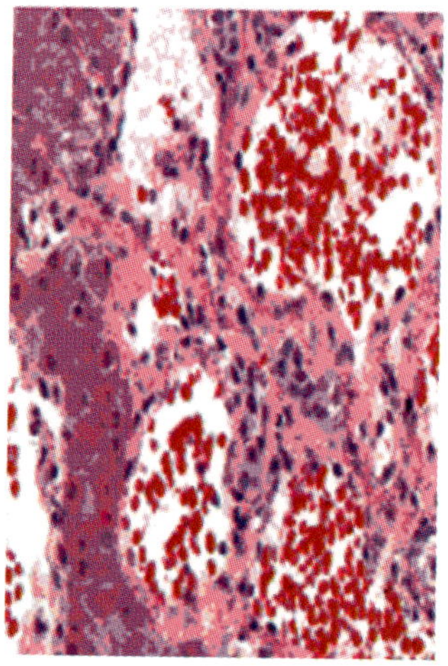

Fig. 121.45: Infantile hemangioendothelioma: Micrograph shows vascular cavities lined by benign endothelium intermingled with aggregates of liver cells

    - ☐ Type 2:
      - ✓ Nuclear atypia and pleomorphism in multilayered endothelium.
        Intravascular papillary projections and budding of the neoplastic endothelial lining.
      - ✓ In cases, solid growth pattern with mitosis.
      - ✓ It does not metastasize.

Acknowledgements

The author is grateful to Dr Katrina Conard for providing some of the photos for this chapter, Doris Warren for the drawings and Linda Krawczuk for her secretarial assistance.

KEY LEARNING POINTS

- The pathologic investigations are dictated by the characteristics of the developmental, inflammatory and neoplastic disorders of the gastrointestinal tract, pancreas, liver and biliary tract.
- Biopsy is crucial for diagnosis of inflammatory disease of the esophagus.
- The diagnosis of H. pylori is confirmed by endoscopic biopsy.
- Small intestinal biopsy is important for diagnosis of celiac disease and tropical sprue.
- Sweat chloride estimation is the most important screening test for cystic fibrosis.
- The diagnosis of the antibiotic-related form of C. difficile is made by detection of C. difficile toxin in feces.
- Suction rectal biopsy is the most accurate test for Hirschsprung's disease, having a mean 93% sensitivity and mean 98% specificity.
- Positive immunohistochemical markers for hepatoblastoma are:
  - AFP
  - HepPar 1
  - CEA-p
- Positive immunohistochemical markers for hepatocellular carcinoma are:
  - AFP
  - HepPar1
  - CEA-P
  - CD10

FURTHER READINGS

1. Diefenbach KA, Breuer CK. Pediatric inflammatory bowel disease.*World J Gastroenterol* 2006;12:3204-3212.
2. Huff D.S. Developmental anatomy and anomalies of the gastrointestinal tract with involvement in major malformative syndromes. In Russo, *et al.* (ed) *Pathology of Pediatric Gastrointestinal and Liver Disease*. New York: Springer-Verlag 2004: 3-36.
3. Kato S, Sherman P.M. What Is New Related to Helicobacter Pylori Infection in Children and Teenagers? *Arch Pediatr Adolesc Med* 2005:159:415-421.
4. Koh EP, *et al.* A report of 6 children with small bowel intussusception that required surgical intervention. *J Pediatr Surg* 2006:41:817-20.
5. Liu C *et al.* The gastrointestinal tract. In Kumar V *et al.* (ed) Robbins and Cotran; *Pathologic bases of diseases.* 7th ed., Philadelphia: Saunders 2005:794-874.
6. Lorijn F de. Diagnostic test in Hirschprungs Disease: A systemic review. *J Pediatr Gastroenterol Nut* 2006: 42, 490-505.
7. Ludvigson JF, *et al.* Effect of HLA DQ2, dietary exposure and coeliac disease on the development of antibody response to gliadin in children. *Scand J Gastroenterol* 2006:41:919-928.
8. Ocku-Heper A, *et al.* Nonobstructive neonatal cholestasis: Clinical outcome and scoring of the histopathological changes in liver biopsies. *Pediatr Dev Pathol* 2006:9:44-51.
9. Pall H, Jonas MM. Pediatric hepatobiliary disease. *Curr Opin Gastroenterol* 2005:21:344-347.
10. Panigrahi P, Necrotizing enterocolitis: A practical guide to its prevention and management. *Paediatr Drugs* 2006:8:151-165.
11. Pawel BR. Polyps and tumors of the gastrointestinal tract in childhood. In: Russo, *et al.* (eds) *Pathology of Pediatric Gastrointestinal and Liver Disease*. New York: Springer-Verlag 2004:3-36.
12. Satapathy S, *et al.* Profile of chronic hepatitis B virus in children in India: Experience with 116 children. *J Gastroenterol Hepatol* 2006:21:1170-1176.
13. Schweizer P, *et al.* Pathogenesis of extrahepatic bile duct atresia (EHBA): Comprehension from a surgical point of view. *Eur J Pediatr Surg* 2005:154:248-257.
14. Sempoux C. Role of the pathologist in the differential diagnosis of malabsorption. *Acta Gastroenterol Belg* 2006:69:49-51.
15. Sokol RG, *et al.* "Let there be bile"–understanding hepatic injury in cholestasis. *J Pediatr Gastroenterol Nutr* 2006:43 (1 Suppl):S4-9.
16. Suskind DL, Rosenthal P. Chronic viral hepatitis. *Adolesc Med Cli* 2004:151:145-158.
17. Tursi A, *et al.* Endoscopic and histological findings in the duodenum of adults with celiac disease before and after changing to a gluten-free diet: A 2-year prospective study. *Endoscopy* 2006:38:702-707.
18. Villa-Carbo JJ, *et al.* Choledocal cyst: Analysis of 29 cases and review of the literature. *Cir Pediatr* 2006:19:33-8.
19. Zambrano E, *et al.* Total parenteral nutrition induced liver pathology: An autopsy series of 24 newborn cases. *Pediatr Dev Pathol* 2004:425-432.

122 Imaging Studies

Chandra Mohan Kumar

INTRODUCTION

Over the past 3 decades, significant changes and advances have been made in diagnostic approach to gastrointestinal tract (GIT). Imaging studies have emerged as one of the most rapidly advancing fields and have revolutionized diagnostic as well as therapeutic approaches in pediatric gastroenterology. The high-resolution real-time imaging modalities like ultrasonography (USG), computerized tomography (CT) and magnetic resonance imaging (MRI) have provided increasingly sophisticated and accurate diagnostic techniques.

This chapter aims to analyze various imaging modalities being used in pediatric gastroenterology with special reference to their best application, utility, limitations, associated risks and cost-effectiveness.

IMAGING MODALITIES

The various imaging modalities used in pediatric practice are as following:

1. Plain X-ray
2. Fluoroscopy
3. Ultrasonography (USG)
   - Endosonography
4. CT
   - Plain
   - Contrast Enhanced
   - Spiral
5. Magnetic Resonance Imaging (MRI)
6. Nuclear Scan
7. Angiography and
8. Interventional imaging
   - Endoscopic retrograde cholangiopancreatography (ERCP)
   - Endosonography.

1. Plain X-ray

It is the oldest and cheapest imaging modality. Ionizing radiation X-ray beam is used for generation of image. The X-ray beam passes through the patient's body and the film is exposed to radiation. The resultant image reflects the differences in the density of structures through which the beam passes. Its advantages are:

a. Available everywhere.
b. Inexpensive; and
c. Fast.

But at the same time it has some limitations and disadvantages also. These are:

a. Uses radiation.
b. Limited information regarding soft tissues.

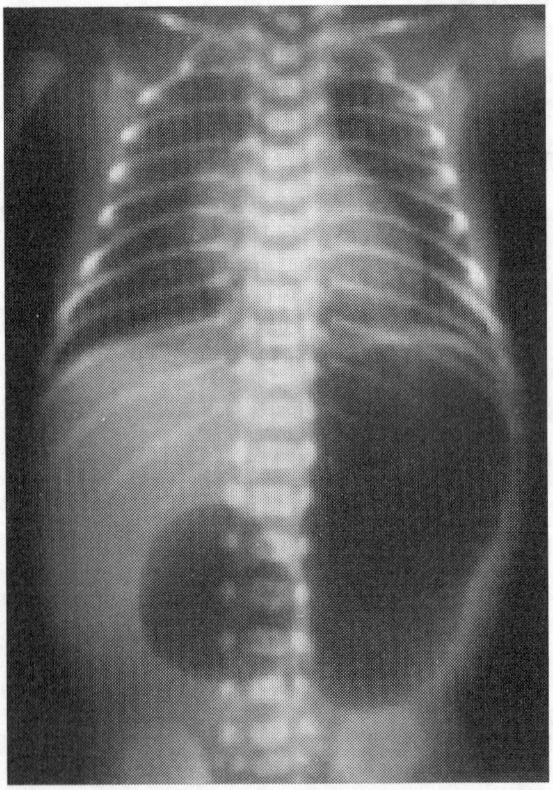

Fig. 122.1: Plain X-ray showing double-bubble appearance in duodenal atresia

c. Cannot distinguish between soft tissues of similar consistency very well.

As an imaging modality in pediatric gastroenterology it is best suited for diagnosis of:

1. Intestinal obstructions.
2. Peptic perforations.
3. Renal calculi.
4. Ingestion of radio-opaque foreign bodies.

2. Fluoroscopy

Fluoroscopy technique uses real time X-ray beam. Child lies on the table and a moving X-ray beam is used to visualize structures real time. Contrast media like barium is used to delineate GI tract, e.g. barium swallow, barium meal, barium enema, etc.

Advantages of barium studies are:

1. Real time visualization of GI tract.
2. Delineate well the inner mucosal lining of GI tract.
3. Relatively inexpensive.

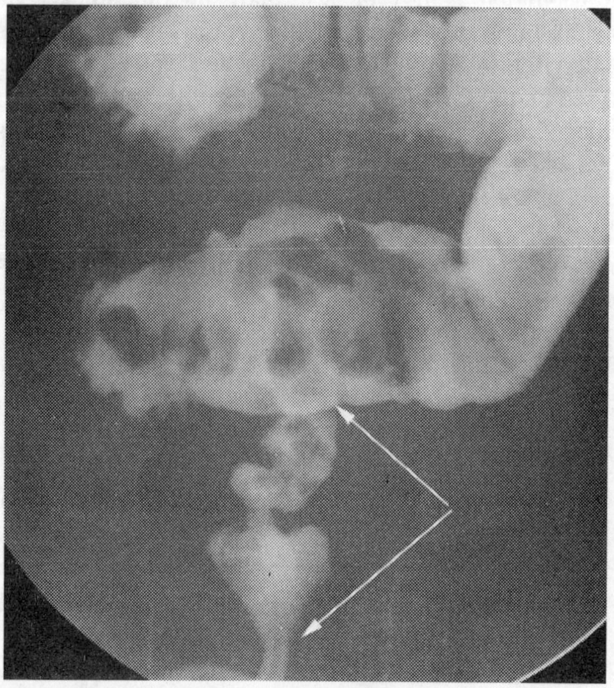

Fig. 122.2: Barium X-ray showing aganglionic segment in Hirschsprung's disease

Disadvantages are:

1. Significant radiation exposure to patients as well as doctors.
2. Limited utility.
3. Ultrasonography.

3. Ultrasonography

This real time, high resolution, non-invasive and non-ionizing imaging modality has revolutionized the investigations in pediatric gastroenterology. It uses high frequency sound waves which travel through human tissue and are reflected from the traversing interfaces. A transducer which emits high frequency sound is rubbed over the patient; based on information which is returned to the transducer, an image is generated by the computer within the machine. Its advantages are:

1. Portable, inexpensive equipment.
2. Cheaper than other cross-sectional imaging techniques.
3. Real-time.
4. Can perform interventional procedures.
5. No radiation.
6. No contrast agents and their risks.
7. Allows multi planar imaging.
8. Good at deciding cystic vs solid.
9. Doppler evaluation allows analysis of blood flow.

However it has some disadvantages also. These are:

1. Doesn't show function, only anatomy.
2. Hard to see deep structures.
3. Can't see through bone or air.
4. Needs specialized and trained professionals.

As a diagnostic tool this is the most useful radiological investigation in pediatric gastroenterology. It is best suited for diagnosis of

a. Acute abdomen
b. Appendicitis and appendicular lump
c. Intussusceptions
d. Cholecystitis and cholelithiasis
e. Pancreatitis and pseudopancreatic cyst
f. Hypertrophic pyloric stenosis
g. Meckel's diverticulum
h Duodenal atresia
i. Ascites
j. Biliary atresia
k. Choledochal cyst
l. Trauma to liver, spleen, pancreas and intestine
m. Malrotation and volvulus
n. Mesenteric adenitis
o. Lymphoma
p. Mesenteric cyst
q. Hydatid cyst
r. Amebic liver abscess
s. Apart from conventional ultra sonography (USG) color doppler study may augment its diagnostic value by showing relative positions of blood flow in arteries and veins. For example duodenal obstruction.
   - Malrotation and volvulus – Color doppler studies aid in the diagnosis by demonstrating SMV anterior or to the left of SMA. The other uses of **Doppler study** are:

   1. Evaluation of the splanchnic venous system in the child with portal hypertension.

2. Determination of patency of vessels (aorta and inferior vena cava), especially following surgery or in the presence of tumours (e.g. Wilm's).
3. Assessment of vascularity and rejection of transplant organs e.g. liver.
4. Identification of unknown structure (tortuous portal vein versus dilated bile duct, dilated vein versus dilated ureter or lymphatic channel).
5. Defining malignant nature of a mass by its abnormal vascularisation.

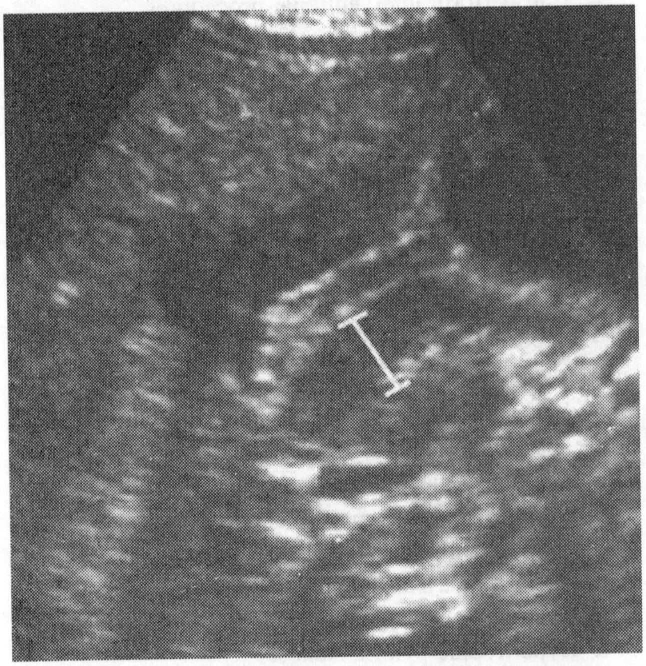

Fig. 122.3: Endosonography showing thickening of pyloric muscle and elongated pyloric canal in congenital hypertrophic pyloric stenosis

Endosonography is a new and potentially very useful tool for studying the morphology and motor function of the gastrointestinal tract. Intraluminal ultrasonography is the common denomination of ultrasound examinations using intracorporal transducers which are inserted into the GI tract. Thus, the visceral wall and adjacent structures can be imaged in detail. This technique employs endoscope combined with integrated ultrasound transducer. US mini probes have a diameter which allows the probe to be inserted through the biopsy channel of a conventional endoscope or a suitable catheter.

Ultrasound elastography is a new method with the potential of separating normal from pathological tissue. Recently, elastography and contrast enhanced ultrasound have been applied also in endosonographic imaging. Doppler sonography may provide important information about vascular flow and separate vessels from other echo-poor structures.

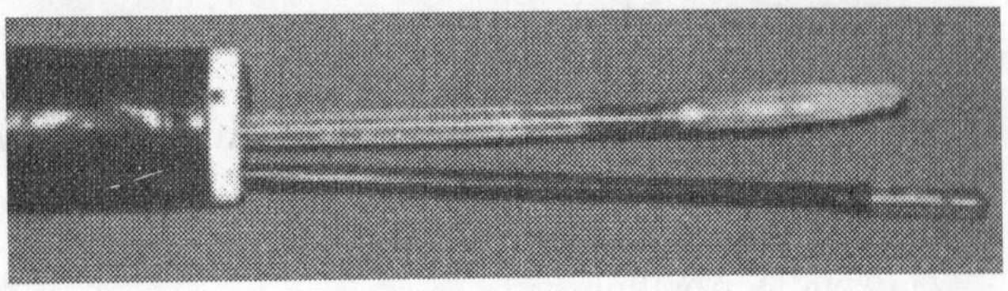

Fig. 122.4: Intracorporal transducers

As an imaging modality it is best suited for studying motility.

4. Computed Tomography

A computed tomography (CT) scan uses X-rays to make detailed cross-sectional pictures of structures inside of the body. The CT scanner sends X-ray pulses through the body area being studied. Each pulse lasts less than a second and takes a picture of a thin slice of the organ or area. One part of the scanning machine can tilt to take pictures from different positions. The patient should lie still holding breath in inspiration as movement of body blurs the image. The pictures are saved on a computer. An iodine dye (contrast material) is often used to make structures and organs easier to see on the CT pictures. The dye may be used to check blood flow, find tumors, and look for other pathologies. Dye can be put in a vein (IV) in arm, or orally for some tests, or the dye may be put into the rectum, to see those areas better. CT pictures are taken before and after the dye to have comparative studies of **plain** and **contrast enhanced** anatomical details.

Advantages of CT scanning in gastroenterology are:

1. Excellent soft tissue contrast and discrimination.
2. Readily displayed.
3. Allows deep structures to be visualized.
4. Widely available.
5. Interventional procedures can be performed using CT.

Disadvantages are:

1. Relatively expensive.
2. Radiation hazards are more compared to USG, MRI and X-ray.
3. Requires contrast enhancement with risks of nephrotoxicity and anaphylaxis.

CT scan may be very useful in diagnosis of following conditions:

1. Abscesses.
2. Acute cholecystitis.
3. Amebic liver abscess.
4. Appendicitis.
5. Bowel wall thickness.
6. Chronic cholelithiasis.
7. Choledocholithiasis.
8. Chronic pancreatitis.
9. Chronic cholecystitis.
10. Choledochal cyct.

11. Hydatid cyst.
12. Mesenteric adenitis.
13. Enlarged organs.
14. Gastrointestinal or bowel obstruction.
15. Hepatitis and chirrhosis.

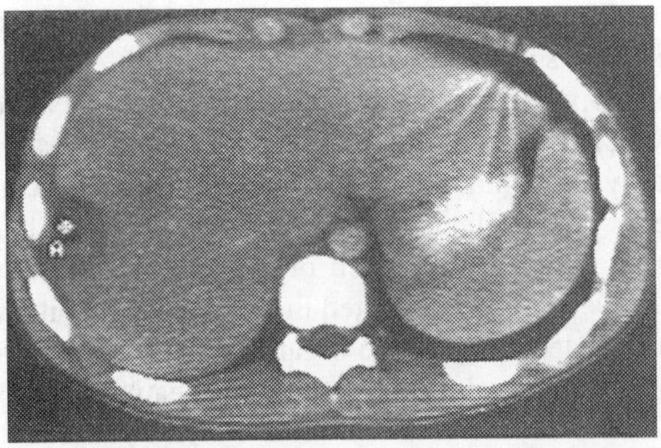

Fig. 122.5: CT scan showing amebic liver abscess

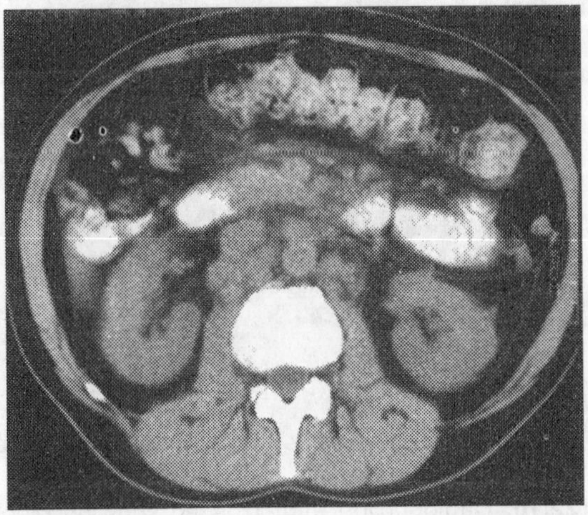

Fig. 122.6: CT scan showing mesenteric lymhadenitis

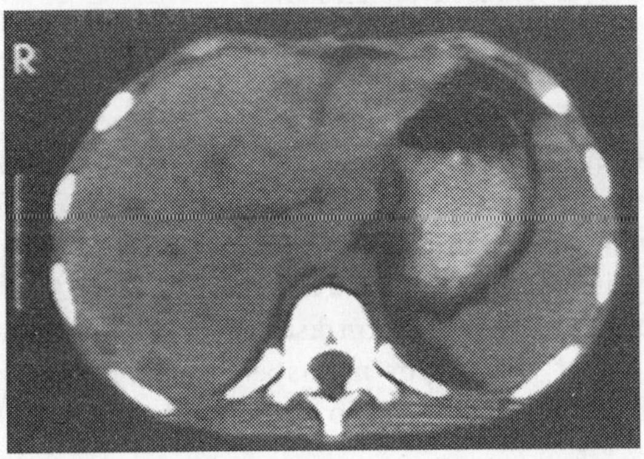

Fig. 122.7: CT scan showing multiple microabscesses in liver

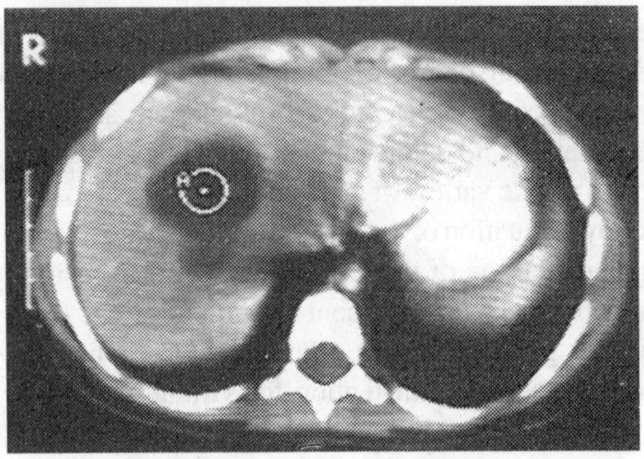

Fig. 122.8: CT scan showing hydatid cyst of liver

Spiral CT

Spiral (helical) CT scanning is a method of CT imaging which enables rapid acquisition of truly volumetric CT data.In this technology, a series of projections is obtained in helical spatial distribution. This helical data set is obtained by moving the table on which the patient lies at constant speed while the X-ray tube continuously rotates and a sustained exposure is made.

Scanning time for helical CT is very short compared to conventional CT.

With conventional 1 cm collimation, a 30 sec helical exposure would cover 30 cm of tissue in the z direction (from head to foot). A slip-ring scanner in the nonhelical mode would require 60 sec to cover the same 30 cm. A non slip-ring scanner would take 3-4 minutes for the same number of slices. Thus advantages of spiral CT are:

1. Rapid scanning.
2. Scanning at the peak of contrast.
3. Requires less contrast.
4. Easy to perform as it requires breath holding for shorter period 30 secs.
5. Retrospective reconstruction of overlapping areas can be done to identify small lesions.

Disadvantages are:

1. It's expensive.
2. Helical artifact.
3. Vascular flow artifact.

Virtual Endoscopy

Virtual endoscopy (or computed endoscopy) is a new method of diagnosis using computer processing of 3-D image datasets (such as spiral CT or MRI scans) to provide simulated visualizations of patient specific organs similar or equivalent to those produced by standard endoscopic procedures.

A very interesting and very promising application of spiral CT imaging is virtual endoscopy. This is due to its capability for reconstruction of GI segments. Virtual endoscopy can assist in preoperative planning as well as in planning actual endostions can depict abnormalities in a format that is easier to interpret than are the corresponding axial images. The technique can also provide endoscopic views of areas otherwise inaccessible to endoscopy and can assist in the characterization and delineation of the extent and anatomic location of a wide variety of gastrointestinal diseases. Virtual endoscopy evaluation of the gastrointestinal system requires complete distention of the viscus being studied, using oral contrast material, effervescent granules, rectal contrast material, or gas insufflation. Methylcellulose enteroclysis may provide adequate distention for virtual endoscopy of the small bowel, otherwise a difficult area to evaluate.

It is best suitable for diagnosis wall thickening, polyps in bowel lumen as well as choledocolithiasis, choledochal strictures and duplications in biliary tree.

This is a very useful investigation in evaluation of filling defects in barium studies and helps differentiating between extrinsic, intramural, mucosal and submucosal causes.

5. Magnetic Resonance Imaging (MRI)

MRI is application of radio-frequency pulses in a magnetic field. It uses hydrogen ions to move and uses its deflection in the magnetic field to generate images. Like CT it is also a very important tool for detailed cross-sectional pictures of structures inside of the body. However it has the advantage of providing multiplanar images and being free from radiation hazards.

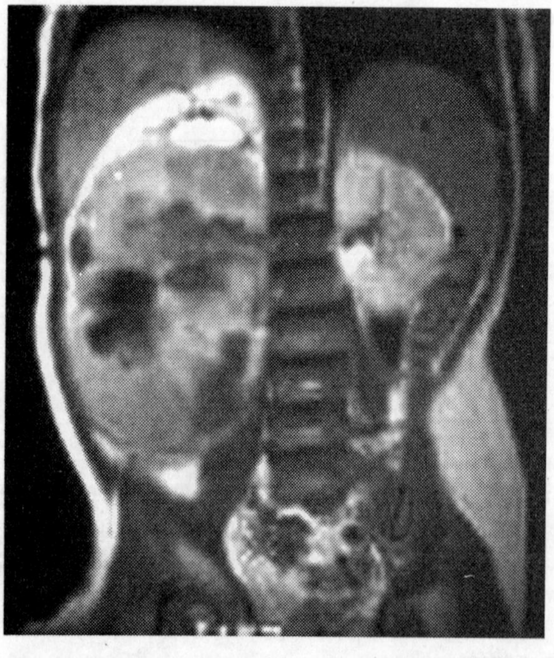

Fig. 122.9: MRI showing bilateral Wilms tumor

Its disadvantages are its high costs and unavailability at most of the centers.

For GI imaging this modality is best suited for evaluation of pancreatic and mesenteric pathology.

6. Nuclear Scan

Nuclear imaging is different from radiological imaging and the primary difference being that it is emission imaging in contrast to transmission imaging. Radioisotope imaging centers on the recording radiation emitted when atoms of an unstable element disintegrate spontaneously to a stable form. The source of radiation (a suitable non-toxic radioisotopes injected into the patient) gets localized at desired sites as per functional status and emits radiation primarily the gamma radiation from within the cells. Gamma cameras can collect energy from the emitted beams, showing areas of increased or decreased activity. The radioactive isotope is selected in such a way that it will be taken up selectively by the organ under evaluation. It has the advantage that it is excellent in delineating functions.

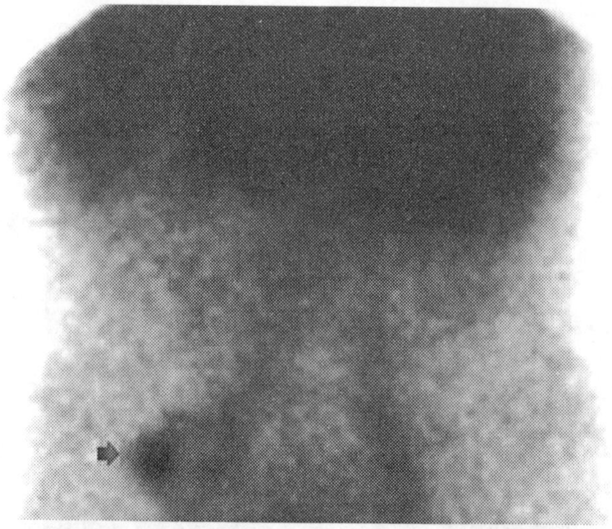

Fig. 122.10: Radionuclide 99m-Tc scan showing Meckel's diverticulum through increased uptake of 99m-Tc labeled pertechnetate in ectopic gastric mucosa

However its disadvantages are:

1. Weak anatomical analysis.
2. Relatively expensive.
3. Not good for interventional procedures.

It is very useful tool in evaluating a child with GI bleeding as well as in assessment of hepatobiliary and pancreatic functions in Pediatric Gastroenterology. Liver scans are done using technitium bound to sulphur colloid. A scan of a normal liver shows uniform distribution of isotope whereas in cases of abscess or metastasis in liver devoid of reticuloendothelial tissue shows hole in the scan.

7. Angiography

Angiography can also be very useful in certain conditions of GI tract. Angiography shows the vascular architecture of the target organ and thus helps in identifying the location of the pathology.

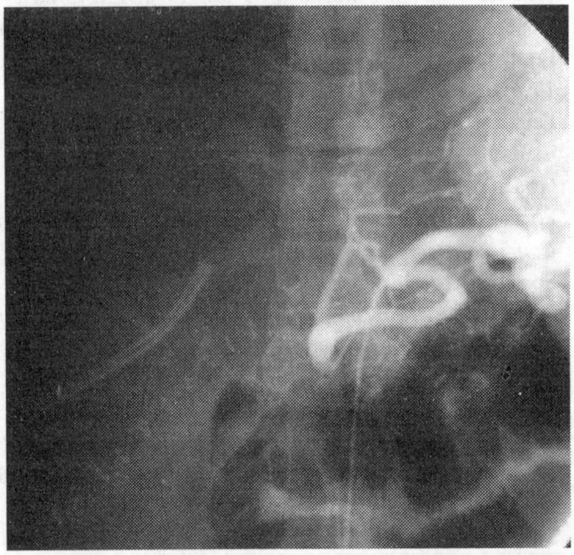

Fig. 122.11: Angiography showing hepatic artery thrombosis leading to hepatic infarction

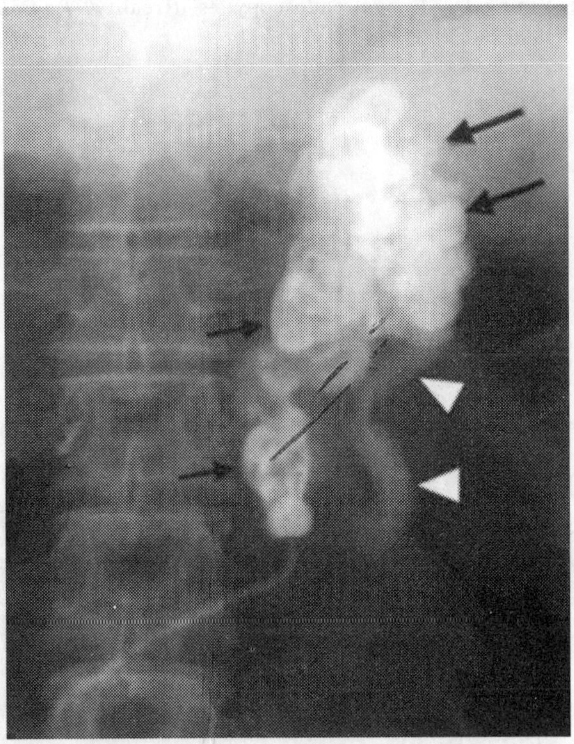

Fig. 122.12: Portal venogram showing esophageal varices

For example in portal venography the dye injected into the spleen delineates the portal system and helps localizing esophageal varices. Hepatic angiography can help in diagnosis of hepatic malignancy.

8. Endoscopic Retrograde Cholangiopancreatography (ERCP)

ERCP is an invasive interventional imaging technique for biliary tree and pancreatic duct. It provides more definitive information about the site and nature of biliary obstruction in patients in whom ultrasonagraphy is inconclusive.

In ERCP, the fiberoptic endoscope is positioned within the tip of the second part of duodenum and a catheter is passed through it into the ampulla of Vater. Contrast medium is injected into it to opacify the biliary tree and pancreatic duct. Stones as well as any growth within the CBD or pancreatic duct appear as filling defects.

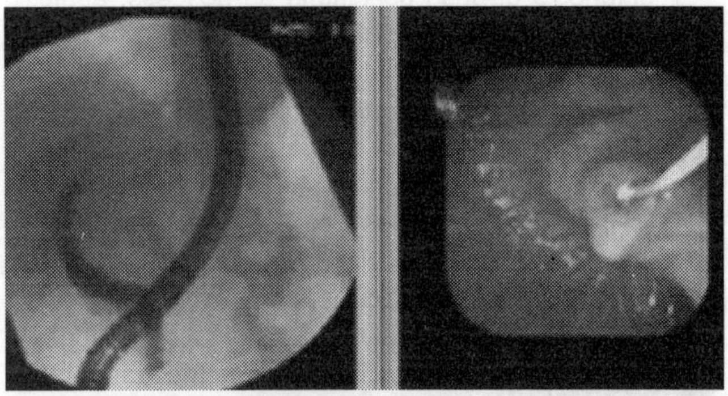

Figs. 122.13 and 122.14: ERCP procedure (See for colour figure Plate 10)

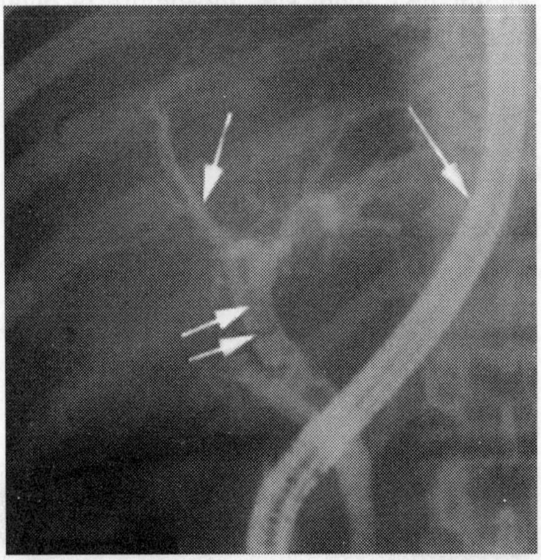

Fig. 122.15: ERCP image showing filling defects (stones) in CBD

Disadvantages of ERCP are:
1. Its invasive.
2. Lengthy procedure.
3. Difficult to perform and needs specialized training.

Thus, these imaging modalities provide a diverse range of techniques and a plethora of useful information for diagnostic as well as therapeutic purposes.

KEY LEARNING POINTS

- Imaging studies have brought about a breakthrough in diagnostic and therapeutic gastroenterology.
- Despite availability of new sophisticated imaging studies, plain X-ray and fluoroscopy still occupy a space in diagnosis in pediatric gastroenterology.
- Ultrasonography is most suited in situations such as acute abdomen, appendicular lump, intussusception, cholelithiasis, pseudopancreatic cyst, etc.
- Endosonograhpy is best suited for studying morphology and motor function of GIT.
- Computed tomography is of special value in diagnosis of such conditions as abscess, acute cholecystitis, appendicitis, etc.
- Though more expensive, spiral (helical) CT is superior to conventional CT.
- Virtual endoscopy is of special value in evaluation of filling defects in barium studies.
- MRI not only provides detailed cross-sectional images but also multiplanar images.
- Nuclear scan is of particular help in evaluation of GI bleed, and hepatobiliary and pancreatic functions.
- Angiography assists in showing the vascular architecture of the target organ.
- ERCP, though invasive, provides quite dependable information about site and nature of biliary obstruction.

FURTHER READINGS

1. Barr LL. Sonography in the infant with acute abdominal symptoms. *Semin Ultrasound CT MR* 1994; 15:275-289.
2. Donoghue V. Neonatal gastrointestinal tract. In: Carty H, Brunelle F (eds): *Imaging Children*. New York: Churchill Livingstone 1994: 250-260.
3. Fenlon HM, Femicci JT. Virtual colonoscopy:What will the issues be?*AJR* 1997:169:453-458.
4. Griscom NT. Gastrointestinal problems in the neonate. In: Poznanski AK, Kirkpatrick JA, Jr (eds) *Syllabus: A Categorical Course in Pediatric Radiology*. Oak Brook, Ill: Radiological Society of North America1989:27-37.
5. Hayden CK, Jr. Advances in the ultrasonographic evaluation of the pediatric gastrointestinal tract. *Ultrasound Quatr* 1991; 9:139-169.
6. Hayden CK, Jr. Ultrasonography of the gastrointestinal tract in infants and children. *Abdom Imaging* 1996; 21:9-20.
7. Merten DF. Practical approaches to pediatric gastrointestinal radiology. *Radiol Clin N Am* 1993; 31:1395-1407.
8. Singleton EB, Wagner ML, Dutton RV. *Radiology of the Alimentary Tract in Infants and Children.* 2nd edn. Philadelphia: Saunders 1977.
9. Odegaard S, Birger L N, Hoff DAL, Gilja OH, Morphology OH.Motor function of the gastrointestinal tract examined with endosonography; *World J Gastroenterol* 2006; 12: 2858-2863.
10. Vining DI. Virtual endoscopy: Is it reality? *Radiology* 1996;200:30-36.

123 Upper Gastrointestinal Endoscopy

Jeremy King • Raman Sreedharan

INTRODUCTION

Examination of the upper gastrointestinal tract by esophagogastroduodenoscopy (EGD) is the most frequently performed endoscopic procedure in children.

This chapter reviews the diagnostic applications, including indications for and risks of upper gastrointestinal endoscopy. It also describes the fiberoptic and video systems, procedure techniques, tissue sampling (biopsy and cytology), and some new approaches to diagnosis. Preparation for the procedure, sedation and potential complications are also covered. However, it does not focus on therapeutic endoscopic procedures, such as foreign body removals, dilatations and polypectomies.

BASIC EQUIPMENTS

Two distinct types of flexible endoscopes are commonly used and commercially available from three major manufacturers (Olympus, Pentax and Fujinon). The two types are the standard fiberoptic endoscope and the electronic or video endoscope. Since we are in the digital era, most of the new endoscopes are video endoscopes, which allow digital image capturing. The size of the pediatric upper GI endoscopes varies from 5.3 mm to 11 mm.

Although fiberoptic endoscopes are still around, since the late nineteen nineties, they have been almost universally replaced by the more technologically advanced electronic endoscopes. These new endoscopes contain a charge-coupled device that is able to convert light to an analog signal. This signal is then converted into a digital signal in a digital video processor. Once digitized, the signal is transferred to a video monitor and stored in computer memory as captured images. Videoendoscopes can project large, high-resolution images onto television monitors, allowing the examiner to detect subtle mucosal abnormalities that might not be seen with a conventional fiberoptic endoscope. A variety of computerized storage devices offer virtually limitless storage capacity for images and patient information that may be recalled for later review. Updated computer software offers not only advanced image storing but also patient database searching capabilities. Hard-copy images can be embedded into an endoscopy report or patient chart, given to the family, or sent to a referring physician.

Videoendoscopy sessions can be electronically transmitted offsite for live or recorded video-conferences, greatly enhancing the educational value of endoscopy to training endoscopists and physicians. This technology also enhances communication between endoscopist, endoscopy assistants, and endoscopy trainees by virtue of simultaneous, real-time viewing. This is especially beneficial during technically challenging procedures. The hard-copy data, in the form of images obtained during the procedure, also may greatly enhance a patient's, family's, or referring physician's understanding of abnormal endoscopic findings.

THE ENDOSCOPE

Regardless of the type, each endoscope includes several important components to allow it a multitude of diagnostic and therapeutic options. First, there is an objective lens system, which allows the target to be focused into the fiberoptic image bundle. The endoscope contains a light source at the scope's tip. Two buttons are present on the endoscope head (Fig. 123.1), the first of which provides both a jet of water to clean the objective lens and air insufflations. The upper button connects to a suction channel and is used to remove both liquids and gases from the upper intestinal tract. The suction channel is used to pass endoscopic accessories that may be used for diagnostic or therapeutic purposes, such as biopsy forceps, snares, injecting catheters and coagulation probes.

The control wheels connect to wires that run to the tip of the scope and allow manipulation. The wheels are seen in Fig. 123.1. Maneuvering these buttons the deflectable tip of the endoscope moves up and down or right to left directions makes possible a complete inspection of entire luminal surfaces and gastrointestinal organs. Deflection of the scope tip can be coupled with a clockwise or counter

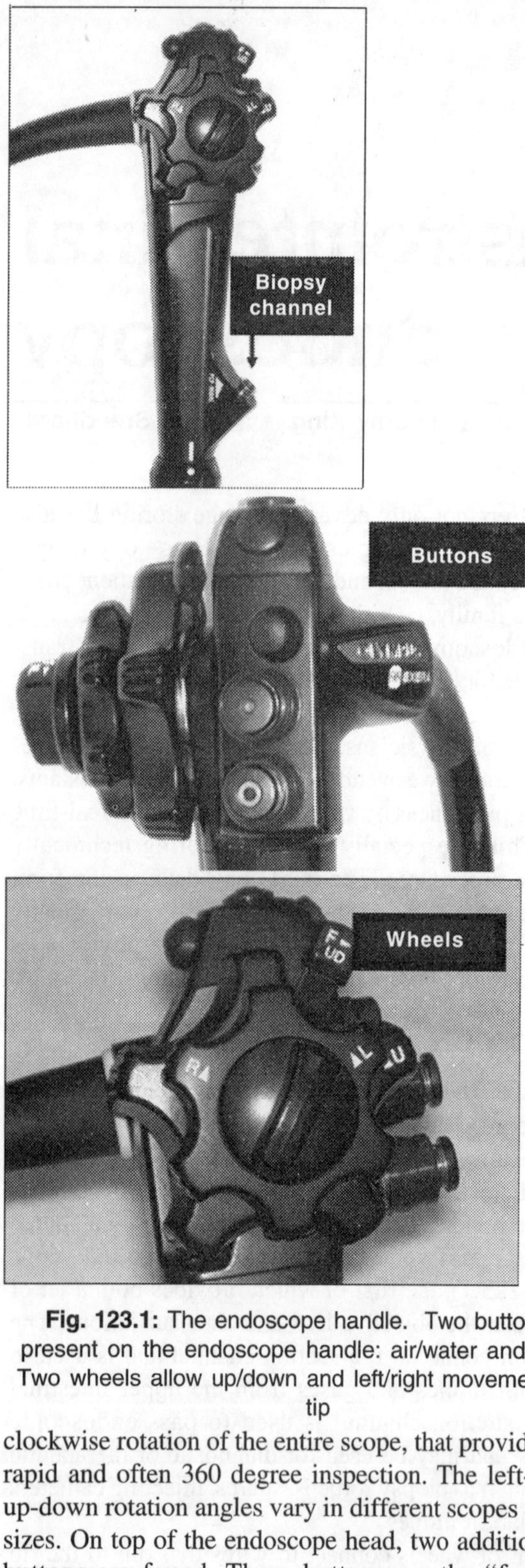

Fig. 123.1: The endoscope handle. Two buttons are present on the endoscope handle: air/water and suction. Two wheels allow up/down and left/right movement of the tip

clockwise rotation of the entire scope, that provides a more rapid and often 360 degree inspection. The left-right and up-down rotation angles vary in different scopes and scope sizes. On top of the endoscope head, two additional small buttons are found. These buttons are the "freeze" and "capture" buttons that allow still photographs to be taken during the procedure. The biopsy channel is located on the lower front of the scope.

Figure 123.2 shows the endoscope attached to the box containing the lighting source, water bottle and digital unit.

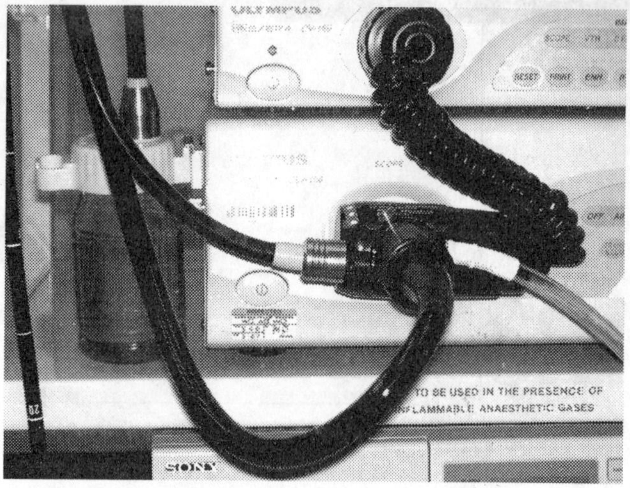

Fig. 123.2: The endoscope attached to the box containing the lighting source, water bottle and digital unit

FACILITIES AND EQUIPMENT

Procedures must be performed in a location that is adequate in size and equipped to deal with a cardiopulmonary emergency, usually a designated endoscopy suite or hospital or surgical center operating room. A pediatric "crash cart" should be immediately available in the endoscopy suite. Necessary equipment includes appropriate lighting, an operating table or trolley, oxygen supply with self-inflating bag-mask, intubation kit, suction source and supplies, and suitable vital sign monitoring instruments. Furthermore, intravenous fluid and equipment, as well as appropriate drugs for cardiopulmonary resuscitation and reversal of benzodiazepines and opiates should be readily available.

INDICATIONS FOR ENDOSCOPY

The indications for upper endoscopy are too numerous to cover and must be individualized in the context of each patient's complete presentation. The major indications and contraindications for diagnostic upper endoscopy are listed in Table 123.1.

PATIENT PREPARATION

Prior to the procedure, usually at the time of scheduling, preparation instructions, including the importance of fasting (generally 4-8 hours), should be reviewed. The patient should be provided with written information including a description of the nature, risks and benefits of the procedure. He should also be informed of what to expect during the immediate and long-term recovery period following discharge. Informed consent for sedation or anesthesia should also be obtained.

PATIENT ASSESSMENT

All patients should be assessed before sedation for

Table 123.1: Indications and contraindications for endoscopy

Indications
- To evaluate abdominal pain, dysphagia, odynophagia, or dyspepsia
- To establish the site of upper GI bleeding
- To evaluate healing of treated gastric or duodenal ulcers
- To determine the extent of damage following caustic ingestion
- To visually define an abnormality seen on upper GI series

Absolute Contraindications
- Shock
- Acute myocardial infarction
- Severe dyspnea with hypoxia
- Coma
- Seizures
- Acutely perforated ulcer or esophagus
- Atlantoaxial subluxation

Relative Contraindications
- Uncooperative patient
- Coagulopathy
- Zenker's diverticulum
- Upper esophageal stricture
- Myocardial ischemia
- Thoracic aortic aneurysm

endoscopic procedures. The assessment should include details of the current problem, indication for the procedure, past medical and surgical history including previous response to anesthesia or sedation, current medications, allergies, fasting status and prior upper endoscopic results. A focused physical examination should be performed and include examination of the systems related to the procedure or identified during the history. Also, evaluation of the airway, respiratory system, and cardiovascular system should be covered at minimum. If general anesthesia is indicated, both the endoscopist and anesthesiologist will generally perform assessments.

ANTIBIOTIC PROPHYLAXIS

Prophylaxis is probably indicated for prosthetic heart valves in patients undergoing diagnostic endoscopy. Below, a list of the indications for antibiotic prophylaxis as recommended by the American Heart Association is provided in Table 123.2.

POSITIONING AND MONITORING

Usually prior to transporting the patient to the operating suite, reliable venous access is obtained. The patients should partly undress and put on a gown. Spectacles or contact lenses should be removed and stored safely. The patient lays either supine for general anesthesia or on his left side for sedation, ideally with intravenous access in the right arm. The head is supported with a small firm pillow. Monitoring sensors are placed and supplemental oxygen is provided. If sedation is being used, rather than general anesthesia, a topical pharyngeal anesthetic (2% viscous xylocaine or cetocaine or hurricaine spray) is administered. Parenteral sedatives, the choices of which vary greatly among endoscopists, are then given. A mouth guard is placed to protect both the endoscope and the patient's dentition.

A "surgical pause" in which the patient and procedure are identified, matched, and with the patient identification bracelet, should be completed prior to the start of the procedure. All patients must be monitored continuously with pulse oximetry. Regular recording of heart rate, respiratory

Table 123. 2: Cardiac conditions and endocarditis prophylaxis

Endocarditis prophylaxis recommended

High-risk category
- Prosthetic cardiac valves, including bioprosthetic and homograft valves
- Previous bacterial endocarditis
- Complex cyanotic congenital heart disease (e.g., single ventricle states, transposition of the great arteries, tetralogy of Fallot)
- Surgically constructed systemic-pulmonary shunts or conduits

Moderate-risk category
- Congenital cardiac malformations other than those listed in the high-risk and negligible-risk categories
- Acquired valvular dysfunction (e.g., rheumatic heart disease)
- Hypertrophic cardiomyopathy
- Mitral valve prolapse with valvular regurgitation and/or thickened leaflets

Endocarditis prophylaxis not recommended

Negligible-risk category (no greater risk than the general population)
- Isolated secundum atrial septal defect
- Surgical repair of atrial septal defect, ventricular septal defect or patent ductus arteriosus (without residua beyond six months)
- Previous coronary artery bypass graft surgery
- Mitral valve prolapse without valvular regurgitation
- Physiologic, functional or innocent heart murmur
- Previous Kawasaki disease without valvular dysfunction
- Previous rheumatic fever without valvular dysfunction
- Cardiac pacemakers (intravascular and epicardial) and implanted defibrillators

Adapted Dajani AS, Taubert KA, Wilson W, Bolger AF, Bayer A, Ferrieri P, *et al.* Prevention of bacterial endocarditis. Recommendations by the American Heart Association *JAMA* 1997;277:1794-1801.

rate, and blood pressure should be performed throughout the procedure.

SEDATION FOR THE PROCEDURE

Sedation for gastrointestinal endoscopic procedures is variable and often depends upon the patient's age, risk factors, the indication for endoscopy, and the physician comfort level and preference. Endoscopy can be performed with little or no sedation in the first year of life. Fasted babies often will swallow the endoscope upon introduction into the mouth and "suck" on it throughout the procedure. Many endoscopists prefer to use general anesthesia beyond one year and through the teen-age years.

Risks of sedation result from depression of the central nervous system and include depression of protective reflexes, respiration, and the cardiovascular system. One must also keep in mind the potential for adverse drug reactions, including anaphylaxis, and the wide individual variation in response to the sedative drugs.

During sedation, a minimum of three appropriate staff members must be present during an endoscopy, including the endoscopist, an assistant, and the person monitoring the patient's level of consciousness and cardiopulmonary status during the procedure.

STANCE AND INSTRUMENT HANDLING

The endoscopist should stand in a comfortable position and hold the scope in a way that it runs in a gentle curve directly into the patient's mouth. The endoscopist and the assistant should wear safety glasses, a protective gown, and latex-free examination gloves.

The instrument head should be placed in the palm of the left hand. The thumb should rest on the up/down control wheel and the forefinger on the air/water button. The second finger can assist the thumb during major up/down movements. Remaining free, the right hand is used to hold, push, pull and torque the scope.

Prior to beginning any endoscopic procedure, the scope should be checked to assure proper function. The light source, video transmission, air insufflator, water, and suction should be tested, as should each directional dial.

UPPER ENDOSCOPIC BASICS

It is usually appropriate to survey the entire esophagus, stomach, and proximal duodenum, regardless of the indication for upper endoscopy. Development of a systematic method to reduce the possibility of missing any area is necessary. Endoscopic movements should be precise and a mental map of what is being seen should be processed. Mucosal views are often better during instrument withdrawal, after the scope has reached the duodenum and the organs are fully distended with air. For this reason, many endoscopists prefer to perform detailed surveillance, take photographs, and retrieve biopsies upon endoscope withdrawal. Regardless of position during any procedure, two simple rules of endoscopy apply. The first is to never push or advance the scope if there is no clear mucosal view. Next, an adjunct of the first rule is that if in doubt pull it back. Keeping these rules in mind throughout any endoscopic procedure helps assure the test will be as safe and minimally traumatic as possible.

PASSING THE INSTRUMENT INTO THE ESOPHAGUS

The safest and most exact method is to introduce the scope into the esophagus under direct vision. The instrument should be held at about the 30 cm mark while angling the scope upward appropriately. Often, it is helpful to first "prerehearse" tip angulation to assure the correct axis is found before insertion. The tip of the scope is passed over the curve of the tongue in the midline, past the uvula. As the tip is advanced, the epiglottis and cricoarytenoid cartilage becomes visible. The tip of the scope is next angled slightly downward so the tip passes inferior to the cricoarytenoid cartilage. It is usually necessary to pass slightly right or left of midline to avoid the bulge of cartilage against the cervical spine. At this point, with gentle inward pressure and insufflations of air, the scope usually slides into the esophagus safely and rapidly.

Esophagus

The endoscope is steadily advanced along the length of esophagus with the assistance of air insufflations while the examiner takes notice of normal and abnormal features. Major landmarks include the indentation from the left main bronchus, pulsation from the left atrium and aorta, and the Z-line. The location of the gastroesophageal junction is recorded in centimeters from the incisors or lips. It is identified by the tops of the gastric folds, the Z-line or squamocolumnar epithelium junction, and diaphragmatic pinch. The Z-line is the jagged, irregular zone where pale pink squamous mucous meets darker red gastric mucosa.

The squamous epithelium of the esophagus should have a glistening pink surface with a visible network of tiny blood vessels (Fig. 123.3). Loss of this visible vascular pattern is often suggestive of inflammation or edema. Columnar epithelium, though, has a slightly rougher surface and deeper red color. Tissue of this sort in the esophagus suggests ectopic gastric mucosa, Barrett's metaplasia, or a hiatal hernia. A hiatal hernia may be distinguished from Barrett's metaplasia by finding the origin of the gastric folds, usually 2 cm above the diaphragm. Barrett's esophagus appears as an irregular Z-line with "fingers" of red gastric epithelium extending up into the normal esophageal mucosa.

Stomach

With slight angulation to the left and anteriorly, the endoscope is passed into the stomach. As the tip of the

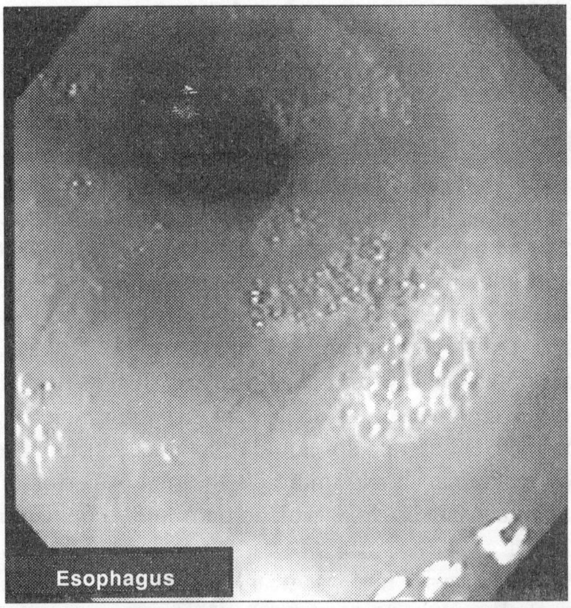

Fig. 123.3: Endoscopic view of the normal esophagus (See for colour figure Plate 10)

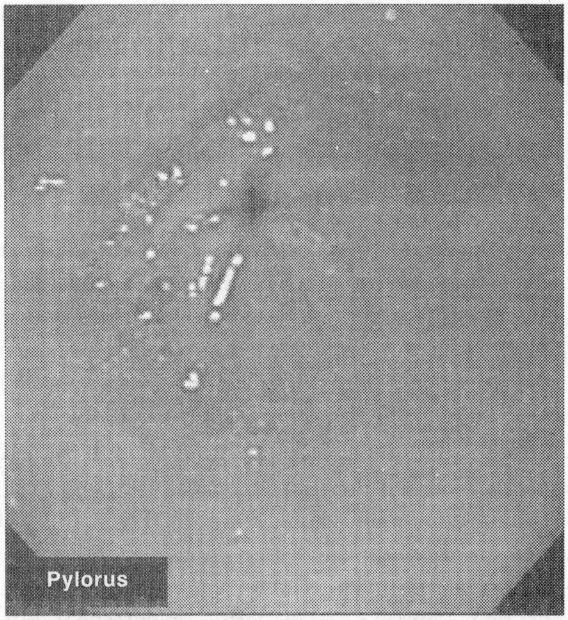

Fig. 123.4: Endoscopic view of the normal antrum (See for colour figure Plate 11)

scope is passed into the stomach, it is necessary to rotate the tip left or counterclockwise, to reach the cardia. The fluid sitting in the gastric pool should be aspirated to improve endoscopic inspection and to reduce the likelihood of regurgitation and aspiration during the procedure. The stomach should then be inflated sufficiently. The gastric mucosa is inspected, and observations are made regarding mucosal appearance, presence of erythema, gastric contractions, and any defects or abnormalities. Peristalsis begins in the mid body and progresses downward to the pylorus. The frequency is approximately three contractions per minute.

With the stomach inflated, the scope should be rotated clockwise and the tip angled upward to allow the scope to follow and be advanced along the longitudinal folds of the greater curvature of the stomach toward the antrum. The antrum and pylorus should be inspected, first from a distance, and then more closely (Fig. 123.4). The incisura angularis is a fold that marks the entrance to the antrum. The pylorus is usually open at rest, but it closes as the contraction wave reaches it.

Endoscopy of the stomach is not complete without retroflexion while at the antrum, allowing inspection of the lesser curvature, cardia, and fundus. To perform a retroflexion, the tip of the endoscope is flexed upward more than 180 degrees as the scope is slowly advance into the wall of the antrum. The endoscopist next rotates the scope clockwise and counterclockwise and gently moves the shaft in and out to inspect the entire area of the cardia, lesser curvature, and fundus. Without retroflexion, certain abnormalities such as Mallory-Weiss tears or ulcers, as well as complete inspection of a hiatal hernia, may be missed. The stomach must be fully inflated during this maneuver to ensure complete inspection of the fundus, the gastroesophageal junction and the lesser curvature of the stomach (Fig. 123.5).

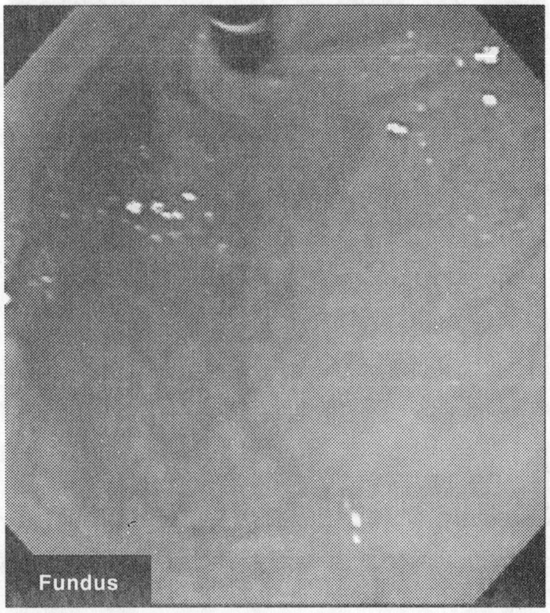

Fig. 123.5: Endoscopic retroflexed view of the cardia of the stomach (See for colour figure Plate 11)

Duodenal Bulb

The pylorus is entered with the tip deflected slightly downward and to the right. The duodenal bulb should be examined upon initially entering the duodenum to avoid misinterpreting lesions on withdrawal that may result from endoscope trauma. The bulb is scanned circumferentially by manipulation of the scope tip. The surface of the duodenal bulb is generally smooth, though fine nodularity may be present, representing lymphoid or Brunner gland hyperplasia.

Duodenum

The endoscope is passed beyond the apex of the duodenal bulb into the second descending portion of the duodenum. Passage from the tip of the bulb into the descending duodenum is often possible under direct vision but occasionally the following maneuver allows further advancement into the second and third portions of the duodenum. While gently advancing the endoscope, the tip is initially deflected downward and to the right, then upward and to the left. A tunnel view of the circular (Kerckring's) folds of the descending duodenum should be seen (Fig. 123.6). The mucosal surface of the duodenum appears slightly granular due to the underlying villus architecture. Introducing water into the bowel lumen often magnifies the intestinal villi for better viewing. A tangential view of the papilla of Vater on the convex wall of the descending duodenum is often also possible.

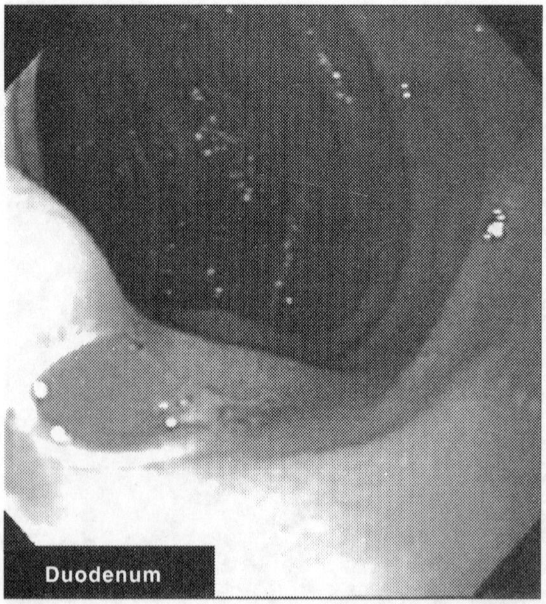

Fig. 123.6: Endoscopic view of the normal duodenum (See for colour figure Plate 11)

Removing the Scope

The duodenum, stomach, and esophagus should be surveyed again during scope withdrawal. Biopsies may be obtained at this point and upon further withdrawal of the endoscope. Routine biopsies are often taken from each part of the upper gastrointestinal tract, even when no gross abnormalities are detected, because visual inspection alone is not sensitive enough to determine histopathology.

It is important to aspirate air and fluid from the stomach upon scope withdrawal to minimize post-operative risks of aspiration.

Biopsies

A variety of biopsy forceps are available, and the choice of biopsy forceps is largely based on personal preference. Biopsy technique involves the forceps being gently opened onto the mucosal surface under direct vision. The tip of the forceps is closed around the mucosal tissue. Upon closure, the forceps should cut the tissue clearly as the endoscopist briskly pulls the forceps away from the mucosa. Excessive tenting of the mucosa by grasping tissue far from the endoscope tip should be avoided. A controlled biopsy technique should minimize the risk of perforation and submucosal shearing, which contribute to hematoma formation.

Most endoscopic forceps are able to obtain mucosa and, occasionally, a small amount of submucosa. The tissue sample is gently recovered from the biopsy forceps, often with the use of a toothpick, and placed immediately into a fixative such as formalin. Orientation of tissue for mounting and section may be deferred to the histopathology technician. Preferred sites for biopsy include the distal duodenum, duodenal bulb, gastric antrum and corpus, and distal and proximal esophagus.

In addition to biopsies, diagnostic fluid samples may be obtained from the duodenum or stomach for bile, pancreatic enzymes (usually after pancreatic stimulation with secretin), quantitative bacterial culture, and parasite analysis. Cytology brushes are used to obtain cell samples from the surface of a lesion for cytological study or for examination of an exudate to detect, for example, the presence of *Candida*. These brushes are often protected by a plastic overtube or sheath, which allows the examiner to advance the brush out and pull it back into the sheath to prevent contamination of the recovered sample.

RECOVERY AND DISCHARGE

Recovery should take place under appropriate supervision in the procedure room or post-anesthesia care unit. Oxygen, suction and resuscitative drugs and equipment should be immediately available. Discharge should occur only after an appropriate period of recovery and observation by an authorized practitioner. The patient should be discharged into the care of a responsible adult, and written instructions regarding eating and drinking and prohibition of driving should be provided.

COMPLICATIONS

Diagnostic endoscopy with mucosal biopsy confers a very low risk of serious complications. A single prospective survey published in the form of an abstract provides the only large-scale data in pediatrics. A complication rate of 1.7 percent was reported in 2,046 upper gastrointestinal endoscopies. This included a single bowel perforation and one incident of post procedure bleeding. Most adult data have been derived from retrospective studies, although some prospective data are available. Fleischer, Al-Kawas, and Benjamin reported prospective data collected over 1 year including 3,287 procedures. The overall complication rate was 1.9 percent. This included 2 deaths (0.06%), 3 bowel perforations (0.09%), 6 patients requiring surgical intervention (0.18%), and 16 patients with cardiopulmonary problems (0.49%).

Obviously, major negative events like bowel perforation can be viewed as a complication, but minor events such as transient odynophagia, nausea, or transient oxygen desaturation might rather be better described as negative outcomes. Complications and negative outcomes associated with upper gastrointestinal endoscopy can be categorized as either sedation or procedure related, with sedation-related problems being far more common. These range from inadequate sedation with patient agitation to hypoventilation, oxygen desaturation, airway obstruction, and cardiac dysrhythmias.

Procedure-related complications rarely occur during diagnostic endoscopy. Duodenal hematoma (Fig. 123.7) has been reported in children following routine diagnostic endoscopy. Fatal air embolism has also been reported. Most complications in children have been related to therapeutic rather than diagnostic procedures, such as percutaneous gastrostomy, esophageal dilation, variceal sclerotherapy, and foreign body removal.

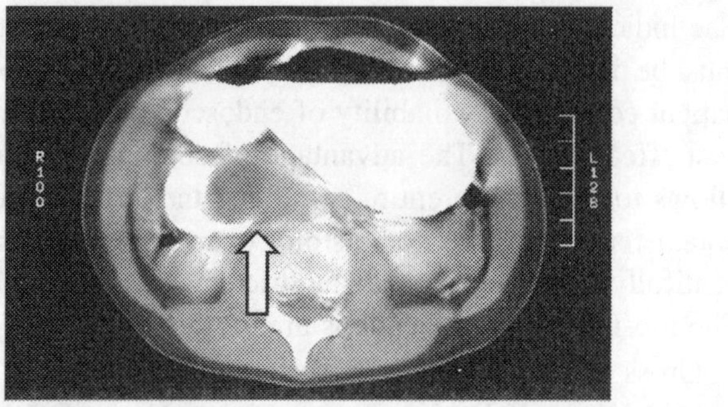

Fig. 123.7: Endoscopic view of the duodenojejunal hematoma, a complication of upper endoscopy, with complete obstruction of the third part of duodenum

DOCUMENTATION

The clinical record should include the names of the patient and procedure, all staff members involved, details of medications and fluids administered, as well as monitoring data obtained. Resulting endoscopic findings, specimens taken, and complications should also be recorded. With video endoscopes, photographic documentation of both normal and abnormal endoscopic features can be saved and printed to share with the patient, family, and medical record.

KEY LEARNING POINTS

- Examination of the upper gastrointestinal tract by esophago-gastro-duodenoscopy (EGD) is the most frequently performed endoscopic procedure in children.
- The indications for upper endoscopy are numerous and include evaluation of abdominal pain and dysphagia. Therefore, the decision to perform and upper endoscopy must be individualized in the context of each patient's complete presentation.
- Development of a systematic method to reduce the possibility of missing any area is necessary in upper endoscopy.
- Two simple rules of endoscopy apply, never push or advance the scope if one cannot clearly see a lumen or open area, and, if in doubt, inflate and pull back. Keeping these rules in mind, one can assure the safest and best possible outcome for any endoscopic procedure.

FURTHER READINGS

1. Ament, ME: Prospective study of risks of complication in 6,424 procedures in pediatric gastroenterology [abstract]. *Pediatr Res* 1981;15:524.
2. Fleischer DE and others: Prospective evaluation of complications in an endoscopy unit: Use of the A/S/G/E quality care guidelines, *Gastrointest Endosc* 1992;38:411-414.
3. Squires RH, Colletti RB. Indications for Pediatric Gastrointestinal Endoscopy: A Medical Position Statement of the North American Society for Pediatric Gastroenterology and Nutrition. *J Pediatr Gastroenterol Nutr* 1996;23:107-110.

124 Colonoscopy

Jeremy King • Raman Sreedharan • Karoly Horvath

INTRODUCTION

Colonoscopy involves examination of the entire colon and terminal ileum using a fiberoptic or video endoscope. Though the majority of principles of diagnostic colonoscopy are similar to that of upper gastrointestinal endoscopy, there are several distinct differences between upper endoscopy and colonoscopy. This includes differences in instrumentation, patient preparation, technique, risk and skill level.

Initial reports of pediatric colonoscopy appeared in the literature during the late 1970s and extended into the 1980s. Experience and skill have since advanced to the point that colonoscopy is now routinely performed by most clinical pediatric gastroenterologists for children of all ages.

THE COLONOSCOPE

Much of the technology and mechanics of the colonoscope are similar to the upper gastrointestinal endoscope. This is reviewed in Chapter 123, which describes, in detail, the mechanics of the upper endoscope. Compared to the upper endoscope, the colonoscope is longer, has a larger channel, and is modified to allow greater torque responses. This is necessary because colonoscopy is a more challenging and technically difficult procedure due to the various colonic bends encountered.

The lengths of the scopes range from the 65 cm flexible sigmoidoscope to the 165 cm colonoscope, and shaft diameters vary from the 10 mm pediatric colonoscope to the 15 mm adult instruments. The diameter of the suction channel ranges from 2.7 to 4.2 mm permitting aspiration of thick or fibrous stool and food residue. Tip angulations in four directions by 160 to 180 degrees allow passage around the most acute curves. Pediatric colonoscopes tend to have a less "stiff" and more "floppy" shaft than do adult scopes. The floppier shafts conform more easily to the colon, cause less stretch pain, and respond more easily to dexterity in handling. Latest pediatric colonoscopes have a rotating ring below the handle that allows the endoscopist to "stiffen" the shaft, that is often helpful when advancing through a very redundant colon. Magnifying colonoscopes which give high resolutions views of the mucosa with 20- to 30-fold magnification provide more details of the mucosal surface. These scopes are often used in combination with various tissue stains for early detection of dysplasia or malignancy.

Although there is no ideal colonoscope, availablity of several instruments allows the endoscopist to choose the best endoscope based on the patient's age, procedure indication and personal preference.

All the standard accessory equipment used in upper endoscopy is available for colonoscopy, including biopsy forceps, retrieval baskets, injector needles, cytology brushes, washing catheters and dilating balloons.

INDICATIONS FOR COLONOSCOPY

The indication for colonoscopy or flexible sigmoidoscopy must be determined individually based on clinical problem, patient condition, availability of endoscopic expertise and cost-effectiveness. The advantage of colonoscopy that it allows to inspect the entire colon and the terminal ileum, obtain tissue biopsies for histology, and intervene therapeutically to stop bleeding, dilate strictures or remove polyps. The most common indications are:

- Gross lower GI bleeding.
- Occult lower GI bleeding or unexplained iron deficiency anemia.
- Abnormality on barium enema requiring further evaluation.
- Acute or chronic colitis.
- Chronic diarrhea.
- Suspected disease of the terminal ileum.
- Suspected polyposis disorder or surveillance.
- Dilation of stricture.
- Decompression of obstructed colon.
- Removal of foreign body.
- Cancer surveillance.

CONTRAINDICATIONS

Contraindications for colonoscopy are similar to those for upper gastrointestinal endoscopy, including cardiovascular, respiratory, or neurologic instability. Colonoscopy is absolutely contraindicated when bowel perforation is suspected. Similarly, colonoscopy should not be performed if marked abdominal tenderness or peritonitis are present. The procedure, during any acute and severe inflammatory process, such as Crohn's disease or ulcerative colitis, should be undertaken with extreme caution.

Neutropenia and immunodeficiency are relative contraindications because of the increased risk of sepsis due to the bacterial translocation during the procedure. Coagulopathy, though not an absolute contraindication, should be corrected before proceeding with colonoscopy because of bleeding risk, especially with biopsies. Inadequate bowel preparation is another relative contraindication since diagnostic lesions may be overlooked and the endoscope may not be able to be advanced through the lumen under direct visualization.

RISK/BENEFIT

Colonoscopy has become the procedure of choice for most colonic investigations. The technical difficulties of colonoscopy in patients with severe constipation and megacolon make a contrast study more appealing in these patients. On the other hand, patients who have reduced mobility, rectal incontinence, prolapse, or stomas are best examined by colonoscopy.

Because of its technical challenge, failure to perform a complete examination due to the inadequate bowel preparation or inability to reach the cecum/terminal ileum is a limitation of colonoscopy. Poor bowel preparation may result in a failure to identify small lesions or areas of pathology if they are under or behind pools or pieces of stool. Also, because blind spots may fall around sharp bends, at the flexures, and even fairly large lesions may be missed.

Colonoscopy is able to identify specific diseases and provide definitive treatment. Colonoscopy is useful when initial stool tests are negative for infectious etiologies. Gross inspection of the colon may reveal findings that suggest an infectious etiology (e.g., pseudomembraneous exudate), identify unusual focal lesions, or find the source of a lower gastrointestinal bleed, such as juvenile polyp or anastomosis ulceration. Mucosal biopsies obtained during colonoscopic procedures allow further characterization of infectious, ischemic, allergic, neoplastic, or inflammatory diseases that induce bleeding.

Colonoscopies have a higher complication rate than the contrast barium enema studies (1 per 1700 vs. 1 per 2500). Again, the clinical indication and risk/benefit must be weighed in each individual scenario when deciding the appropriate test for diagnostic purposes.

SEDATION

Sedation for colonoscopic procedures is variable and often depends upon the patient's age, risk factors, and the physician comfort level. Flexible sigmoidoscopies can be performed with little or no sedation, especially in young infants. Similarly, skilled adult gastroenterologists will perform colonoscopies in adult patients with little or no sedation. Pediatric endoscopists usually prefer to use general anesthesia for full colonoscopies. The use of sedation/anesthesia has its advantages and disadvantages. Without sedation, the bowel is often shorter, more tonic, and easier to examine. The patient can also cooperate in position changes that may provide technical ease. On the other hand, sedation (and especially general anesthesia) makes the examination much more tolerable and amenable to anxious patients.

Risks of sedation result from depression of the central nervous system and include depression of protective reflexes, the respiratory system, and the cardiovascular system. One must also keep in mind the potential of adverse drug reactions, including anaphylaxis, and the wide individual variation in response to the sedative drugs used for the procedure.

PATIENT PREPARATION

Prior to the procedure, usually at the time of scheduling, dietary and bowel preparation instructions should be thoroughly reviewed. Also, the parents and older children should be provided with written information including a description of the nature, risks, and benefits of the procedure and informed consent for the procedure and sedation should be obtained. Patients and families should have an understanding of what to expect during the immediate and long-term recovery period following discharge.

Bowel Preparation

The bowel preparation depends on the procedure being performed (sigmoidoscopy or full colonoscopy), patient's age, stool pattern (i.e. regular, chronic diarrhea, constipation), concerns of compliance, presence of other systemic disorders (cardiac, hematological etc.) and finally the endoscopist preference. Full compliance with bowel preparations in children is often difficult and impacts the effectiveness and success of the procedure. Being able to perform the bowel clean-out at home is not only cost-effective but often more comfortable and preferable to patients. The ideal preparation cleanses the whole colon, has few side effects such as pain, nausea or vomiting, and does not cause dehydration or fluid shifts.

For some children, combination stimulant laxative (bisacodyl) and series of enemas alone may be sufficient, especially for sigmoidoscopy. Colonic lavage using commercially available polyethylene-glycol (PEG) based solutions with (GoLytely, Nulytely, HalfLytely) or without electrolytes (Miralax, Glycolax) ensures a safe, effective, and rapid cleansing of the colon in most children. However, hospitalization and nasogastric (NG) tube placement may be required. In general, smaller volume cleansing preparations are better tolerated and equally effective compared to large-volume lavage solutions. If combined with a 24 to 48-hour clear liquid diet, several of these preparations can effectively be employed and tolerated in children and can be easily performed at home. Several cleanout methods used in children are outlined below. The used doses should be adjusted to the individual child, e.g. in the case of chronic diarrhea less preparation is needed than in those with firm stools. Infants typically need less volume and shorter preparation than older children.

PEG based Clean-outs

GoLytely is used for inpatient clean-out after NG-tube placement. It can be started at a rate of 10cc/kg/hr and increase by 10cc/kg/hr per hour until 300-400cc/hour and run until stools are clear. However, many children due to nausea, vomiting, and abdominal distention will not tolerate this prep. Because Reglan helps gastric emptying, some centers administer one dose of Reglan 0.1mg/kg via NG, and others give it every 3 hours during the infusion. The diet is restricted to sips of water only while the infusion is running. An enema is given before the preparation usually only in the case of significant fecal impaction. Again, this depends on the physician's preference.

Miralax has been widely used as a home clean-out regimen in the last few years. The principles of this clean-out are the same as the other PEG protocols, but the prescribed dose depends on the age rather than weight of the child. The advantage of Miralax (Glycolax) is that it can be mixed into a clear or flavored fluid without altering smell or taste. Also, it does contain electrolytes like GoLytely. The procedure usually starts in the night 2 days prior the procedure by giving a Bisacodyl tablet or suppository. The dose is 5 mg for younger children (<10 years) and 10 mg for those older (>10 years). A clear liquid diet is started next morning, the day prior the procedure, and by noon Miralax is started. A *Clear liquid diet* means that the children may take strained fruit juices without pulp (i.e. apple, white grape, lemonade), water, clear broth or bouillon, tea without milk or non-diary creamer, Gatorade, carbonated and non-carbonated soft drinks, Kool-Aid or other fruit flavored drinks. Plain jell-O without added fruits or toppings and ice popsicles are also allowed.

The protocol used by our group has age dependent doses: 4 capfuls (68 grams) in 20 oz of fluid for patients 3-5 years of age, 6 capfuls (102 grams) for ages 6-11 years and 10 capfuls (170 grams) for children over 11 years in 32 oz of fluid. This mixture should be offered in 4-6 oz of portions every 30-60 minutes. Another bisacodyl tablet or suppository can be given later that day that to help eliminate the excess fluid. For children younger than 3 years, a modified Miralax protocol with smaller doses and without the bisacodyl stimulant is appropriate.

Many centers and gastroenterologists opt to use slightly higher Miralax doses than outlined above to achieve better cleanout results. Parents should be instructed to contact the procedure nurse or physician if the child is not compliant or tolerating the preparation. For example, if the parent happens to call the morning of the procedure stating that the child "only drank half of the prep is still stooling brown and solid stool", it may be advisable to give an enema before or postpone the procedure.

Magnesium citrate is also commonly used for clean-out. Solid foods are restricted starting the morning 2 days prior to procedure and only clear liquids are allowed in this protocol. The typical dose is 1 ounce/year (age), upto 10 ounces total per day for 2 days. Patients may mix magnesium citrate with the clear liquid of choice and continue taking clear liquids until 4 hours prior to procedure.

Oral phospho-soda solutions are also used for colonic preparation in older children and adults. These preparations are advantageous because they involve drinking far less volume and are relatively inexpensive compared to many of the other preparations. The protocol involves drinking 1-1/2 ounces of the phospho-soda oral solution twice along with a lot of clear liquids the day before the test to clean out the colon. Since the phospho-soda tastes salty, mixing it with white grape juice or another flavored beverage is recommended. Despite its relative ease of administration, oral phospho-soda may cause significant gastric discomfort and sometimes vomiting, as well as superficial apthous ulcers in the stomach and rectum.

SUBACUTE BACTERIAL ENDOCARDITIS PROPHYLAXIS

Prophylaxis is probably indicated for patients with cardiac problems. The patients who need and do not need prophylaxis are listed in the guidelines of the American Heart Association as described in Chapter 123.

PATIENT ASSESSMENT, STAFFING, FACILITIES AND EQUIPMENT, POSITIONING AND MONITORING

The patient assessment, procedure staffing, facilities, equipment and patient monitoring are similar to those reviewed in detail in Chapter 123. Patient positioning can be individualized by the physician's preference. Most commonly, patients are positioned in either the left lateral recumbent position with knees partially bent or the supine frog-leg position. The patient's position may be changed to supine, right lateral decubitus, and very rarely prone to facilitate successful and comfortable passage of the scope around challenging loops or into the cecum and distal ileum.

STANCE AND INSTRUMENT HANDLING

The endoscopist and the assistant should wear safety glasses, a protective gown, preferably latex-free examination gloves, and stand in a comfortable position. Prior to beginning any endoscopic procedure, the scope always should be checked to assure proper functioning. The light source, video transmission, air insufflator, water, and suction should be tested, as well as the directional dials.

The majority of gastroenterologists favor a "one-man approach", though some prefer a "two-men" method with the assistant pushing and manipulating the shaft. The instrument head should be placed in the palm of the left hand. The thumb should rest on the up/down control wheel and the forefinger on the air/water button. The second finger can assist the thumb during major up/down movements. The right hand again is free to hold, push, pull, and torque the scope. The shaft should be gripped at all times with a gauze pad for reasons of hygiene and better grip.

COLONOSCOPY BASICS

The fundamentals of colonoscopic technique are the basis of providing a rapid, relatively pain-free, and accurate total colonoscopy. During a technically difficult colonoscopy, there are only a limited number of options available to assist in providing a non-traumatic, thorough examination. Using these strategies logically, quickly, and sequentially is the key to successful maneuvering.

A cardinal principle of colonoscopy is to shorten and telescope the colon rather than stretch it out. Only a light touch is needed on the instrument which has a 1:1 correspondence between shaft and tip during shaft manipulations. Another principle is to insufflate as little as possible. Overinflation cannot only lead to significant patient discomfort both during and following the procedure, but stretch the colon resulting in sharp, difficult to maneuver curves. Constant air suctioning throughout the colonoscopy will also help in shortening the bowel. Keeping in mind these principles, one can effectively improve colonoscopic efficiency.

Similar to upper endoscopy, the scope should only be advanced under direct visualization. More so, pulling back is the most important maneuver in colonoscopy. This maneuver is virtually inevitable during a colonoscopy, because of the colon has many bends and curves. By pushing the instrument, the colon is stretched and unwanted loops form. To prevent this during advancing, suctioning should be applied, allowing the scope to telescope into the lumen visible. Pulling back is necessary when the luminal view is lost, usually because the scope is against the colon wall. During the pulling back process, the colon can also be effectively shortened. In the shortened colon, looping is less likely, allowing sequential, effective advancement of the scope on a "two-steps-forward-and-one-step-back" basis.

In addition to techniques involving torquing and steering, as covered in Chapter 123, specialized techniques must be mastered to remedy looping or other difficult situations incurred. When no lumen is seen, withdrawing and "jiggling" the scope with a series of short and rapid in-and-out movements while simultaneously applying torque helps to straighten the scope and shorten the colon over it. If a colonic bend or flexure cannot be passed, changing the position of the patient can be helpful. For example, placing the patient in the right lateral recumbent position can help pass a stubborn splenic flexure.

Advancing Through the Colon

Anus and rectum: Prior to insertion of the colonoscope into the anus, it is recommended to perform a thorough examination of the perianal region (Fig. 124.1) and a rectal examination using two gloves on the right hand. Digital examination of the anorectum is used to pre-lubricate and relax the anal canal as well as palpate any potentially blind lesion. The outer glove is then removed. After lubrication of the scope, the tip is introduced through the anus. This is best accomplished by placing the index finger alongside the tip while applying steady pressure.

After the scope enters the rectum, a "red-out" is usually seen as the lens presses against the mucosa. To counteract this, simultaneous air insufflation and instrument withdrawal should be used. Attempts at rotary or angulation movements, made more easily in a dilated, capacious rectum to

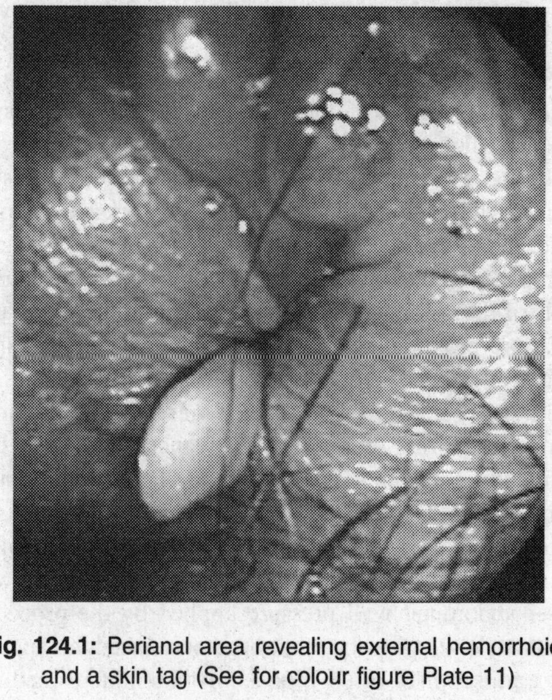

Fig. 124.1: Perianal area revealing external hemorrhoids and a skin tag (See for colour figure Plate 11)

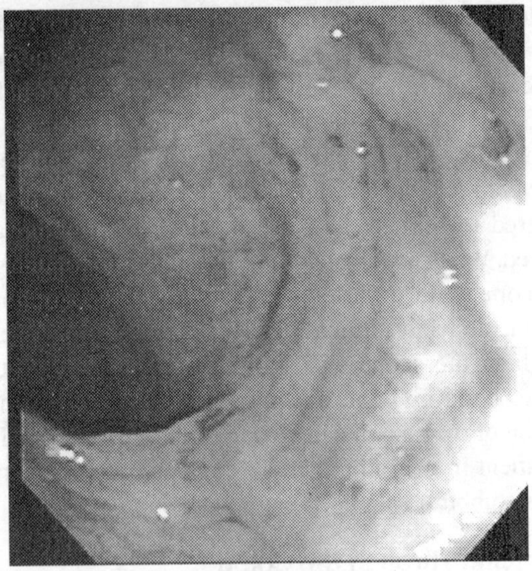

Fig. 124.2: Photograph of the rectum obtained during colonoscopy showing erythema and edema (See for colour figure Plate 11)

find the lumen (Fig. 124.2). Once the lumen is located, it is often necessary to aspirate fluid or residue that has accumulated in the rectum. With the lumen in view, the colonoscope can be advanced under direct visualization. The three valves of Houston, which lie on alternating sides of the lumen, appear as semilunar folds.

A retroflexed view of the rectum also can be accomplished to sufficiently examine potential blind spots that fall behind major folds or valves, as well as inspection for hemorrhoids, fissures, or other anorectal disorders. Angulating the tip fully and then pushing the scope inward into the rectal wall will flex the scope backward. Clockwise and counterclockwise torques will allow a 360-degree view of the rectum.

Sigmoid and descending colon: Passing through the very flexible sigmoid colon is often the most daunting aspect of a full colonoscopy (Fig. 124.3). It is here that adherence to the basic procedure principles and techniques must be utilized while attempting to slalom and corkscrew around bends in order to successfully navigate this region. Visually, within the sigmoid and descending colon the classic haustral folds of the colon appear, though less prominently than in the more proximal segments. The sigmoid colon is quite mobile and may be redundant, resulting in difficult passage. Furthermore, this is the area where the scope most commonly forms loops during advancement. Each loop formation is named by a letter (e.g., N, U, alpha, double alpha, gamma), which physically illustrates the shape into which the scope has "looped". Using a combination of the above techniques, position changes, and direct, downward lower abdominal wall pressure applied by the procedure assistant, looping can be minimized or reduced. Inexperienced endoscopists often mistakenly attempt to push the

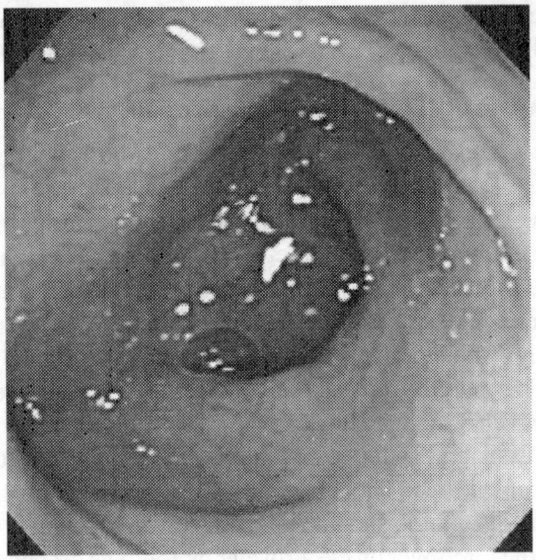

Fig. 124.3: Normal sigmoid colon (See for colour figure Plate 11)

looped scope toward the descending colon because they have a clear view of the lumen. This generally results in an expanding sigmoid loop without progression of the scope tip, and it causes profound discomfort in unsedated or minimally sedated patients. After passing a sometimes hairpin bend at the sigmoid junction, the descending colon is normally found held down retroperitoneally and generally runs a long and tubular straight line (Fig. 124.4).

Splenic flexure and transverse colon: The splenic flexure is encountered at the end of the descending colon, and the spleen can often be seen as a dark blue impression

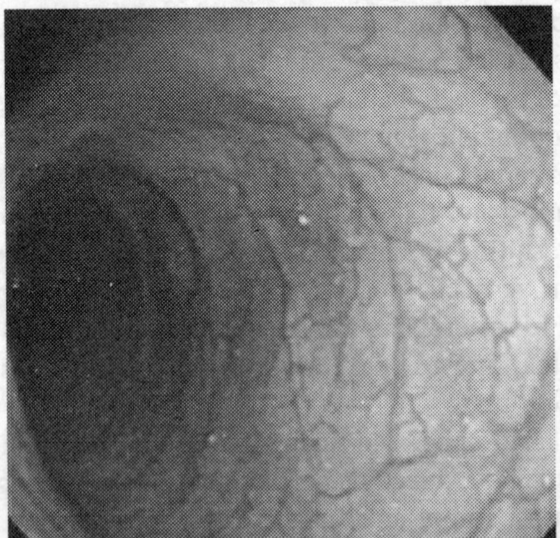

Fig. 124.4: Normal descending colon (See for colour figure Plate 12)

along the bowel wall. The flexure is often traversed easily, if the sigmoid has been straightened and held straight. Combining gentle shaft advancement with clockwise twist and sometimes simultaneous abdominal pressure over the sigmoid, the scope can be passed through the flexure.

Overangulation tends to impact the tip into the flexure, while overaggressive pushing tends to re-form a loop in the sigmoid. Placing the patient in the right lateral position almost invariably causes the splenic flexure to drop downward, allowing the instrument to slide more easily around it. Entrance into the *transverse colon* is often recognizable by the characteristic, thin, triangular folds formed by the taeniae coli. The colonoscope can often be advanced easily toward with its straight lumen in view the hepatic flexure, again if the endoscopist was careful to avoid any sigmoid loops.

Hepatic flexure and ascending colon: The hepatic flexure recognized by the dark shadowing of the liver through the bowel wall, and it is the next bend to pass. The endoscopic view of a capacious hepatic flexure sometimes can be mistakenly identified as cecum. However, the absence of light illuminating through the skin in the left lower quadrant of the abdomen can warn that the ascending colon has not been entered. While rotating the shaft, passage around the hepatic flexure is usually achieved by suctioning to collapse the bowel toward the tip of the scope. Deflation is extremely helpful in advancing the instrument and shortening the distance to the cecum through the large, asymmetric folds of the ascending colon.

Ileocecal region: Arrival at the cecum is suggested by the illumination of the colonoscope light in the right lower quadrant of the abdomen. However, identification of the appendiceal orifice and ileocecal valve, and the visualization of sling fold of the caput cecum, forming the "Mercedes Benz" sign, confirms it.

The *ileocecal valve* (Fig. 124.5) appears as a smooth, asymmetric fold with a lips-like appearance on the medial wall of the cecum. It is important to collapse the cecum as much as possible before intubation, as overinflation makes it difficult to find and maneuver into the ileocecal valve. Because the valve is typically 90 degree from the lumen, intubation requires skillful and often careful manipulation of the colonoscope tip. Advancement of the tip just beyond the valve is the first step. The endoscope is then slowly withdrawn while insufflating with air and turning the tip into the fold, hooking it into the ileocecal valve. Often, small, controlled movements are needed, and the valve will "pop" open allowing the scope to be advanced into the ileum. In some instances, a closed biopsy forcep is used to push downward on one edge of the ileocecal valve and assist intubation.

Terminal Ileum: Small bowel mucosa is recognized by the presence of a bright and shiny mucosa covered with lymphoid nodules (Peyer patches) (Fig. 124.6). These nodules and the surrounding mucosa are covered with a granular appearing surface, and the usually visible villi clearly distinguish the ileum from colon. However, the villi may disappear as a result of inflammation in cases of "blackwash ileitis".

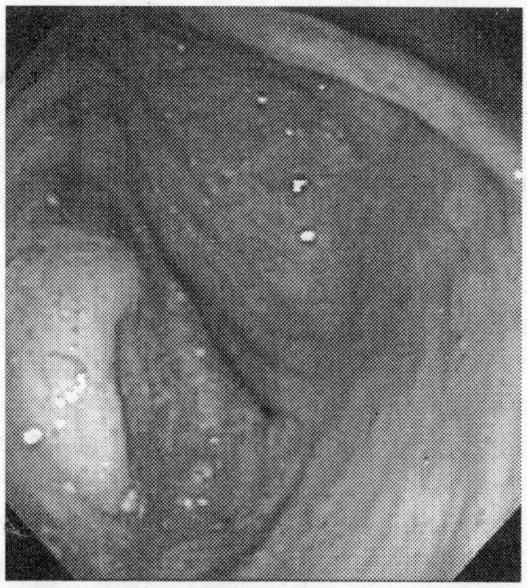

Fig. 124.5: Normal cecum with apparent appendiceal orifice (See for colour figure Plate 12)

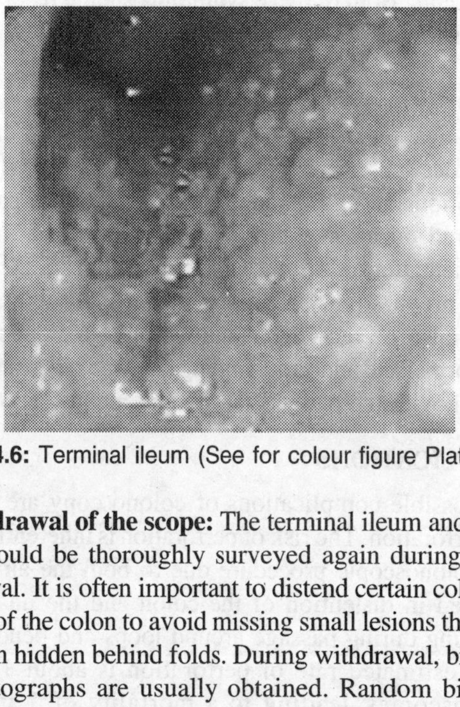

Fig. 124.6: Terminal ileum (See for colour figure Plate 12)

Withdrawal of the scope: The terminal ileum and entire colon should be thoroughly surveyed again during scope withdrawal. It is often important to distend certain collapsed portions of the colon to avoid missing small lesions that may have been hidden behind folds. During withdrawal, biopsies and photographs are usually obtained. Random biopsies should be obtained from the terminal ileum and each segment of the colon, as well as the rectum, even when no gross abnormalities are visualized. The techniques of biopsy are discussed in the upper endoscopy chapter. One distinct difference in biopsy technique is that a "spiked" biopsy forceps is often used. These forceps are constructed similarly to upper endoscopy forceps and function the same way. However, they contain a pointed pin or "spike" at the base that is capable of securing a piece of biopsy tissue. This allows a second biopsy to be obtained, keeping the first in place on the spike. This prevents the need to withdraw the forceps after each biopsy and saves procedure time. As discussed in the chapter on upper endoscopy, visual inspection alone not sensitive enough to determine histopathology of the tissue, warranting biopsies be obtained.

It is also important to aspirate as much air as possible from the colon during withdrawal to minimize post-operative discomfort from colonic and abdominal distention.

RECOVERY AND DISCHARGE

Recovery should take place under appropriate supervision in the procedure room or post-anesthesia care unit. Oxygen, suctioning catheters and resuscitative drugs and equipment should be available. After an appropriate period of recovery and observation by an authorized practitioner, the patient can be discharged. Children should be discharged into the care of a responsible adult. Teenagers with a driver license should be restricted from driving following the procedure. Patients should be informed that residual cramping and flatulence from air insufflated into the colon is common. Streaks of blood may also be seen in subsequent bowel movements. Both of these symptoms should resolve within 24-48 hours.

DOCUMENTATION

The clinical record should include the names of the patient and procedure, all staff members involved, details of medications and fluids administered, and vital parameters measured during the procedure and until the discharge. Documentation of all colonoscopic findings, adequacy of bowel preparation, specimens taken, and complications should also be recorded. Photographic documentation of both normal and abnormal findings may be saved and printed to share with the patient, family and medical record.

COMPLICATIONS

The possible complications of colonoscopy are bleeding and perforation. The risk of perforation is inherently present in a colonoscopic procedure due to both the air pressure involved in distention of the colon and the unavoidable stretching during passage around loops and bends.

An estimated rate of perforation is about 1 in 2500 colonoscopies, leading to a mortality of 1 in 15,000 colonoscopies in the adult literature. The majority of deaths, however, usually are the result of inappropriate conservative management of suspected perforation. The complication rate is inevitably higher in therapeutic colonoscopy (polypectomy, stricture dilation) than in diagnostic colonoscopy.

Following any colonoscopy perforation is suspected, it is important to obtain immediately an X-ray film and request surgical consultation. In the instance of a technically difficult procedure requiring a great deal of manipulation, it is often reasonable to have a low threshold to suspect possible perforation. In an asymptomatic patient with a small amount of free air on a post-procedure X-ray, it is safe to treat the patient conservatively with antibiotics. A surgical consultation again is warranted.

A small amount of bleeding should be expected during diagnostic colonoscopy biopsies. The bleeding rate following the procedure, however, is extremely low. In fact, the bleeding rate after therapeutic polypectomy is only estimated to occur 0.26% to 1.5% of the time.

KEY LEARNING POINTS

- Colonoscopy needs more preparation by the patients and more expertise by the gastroenterologist than upper endoscopy.
- Colonoscopy is a technically more challenging procedure than upper endoscopy, something that can be compounded further by inadequate bowel preparation, sedation, or physician skill level.
- Following the fundamentals of colonoscopic technique allows rapid and accurate total colonoscopy and terminal ileum intubation with minimal risk or postoperative discomfort.

FURTHER READING

1. Squires RH, Colletti RB. Indications for pediatric gastrointestinal endoscopy: A medical position statement of the North American Society for Pediatric Gastroenterology and Nutrition. *J Pediatr Gastroenterol Nutr* 1996; 23: 107-110.

Index

D

Index

D

E

F

G

H